OXFORD MEDICAL PUBLICATIONS

# BRAIN DAMAGE, BRAIN REPAIR

# Brain Damage, Brain Repair

by

JAMES W. FAWCETT

*Department of Physiology,*
*Cambridge University, UK*

ANNE E. ROSSER

*School of Biosciences,*
*Cardiff University, UK*

and

STEPHEN B. DUNNETT

*School of Biosciences,*
*Cardiff University, UK*

with additional contributions from:

Harry Baker, Roger Barker, Charlotte Behan, German Berrios,
Stacey Efstathiou, Robin Franklin, Joe Herbert, Andrew Lawrence,
Ian H. Robertson, Barbara J. Sahakian, Neil Scolding,
Steve Wharton and Barbara Wilson

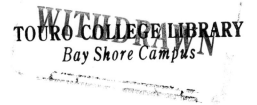
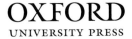

**OXFORD**

UNIVERSITY PRESS

BS

# OXFORD
## UNIVERSITY PRESS

Great Clarendon Street, Oxford OX2 6DP

Oxford University Press is a department of the University of Oxford.
It furthers the University's objective of excellence in research, scholarship,
and education by publishing worldwide in

Oxford New York

Auckland Bangkok Buenos Aires Cape Town Chennai
Dar es Salaam Delhi Hong Kong Istanbul Karachi Kolkata
Kuala Lumpur Madrid Melbourne Mexico City Mumbai
Nairobi São Paulo Shanghai Taipei Tokyo Toronto

Oxford is a registered trade mark of Oxford University Press
in the UK and in certain other countries

Published in the United States
by Oxford University Press, Inc., New York

A catalogue record for this title is available from the British Library

Library of Congress Cataloging in Publication Data

(Data available)

ISBN 0 19 852338 6 (hbk)

ISBN 0 19 852337 8 (pbk)

Typeset by
Best-set Typesetter Ltd., Hong Kong
Printed in Great Britain on acid free paper by
Antony Rowe Ltd, Chippenham, Wiltshire

5/22/06

# Contents

List of contributors      ix
List of abbreviations      x

**Section I    Mechanisms of Brain Damage**

1   Death and Survival in the Nervous System      3

2   Axotomy and Mechanical Damage      15

3   Metabolic Damage      26

4   Inflammation and Demyelination      45

5   Infection      57

6   Neurodegenerative Disease      79

**Section II    Damage Limitation**

7   Neuroprotection      107

8   Steroids      121

9   Trophic Factors      127

10   Control of Inflammation      139

**Section III    Intrinsic Mechanisms of Recovery**

11   Peripheral Nerve Regeneration      145

12   Failure of CNS Regeneration      155

13   Anatomical Plasticity      171

14   Biochemical Plasticity      196

15   Remyelination      205

**Section IV    Clinical Assessment of Brain Damage**

16   Coma      217

17   Motor, Sensory, and Autonomic Function      223

18   Cognition      243

19   Psychiatric Assessment      255

## Section V  Pharmacology and Rehabilitation

20  Pharmacological Management 275

21  Neuropsychological Rehabilitation 289

## Section VI  Structural Repair

22  Axon Regeneration in the CNS 301

23  Primary Neuronal Transplantation 313

24  Glial Transplantation 335

25  Stem Cells 344

26  Gene Therapy 357

## Appendicies: Specific Diseases

Appendix 1: Alzheimer's Disease 385

Appendix 2: Amyotrophic Lateral Sclerosis/Motor Neurone Disease 387

Appendix 3: Creutfeldt–Jakob Disease (CJD) 389

Appendix 4: Epilepsy 391

Appendix 5: Huntington's Disease 393

Appendix 6: Multiple Sclerosis 395

Appendix 7: Parkinson's Disease 397

Appendix 8: Spinal-cord Injury 399

Appendix 9: Stroke 401

*Reference List* 403

*Subject Index* 457

# Contributors

Harry Baker — MRC Cognition and Behaviour group, Department of Experimental Psychology, University of Cambridge

Roger Barker — Department of Neurology, University of Cambridge Medical School

Charlotte Behan — Department of Neurology, University of Cambridge Medical School

German Berrios — Department of Psychiatry, University of Cambridge Medical School

Stacey Efstathiou — Department of Pathology, University of Cambridge

Robin Franklin — Department of Clinical Veterinary Medicine, University of Cambridge

Joe Herbert — Department of Anatomy, University of Cambridge

Andrew Lawrence — Wolfson Brain Imaging Centre, University of Cambridge Medical School

Ian H. Robertson — MRC Cognition and Brain Sciences Unit, Cambridge

Barbara J. Sahakian — Department of Psychiatry, University of Cambridge Medical School

Neil Scolding — Institute of Clinical Neurosciences, University of Bristol

Steve Wharton — Neuropathology Laboratory, University of Edinburgh

Barbara Wilson — MRC Cognition and Brain Sciences Unit, Cambridge

# Abbreviations

| | |
|---|---|
| 2VO | 2-vessel occlusion |
| 3-NP | 3-nitropropionic acid |
| 4VO | 4-vessel occlusion |
| 5,7-DHT | 5,7-dihydroxytryptamine |
| 5-HIAA | 5-hydroxyindoleacetic acid |
| 5-HT | serotonin, 5-hydroxytryptamine |
| 6-OHDA | 6-hydroxydopamine |
| 7-NI | 7-nitroindazole |
| A2B5 | A ganglioside marker for oligodendrocyte precursors |
| AADC | aromatic amino acid decarboxylase (= DDC) |
| AAV | adeno-associated virus |
| ACh | acetylcholine |
| AChE | acetylcholinesterase |
| ACTH | adrenocorticotrophic hormone |
| AD | Alzheimer's disease |
| ADEM | acute disseminated encephalomyelitis |
| ADH | antidiuretic hormone |
| ADL | activities of daily living |
| ADP | adenosine diphosphate |
| AHLE | acute haemorrhagic leukoencephalitis |
| AIDS | acquired immune deficiency syndrome |
| Akt | a protein kinase, an effector of PI3 kinase |
| ALS | amyotrophic lateral sclerosis |
| AMPA | $\alpha$-amino-3-hydroxy-5-methyl-4-isoxazole proprionic acid |
| ANCA | anti-neutrophil cytoplasmic antigen |
| ANNA (-1, -2, etc.) | anti-neuronal nuclear antibodies |
| AOAA | aminooxyacetic acid |
| apaf-1 | apoptotic protease activating factor-1 |
| APC | antigen presenting cell |
| APCA | anti-Purkinje cell cytoplasmic antibodies |
| APD | atypical prion disease |
| ApoE | apolipoprotein |
| APP | amyloid precursor protein |
| APV, AP-5 | 2-aminophosphonohaptanoic acid |
| ATP | adenosine triphosphate |
| ATPase | adenosine triphosphatase |
| AV | adenovirus |
| $A\beta$ | alternate name of $\beta$/A4 amyloid protein |
| Bad | Bcl-2-associated protein |
| Bak | Bcl-2-associated killer protein |
| Bax | Bcl-2-antagonist x protein |
| BBB | blood-brain barrier |
| Bcl-2 | B cell lymphoma leukaemia 2 protein |
| BDNF | brain derived neurotrophic factor |
| BHK | baby hamster kidney cells |
| BPRS | Brief Psychiatric Rating Scale |

| | |
|---|---|
| BSE | bovine spongiform encephalopathy |
| *C. elegans* | species of nematode worm, Caenorhabditis elegans |
| CA (1–4) | Ammon's horn fields 1–4, of the hippocampus |
| CADASIL | cerebral autosomal dominant arteriopathy with subcortical infarcts and leukoencephalopathy |
| CAG | DNA trinucleotide encoding glutamine |
| CALT | Conditional Associative Learning Test |
| CAMBS | Cambridge Multiple Sclerosis Basic Score |
| cAMP | adenosine-3′,5′-cyclic monophosphate |
| cANCA | cytoplasmic anti-neutrophil cytoplasmic antigen |
| CANTAB | Cambridge Neuropsychological Test Automated Battery |
| CANTAB | Cambridge Automated Neurological Test Battery |
| CAP-23 | cytoskeleton-associated protein-43 |
| CAPIT (-PD, -HD) | Core Assessment Protocol for Intracerebral Transplantation in Parkinson's and Huntington's diseases |
| CARE-HD | coenzyme $Q_{10}$ and remacemide evaluation in Huntington's disease |
| CAT | chloramphenicol acetyltransferase |
| CAT | computed axial tomography |
| CBG | corticoid-binding globulin |
| CBP | CREB binding protein |
| CCA | common carotid artery |
| CCK | cholecystokinin |
| CDF | cholinergic differentiation factor |
| CDK | cyclin-dependent kinase |
| ced (-3, -4, etc.) | *drosophila* cell death abnormal genes (= mammalian ICE, apaf-1, etc.) |
| *c-fos* | an immediate early gene |
| CGRP | calcitonin gene related peptide |
| CGS-19755 | *cis*-4-(phosphonomethyl)-2-piperidine carboxylic acid |
| ChAT | choline acetyltransferase |
| CHO | Chinese hamster ovary cells |
| CJD | Creutzfeldt-Jacob disease |
| *c-Jun* | an immediate early gene |
| CMUA | continuous motor unit activity |
| CMV | cytomegalovirus |
| CN | caudate nucleus |
| CNS | central nervous system |
| CNTF | ciliary neurotrophic factor |
| CoST | corticospinal tract |
| COX | cytochrome oxidase |
| CPP | 4-(3-phosphonopropyl)-2-piperazine-carboxylic acid |
| CPu | caudate-putamen |
| CREB | cAMP response element binding protein |
| CSF | colony stimulating factor |
| csf | cerebrospinal fluid |
| CSPG | chondroitin sulphate proteoglycan |
| CVA | cerebrovascular accident (stroke) |
| DA | dopamine |
| DA | dopamine, dihydroxyphenylalanine |
| DAF | decay accelerating factor |
| DARPP-32 | dopamine and adenosine-3′,5′-monophosphate regulated phosphoprotein, of 32 kD molecular weight |

| DATATOP | Deprenyl and tocopherol antioxidant treatment of parkinsonism |
|---|---|
| DBH | dopamine-$\beta$-hydroxylase |
| DC | dorsal column |
| DDAVP | desmopressin acetate |
| DDC | DOPA-decarboxylase |
| DHEA | dehydroepiandrosterone |
| DHEAS | dehydroepiandrosterone sulphate |
| DIS | NIMH Diagnostic Interview Schedule |
| DLBD | diffuse Lewy body disease |
| DNA | deoxyribonucleic acid |
| DOPA | dihydroxyphenylalanine |
| DOPAC | dihydroxyphenylacetic acid |
| DRG | dorsal root ganglia |
| *drosophila* | species of fruit fly, *drosophila melanogasta* |
| DRPLA | dentorubral-pallido-luysian atrophy |
| DRS | Mattis Dementia Rating Scale |
| DSD-1 | A chondroitin sulphate proteoglycan, the mouse homologue of phosphacan |
| DSM (-III, -IV) | Diagnostic Statistical Manual of the American Medical Association (versions III, IV) |
| *E. coli* | bacterium *Escherichia coli* |
| EAA | excitatory amino acid |
| EAE | experimental allergic encephalomyelitis |
| EC | entorhinal cortex |
| ecf | extracellular fluid |
| ECT | electroconvulsive therapy |
| EDSS | Expanded Disability Status Scale |
| EEG | electroencephalography |
| EGF | epidermal growth factor |
| Erk | extracellular-signal-regulated protein kinase |
| E-W | Ehringer-Westphal nucleus |
| F3/F11 | An adhesion molecule linked to the membrane by GPI |
| FADD | Fas-associated death domain protein (= MORT-1) |
| FADH2 | flavin adenine dinucleotide (reduced form) |
| FF | fimbria-fornix |
| FFI | fatal familial insomnia |
| FGF (1–5) | fibroblast growth factor |
| FLIP | FL-ICE (caspase 8) inhibitory protein |
| fMRI | functional magnetic resonance imaging |
| FTDP-17 | frontotemporal dementia with parkinsonism linked to chromosome 17 |
| GABA | $\gamma$-amino butyric acid |
| GAD | glutamic acid decarboxylase |
| GAG | glycosaminoglycan |
| GAL | galactose-$\alpha$-(1,3)-galactose |
| Galactocerebroside (GalC) | Cerebroside found on oligodendrocytes |
| GAP-43 | growth associated protein of 43 kD molecular weight |
| GCS | Glasgow coma scale |
| G-CSF | granulocyte colony-stimulating factor |
| GD3 | GD3 ganglioside |
| GDNF | glial cell line-derived neurotrophic factor |
| GDP | guanidine diphosphate |
| GFAP | glial fibrillary acidic protein |

| | |
|---|---|
| GFP | green fluorescent protein |
| GFR (-$\alpha$, -$\beta$, etc.) | GDNF family receptors |
| GGF (1, 2, 3, . . .) | Glial growth factor |
| GluR (1–6) | glutamate receptor subunits |
| GM-CSF | granulocyte-macrophage colony-stimulating factor |
| GnRH | gonadotrophin releasing hormone |
| Gpe | globus pallidus external segment |
| Gpi | globus pallidus internal segment |
| GR | glucocorticoid receptor |
| GRE | glucocorticoid regulatory element |
| GSS | Gerstmann-Sträussler-Scheinker syndrome |
| GTP | guanidine triphosphate |
| HAM | HTLV-1 associated myelopathy |
| HAP (-1, -2, etc.) | huntingtin-associated protein |
| HARS | Hamilton Anxiety Rating Scale |
| HCF | human host cell factor, a transcription co-factor for HSV |
| HCMV | human cytomegalovirus |
| HD | Huntington's disease |
| HDRS | Hamilton Depression Rating Scale |
| HIP (-1, -2, etc.) | huntingtin interacting protein |
| HIV | human immunodeficiency virus |
| HNK-1 | human natural killer cell epitope (= CD57) |
| hpg | hypogonadal |
| HRP | horseradish peroxidase, an axonal tracer |
| hsp | heat shock protein |
| HSV | herpes simplex virus |
| HSVc | hyperstriatum ventrale (in chick) |
| HSVc | hyperstriatum ventrale, pars caudalis (in chick) |
| HSVE | herpes simplex encephalitis |
| HTLV-1 | human T-cell lymphotrophic virus, type 1 |
| HVLT | Hopkins Verbal Learning Test |
| ICAM (-1, -2) | intercellular adhesion molecules |
| ICE | interleukin 1$\beta$ converting enzyme |
| IEG | immediate early gene |
| IFN-$\gamma$ | interferon-$\gamma$ |
| IGF (-I, -II, etc.) | insulin-like growth factors |
| IL (-1, -2, -4, -6, -10, -11, etc.) | interleukins |
| IN-1 | antibody against myelin inhibitory molecules |
| iNOS | inducible nitric oxide synthase |
| ISC | intermittent self-catheterisation |
| IT15 | 'interesting transcript' 15, the locus of the HD mutation |
| ITR | inverted terminal repeats |
| Jak (-1, -2, etc.) | Janus kinases |
| JAK/STAT | Janus kinase/signal transducers and activators of transcription |
| JNK | c-Jun N-terminal kinase |
| JPS | joint position sense |
| KA | kainic acid |
| L1 | Cell surface adhesion molecule L1 |
| lacZ | *E. coli* $\beta$-galactosidase gene |
| LAP | latency associated promoter |
| LAT | latency associated transcript |

| | |
|---|---|
| LCMV | lymphocytic choriomeningitis virus |
| L-DOPA | l-dihydroxyphenylalanine |
| LEMS | Lambert-Eaton myasthaenic syndrome |
| LFA-1 | lymphocyte function associated antigen 1 |
| LHA | lateral hypothalamic area |
| LIF | leukaemia inhibitory factor |
| LMN | lower motor neurone |
| L-NAME | nitro-L-arginine methyl ester |
| LTP | long term potentiation |
| LTR | long terminal repeat |
| LV | lentivirus |
| MAC-1 | A mouse macrophage marker |
| MAG | myelin-associated glycoprotein |
| MAO (-A, -B) | monoamine oxidase |
| MAOI | monoamine oxidase inhibitor |
| MAP | microtubule associate protein |
| MAPK | mitogen-activated protein kinase |
| MBP | Myelin basic protein |
| MCA | middle cerebral artery |
| M-CSF | macrophage-colony stimulating factor |
| MD | mediodorsal nucleus (of thalamus) |
| MEK | mitogen-activated/Erk-activating kinase |
| MG | myasthaenia gravis |
| MHC (class, 1, 2, etc.) | major histocompatibility complex molecules |
| MID | multi-infarct dementia |
| MIF | macrophage inhibitory factor |
| MIP | macrophage inflammatory protein |
| MJD | Machado-Joseph disease |
| MLV | murine leukaemia virus |
| MMLV | Moloney murine leukaemia virus |
| MMSE | Mini Mental State Exam |
| MND | motor neurone disease (= ALS) |
| MOG | myelin/oligodendrocyte glycoprotein |
| MOBP | Myelin/oligodendrocyte basic protein |
| MPO | myeloperoxidase |
| MPP+ | methylphenylpiridinium ion |
| MPTP | 1-methyl-4-phenyl-1,2,3(5),6-tetrahydropyridine |
| MR | mineralocorticoid receptor |
| MRI | magnetic resonance imaging |
| MS | medial septum |
| MS | multiple sclerosis |
| Ms1 | Primary motor cortex |
| MSA | multiple system atrophy |
| NA | noradrenaline |
| NAC | N-acetyl cysteine |
| NADH | nicotinamide adenine dinucleotide (reduced) |
| NADPH | nicotinamide adenine dinucleotide phosphate |
| NAME | nitro-arginine methyl ester |
| NART | National Adult Reading Test |
| NBM | nucleus basalis magnocellularis |
| N-CAM | neuronal cell adhesion molecule |

| | |
|---|---|
| NECTAR | Network for European CNS Transplantation and Restoration |
| NEST-HD | Network for European Striatal Transplantation in Huntington's Disease |
| NFT | neurofibrillary tangle |
| NF-$\kappa$B | transcription factor |
| NG2 | Neuron-Glia antigen, a chondroitin sulphate proteoglycan |
| NGF | nerve growth factor |
| Ng-CAM | Neuron-glial cell adhesion molecule |
| NIH | National Institutes of Health |
| NIMH | National Institute of Mental Health |
| NK cells | natural killer cells (immune system) |
| NMDA | N-methyl-D-aspartic acid |
| NO | nitric oxide |
| NOS | nitric oxide synthase |
| NP | neuritic plaques |
| NSE | neurone-specific enolase |
| NT (-3, -4/5, 6) | neurotrophins |
| nvCJD | new variant Creutzfeldt-Jacob disease |
| O1 | A ganglioside marker for oligodendrocytes |
| O4 | A ganglioside marker for immature oligodendrocytes |
| O-2A | oligodendrocyte and type 2 astrocyte precursor |
| OCD | obsessive-compulsive disorder |
| OH | hydroxyl ion |
| ONOO$^-$ | peroxynitrite |
| OPN | olivary pretectal nucleus |
| OX42 | an antibody against macrophages and microglia |
| P(S) | pregnenolone (sulphate) |
| p53 | a tumour suppressor protein |
| p75 | low affinity NGF receptor |
| PAF | platelet activating factor |
| PAK (-2) | p21-activated kinase |
| pANCA | perinuclear anti-neutrophil cytoplasmic antigen |
| PBN | $\alpha$-phenyl-*tert*-butyl-nitrone |
| PBS | phosphate buffered saline |
| PC12 | a phaeochromocytoma-derived cell line |
| PD | Parkinson's disease |
| PDGF | platelet derived growth factor |
| PEG | percutaneous endoscopic gastrostomy |
| PET | positron emission tomography |
| PI3 | phosphatidylinositol 3 |
| PKC | protein kinase C |
| PLP | proteolipid protein |
| PMC | premotor cortex |
| PML | progressive multifocal encephalopathy |
| PNS | peripheral nervous system |
| polyQ | poly glutamine repeats |
| PR3 | proteinase 3 |
| PrP | prion protein |
| PSA-N-CAM | polysialyated neuronal cell adhesion molecule |
| PSE-CATEGO | Computerised categorisation algorithm for the Present State Examination |
| PTA | post-traumatic amnesia |
| PVS | persistent vegetative state |

| Quin | quinolinic acid |
| Quis | quisqualic acid |
| RA | nucleus robusus archistriatalis (in chick) |
| Raf | a small GTPase |
| Ras | a small GTPase |
| RBMT | Rivermead Behavioural Memory Tests |
| REM | rapid eye movement |
| ReST | reticulospinal tract |
| RNA | ribonucleic acid |
| ROC | receiver operating characteristic |
| RSV | Rous sarcoma virus |
| RuST | rubrospinal tract |
| SACD | subacute combined degeneration of the cord with vitamin B12 deficiency |
| SAF | scrapie-associated fibrils |
| SAH | subarachnoid haemorrhage |
| SAPK | stress activated protein kinase |
| SBMA | spinal and bulbar muscular atrophy |
| SCA (-1, -2, etc.) | spinocerebellar atrophy, types 1, 2, etc. |
| SCG | superior cervical ganglia |
| SDH | succinate dehydrogenase |
| SDMT | Symbol Digit Modalities Test |
| SDT | signal detection theory |
| SGF | sweat gland factor |
| SLE | systemic lupus erithematosus |
| Sm1 | primary somatosensory cortex |
| SMA | supplementary motor area |
| SmII | secondary somatosensory cortex |
| SN | substantia nigra |
| SNc | substantia nigra pars compacta |
| SNr | substantia nigra pars recticulata |
| SOD | superoxide dismutase |
| S-PBN | n-tert-butyl-$\alpha$-(2-sulfophenyl)-nitrone |
| SPECT | single protein emission computed tomography |
| SSPE | subacute sclerosing panencephalitis |
| STAT | signal transducer and activator of transcription factor |
| STN | subthalamic nucleus |
| STT | spinothalamic tract |
| Sv40T | simian virus temperature sensitive proto-oncogene |
| SVZ | subventricular zone |
| Tag1/axonin1 | An axonal cell surface adhesion molecule |
| TCR | T cell antigen receptor |
| TCR | T cell receptor |
| TeST | tectospinal tract |
| TGF (-$\alpha$, -$\beta$, etc.) | transforming growth factor |
| TH | tyrosine hydroxylase |
| Thal | thalamus |
| TMT | Reitan Trail Making Test |
| TNF (-$\alpha$, -$\beta$, etc.) | tumour necrosis factor |
| tPA | tissue plasminogen activator |
| *trans*-ACPD | *trans*-1-aminocyclopentane-1,3-dicarboxylic acid |
| trk (A, B, C, etc.) | tyrosine kinase (neurotrophin) receptor |

| | |
|---|---|
| TRS | tetracycline regulatable system |
| Tta | tet transactivator protein |
| TUNEL | TdT-mediated dUTP-biotin nick end labelling |
| UHDRS | Unified Huntington's Disease Rating Scale |
| UMN | upper motor neurone |
| UPDRS | Unified Parkinson's Disease Rating Scale |
| VA-VL | ventral anterior and ventral lateral nuclei (of thalamus) |
| VCAM | vascular cell adhesion molecule |
| VER | visual evoked response |
| VeST | vestibulospinal tract |
| VIP | vasoactive intestinal polypeptide |
| VMA | ventromedial area (of hypothalamus) |
| VOSP | Visual Object and Space Perception Battery |
| VP | ventral pallidum |
| VPT | vibration perception threshold |
| VSV | vesicular stomatitis virus |
| VTA | ventral tegmental area |
| WAIS (-R) | Wechsler Adult Intelligence Scale (— revised form) |
| WCST | Wisconsin card Sorting Test |
| WGA-HRP | wheat germ agglutinin — horseradish peroxidase conjugate, an axonal tracer |
| X-gal | 5-bromo-4-chloro-3-indolyl-$\beta$-D-galactopyranoside |
| *xenopus* | acquatic frog, *xenopus laevis* |
| YVAD-cho | N-acetyl-Tyr-Val-Ala-Asp-aldehyde |
| YVAD-cmk | N-acetyl-Tyr-Val-Ala-Asp -chloromethyl ketone |
| zDCB | carbobenzoxy-Asp-1-yl-[(2,6-dichlorobenzoyl)oxy]methane |
| zVAD-cmk | benzyl-oxycarbonyl-Val-Ala-Asp-chloromethyl ketone |
| zVAD-fmk | benzyl-oxycarbonyl-Val-Ala-Asp-fluoromethyl ketone |
| $\alpha$-MCPG | $\alpha$-methyl-4-carboxyphenylglycine |
| $\alpha$-MT | $\alpha$-methyl tyrosine |
| $\beta$/A4 | alternate name of A$\beta$ amyloid protein |
| $\beta$-gal | $\beta$-galactosidase |
| GSH | glutathione |

# Section I
# Mechanisms of brain damage

# 1 | Death and survival in the nervous system

It is only in recent years that we have come to realise how important is the part played by cell death in the development, homeostasis, and injury responses of the nervous system. During development excess neurones and glia are produced, and many then die to leave behind the required number of cells. In the mature nervous system there are progenitor cells constantly dividing, the progeny either dying or differentiating, and following injury there is extensive neuronal and glial cell death. In the following sections of this book these events will be referred to in many places. This section covers the basic biology of cell survival and death, providing a background for the other chapters of this book.

## Mechanisms of cell death

Cells can die by two basic processes. The first, *necrosis*, involves a catastrophic failure of cellular homeostasis following some form of insult such as mechanical damage or anoxia, and is essentially the result of a damaging outside influence of such magnitude that the cell's homeostatic machinery is unable to compensate. The cell splits open, spilling its contents into the extracellular space. The second cell death process is called *apoptosis* and is an active suicide, in which the cell uses its own cellular mechanisms to initiate a series of molecular events that lead to the cell digesting away many of its components from the inside: the cell membrane is not disrupted, and the cell is reduced to small packages of cellular remains that can be removed by macrophages and microglia. Apoptosis can be initiated by a wide variety of extracellular events. An extreme view would be that all the cells in the body are trying to commit apoptosis all the time, but are only prevented by the action of various trophic and other molecules that suppress the necessary molecular machinery.

## Necrosis

Death by necrosis follows a complete overwhelming of the homeostatic processes in the cell, and is associated with swelling and then disruption of the nuclear, endoplasmic reticular and cell surface membranes. Necrosis is therefore always an abnormal event following damage, and is not part of the normal process of development or adult life. Any form of damage or metabolic disruption to the nervous system that leads to a challenge to cellular homeostasis which cannot be compensated, will lead to necrotic cell death. The simplest routes to necrosis are therefore events such as mechanical damage causing disruption of the cell membrane, or anoxia leading to stopping of the membrane ion pumps, cellular swelling and membrane disruption. However, necrosis occurs following events that do not kill the cell immediately, but initiate a series of intracellular and extracellular events that lead inexorably to necrotic cell death. This is particularly seen in regions of brain that are ischaemic, or in which toxic concentrations of glutamate have been released following ischaemia or trauma (see Chapter 3).

Ischaemia leads to the slowing or stopping of ATP production, and this in turn leads to the membrane pumps that use ATP directly, particularly the sodium/potassium exchange pump and the calcium/hydrogen ion exchange pump, slowing or stopping. Most other membrane pumps use the sodium ion concentration and potential gradient across the membrane established by the sodium/potassium exchange pump to power co-or counter-transport, and they will also stop. Where ATP production has stopped completely, it will lead rapidly to swelling of the cells, and disruption of the membrane and death. In regions where ischaemia is not complete, slowing of the membrane pumps leads to an influx of sodium, calcium and water, and lowering of the membrane potential. It is the rise in intracellular calcium that is responsible for initiating much of the damage that now results.

Toxic levels of glutamate are released from both neurones and glial cells following ischaemia or trauma (see Chapter 3 for details). Glutamate acts on NMDA and some AMPA channels to greatly increase their permeability to calcium, and the result is again a rise in intracellular calcium, which initiates further damage.

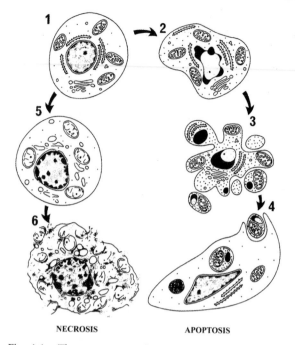

NECROSIS          APOPTOSIS

**Fig. 1.1.** The appearance of necrosis (*left*) and apoptosis (*right*). 1 is a normal cell. At the onset of apoptosis in 2, there is compaction of chromatin around the outside of the nucleus and condensation of the cytoplasm. In 3 the cell surface has become convoluted, and some convolutions separate off as apoptotic bodies; the nucleus fragments. The apoptotic bodies are ingested by neighbouring cells in 4. Necrosis begins in 5 with mitochondrial swelling and clumping of chromatin. This is followed in 6 by disruption of the membrane and breakdown of the cell. (From Kerr and Harmon 1991, with permission.)

A moderate rise in intracellular calcium in neurones will lead to apoptosis (see later), a larger rise will lead to necrosis. A demonstration that glutamate toxicity can cause both necrosis and apoptosis was made by Ankarcrona *et al.* in 1995. They found that on exposure to glutamate *in vitro*, some neurones lost their mitochondrial membrane potential and immediately underwent necrosis. However, some neurones survived this and their mitochondria recovered their membrane potential, but many of these surviving neurones underwent apoptosis a few hours later (see Fig. 1.2).

A massive rise in intracellular calcium, sufficient to induce necrosis, activates a wide range of enzymes, particularly endonucleases, calpains, lipases, and other proteases, and also leads to the production of arachidonic acid derivatives. A crucial event may be free radical production within the cell, particularly due to damage to the mitochondria. Mitochondria act as a short-term calcium buffer within the cell, taking in calcium via their membrane ATPase. The consequent large rise in mitochondrial calcium can inhibit and uncouple oxidative phosphorylation, leading to massive release of free radicals. In addition, large rises in intramitochondrial calcium can cause the opening of large non-specific channels in the membrane, known as the permeability transition pore, and this in turn leads to a loss in the mitochondrial membrane potential (as seen in the experiment by Ankarcrona *et al.* mentioned above), and this leads to swelling and dysfunction, with loss of ATP production. Mitochondrial dysfunction leads to the production of large quantities of free radicals and these can combine with nitric oxide, whose production is also increased by raised intracellular calcium, to produce the particularly toxic peroxynitrite radical, or act by themselves to cause severe damage to many aspects of neuronal function, including further damage to mitochondrial function. All of these together are sufficient to overwhelm neurones or glial cells, and lead to their rapid and messy demise.

## Apoptosis

That damaged adult neurones could die by a process radically different to necrosis is a relatively recent finding, although the idea has its roots in Clarke's writings in the nineteenth century. It has been recognised for some time that developmental cell death in the nervous system and elsewhere has different morphological features from necrosis, and this led to the process being christened 'apoptosis' by Wylie. Vertebrate neurobiologists were rather slow to grasp the significance of this, although apoptotic cell death in the development of the nervous system of invertebrates was well established. A key experiment in demonstrating that apoptosis was an important mechanism came from studying the death of neurones in tissue culture following the withdrawal of nerve growth factor. Eugene Johnson and his colleagues noted that this form of cell death could be greatly delayed by inhibiting RNA synthesis (Martin *et al.* 1988a). The implication was that cell death caused by trophic factor withdrawal was an active process that required the transcription of new genes, the synthesis of new proteins, and might therefore be apoptosis. While it is now clear that there are pathways to apoptosis that require synthesis of new proteins and also pathways that use proteins already present in the cell, this was a key insight. Apoptosis in its pure form, as is generally seen in developmental cell death, is anatomically and bio-

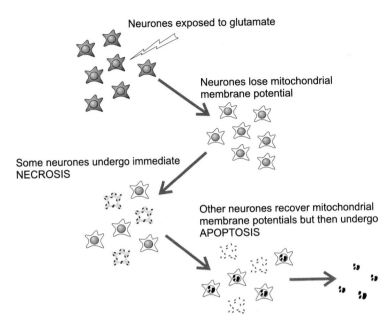

**Neurones exposed to glutamate**

**Neurones lose mitochondrial membrane potential**

**Some neurones undergo immediate NECROSIS**

**Other neurones recover mitochondrial membrane potentials but then undergo APOPTOSIS**

**Fig. 1.2** Exposure of neurones to glutamate can lead to immediate loss of mitochondrial membrane potential, after which some cell death by necrosis. However, some neurones can recover their mitochondrial membrane potential, but still die later by apoptosis.

chemically quite different from necrosis, its hallmarks being chromatin condensation with nuclear pyknosis, DNA fragmentation, and cytoplasmic shrinkage (see Fig. 1.1). However, apoptosis as seen following damage to the adult CNS may have the classical appearance, but may equally have some features that are also seen in necrosis. The morphological appearance of apoptosis has therefore been subdivided into three main types. Type 1 is the classical appearance: dense chromatin condensations appear in the nucleus and increase in number, rendering it pyknotic (condensed and electron-dense), while the cell membrane undergoes blebbing, giving a star-shaped appearance, and the blebs then detach and are phagocytosed, as eventually is the whole condensed cell. Type 2 apoptosis is characterised by the formation of autophagic vacuoles, sometimes with dilation of mitochondria and endoplasmic reticulum. The nucleus shows some pyknosis, and there may be some membrane blebbing. In type 3 apoptosis there is dilation and disintegration of greatly dilated mitochondria, Golgi, and endoplasmic reticulum, no membrane blebbing and no chromatin clumping. The vesiculated degenerating cell is eventually phagocytosed. Overall, type 3 apoptosis is anatomically rather similar to necrosis.

The practical determination of what is necrosis and what is apoptosis is sometimes straightforward, sometimes very difficult. There are two main sets of criteria: observational and interventional. The observational criteria are anatomical, as described above, and biochemical. The biochemical criteria depend on the fragmentation of DNA, which can be detected on tissue sections by the TUNEL (TdT-mediated dUTP-biotin nick end labelling) technique, or on agarose gels by DNA laddering, both demonstrating the break-up of DNA into small segments. However, both of these tests can be positive at least transiently in cells undergoing necrosis. There has therefore been something of a switch to interventional criteria. These rely on the fact that apoptosis can be blocked in most cells by inhibiting protein synthesis with agents such as cyclohexamide (although apoptosis in a few cell types does not require new protein synthesis) or more specifically by inhibiting caspases (also known as ICE-like proteases) (see below). Prevention of cell death by administering neurotrophins, or by increasing Bcl-2 (see below) expression, also point to apoptosis.

Apoptosis can be initiated in many ways, as we will now describe, but most share a final common path via a family of proteolytic enzymes called the caspases. There are, however, cellular processes with most of the features of apoptosis that do not depend on caspases, and can occur in the presence of caspase inhibitors. We will describe the molecular mechanisms and control of apoptosis after considering the way in which it is initiated and prevented.

All cells are teetering on the edge of apoptosis, with most of the necessary molecules in their cytoplasm in an inactive form. The process can be initiated by outside events, or by some malfunction of intracellular mechanisms. The sensitivity of all cells to apoptosis shows that this process is used to get rid of cells that have malfunctioned in some way, or are excess to requirements.

## Control of apoptosis

### Developmental control via trophic factors

Apoptosis was first recognised as a normal developmental event in the development of invertebrate nervous systems, particularly in that of the nematode *Caenorhabditis elegans*. This tiny nematode was originally developed as a developmental biology model in Cambridge by Brenner, White, Sulston, and many collaborators. The first work involved creating a complete anatomical cellular map of the animal at different developmental stages using electron and light microscopy. It soon became clear that during the creation of the simple nervous system there were many asymmetrical cell divisions, some of which led to two different neuronal cells but many of which led to one cell that lived, and one that committed programmed cell death (for review see: Driscoll and Chalfie 1992). Mutant nematodes, in which cell death does not occur normally, have been, as we will see later, a hugely important source of information about the molecular mechanisms of cell death. It had long been known that cell death was a normal feature of the development of the vertebrate nervous system. Almost all types of neurone are created in excess, and then around half of them die during a short period of ontogenetic cell death that occurs just after the beginning of synaptogenesis. However, the general view was that these neurones were withering away due to lack of a target-derived trophic factor. Only recently has it become clear that these excess neurones are dying by apoptosis, using a molecular mechanism very similar to that found in invertebrates.

The period of developmental cell death in neuronal populations in vertebrates occurs after axons have grown to their targets, and during or after the formation and refinement of connections. Two pioneer investigators who first worked out the rules behind the control of cell death were Viktor Hamburger, who worked on motor neurones, and Rita Levi-Montalcini, who worked on sensory neurones (Levi-Montalcini 1982; Cowan *et al.* 1984). Both left Europe around the time of the Second World War, and both ended up as colleagues in St Louis. The crucial findings were:

- Cell death only occurs in a short developmental time window, just after neurones have made their connections.

- Neuronal survival depends on making connections with an appropriate target structure. Removing the normal target leads to death of all the neurones that would normally supply it, while adding extra target reduces cell death.

Rita Levi-Montalcini, Stanley Cohen, and others were able to identify the target derived factor for sensory neurones as Nerve Growth Factor (NGF), for which work they received the Nobel Prize. NGF belongs to a family of molecules, the neurotrophins, that include NGF, NT-3, BDNF, and NT-4/5, and they in turn act on a family of tyrosine kinase receptors: trkA, trkB, and trkC. Many other growth factors can also act to promote neuronal survival via a variety of receptor types. The general principle that neurones must receive survival signals from trophic factors, most of which will be target-derived, has held up almost universally for all classes of neurone, and of course the number of trophic factors is now large. In the sensory neurones that were originally studied by Levi-Montalcini there are populations that require one of the neurotrophins (NT-3, BDNF, GDNF, or NGF) to survive, and most neurones only have receptors for one of these molecules. If these trophic factors are lacking, or if their receptors are absent, all the neurones that normally require these factors will die. This was originally shown by Cohen and Levi-Montalcini for NGF by injecting neutralising antibodies into newborn animals, and seeing that all the sympathetic neurones were lost. In a subsequent experiment, neutralising antibodies that cross the placenta were injected into the maternal circulation, again leading to the loss of sensory neurones. These findings have been confirmed in genetic knockouts, which have been made for all the neurotrophins and their receptors: thus NGF or trkA knockouts lack small pain-sensitive sensory axons and sympathetic fibres, NT-3 or trkC knockouts lack large proprioceptive axons (Carroll *et al.* 1992). In all cases, the neurones initially develop normally but then die during the period of developmental cell death, during which their survival is completely dependent on the presence of the appropriate trophic factor.

In most other neurones the situation is less straightforward because they can respond to multiple trophic factors, although the general principle that neuronal survival requires the presence of trophic support holds good. Motor neurones, for instance, receive trophic support from muscles, but have receptors and survival responses for large numbers of potential trophic molecules (Henderson 1996).

Neurones become susceptible to the absence of target-derived trophic factors once they have made connections. Clearly it would make little sense for them to be sensitive to the absence of these factors while they are still growing their axons towards that target. It is essential, therefore, that they switch on the relevant machinery only after target contact. Alun Davies and his colleagues have studied the sensitivity of neurones to lack of trophic factor and the appearance of trophic factor receptors in developing sensory and sympathetic neurones. They find that neurones placed into culture at the time when they are growing their axons, do not die when there is no trophic factor in their culture medium. However, after a period of time in culture, which corresponds to the time it would normally take the axons to make contact with their targets, the neurones start to produce trophic factor receptors, and shortly thereafter become sensitive to absence of an appropriate ligand, and die unless given the correct trophic

support (Davies 1994). This would imply that in each developing neurone there is an intrinsic genetic programme that times the appearance of trophic factor receptors and shortly thereafter initiates sensitivity to absence of trophic factor stimulation. However, there is also evidence for target-derived influences that switch neurones from dependency on one trophic factor to another and initiates production of receptors for the new factor.

After the period of developmental cell death, neurones are less sensitive to trophic factor withdrawal. For instance, as shown by Eugene Johnson, it is possible to neutralise NGF in an adult animal by injecting an antibody, and this does not result in the death of sensory and sympathetic neurones, although there is some atrophy. However the ability of adult neurones to survive stressful and damaging events and their ability to regenerate their axons is generally much improved by the presence of an appropriate trophic factor (this subject is covered in detail in Chapters 9 and 11)

Some glial cells also require trophic support at critical times. This is seen particularly during myelination,

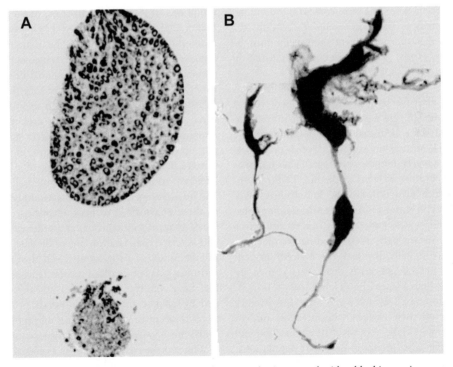

**Fig. 1.3** A comparison of sympathetic ganglia from control mice, and mice treated with a blocking antiserum to nerve growth factor for 9 days after birth. In A there are control (*top*) and experimental (*bottom*) superior cervical ganglia. In B there are whole mounts of the stellate ganglia and sympathetic chains from control (*right*) and experimental (*left*) animals. (From Levi-Montalcini 1972, with permission.)

where the number of myelinating cells is controlled by apoptosis. Extensive apoptosis in the myelinating oligodendrocyte population was first described by Barbara Barres and Martin Raff in the rat optic nerve (Barres *et al.* 1992). In a series of experiments combining tissue culture and *in vivo* experiments, they and others then went on to find out which trophic factors were necessary to keep oligodendrocytes alive. The results are complicated, in that a large number of trophic molecules can act on oligodendrocytes and their precursors, to regulate their multiplication, differentiation, and survival. The factors that have been shown to inhibit apoptosis in oligodendrocytes are: IL-1, IGF-1, CNTF, LIF, NT-3, and PDGF.

After development is complete, apoptosis in most neuronal and glial cells occurs only in pathological conditions. However, the normal adult brain does contain cells that are continually being renewed and undergoing apoptosis. The olfactory lobe contains neurones that are constantly dying and being replaced by the progeny of a precursor population that migrates from the subventricular zone of the forebrain. Several groups have recently shown that there are a small number of cells throughout the adult CNS, which are probably oligodendrocyte precursors, that are constantly dividing. Since the numbers of these cells remain constant, the implication is that the progeny of these cells must be undergoing apoptosis. These issues are discussed in detail in Chapters 13, 15, and 24.

A variety of stimuli can initiate apoptosis in adult neurones and glia. We have already described trophic factor withdrawal during development as a stimulus to apoptosis, and some neurones in the adult brain die when deprived of trophic support. Some cytokines, however, can actively initiate apoptosis. This happens when ligands bind to receptors of the fas, TNFα receptor family, which also includes the low-affinity NGF receptor, p75. TNFα, for instance, can initiate apoptosis in oligodendrocytes, and fas can initiate apoptosis in astrocytes. Surprisingly, NGF binding to the low-affinity receptor in cells that lack the high-affinity trk receptors can initiate apoptosis. This was shown by Casaccia-Bonnefil in Moses Chao's laboratory for oligodendrocyte precursors, which carry the low-affinity NGF receptor on their surface without trkA, and in which NGF can initiate apoptosis (Casaccia-Bonnefil *et al.* 1996). This also occurs in neuronal populations, where NGF secreted by microglial cells is a stimulus to the death of retinal ganglion cells following axotomy due to an optic nerve crush (Frade and Barde 1998). Other initiating stimuli are pathological challenges that

are able to initiate apoptosis in any cell type. As described earlier, a rise in intracellular calcium insufficient to cause instant necrosis can cause apoptosis. Other deleterious cellular events such as DNA damage and free radical damage may also initiate neuronal apoptosis.

## Molecular pathways in apoptosis

The molecular pathways leading to, and controlling, apoptosis are not fully worked out, although this is at present an extremely active area of research and progress is rapid. It is clear that there are many ways of initiating apoptosis, but there is in most cases a final common pathway for actually killing the cell. This usual final common pathway involves a family of molecules called ICE-like proteases, standing for interleukin 1β converting enzyme, or caspases. The involvement of these molecules was suggested by experiments in R. Horwitz's laboratory. These involved mutants of the nematode *Caenorhabditis elegans* in which programmed cell death failed to occur in the expected neurones. These mutants were found to have mutations in one of two proteins, ced-4 and ced-3, the mammalian homologue of ced-3 being ICE. Ced-4 regulates the activity of ced-3, and has a mammalian homologue apaf-1 (see later). The possible role of ICE in mammalian cells was then examined in several laboratories, and it was found that increasing the levels of ICE in cells by direct injection leads to their death by apoptosis. However, ICE itself is not crucial for neuronal apoptosis, because knockout mice have a normal pattern of programmed cell death in their nervous system. ICE, however, is a member of a large family of similar proteases, initially called the ICE-like proteases and now renamed the caspases. A number of inhibitors to these enzymes have been identified, and these can block apoptosis in neuronal and other cells both *in vivo* and *in vitro*. For instance, one of the first model systems for the study of programmed cell death in vertebrate neurones was the death of motor neurones shortly after they have connected to muscles, and this death is inhibited by caspase inhibitors. However, it is possible for death to occur in ways that resemble apoptosis anatomically, but apparently without caspase involvement.

What do the caspases do? As expected with enzymes with such dramatic and widespread effects on cells, their effects are several. A key event in apoptosis is the breakdown of nuclear DNA, which is chopped into small pieces. This is achieved because caspases modify the

DNA-cleaving enzyme, endonuclease, altering it so that it can enter the nucleus. A second key event is the breakdown of the cytoskeleton. Caspases attack gelsolin, an actin-binding protein, and the gelsolin pieces then in turn cut actin filaments. Finally, apoptosing cells break up into small membrane-covered pieces called apoptotic bodies, which are engulfed by macrophages or microglia. The kinase PAK2 is involved in this process, and is activated by caspases. Another target of caspases are caspases themselves. The caspases are present in many cells in an inactive form, and will only become active if cleaved by another protease. The cleavage site is recognised by caspases, which are therefore self-activating. Once some caspases are activated there is therefore a feedback loop leading to increasing activation.

There are many caspases: why so many? There is evidence that different caspases are involved in different apoptosis pathways. In a recent collaborative experiment from the Shelanski, Geller, and Greene laboratories, the involvement of caspases in neuronal cell death caused by trophic factor withdrawal, oxidative stress, and DNA damage was examined. All three processes could be blocked by caspase inhibitors, but not by the same ones. The implication is that the three pathways activate different caspases (see Fig. 1.4).

Apoptosis is an important mechanism for removing unwanted cells from the body, but it is of crucial importance that it is precisely controlled. Damaged and unwanted cells must be removed quickly but, since all cells have caspases and other elements of the apoptotic machinery poised to kill the cell at all times, there must be effective mechanisms for suppressing caspase activity and apoptosis, and for controlling its initiation. As we have already seen, different causes of apoptosis may activate different caspases, so it is not surprising that different control mechanisms are involved. These are far from fully worked out, but the broad picture is understood, and we outline it below.

## Cell death caused by Fas and TNFα

Fas, the TNFα receptor, and p75, the low-affinity NGF receptor, all belong to a receptor family that includes other cell death receptors found in the immune system. The activation of the cell death process relies on an adapter protein, named MORT-1/FADD (see Fig. 1.5).

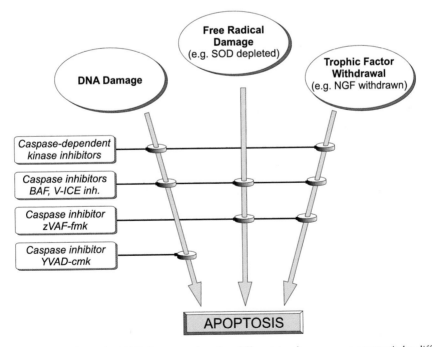

**Fig. 1.4** An experiment by Park *et al.* (1998) demonstrating that different insults can cause apoptosis by different pathways. Apoptosis can be inhibited by blockers of the cell cycle-regulating cyclin-dependent kinases (a ring across the arrow indicates the ability to block the process), but not if it is initiated by free-radical damage. Different caspase inhibitors show differential blocking of the three pathways.

This protein contains two crucial domains. The first is the death domain, which is shared with the receptor itself and allows the adapter to bind to the activated receptor. The other domain found in the adapter protein is the death effector domain, which is also found in caspases 8 and 10, and allows adapter and caspase to bind to one another. When MORT-1/FADD and the caspase are bound together, cleavage of the caspase, possibly by other caspases in the same complex, results in caspase activation, and then apoptosis. Also in the pathway are regulatory proteins, one of which is called FLIP, which may block caspase-adapter binding: viral inhibitors of apoptosis exist that act in the same way as FLIP. Paradoxically, activation of the transcription factor NF-κB by Fas activation also turns on genes that may protect against cell death.

## Cell death caused by calcium and free radical damage

The key to this pathway to cell death is the release of cytochrome c from mitochondria. The part played by cytochrome c was worked out by Wang and his colleagues, who started looking for the mechanisms of caspase activation. They found two molecules that had to be present simultaneously to activate caspases 3 and 9. One of these turned out to the be mammalian homologue of the nematode ced-4, which they named apaf-1, and the second turned out to be the mitochondrial enzyme cytochrome c. A probable mechanism (see Fig. 1.6) of activation is for cytochrome c to bind to apaf-1, inducing a conformational change which allows it to bind to pro-caspases, which in turn allows the pro-

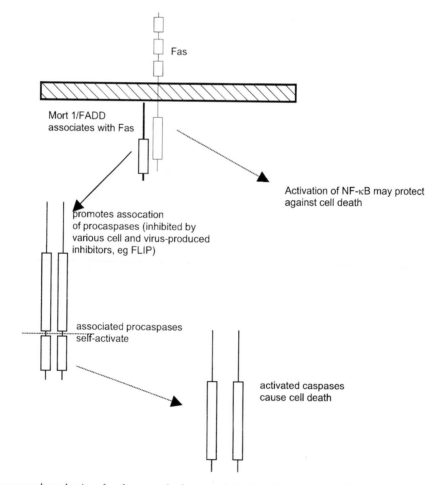

**Fig. 1.5** The proposed mechanism for the control of apoptosis by Fas. Fas is activated by the Fas ligand (or the TNFα receptor by TNFα, or p75 by NGF). This allows activation of Mort1/FADD, which can then associate with caspases, bringing them together to allow self-activation by cleavage. The activate caspases can then cause apoptosis.

caspases to autoactivate one another. Apaf-1 is present constitutively, so the key regulatory molecule turned out unexpectedly to be a mitochondrial enzyme. What then might regulate the release of mitochondrial contents? The general answer is any stressful event that sufficiently challenges cellular and mitochondrial homeostasis. Into this category would come free radical damage, anoxia, and raised intracellular calcium. Why calcium? The mitochondria act as a calcium buffer, rapidly taking up calcium when cytoplasmic levels rise. At moderate mitochondrial calcium levels both Krebs' cycle and the respiratory chain are inhibited, with an increase of free radical production and some mitochondrial rupture and damage. At higher calcium levels a non-specific mitochondrial membrane pore (named the permeability transition pore) may open, leading to depolarisation of the mitochondrial membrane, mitochondrial dysfunction and swelling, and cytochrome c release. In addition to these directly challenging events, caspases themselves promote mitochondrial cytochrome c release, setting up yet another positive feedback loop, where caspase activation leads to further caspase activation. The other major control of cytochrome c release from mitochondria is via molecules of the Bcl-2/Bax family (see next paragraph).

## Cell death caused by trophic factor withdrawal

The molecular links between the known cell-signalling events initiated by trophic factor binding and the control of cell death are not fully in place. Many of the first steps in the signalling pathways following trophic factor binding are now known, as are some of the various ways in which trophic factors inhibit apoptosis. Some of the effects of trophic factor withdrawal are also understood, and it is important to realise that the question, 'What effects do trophic factors have on neurones?' may have a very different answer to the question, 'What causes cell death when trophic factors are withdrawn?'. There are three main signalling pathways that are activated by trophic factors binding to their receptors, as shown in Fig. 1.7.

1. Binding of a neurotrophin to one of the trk receptor tyrosine kinases initiates a cascade of phosphorylation events. The first kinase is Ras, activated via three membrane proteins by replacing a GDP with GTP. Ras activates sequentially Raf, MEK, Erk kinase, and MAP kinase. MAPK translocates to the

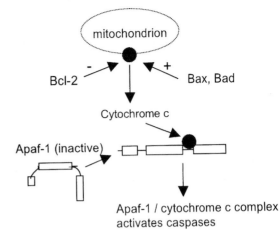

**Fig. 1.6** A probable mechanism for the control of apoptosis by Bcl-2 and Bax. Bcl-2 and Bax have opposing actions on the release of cytochrome c from mitochondria. If released, cytochrome c activates apaf-1, which in turn activates caspases. In addition, Bcl-2 may directly inhibit the activation by apaf-1 of caspases.

nucleus, where it phosphorylates several transcription factors.

2. Trk activation also activates a survival-promoting pathway, leading to the activation of PI3 kinase either directly by trk or by Ras, and its downstream target the serine-threonine kinase Akt.

3. CNTF receptor, and related receptors for LIF, IL-6, and IL-11, signal via a pathway in which the first event is the activation of the kinases Jak1 and Jak2, which in turn phosphorylate and activate two members of the STAT family of transcription factors: MAP kinase is also activated. These in turn activate the CNTF-responsive genes, which are not identical to those regulated by trk activation.

These three signalling pathways, or rather absence of signalling down these pathways, must be responsible for the initiation of apoptosis. However, only in one case is a plausible mechanism known that goes all the way from loss of trophic factor to caspase activation (see below). In general it is possible to say that trophic factor binding has many different effects on cell survival, each of which by itself may not be critical in initiating or preventing apoptosis. Also, in general, trophic factor binding can have long-term effects on cells via changes

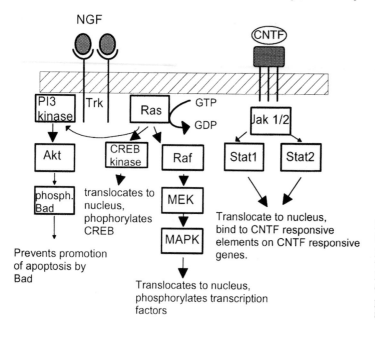

Fig. 1.7 Signalling pathways from trophic factor receptors. The kinase Ras plays a central part in the response from Trk receptors, controlling the activity of Raf and thus MAP kinase, and of CREB kinase and thus of the CREB (cyclic AMP response element binding protein), which activates transcription of many immediate early genes.

in gene expression, but also much shorter term effects through phosphorylation events, and both types of mechanism have effects on cell survival. Amongst the potentially apoptosis-inhibiting effects of trophic factor binding are suppression of stress-activated kinase (JNK) activity, effects on the intracellular calcium set-point, and suppression of free radical production.

In order to understand the control of apoptosis, it is first necessary to describe its control by molecules of the Bcl-2/Bax family of molecules. Bcl-2 and its role in the control of apoptosis was first identified in two ways. First, it is homologous to yet another nematode cell death gene, ced-9, and second, it plays an important part in the control of lymphocyte cell death in the immune system. Increasing Bcl-2 levels in lymphocytes inhibits cell death, and the same turned out to be broadly true for neurones. Thus, Alun Davies and others were able to show that increasing Bcl-2 levels in cultured neurones protected them from the cell death that normally occurs after trophic factor withdrawal, while decreasing Bcl-2 levels increased cell death, and this increased death could not be prevented by trophic factor treatment. However, the involvement of Bcl-2 in preventing cell death on trophic factor withdrawal was not universal because some neurones that die on with-

drawal of CNTF were not protected by Bcl-2. Subsequently equivalent experiments have been done by producing transgenic mice in which Bcl-2 is either overexpressed in neurones or knocked out, resulting in increased neuronal survival in the former case, and increased death in the latter. Bcl-2 is a member of a family of proteins, which include Bcl-2, Bcl-x, Bax, and Bad, all of which can dimerise with one another. While Bcl-2 and Bcl-x are neuroprotective in most neurones, increased levels of Bax and Bad lead to increased neuronal death. Bcl-2 binds to several proteins, but two mechanisms by which it can prevent cell death have been identified. The first involves mitochondria (see Fig. 1.6), as mentioned above. Bcl-2, in ways that are not fully understood, can prevent the release of cytochrome c from mitochondria, possibly by blocking a membrane channel, while the presence of Bax dimerising with Bcl-2 prevents the Bcl-2 performing this function. Thus Bcl-2 and Bcl-x are yet another way of regulating apoptosis through cytochrome c levels in the cytoplasm. However, Bcl-2 also has another function in binding to apaf-1, the protein that co-operates with cytochrome c to activate caspases. By binding to apaf-1, Bcl-2 is able to prevent caspase activation, and thus promote cell survival. Apart from caspase-dependent apoptosis there are also other apoptosis-like forms of cell death that are caspase independent, and these are also controlled by Bcl-2.

Bcl-2 and its homologues are therefore able to influence cell survival, but does this have anything to do with trophic factors, or is it just providing yet another independent regulator of apoptosis? There is little evidence that trophic factors can regulate Bcl-2 or Bax levels directly. There is, however, one experiment that directly links trophic factors to Bax. M. Greenberg (Datta *et al.* 1997) was looking for the mechanism by which the PI3 kinase/Akt signalling pathway, which is trophic factor controlled by IGF-1, was able to influence cell death. He was able to show in cerebellar granule cells that Akt phosphorylates Bad, blocking Bad-induced neuronal death. Moreover, mutagenising Bad so that it cannot be phosphorylated by Akt prevented cell death being rescued by IGF-1.

However, it is almost certainly incorrect to ascribe the prevention of apoptosis to a single metabolic pathway. Trophic factors have many different effects within neurones, and trophic factor withdrawal therefore probably tips cells towards apoptosis in several different ways. Some trophic factor effects are long-term, via changes in gene expression, others shorter term via post-translational mechanisms. At present it is far from clear how these various parallel mechanisms might act. In sympathetic neurones in culture, A. Tolkovsky (Nobes and Tolkovsky 1995) has shown that the crucial NGF-activated mediator of cell survival is Ras, but this molecule can phosphorylate a large number of other proteins, leading amongst other things, as discussed earlier, to MAP kinase activation and to PI3 activation. Some ways in which NGF binding could suppress cell death are via PI3/Akt as above, via the suppression of JNK (c-Jun N-terminal kinase) activity and via regulation of the intracellular calcium set-point concentration. In addition, trophic factors may suppress free radical formation in the neurone. The first suggestion of this was the finding that NGF withdrawal from sympathetic neurones causes a short-lived increase in reactive oxygen intermediates, insufficient to kill the cells by itself. It has now been shown that motor neurones deprived of trophic support and induced to undergo apoptosis by withdrawal of BDNF, upregulate the enzyme nitric oxide synthase. Nitric oxide is somewhat toxic to cells by itself, but much more toxic when it combines with superoxide radicals to make peroxynitrite (ONOO$^-$) Apoptosis would then be initiated by the mechanism we outlined above for free radical-induced cell death. That the nitric oxide production might be playing an impor-

tant part in causing apoptosis was suggested by the fact that death was reduced by application of a nitric oxide synthase inhibitor. Also implicated in cell death due to NGF deprivation are the cell cycle control molecules, cyclins, and cyclin-dependent kinases. Loss of trophic factor leads to the upregulation of two early cyclins, which must normally be repressed by the trophic factor. Inhibition of the cyclin-dependent kinases that interact with these molecules can suppress apoptosis. This suggests that after loss of a trophic signal, a cell cycle-related pathway involving the cyclin-CDK machinery is turned on inappropriately, and this improper signal ultimately serves to activate the apoptotic pathway

## Cell death caused by DNA damage

Apoptosis due to DNA damage involves components of the cell cycle machinery. Cell cycle progression is largely determined by the interactions of the various cyclins with their specific cyclin-dependent kinases, and DNA damage can upregulate some cyclins. Also involved is the tumour suppressor protein, p53, which mediates the apoptotic responses of most cell types to DNA damage. A variety of experiments have used inhibitors of cyclin-dependent kinases and cell-cycle progression to modulate apoptosis induced by various DNA damaging agents. The general finding is that inhibiting the early stages of the cell-division cycle, before S phase, stops apoptosis. The G1/S phase inhibitor mimosine prevents DNA damage-induced death, while the S phase inhibitor aphidicolin does not. In addition cyclin-dependent kinase inhibitors can prevent apoptosis. The conclusion is that DNA damage activates the early stages of the cell-cycle machinery, and the combination of this and damage to the genetic material puts the neurones into apoptosis.

There are many ways for a neurone to die, and many different molecular pathways. In later sections of this book many different ways of initiating neuronal death are described. Clearly there cannot be a single simple way of preventing cell death, and if a neurone is badly damaged it may not even be advantageous to do so. Inhibition of necrotic cell death is particularly difficult, because the insult to the cell is in most cases simply not survivable. However apoptosis is largely an active process, initiated and mediated by machinery within neurones themselves. As can be seen from the preceding paragraphs, there is more than one path to apoptosis.

However, most forms of apoptosis end with the activation of caspases, and it is largely the caspases that finally destroy the cell. These molecules are therefore attractive pharmacological targets. However, the design of caspase blockers is complicated by the number of different caspases that are found in neurones, and by the fact that different routes to apoptosis appear to activate different caspases.

# Further reading

Pettmann, B. and Henderson, C.E. (1998). Neuronal cell death. *Neuron*, **20**, 633–647.

Rubin, L.L. (1998). Neuronal cell death: an updated view. *Progress in Brain Research*, **117**, 3–8.

Wyllie, A.H. (1997). Apoptosis: an overview. *British Medical Bulletin*, **53**, 451–465.

*Axotomy and mechanical damage*

Almost any form of damage to the nervous system will damage axons. Axons are in a uniquely vulnerable position compared with most other cell components in that they are long and, therefore, for the most part physically far removed from their cell body. Yet they are entirely dependent on the cell body for the provision of the proteins required for homeostasis and function. Cutting an axon disconnects that part of it distal to the lesion from its source of protein synthesis and eventual death is, therefore, inevitable. The myelin that surrounds a dying axon is also inevitably compromised. The degeneration of the distal portion of a cut axon, together with the degeneration of its myelin, was originally described by Waller in 1850, and is now termed Wallerian degeneration.

The mechanism of axonal degeneration is not, as might be supposed, a gradual withering away due to protein malnutrition, but an active process. The most direct demonstration of this comes from comparing axonal degeneration in normal animals with degenera-

tion in the mutant Ola mouse (see Fig. 2.1). In normal animals, after axotomy the axonal cytoskeleton starts to fragment and degenerate, and the axon starts to break up within a few days, the exact timing depending on which axon has been cut and how far from the cell body it is sectioned. However, in the Ola mouse, cut axons, which are just as disconnected from the cell body and just as starved of newly synthesised proteins, may survive and appear quite normal for as long as a month after being cut (Lunn *et al.* 1989). This shows that the process of axonal death due to starvation is slow, and that normal axons have an active mechanism that causes their death, which must be blocked in the Ola mouse due to a mutation in one of the proteins in the pathway.

Experiments examining axonal degeneration following axotomy in tissue culture have identified the key mechanisms. Axons can be grown in a tissue culture dish and cut with a microknife, and this is followed by a process of axonal dissolution that appears to be

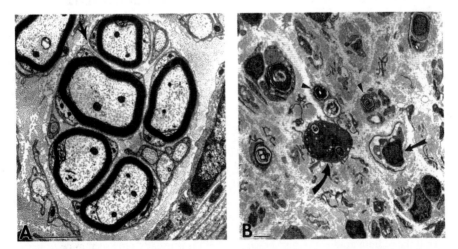

**Fig. 2.1** Degeneration of axons in the normal and Ola mouse. A, Ola peripheral nerve axons 7 days after nerve transection, showing no signs of degeneration. The *arrow* points to a basal lamina sheath. B, axons from wild-type mice 7 days after transection, showing complete degeneration. The *bent arrow* shows a macrophage, the *straight arrow* shows myelin debris. Prolonged survival of transected nerve fibres in C57BL/Ola mice is an intrinsic characteristic of the axon. (From Glass *et al.* 1993, with permission.)

identical to that seen *in vivo*. There is a delay of 24–48 h during which the cut axon appears normal, then there is blebbing of the axon surface, disruption of the cytoskeleton, and eventually almost complete dissolution of the axon. This shows that axonal degeneration does not require the intervention of other cells outside the axon — neither Schwann cells, oligodendrocytes, astrocytes, nor microglia are required for the basic degenerative process.

An important experiment in elucidating the mechanism behind this process was performed by Schlaepfer and Bunge in 1973, investigating the role of calcium ions in axonal degeneration. By culturing axons in low-calcium media, or in the presence of calcium-chelating agents, they were able to show that the sudden dissolution of axotomised axons, after a 1- or 2-day, delay was completely prevented by the absence of extracellular calcium concentrations above about 200 μM. The subsequent sequence of events has now largely been worked out by Schlaepfer and other authors (see George *et al.* 1995). Calcium entry into a cut axon happens in two phases. Immediately after cutting the axon there is diffusion of calcium from the high-concentration extracellular pool (around 1.8 mM) through the disrupted membrane into the low-concentration intracellular pool. This ceases as soon as the axonal membrane reseals, which happens rapidly unless the axon is cut very close to the cell body causing major damage to the neurone itself. Intracellular calcium in the cut axon is then well controlled until a second phase of calcium entry, which immediately precedes the onset of degeneration. This second phase of entry can probably occur through two routes. One route is voltage gated calcium channels, particularly the L-type channels. Thus degeneration in sensory axons in culture can be blocked by L-type calcium channel blockers. Entry of calcium is probably triggered by depolarisation of the axon, which implies that at some point after axotomy the axon loses its ability to maintain a normal resting membrane potential. A second route of calcium entry, which has been implicated in axonal degeneration in the CNS following anoxia, is through the sodium–calcium exchange pump running in reverse. Normally the energy produced by allowing sodium ions to pass down the concentration and potential gradient across the membrane is used to drive an exchange pump that removes calcium from the cell. However, if the sodium gradient diminishes and the membrane becomes partially depolarised due to intense action potential activity, or due to failure of the ATP-driven sodium–potassium exchange pump, then the calcium gradient, with high extracellular and low

intracellular calcium, can drive the sodium–calcium counter-transport pump in reverse. In either case, the result is a sudden major increase in the calcium concentration within the axon. This rise in calcium, if the intracellular concentration exceeds 200 μM, is sufficient to trigger the activity of the calcium-activated enzymes, the calpains, and possibly other mechanisms as well. The main enzymatic substrates of the calpains are cytoskeletal molecules and, therefore, calpain activation leads to degradation of the axonal cytoskeleton. Inhibition of calpains is sufficient to prevent axonal degeneration in tissue culture.

## Neuronal responses to axotomy

Cutting an axon not only affects the axon distal to the cut, it also affects the neurone itself. The most extreme effect is neuronal death, which may occur by apoptosis or necrosis (see Chapter 1). In those neurones that are not killed immediately by the lesion, there is a well-described set of changes that occur, many of which are associated with re-initiating synthesis of the proteins that are needed for axon growth and regeneration. In terms of the anatomical appearance of the neurone, these changes take the form of chromatolysis. This is the dispersal of the large granular condensations of Nissl stained material, which represent condensations of rough endoplasmic reticulum, coupled with changes in the appearance of the nucleus (Lieberman 1971). In molecular terms this process underlies major changes in the pattern and quantity of protein synthesis. The initiation of these changes requires some information to reach the cell body via axonal transport, since inhibition of rapid axonal transport with colchicine prevents the onset of chromatolysis following axotomy. Many genes are upregulated or down-regulated after axotomy, and far from all of them have been identified. Those that have been identified fall into the following categories.

- *Transcription factors.* At around 24 h after axotomy, c-jun and jun D are upregulated in most neurones, and Krox-24 may also be expressed, as may some heat-shock proteins. There is differential control of immediate early gene expression, since c-fos is usually only seen in neurones very close to the lesion that may be fatally injured. The position of the lesion is also a factor. In peripheral nervous system (PNS) neurones, cutting the axon at any point can upregulate c-jun, while in the rubrospinal tract, and probably other central nervous system (CNS) pathways, lesions made near the neuronal cell body lead to upregulation, while more distal lesions do not. Expression may continue in the PNS during the time when axons are regenerating, but also persists in the CNS for months in neurones whose axons will not regenerate (De Felipe *et al.* 1993) (see Chapters 11, 12, and 22).

- *Growth associated proteins.* GAP-43 is a protein found on the inner surface of the growth cones of all growing and regenerating axons, and is probably involved in the dialogue between axonal growth mechanisms and the outside environment. Its pattern of expression is similar to that of c-jun, in that it is upregulated rapidly in PNS neurones wherever they are axotomised, but in CNS neurones only when the axon is cut near the cell body (Tetzlaff *et al.* 1994) (see Chapters 11, 12, and 22).

- *Cytoskeletal proteins.* After axotomy there is a large increase in tubulin synthesis, and a decrease in neurofilament synthesis. The tubulin gene activation is not general to all the tubulin genes, but is specific to the $T\alpha1$ gene, the major tubulin gene expressed in neurones during embryonic axon growth. However, while most of the changes in cytoskeletal gene expression recapitulate the pattern seen during development, there is one important class of proteins that retain their adult pattern of expression. The microtubule associated proteins (MAPs) are centrally involved in the stabilisation of the microtubules and construction of the axonal cytoskeleton during growth. The types of MAPs expressed change at the end of development, and after axotomy there is little change in the level of MAP synthesis and reversion to expression of the types of MAP expressed during development (Fawcett *et al.* 1994). This may be an important reason for the relatively poor growth of axons during regeneration (see Chapters 11, and 12).

- *Growth factor receptors and growth factors.* In general, neurotrophin receptors are upregulated on axotomised neurones. mRNA levels for the trk family of receptors for the neurotrophins NGF, BDNF, and NT-3 are reported to increase two- or three-fold within 2 days of axotomy in several neuronal types, and expression of the-low affinity NGF receptor, p75, is also increased. In some neurones there is also an increase in synthesis of the neurotrophins; for instance, both BDNF and trkB pro-

duction are increased in facial nerve nucleus motor neurones after axotomy (Kobayashi *et al.* 1996; Verge *et al.* 1996).

- *Cytokines.* Axotomised sensory neurones increase expression of IL-6, IL1$\beta$, and TNF$\alpha$.

# Neuronal death following axotomy

Death may be via the apoptosis pathway and delayed, in which case it is probably due to loss of support from target-derived trophic factors (see later), or due to calcium influx. Rapid necrotic cell death after axotomy occurs mainly when the axon is damaged very close to the cell body, for instance, motor neurones may be killed in injuries in which the ventral roots are avulsed from the spinal cord due to traumatic stretching of the brachial plexus. This immediate death is probably due to a combination of physical trauma to the neurone, which disrupts the membrane and cytoskeleton, and to the massive calcium influx that occurs when the axonal membrane is disrupted.

Many neurones do not die immediately when their axons are cut, but may die days later. Some of these neurones are close to the site of injury, but many may be some distance away. In addition to this retrograde cell death of neurones whose axons have been cut, there is also in some situations anterograde cell death, with death of the neurones to which those axons connect, also by apoptosis. Both anterograde and retrograde neuronal death are at least partly due to loss of access to trophic factors. Neurones can gain access to trophic support from several sources. These include the target neurones with which they synapse, from neurones which make synapses with them, from Schwann cells, astrocytes, and oligodendrocytes that contact the neurone at different points, and from microglia that cluster around damaged neurones (see Fig. 2.2). When its axon is cut, a neurone clearly loses contact with its target cells and loses trophic support from that source. In addition, as Kreutzberg and his collaborators have shown in the facial nerve nucleus, when a neurone has its axon cut there is a retrograde reaction that leads to most of the synapses on the cell soma retracting, their place being taken initially by microglia and, later, by astrocytes (Kreutzberg 1996).

Therefore, an axotomised neurone will lose much of the trophic support it would have received from the synapses impinging on it, although this may be replaced

sources of neuronal trophic support

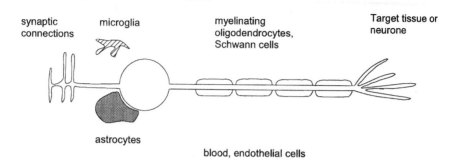

**Fig. 2.2** Neurones can in principle gain trophic support from many different sources. Possible sources are target structures, myelinating cells, astrocytes, input synapses, blood, endothelial cells, microglia.

by a different set of trophic factors secreted by microglia and astrocytes (see later). While the neurone may lose trophic support from its efferent and afferent connections, a new source of support arises from the glial cells surrounding the area of damage. In the CNS, astrocytes in areas of damage become reactive, in which state they secrete several potentially trophic molecules (see later). Also, microglia migrate to areas of damage and undergo mitosis and also become activated, again leading to the production of a variety of cytokines, some with neurotrophic activity, some which may be toxic (see later). In the PNS, Schwann cells become activated after axotomy and there is a rapid accumulation of macrophages. Again, these cells secrete molecules that are trophic to neurones with appropriate receptors, but macrophages may, in addition, secrete toxic molecules.

There is, therefore, a complex set of changes in the molecules impinging on an axotomised neurone. The overall change that affects neurones after axotomy must be a loss of trophic support, since many neurones die and many others become atrophic. The overall hypothesis that axotomy induced cell death and atrophy is largely due to a loss of trophic factors is supported by the fact that death and atrophy can be greatly attenuated by application of a variety of trophic factors. There are many examples of this (see Chapter 9). For instance, infusion of NGF into the ventricles prevents the death or atrophy of basal forebrain cholinergic neurones that usually follows fimbria fornix transection (Hefti 1986).

The various types of axotomy-induced changes and the effects of trophic factors are particularly well worked out in the rubrospinal pathway of the rat,

largely as a result of experiments by Wolfram Tetzlaff. The changes seen in these neurones are, as with most, dependent on the position of axotomy (see Fig. 2.3). Thus, if the rubrospinal axons are sectioned close to the cell body in the cervical spine, many neurones die, but those remaining upregulate the production of GAP-43, and the axons can exhibit a robust regenerative response provided a permissive environment is provided for them to grow into (see Chapter 22). However, if the axons are sectioned more distally in the thoracic cord there is less neuronal cell death, no upregulation of GAP-43, and the axons will not regenerate even if presented with a permissive peripheral nerve graft. Trophic factors are involved in some aspects of these changes. If rubrospinal axons are cut distally and BDNF applied to the neuronal cell bodies, the atrophy that normally occurs is reduced, GAP-43 expression is upregulated, and the axons attain the ability to regenerate into grafts of peripheral nerve (Tetzlaff *et al.* 1994).

A similar set of conditions applies in the nigro-striatal tract. Here, axotomy close to the substantia nigra eventually leads to the death of almost all the dopaminergic neurones; the closer the lesion to the cell body, the faster the death. However, if only the terminals of the neurones are lesioned, there is much less cell death. Again, cell death and atrophy in the form of the loss of dopaminergic phenotype after axotomy can be much reduced by infusions of an appropriate trophic factor, in this case GDNF. However, the results of axotomy are much less dependent on its position in other pathways. For instance, in sensory neurones the changes in protein synthesis after axotomy are much the same regardless of where the axon is cut. In all these

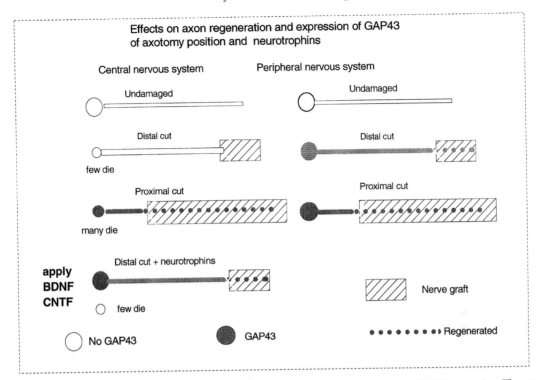

**Fig. 2.3** The regenerative response of CNS and PNS neurones to different environments, and GAP43 expression. The *top pair* show that undamaged neurones mostly express little GAP43. In the *second row*, a PNS axon cut some distance from the cell body upregulates GAP43 expression, and the axon regenerates into a peripheral nerve graft, while a CNS axon, such as a rubrospinal axon, neither regenerates nor expresses GAP43. However, as shown in the *third row*, if cut close to the cell body both PNS and CNS neurones will upregulate GAP43, and regenerate their axons into a peripheral nerve graft. The *fourth row* shows that CNS neurones may have their regenerative response modified by trophic factors: BDNF or CNTF applied to a rubrospinal neurone will alter the regenerative response to distal axotomy, so that when cut far from the cell body the axons will now regenerate, and the neurone upregulates GAP43.

models, cutting the axon at any point will deprive neurones of their source of target-derived trophic factor. However, since the consequences are very different depending on where the axon is cut, there must be mechanisms other than simply the loss of target-derived molecules. Amongst these factors are the delivery of trophic factors by the glial cells along the pathway of the cut axon (see later), and the mechanical damage and calcium entry that result from axotomy close to the cell body. However, even bringing in these two mechanisms does not really explain the differences between proximal and distal axotomy, or the fact that these differences are more pronounced in some pathways than others. There must also be some feature of the signals passing back to the cell body from the cut axon tip that differs depending on distance, and differs from one type of neurone to another.

## Glial responses to axotomy

### Inflammatory cells

An injury anywhere in the body will cause a series of responses that lead to the proliferation and accumulation of inflammatory cells. First to respond are neutrophils, which respond within minutes and remain present at the site of injury for 24–48 h. This is followed by macrophages, which accumulate more slowly but remain for several days until the injury is resolved.

The inflammatory response in the CNS is very different to that seen anywhere else in the body. Neutrophils are not recruited from the circulation unless there is extensive tissue destruction. Unless there is vascular damage and bleeding, the macrophages that accumulate around a CNS injury are largely derived from the resident macrophage population of the CNS, the microglia, and their numbers and rate of accumulation are much slower than elsewhere. These special features of the CNS injury response have several consequences for CNS degeneration and repair.

## Neutrophils

Neutrophils are not a major feature of CNS injuries unless there is damage to blood vessels and extensive bleeding. Where there is haemorrhage, neutrophils will be extravasated along with other blood cells, and there will eventually be a neutrophil response in the organising blood clot. However, there is little or no neutrophil recruitment into the CNS parenchyma itself. This surprising absence of a neutrophil response is also seen in many inflammatory conditions. Some of the reasons why the CNS may be so different in this respect have recently been worked out by Perry and his colleagues (see Foa *et al.* 1997). Outside the CNS, neutrophil recruitment to an injury is caused by the damaged tissue secreting a variety of molecules, particularly bradykinin, kallikrein, arachidonic acid derivatives, and chemokines. These cause the vascular endothelial cells to express a set of adhesion molecules that are adhesive to the circulating neutrophils, and enable them to penetrate the vascular wall. In addition, the molecules secreted by damaged tissue are directly chemotactic towards neutrophils. The vascular responses following CNS inflammatory stimuli are largely normal. The main abnormality of the CNS relative to the rest of the body may lie in the production of chemokines. Outside the CNS the $\alpha$-chemokines are centrally involved in neutrophil recruitment, so if there is no neutrophil recruitment a possible reason is the absence of production of the relevant chemokines. In order to test this possibility Bell, Taub, and Perry injected $\alpha$-chemokines, particularly MIP-2, directly into the CNS, and found that this provokes a massive neutrophil response with breakdown of the blood–brain barrier (Bell *et al.* 1996). The implication is that CNS damage does not lead to chemokine release, and therefore there is little neutrophil recruitment.

## Macrophages/microglia

At the site of an injury to the PNS, macrophages are recruited and respond in much the same way as they would to any injury elsewhere in the body. There is a rapid recruitment of macrophages, partly as a result of local bleeding, but mostly as a result of migration of monocytes through the blood-vessel endothelium. In addition, soon after axotomy, there is macrophage recruitment throughout the distal stump of the nerve, where axons and myelin are degenerating. A variety of factors have effects on the vascular endothelial cells, leading to upregulation of selectins, ICAM-1, on the endothelial surface, allowing macrophages to attach to the blood-vessel wall and migrate into the tissue, where they can respond to a variety of chemotactic stimuli. Macrophages are largely responsible for removing the debris of degenerating axon and myelin from the injury site and the distal part of the nerve, and they are often seen with large vesicles containing degraded myelin. However, the Schwann cells also have some phagocytic activity. Macrophages also accumulate around the neurones whose axons have been cut. In the CNS these cells are microglia, and this process is described later. In peripheral ganglia, macrophages are recruited from the bloodstream, and are found throughout the ganglia, some in perineuronal positions, others near blood vessels or amongst the satellite cells.

In addition to their phagocytic activity, macrophages secrete a large number of molecules, many of which have either positive or negative effects on neuronal survival and development, and on the Schwann cells (see below).

It has been known for many years that there is a conditioning effect on axon regeneration. If a peripheral nerve is crushed it will eventually start to regenerate, but if it is crushed again within a week or so, regeneration will begin sooner and proceed more rapidly. This change affects all the axonal branches of a neurone, not just those that have been cut. Thus when the peripheral branch of a sensory axon is damaged, the branch going towards the spinal cord will, after about 24 h, regenerate with greater vigour. Richardson has shown that part of this conditioning effect may be due to inflammatory changes in the sensory ganglia (Lu and Richardson 1995). He caused inflammation in the ganglia either by injecting bacterial material or by injecting macrophages directly. After both types of injection there was an increase in the number of regenerating axons after dorsal root crushes. This could have been due to a direct action of substances secreted by the macrophages on the neurones, or it could have been a secondary effect via the glial cells.

Macrophages also have direct effects on the Schwann cells of damaged peripheral nerves. Many of the cytokines that are secreted by macrophages may have activity on Schwann cells. A major macrophage cytokine is interleukin 1$\beta$. This acts on Schwann cells to cause them to upregulate their production of NGF, which in turn has positive effects on the survival and regeneration of sensory and autonomic axons. Mitogenic effects of macrophages on Schwann cells have also been shown. Schwann cells can release other neurotrophins in damaged nerves, particularly BDNF and CNTF, but a part played by macrophages in stimulating this has not been proven (see review by Perry and Brown 1992).

In the CNS the response from cells of the macrophage lineage is very different. The CNS has a resident macrophage population, the microglial cells. These enter the CNS from the circulation during embryogenesis. In the adult CNS there is little interchange between the blood monocyte/macrophage population and the microglia. Moreover, even after lesions to the CNS, there is little or no recruitment of macrophages from the vascular system, except where blood vessels are damaged at the site of the lesion. Most of the phagocytic and other macrophage-type activity in the CNS is therefore due to the resident microglial population. In the undamaged CNS these cells have few of the features of macrophages, and express few of the molecules associated with activated macrophages. Where the CNS is damaged they can change into two main states. The first change is that the microglia can become activated, which means that they start to divide, express some new molecules on their surface, such as MHC class 1 and 2, and complement receptors, and secrete a variety of cytokines (see Table 2.1). Where there is degenerated cellular debris or other material microglia can take on a classical macrophage appearance, with vesicles, ruffled membrane, and secretion of the molecules associated with phagocytosis and cell killing.

Where axons are degenerating, and their myelin sheaths are also disrupted, microglial cells accumulate and eventually take on a macrophage-like appearance. However, the number of microglia is very much less than the number of macrophages that would be found in a damaged peripheral nerve. The result is that degenerated axonal and myelin debris is removed very much faster in the PNS than it is in the brain and cord.

Apart from microglial activation, division, and accumulation at the lesion itself, there is also activation around the neurones themselves. This does not require neuronal death. Much of the biology of microglial activation has been worked out in the facial nerve nucleus model, developed by George Kreutzberg and his colleagues, but the actual molecular signals responsible are not fully understood. Following axonal damage microglia around the facial nerve neurones proliferate,

**Table 2.1** Molecules secreted by cells of the monocyte/macrophage lineage

Lysosomal enzymes
Serine proteases
Metalloproteases
Lipases
Serine protease inhibitors
Tissue inhibitors of metalloprotease
Complement components
Coagulation factors
Reactive oxygen intermediates
   superoxide
   hydrogen peroxide
   hydroxyl radical
   nitric oxide
Arachidonic acid intermediates
Cytokines
   IL-1, IL-6, IL-8
   TNF$\alpha$
   IFN$\alpha$, IFN$\beta$
   PDGF
   bFGF
   TGF$\beta$
   GM-CSF
   M-CSF
   erythropoetin
   angiogenesis factor
Other molecules
   thrombospondin
   fibronectin
   glutathione
   apolipoprotein E

but the astrocytes do not (see Fig. 2.4). The microglia become hypertrophic and start to express the various cell surface markers of activation such as complement receptors, MHC class I and II, and start to secrete factors such as TNF$\alpha$ and TGF$\beta$. After a few days the proliferating microglia come to lie all around the cell body, and are involved in the stripping of synaptic terminals from its surface. Eventually, after about 2 weeks, the microglia start to retract and their position around the neuronal cell bodies is taken by astrocytes, which are now interposed between the stripped terminals and the cell body, probably acting as a permanent barrier to re-innervation.

The microglia do not become phagocytic unless the neurones die, in which case microglia are responsible for removing the neuronal debris. It is unusual in the CNS to see microglia transformed into fully activated macrophages of the type that are associated with cytotoxic activity unless there has been a major breach of the cerebral circulation and invasion of blood-borne monocytic cells. It is therefore unusual for

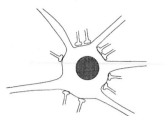

Before axotomy. Neurone receives
many synapses

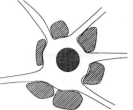

Shortly after axotomy. Most synpases
withdraw, neurone surrounded by
microglia

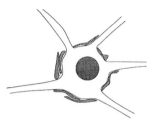

Later microglia withdraw, the neurone
is surrounded by astrocytes. Few synpases
return

**Fig. 2.4** The events following axotomy of facial nerve motor neurones. After axotomy most of the input synapses on the cell soma and proximal dendrites withdraw. Microglia then appear, and surround the neurone. The place of the microglia is then taken by astrocytic processes, which prevent synapses re-establishing their connections to the cell body.

microglia to develop cytotoxic activity against neurones or glia.

While the sequence of microglial events that follows axonal damage is well described, the molecules responsible for those events are only incompletely identified. The complication arises from the fact that astrocytes, neurones, and microglia all have effects on one another, and the microglial reaction is a product of reciprocal neurone/microglial, astrocyte/microglial, and neurone/astrocyte interactions. Some of these interactions are now starting to be worked out, mainly by finding out which factors are released, which cells have receptors for them, and by looking at the abnormalities in the injury response in transgenic mice that lack cytokines.

A major model system for this work is the facial nerve nucleus, in which there is microglial proliferation and activation, and astrocyte activation but not proliferation after damage to the facial nerve. This model was popularised by George Kreutzberg, and the work is continuing in his laboratory and that of Gennadij Raivich. The colony stimulating factors, M-CSF and GM-CSF, are mitogens for macrophages and are released after many types of injury throughout the body. In the CNS, microglia have receptors for M-CSF. A mutant mouse, the osteopetrosis mouse, has a mutation in the M-CSF gene, and has as a result deficient macrophage and osteoclast function. In this mouse, after facial nerve injury there is little microglial activation or proliferation. The M-CSF is probably produced by astrocytes, and its production is therefore dependent on a signal passing from the damaged neurone to the astrocyte.

This molecule is yet to be identified. However, two molecules involved with the astrocyte reaction are IL-6 and TGFβ. In the IL-6 knockout there is a marked decrease in the astrocyte reaction to facial nerve damage. The TGFβ knockout has a reduced microglial response, but the astrocytes are activated even in the absence of nerve damage (Kreutzberg 1996).

## Metabolic changes

A major function of astrocytes in the CNS is to control the composition of the extracellular environment, by controlling ionic concentrations, taking up and metabolising neurotransmitters, and by inducing endothelial cells to form the blood–brain barrier. Following injury this astrocytic control of the CNS extracellular environment is locally lost, with breakdown of the blood–brain barrier and free exchange of molecules with the blood and the colony stimulating factors (CSF). Many of the post-injury changes in astrocytes should be seen in the context of their mission to re-establish control of the brain environment. Some of the changes necessary to do this may have the side-effect of restricting repair by forming a barrier to axon regeneration and to migration of myelinating cells. In addition, astrocytes in the damaged brain are a major source of cytokines, which may have trophic effects on neurones, autocrine effects on astrocytes, effects on microglia and immune cells, and on vascular endothelial cells. Astrocytes define the environment of the damaged CNS, but the complexity of their reactions mean that this environment undergoes many varied changes over time.

The metabolic events that follow acute CNS injury are described in Chapter 3. Many processes are set in train, leading to rising extracellular $K^+$ and $H^+$ concentrations, rising intracellular $Na^+$, calcium entry, and glutamate release. These processes are toxic to astrocytes as well as neurones, and there is generally an area of astrocyte death surrounding any injury, astrocytes dying by necrosis and apoptosis. Any region of the CNS that lacks astrocytes will of course be particularly vulnerable to further damage.

## The macroglial reaction to injury

### Astrocytic reactions

Regions of CNS damage are surrounded by dividing astrocytes, cell division beginning within hours of injury and continuing for many days, depending on the extent of the damage. After some lesions, the amount of cell division may be quite small, while after others it appears that almost all astrocytes around the damaged area divide. The end result is usually an area of astrocytosis in which almost all the cells are astrocytes. Some astrocytes in CNS injuries express nestin, a marker usually associated with progenitor cells. This raises the possibility that some of the astrocytes in regions of gliosis might be derived from progenitors that have migrated into lesions. This question has been examined explicitly in rat spinal cord lesions by Lendahl and his associates. They have used a variety of techniques, including injections of the lipophilic dye DiI into the spinal cord central canal to trace the movements of the periventricular progenitor population after injury. After injury to the dorsal columns there was a stream of progenitors migrating towards the lesion that expressed nestin, but there were also nestin-positive astrocytes that were not labelled with the tracer, and therefore were not stem-cell derived (Johansson *et al.* 1999). The nestin-expressing cells in injuries therefore came from two sources: stem cells and astrocytes at the injury site. Whether the recruitment of stem cells into injuries is common to all CNS lesions is not known, but the distance from the periventricular source of the stem cells to lesions in the cortex is considerable, so it is less likely that they reach so far.

Astrocytes in the injured brain enlarge and change shape, putting out many processes. Since most of the cells around an injury eventually come to be astrocytes, the end result is a tissue made up of many interdigitating astrocyte processes. Many of these processes come to be bound together with junctional complexes and there is also a large amount of extracellular matrix. The result is a dense tissue with the gross morphological appearance of a scar, hence the name of 'glial scar' or 'astrocytic scar' for these reactive areas (see Fig. 2.5). In addition, there is frequently a layer of meningeal cells that migrate in from the surface and divide to form a layer around the inside of an injury, similar to the meningeal layer that surrounds the outside of the CNS. As at the normal meningeal surface, the astrocytes react to the presence of meningeal cells by forming a layer of glial end foot processes adjacent to the meningeal layer. The result is that the meningeal surface of the brain, and the astrocytic processes that underlie it, may form a continuous layer from the outside of the CNS into the region of injury. This presumably also leads to the functional barrier to molecular diffusion being recreated inside the injured region. A reformed glia limitans inside an injury is probably an insuperable barrier to regenerating axons and migrating myelinating cells: one does not see axons or oligodendrocytes passing out of the brain into the meningeal space.

The most studied marker of astrocytes reacting to injury is an increased production of the intermediate filament molecule glial fibrillary acidic protein (GFAP). This type of filament is found only in glial cells, and in the CNS largely in astrocytes. In the normal brain only a proportion of astrocytes can be stained with antibodies to GFAP, but within a day after injury both GFAP message and protein are greatly upregulated in astrocytes surrounding the injury. The increase in GFAP expression is very widespread, extending in the rat brain over both cerebral hemispheres, way beyond the region of actual damage. Much more localised is upregulation of two other intermediate filaments, vimentin and nestin, which are only found directly around the lesion site. The function of these cytoskeletal changes is not known. In GFAP knockout mice, the CNS and its reaction to injury are normal, so presumably the function of GFAP can be replaced by other intermediate filament molecules.

A functionally important astrocytic change following injury is the appearance of many junctional complexes between the cells, with the upregulation of connexin-43 expression. In the normal CNS, tight junctions are found between the astrocytic processes of the glia limitans, but after damage many of the astrocytes throughout the scar region are bound together by tight junctions. This may have the effect of making the tissue mechanically strong, but it may also make it harder for axons and migrating cells to pass through it.

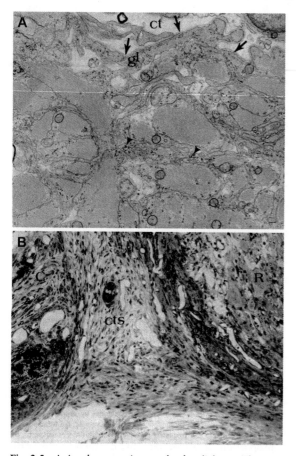

shape of the cells, suggest that they are oligodendrocyte precursors. These cells are seen in injuries after about 4 days, reach peak levels at around 10 days, and then their number starts to decline (Levine 1994). These cells form an important constituent of the glial environment at the time during which axons are trying to regenerate in the CNS. It is therefore extremely important that the cells produce several of the inhibitory chondroitin sulphate proteoglycans that are thought to inhibit axon regeneration in the CNS, of which NG2 is one (see below and Chapter 12).

## Extracellular matrix

Morphologically there is a large quantity of extracellular matrix surrounding many of the astrocyte process in the glial scar. As is described in Chapter 12, some of the matrix molecules, particularly the proteoglycans, are inhibitory to axon regeneration, and may play an important part in preventing axon regeneration in the CNS. Many matrix molecules are upregulated in the glial scar. Some, such as fibronectin, thrombospondin, and laminin, promote axon growth and cell migration. Tenascin-C and the adult-type tenascin-R are also found at injury sites; these large molecules may have several functions. Tenascin-C has both axon growth promoting and inhibitory properties, and also interacts with many of the inhibitory chondroitin sulphate proteoglycans. Tenascin-R is inhibitory to axon growth. The upregulated proteoglycans include decorin, brevican, neurocan, ABAKAN, phosphacan, biglycan, versican, NG2, DSD-1, and probably several others. Their role in axon regeneration is discussed in Chapter 12.

**Fig. 2.5** A An electron micrograph of a glial scar. The tissue consists of many fine interleaving astrocyte processes, some containing glycogen granules (*arrowheads*). A glia limitans (gl) covered with extracellular matrix (*arrows*) adjoins the surrounding connective tissue (ct). B Transected rat spinal cord, with the rostral stump (R) and caudal stump (C) separated by a connective tissue septum (cts) and a reconstituted glial limiting membrane (glm). (From Reier *et al.* 1982, with permission.)

## Regulation of the macroglial CNS injury response

The main astrocytic changes in response to CNS injury are hypertrophy, proliferation, matrix production, and junction formation. These must all be stimulated by molecular changes that occur in the injury site. Because of the large range of cytokine and growth factor receptors on astrocytes, it has been difficult to work out which molecules are involved. There is evidence that FGF-2, interleukin-1, CNTF, and TGF$\beta$ can all cause gliotic reactions when injected into the CNS, and all are present in injuries. In addition, antibodies that neutralise TGF$\beta$ can suppress the upregulation of the cytoskeletal protein GFAP in the injuries. It is probable that the astrocytosis that occurs following injuries is the

Two molecules relevant to the immune system are upregulated following injury: ICAM-1, which is involved in leukocyte migration, and MHC class II.

## Oligodendrocyte precursors

While astrocytes are eventually the major cell type that constitutes the glial scar, early after injury there is recruitment of very large numbers of small cells with a distinctive morphology. These cells express the chondroitin sulphate proteoglycan NG2 and the PDGF$\alpha$ receptor on their surface. This antigenic profile, and the result of a complex set of stimuli provided by several growth factors secreted by astrocytes, microglia, and neurones.

The accumulation of oligodendrocyte precursors must be due to a combination of cell migration and cell proliferation. The migration is probably limited, since it has been shown that following demyelinating injuries, precursors are only recruited from a maximum distance of 2 mm. Much of the increase in number of this cell population must therefore be due to cell proliferation. The mitogens known to stimulate proliferation of oligodendrocyte precursors are PDGF and FGF-2, both of which are released at CNS injuries, and so it is likely that these are the main molecules responsible for recruiting these cells.

## Further reading

Fawcett, J.W. and Asher, R.A. (1999). The glial scar and central nervous system repair. *Brain Research Bulletin*, **49**, 377–391.

Raivich, G., Bohatschek, M., Kloss, C.U.A., Werner, A., Jones, L.L., and Kreutzberg, G.W. (1999). Neuroglial activation repertoire in the injured brain: graded response, molecular mechanisms and cues to physiological function. *Brain Research Reviews*, **30**, 77–105.

# 3 | *Metabolic damage*

Many conditions can cause metabolic damage to the CNS, and they do so through a variety of mechanisms. Stroke, for instance, causes anoxic damage to a region of the brain, the actual cell death being due to excitotoxicity, release of free radicals, release of nitric oxide, and other mechanisms. We therefore describe some of the major mechanisms causing metabolic damage in CNS pathology, and then some of the more common conditions.

## Excitotoxicity

### Excitatory amino acids and cell death

Glutamic acid is an essential amino acid. As such, in the 1950s it was believed to be metabolically useful to the CNS, and monosodium glutamate was administered in large doses as potential treatments for mongoloid idiocy, retardation, and seizures (Kizer *et al.* 1978). In the course of investigating this phenomenon by exploring the capacity of glutamate to alleviate retinal degeneration in mutant rats, Lucas and Newhouse (1957) reported that, far from reducing degeneration, retinal degeneration could be induced even in normal rats within hours of glutamate administration. It was not, however, until 1969 that James Olney made the further observation that peripheral administration of glutamate could also destroy neurones in the brain, in particular in the arcuate nucleus and other ventral cell groups of the hypothalamus (Fig. 3.2). As well as this distinctive profile of neurotoxicity, peripheral injections of glutamate produce a characteristic syndrome in animals, including inducing convulsions and vomiting. Similarly in humans, the 'Chinese restaurant syndrome' of pain and burning sensations about the face, neck, and trunk is associated with ingestion of large quantities of monosodium glutamate as a flavour enhancer.

Olney also demonstrated that similar toxic effects could be induced by a range of other amino acid compounds related to glutamate, such as aspartate, and it was he who introduced the term 'excitotoxicity' to describe this phenomenon. The basis for the 'excitotoxicity' hypothesis lay in the close correspondence between the range of compounds that had seizure-inducing and neurotoxic properties following peripheral administration in experimental animals (Olney *et al.* 1971), and the potency exhibited by the same compounds to depolarise (and hence excite) spinal motor neurones in culture. Whereas a number of compounds (such as aspartate, $\alpha$-aminoadipic acid, $\alpha$-aminophosphonoprionic acid, and $\alpha$-methyl-glutamic acid) all had a similar potency to d- or l-glutamate, others (such as kainic acid, ibotenic acid, quisqualic acid, N-methyl-glutamic acid, and NMDA) were markedly more potent, in both excitatory potential and toxicity (Olney 1978). An important toxin introduced in these early studies was kainic acid, which has potent excitatory effects in culture, and induces seizures and focal damage in the arcuate region of the hypothalamus after peripheral injection (Olney *et al.* 1974).

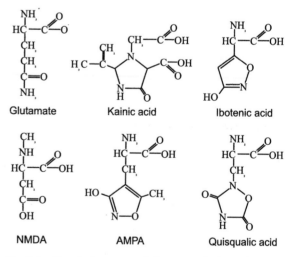

**Fig. 3.1** Chemical structure of glutamate, the ionised form of glutamic acid, and principal agonists at the glutamate receptor. NMDA, AMPA, and Kainic acid define the major pharmacological subclasses of ionotropic glutamate receptors. All agonists are excitatory, i.e. depolarise the post-synaptic neurones, and can be neurotoxic. (Redrawn from Feldman *et al.* 1997.)

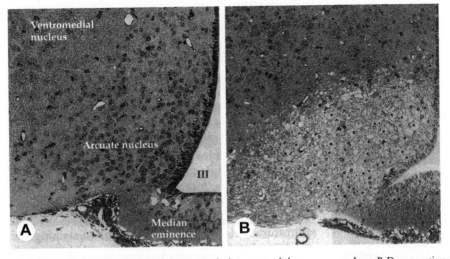

**Fig. 3.2** A Intact ventromedial hypothalamus of the rat, including area of the arcuate nucleus. B Degeneration in the arcuate nucleus after peripheral subcutaneous injection of glutamate into 10 day old mice. (Olney, Ho and Rhee 1971; reproduced from Feldman *et al.* 1997, with permission.)

An important extension of these initial studies with peripheral injections was the specificity of lesion effects when excitatory amino acids (EAAs) are injected centrally into the brain or spinal cord. In close succession, Olney and colleagues (1975) provided preliminary reports that cysteine-S-sulfonic acid, homocysteic acid, n-methyl-aspartic acid, and kainic acid (in increasing order of potency) all induce focal neuronal degeneration when injected into the diencephalon, and Coyle and Schwarcz (1976) demonstrated that small injections of millimolar concentrations of kainic acid into the striatum caused profound and rapid death of striatal neurones. The latter study in particular had great impact, not only because Coyle and Schwarcz offered this lesion as an animal model of Huntington's disease (of which more later) but more generally because they emphasised that the damage was targeted to intrinsic cells within the neostriatum, and spared afferent axons and fibres of passage (Coyle and Schwarcz 1976). This observation was separately confirmed by Simson *et al.* (1977) who showed that glutamate was toxic against hypothalamic neurones after focal injection into the hypothalamus. These studies paved the way for the general use of central injections of EAAs as an experimental tool widely used by neuroscientists for making focal lesions in the CNS.

Kainic acid was the first toxin to receive widespread evaluation: it is highly potent and injections will induce cell death at most sites in the CNS (McGeer *et al.* 1978), although cells vary in their susceptibility to the toxin, and this correlates with the density of kainic acid binding sites on neurones. Other excitatory amino acids (e.g. ibotenic acid, quinolinic acid, NMDA, and glutamate itself) were soon shown to have similar effects (e.g. Schwarcz *et al.* 1979,1983), which was important not only for allowing neuroscientists to produce new animal models of various diseases but also for opening up a strategy for investigating a novel but important mechanism of cell death. An example of kainic acid induced cell death in the hippocampus is shown in Fig. 3.3.

For experimental lesion studies, excitotoxic compounds have the particular advantage over classical lesion methods that the pattern of cell death is specific. Neuronal cell bodies and their dendrites located at the site of injection are killed by excitotoxins, but not the local glial cells nor the axons or terminal processes of remote neurones that pass through the area. Whereas kainic acid is now not widely used as a tool for making experimental lesions, because of the extent of its potent side-effects (remote damage and seizure activity) other more specific EAAs, such as ibotenic acid, quinolinic acid, quisqualic acid, NMDA, and AMPA, have become important experimental tools for neurobiologists, replacing non-specific electrolytic, radiofrequency, or knife-cut lesions to make focal damage in discrete nuclei of the CNS whilst sparing axon pathways '*en passant*' (McGeer *et al.* 1978; Meldrum and Garthwaite 1990).

## Excitotoxicity and glutamate receptors

The demonstration that excitatory amino acids in high concentration could kill neurones with the appropriate receptors was reasonably straightforward. The next step was to find out whether excitatory amino acids were released in pathological conditions in the CNS, and whether these released amino acids were responsible for the observed cell death. This essentially is the hypothesis of excitotoxicity. That large amounts of glutamate and other amino acids are released following brain injury and stroke was soon demonstrated (see later). However, although the hypothesis of excitotoxicity was appealing, direct demonstration that the extensive neu-

ronal death that follows stroke, head injury, and other conditions was due to excitatory action at the glutamate receptor was initially hard to come by. The reasoning was initially based on indirect evidence, such as the observation that the toxicity of a range of EAAs was proportional to their potency to activate glutamate receptors (Olney *et al.* 1971), or that toxicity in the striatum is modified by removal of the corticostriatal inputs. The development of the selective glutamate receptor antagonist MK-801 in the early 1980s opened the way for the direct demonstration that pharmacological blockade of the glutamate receptor dramatically reduced the toxicity of glutamate and kainic acid (Foster *et al.* 1988), both *in vitro* and *in vivo*.

A second line of direct evidence is provided by stimulation of glutamatergic pathways in the brain. For example, sustained electrical stimulation of the perforant path leads to degeneration in the post-synaptic granule cell targets in the dentate gyrus, an effect that is mimicked by inducing seizure activity in the brain. Both of these effects are blocked by treatment with MK-801.

## Other receptors and other glutamate antagonists

As the major excitatory transmitter of the nervous system, most neurones express glutamate receptors, and kainic acid will destroy virtually all neurones of the CNS. Nevertheless, there are several main classes of glutamate receptor. These have traditionally been defined pharmacologically by subtypes of the 'ionotropic' receptors and the metabotropic receptor (see Table 3.1). The three main classes of ionotropic receptors are defined pharmacologically by their preferential sensitivity to kainic acid, NMDA, and AMPA/quisqualate, respectively, as agonists, and have distinctive patterns of distribution in the brain (see Fig. 3.4). Different excitotoxic amino acids have individual

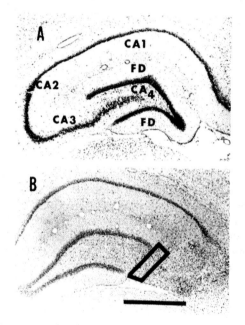

Fig. 3.3 Photomicrographs of kainic acid induced toxicity in the hippocampus. The site of damage depends on site of injection. A Cell death in the CA1 region of hippocampus after kainate injection into the diencephalon. B Cell death in the CA3/4 rein after kainate injection into piriform cortex. Lateral CA3 is most affected after kainate injections into the striatum or intraventricularly. Cresyl violet stain, marker bar = 1 mm. (From Schwob *et al.* 1980.)

**Table 3.1** Glutamate receptors: excitotoxins, antagonists and principle distribution

| Receptor | Properties | Molecular structure | Main agonists | Main antagonists |
|---|---|---|---|---|
| Ionotropic receptors: | | | | |
| AMPA | Na⁺, K⁺ | GluR1-GluR4 | AMPA, quisqualic acid | CNQX, NBQX |
| KA | Na⁺, K⁺ | GluR5-GluR7, KA1, KA2 | kainic acid | CNQX, NBQX |
| NMDA | Na⁺, K⁺, Ca²⁺ | NR1, NR2A-NR2D | NMDA, ibotenic acid | D-AP5, D-AP7, CPP, MK-801 |
| Metabotropic receptors: | | | | |
| Second messengers: | IP3, DAG, cAMP | mGluR1-mGluR7 | quisqualic acid, trans-ACPD* | α-MCPG*, L-AP4 |

*α-MCPG, α-methyl-4-carboxyphenylglycine; *trans*-ACPD, *trans*-1-aminocyclopentane-1,3-dicarboxylic acid.

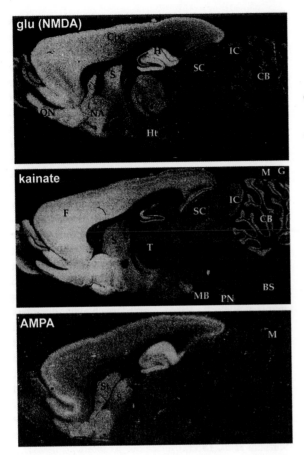

Fig. 3.4 Distribution of the NMDA, kainate, and AMPA sub-types of glutamate receptor in the brain, visualised by receptor-binding autoradiography. (Monaghan *et al.* 1989; reproduced from Feldman *et al.* 1997, with permission.)

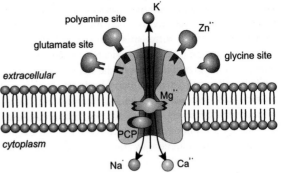

Fig. 3.5. Structure of the NMDA receptor, indicating the ion channel and binding sites of the primary agonists and ions that regulate permeability. (Modified from Feldman *et al.* 1997.)

profiles of action at the three receptors; thus, for example, ibotenic and quinolinic acids act preferentially at the NMDA receptor. Conversely, even the defining ligands are not fully specific; thus, kainic acid can activate the AMPA receptor, and AMPA can activate the kainate receptor, although in each case with a far lower affinity than for their primary targets.

The basic pharmacological features of the primary glutamate receptors has been reviewed by Feldman *et al.* (1997), and may be summarised as follows:

The AMPA receptor gates a fast-acting $Na^+$ channel, which is potentiated by $Zn^{2+}$ and may be influenced by additional modulatory proteins. The widely used neurotoxin quisqualic acid acts preferentially at the AMPA receptor. This channel may also admit $Ca^{2+}$ when it contains the GluR1 subunit.

The kainate receptor also gates a fast-acting $Na^+$

channel that is distinct from the AMPA receptor pharmacologically and is not potentiated by $Zn^{2+}$.

The NMDA receptor gates a channel permeable to both $Na^+$ and $Ca^{2+}$ that is further regulated by both $Zn^{2+}$ and $Mg^{2+}$ in a voltage-dependent manner (see Fig. 3.5). Only after a basal level of depolarisation is reached do $Mg^{2+}$ ions leave the channel and allow passage of $Ca^{2+}$. Opening of this channel therefore requires both the presence of glutamate and depolarisation of the post-synaptic neurone by other synaptic inputs. Calcium entering by this channel will normally act as a signalling molecule, being centrally involved in the induction of long-term potentiation and other forms of synaptic plasticity. However, if very large amounts of calcium enter via this channel it can trigger cell death (see below and Chapters 1 and 2). The widely used neurotoxin ibotenic acid acts preferentially at the NMDA receptor.

The metabotropic receptor is not linked to a particular ion channel, but rather is coupled to inositol triphosphate and diaglycerol, the mobilisation of intracellular $Ca^{2+}$ and the activation of protein kinase C.

More recently, the molecular structures of these receptors have largely been clarified. The first glutamate receptor was cloned and sequenced by Hollman and colleagues in 1989, since when 28 genes encoding glutamate receptor (GluR) subunits have been identified (Hollman and Heinemann 1994). Each receptor is made up of five molecular subunits, with different subsets of subunits contributing to each main class of ionotropic or metabotropic receptors (see Table 3.1). Moreover, identification of the individual receptor subunit cDNA has now enabled traditional receptor-binding autoradiography to be complemented by *in situ* hybridisation of the individual subunits for mapping of glutamate receptor distribution in the CNS. Since these receptors have a differential distribution on neurones, so also are the cells differentially susceptible to EAAs. Thus, in the hippocampus, selective lesions can be induced in the pyramidal cells of the CA3, CA1, and the granule cells of the dentate gyrus by local infusions of kainic acid, ischaemia/colchicine, or ibotenic acid, respectively. Similarly, there are selective antagonists for the main classes of glutamate receptor and excitotoxicity can be blocked by the relevant compounds respectively (Fig. 3.6).

Although *in vitro* studies suggest that homomeric receptors made up of five copies of the same AMPA

subunit can function properly, heteromeric receptors made of combinations of subunits appear to be the more usual situation *in vivo*. Furthermore, 'knockout' mice that fail to express individual receptor subunits are now being investigated. Different lines of knockout mice have been reported to exhibit distinctive patterns of motor and learning impairments (Conquet *et al.* 1994). This highlights the role of glutamate receptors, not only in cell death but also the role of the glutamate (and in particular the NMDA) synapse in the plasticity associated with long-term potentiation and other mechanisms of cellular learning.

In addition to the experimental demonstration that excessive levels of glutamate are neurotoxic, accumulating evidence suggests that glutamate excitotoxicity may play a role in the neurodegeneration seen in specific conditions such as ischaemia (see later) (Choi 1988, 1990; Meldrum and Garthwaite 1990), seizure syndromes (Olney *et al.* 1986; Cain 1989), hypoglycaemia (Wieloch 1985), some psychiatric disorders (Olney 1989), certain forms of trauma (Faden *et al.* 1989), certain idiopathic neurodegenerative conditions such as Huntington's and Alzheimer's diseases (Coyle *et al.* 1978; Beal *et al.* 1986; Maragos *et al.* 1987; Greenamyre and Young 1989; Penney *et al.* 1990), and possibly AIDS dementia complex (Heyes *et al.* 1991). Glutamate toxicity may also play a role in toxicity mediated by other compounds such as metamphetamine (Sonsalla *et al.* 1989).

Since excitotoxic cell death appears to be a receptor-mediated event, receptor blockade with specific antagonist compounds should be able prevent its occurrence (see Fig. 3.7). This is indeed the case and one of the most exciting recent developments in the study of neurodegeneration has been the identification of a variety of antagonist compounds that can protect cells from exposure to excess levels of glutamate or its toxic agonists, either in tissue culture, or in whole animals (Choi 1988, 1990; Meldrum and Garthwaite 1990; Foster *et al.* 1988). Such antagonists are able to provide protection against degeneration in experimental animal models of a number of neurodegenerative conditions, as described below and in Chapter 7.

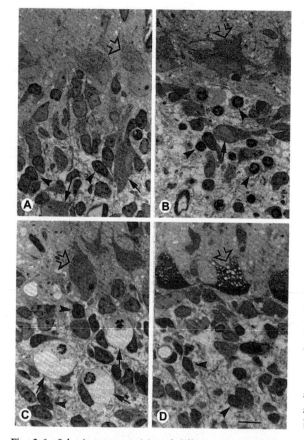

Fig. 3.6 Selective neurotoxicity of different excitotoxins in immature rat cerebellar slice cultures. A Control slices, showing normal healthy Purkinje cells (*open arrows*), granule cells (*filled arrows*) and Golgi cells (*arrowheads*). B NMDA treatment (100 $\mu$M, 30 min) kills granule cells. C Kainic acid treatment (100 $\mu$M, 30 min) kills Golgi cells. D AMPA treatment (30 $\mu$M, 30 min) induces a characteristic 'dark-cell degeneration' of Purkinje cells. (From Meldrum and Garthwaite 1990, with permission.)

## Excitotoxic cell death

What are the mechanisms by which glutamate and other excitotoxins kill cells? As outlined above, the observation of a correlation between the excitatory actions of different classes of glutamate agonists and their toxicity first led Olney to propose the 'excitotoxic' hypothesis,

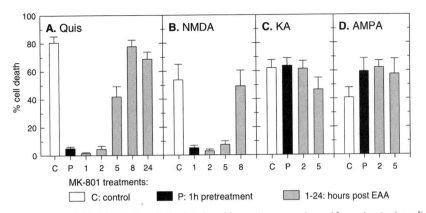

**Fig. 3.7** The NMDA antagonist MK-801 blocks cell death induced by excitatory amino acid agonists (quisqualic acid or NMDA itself) that act primarily at the NMDA glutamate receptor, but not toxins acting at other (kainic acid, AMPA) receptors. (Redrawn from Foster *et al.* 1988.)

encapsulating the idea that sustained depolarisation of the neurone by excitatory amino acids resulted in a lethal exhaustion of cellular energy reserves, collapse of the cell membrane, or disturbance of the internal milieu. Support for this notion came from observations of the morphological changes associated with excitotoxicity. Thus, within 30 min of glutamate application, there may be massive swelling of neuronal cell bodies and dendrites, followed by degeneration of intracellular organelles, and pyknosis of the cell nucleus, leading over a period of several hours to cell necrosis and phagocytosis of the cellular debris (Choi 1992). Rothman and Olney (1987) have described this cell hypertrophy as an 'osmotic explosion'!

However, there are contradictions to the simple hypothesis that glutamate or other glutamate agonists simply excite the cells to death. For example, studies of kainic acid toxicity in the striatum have indicated that toxicity is markedly reduced following lesions of the glutamatergic corticostriatal pathway without changing the direct excitability of the intrinsic striatal neurones (Bizière and Coyle 1978). Detailed analysis of the effects of excitatory amino acids on cortical neurones in tissue culture, experiments particularly associated with the laboratory of Dennis Choi, indicate that other mechanisms may play a major role, in particular related to an excessive influx of calcium (for review see Choi 1992).

## Calcium

In tissue culture, both neurones and glia are rapidly killed by concentrations of glutamate greater that

100 $\mu$M, almost entirely through necrosis. The initial wave of cellular swelling is associated with massive action potential activity, with influx of $Na^+$ and associated changes in membrane permeability in all cells. This acute phase need not be lethal, and under appropriate conditions the majority of cells can recover homeostasis and survive, the sodium–potassium exchange pump restoring the ionic equilibrium across the membrane provided there is sufficient ATP available to drive it. However, large-scale entry of calcium into the cells via NMDA channels, which will open due to the combination of depolarisation and the presence of glutamate, is associated with a slower second phase; it is this that produces irreversible neuronal injury and is the dominant cause of neuronal death. Thus, direct cell death by this second mechanism is mimicked by the calcium channel agonist A23187, the toxicity of glutamate is markedly enhanced by addition of calcium to the culture medium, and removal of calcium from the medium largely prevents glutamate toxicity (Choi 1992). The effects appear to be mediated predominantly via NMDA channels, since glutamate toxicity is largely blocked by the selective antagonist MK-801. Recall that it is the NMDA channel that has been associated with $Ca^{2+}$ as well as $Na^+$ and $K^+$ permeability. Nevertheless, some calcium may also enter cells via AMPA receptors that contain the GluR1 subunit, and blocking these provides additional protection compared with just blocking NMDA receptors. The same conclusion can be drawn from comparisons of the toxicity of selective agonists: 5-min application of NMDA will cause widespread $Ca^{2+}$-dependent cell death in cultured cortical neurones. A similar exposure to kainic acid or AMPA produces only swelling but not cell death, and it requires several

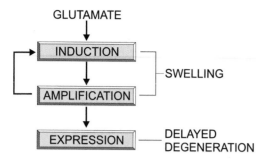

GLUTAMATE

INDUCTION

AMPLIFICATION — SWELLING

EXPRESSION — DELAYED DEGENERATION

**Fig. 3.8** Three phases in the development of glutamate toxicity. Over-stimulation of glutamate receptors induces an initial potentially lethal disturbance of cellular Na+, K+, Ca2+, and other cellular messengers. This disturbance can be augmented by a range of secondary changes, such as the additional release of glutamate from injured excitatory neurones. Finally, sustained calcium overload leads to a cascade of further toxic events that eventually leads to delayed neuronal degeneration. (Reproduced from Choi 1992.)

hours exposure to these agonists to induce comparable lethality (Choi 1992).

Sustained elevation of intracellular calcium triggers a destructive cascade of events and leads to the slow degeneration of the neurone. Choi refers to this third and final wave in the process of excitotoxic cell death as the 'expression of toxicity'. This includes the induction of proteases and phospholipases that can damage cellular constituents, and disturb cellular mechanisms of free radical elimination. These processes are elaborated further in the context of ischaemia, in the following section.

Ionic calcium ($Ca^{2+}$) is an important intracellular second messenger, and cytosolic $Ca^{2+}$ concentrations are carefully regulated in the 50–300 nM range under normal function in most neurones. Substantial evidence now indicates that sustained abnormal elevations of cytosolic $Ca^{2+}$ concentrations lead to cell death (Choi 1988; Siesjö and Bengtsson 1989). The main sources for increased cytosolic $Ca^{2+}$ levels are release from intracellular stores in mitochondria and entry from the extracellular fluid. Cytosolic $Ca^{2+}$ concentrations can be increased to toxic levels in several ways including physical damage to the cell membrane and receptor-mediated events, such as glutamate excitotoxicity. A major toxic consequence of inappropriate activation of the various glutamate receptors appears to be cytosolic $Ca^{2+}$ overload, resulting from a combination of increased entry via the NMDA-receptor linked channel, increased entry via voltage-dependent $Ca^{2+}$ channels, and release from intracellular stores via the phospho-

inositol system (Choi 1988; Siesjö and Bengtsson 1989). $Ca^{2+}$ imbalances may play a role in other forms of neurodegeneration, but this is not yet certain. The mechanisms by which $Ca^{2+}$ overload causes cell death include activation of intracellular proteases, depletion of intracellular energy reserves by activation of $Ca^{2+}$-ATPase, generation of free radicals, and impairment of oxidative phosphorylation (see Chapter 1) (Choi 1988; Siesjö and Bengtsson 1989). Cell death mediated by $Ca^{2+}$ overload is often delayed for hours and possibly days after the triggering insult. This delay may provide a window of opportunity for therapeutic intervention. Although much attention has been focused on the deleterious effects of intracellular $Ca^{2+}$ overload, decreased levels of $Ca^{2+}$ can also put nerve cells at risk of degeneration (Koike *et al.* 1989). It appears that an optimal level of intracellular $Ca^{2+}$ concentration is maintained by appropriate interactions between neurones and extracellular ions, transmitters, growth factors, and other molecules; events that lead to major intracellular $Ca^{2+}$ fluctuations in either direction may be harmful.

## *Metabolic toxins*

A variety of neurodegenerative diseases (such as Huntington's disease) have been associated with a metabolic disturbance in the energy balance of cells (Beal 1992; Browne *et al.* 1997). Conversely, a number of diseases associated with mitochondrial dysfunction and impaired energy balance (such as Leber's disease) are associated with neuronal degeneration. Not surprisingly, therefore, there has been a growing interest in the role of metabolic factors in neuronal dysfunction and as a primary factor in cell death. More recently, many of these metabolic and excitotoxic mechanisms of neurodegeneration have converged on a final common pathway of neuronal cell death via glutamate toxicity and calcium imbalance (Beal *et al.* 1993).

The primary source of cellular energy is via the generation of ATP from ADP at electron transport complexes located in an inner compartment within the mitochondria. NADH and FADH2 are generated by the Kreb's cycle and act as electron donors to the series of electron transport enzymes of the chain (see Fig. 3.9). In parallel, protons are ejected across the inner mitochondrial membrane that provide an electrochemical proton gradient as a potential energy store. Electrons are transferred to oxygen by oxidative phosphorylation coupled to the synthesis of ATP. ATP derived from the mitochondria then provides the main source of energy

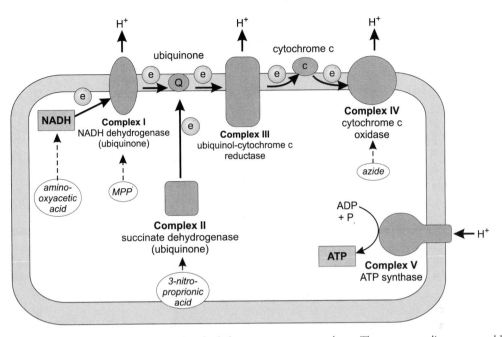

**Fig. 3.9** Schematic diagram of the major mitochondrial electron transport complexes. The proton gradient generated by complexes I, III and IV is used by complex V to for phosphorylation of ADP to ATP. The sites of action of key metabolic toxins are indicated: aminooxyacetic acid (AOAA), the methylphenylpiridinium ion (MPP+), azide and 3-nitroproprionic acid (3-NPA). (Redrawn from Beal *et al.* 1993.)

for driving a multitude of ion pumps to generate and maintain critical voltage gradients across membranes and necessary for all aspects of cell survival and metabolism including neuronal signalling mechanisms (Beal *et al.* 1993).

A variety of 'metabolic toxins' have been identified that interfere with mitochondrial energy production leading to cell death. For example, aminooxyacetic acid (AOAA) is a non-specific transaminase inhibitor and blocks the first step of the electron transport chain in mitochondria (see Fig. 3.9). When injected into the rat brain, AOAA induces degeneration of striatal neurones by a mechanism that involves an excitotoxic process, since it is blocked by MK-801 or decortication (Beal *et al.* 1991). The toxin induces a particular profile of striatal cell death, with the GABAergic medium spiny projection neurones being more susceptible than the somatostatin or neuropeptide Y interneurones. Since this is very similar to the pattern of cell death seen in Huntington's disease, post-mortem studies of which also indicate mitochondrial dysfunction, the metabolic toxin in experimental rodent brain appears to provide a close model of the human disease.

A second toxin acting on cellular energy metabolism

is 3-nitropropionic acid (3-NP). 3-NP is an irreversible inhibitor of succinate dehydrogenase, and blocks both the Kreb's cycle and complex II of the mitochondrial electron transport chain (see Fig. 3.9). It is a potent neurotoxin, derived from both plants and fungi, that produces a pronounced dystonic disorder associated with focal degeneration in the basal ganglia after accidental ingestion by both humans and livestock (Ludolph *et al.* 1991). 3-NP is of interest because even after peripheral administration, the basal ganglia appears to be selectively targeted. When injected intraperitoneally, 3-NP produces an acute down-regulation of succinate dehydrogenase activity throughout the brain, but causes extensive non-specific degeneration only in the neostriatum (see Fig. 3.10). The focal damage is generally a rather non-specific death of all cells, neurones, and glia alike, following a single large dose of 3-NP, but repeated injections of low doses that are individually subtoxic will produce, over several weeks or months, a more specific degeneration of the neostriatal projection neurones without overt generalised neuropil damage, in rats and monkeys alike. Moreover, whereas the acute degenerative response to a large dose that destroys all neurones cannot be blocked by NMDA antagonists, the more

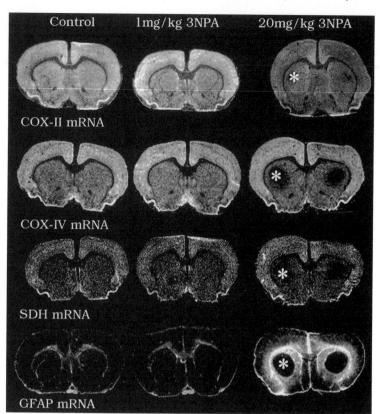

**Fig. 3.10** Peripheral injection of 3-nitropropionic acid in rats induces generalised down-regulation of cellular succinate dehydrogenase (SDH) and cytochrome oxidase (COX) activity, but focal degeneration of striatal neurones and astrocytosis. (From Page *et al.* 1999, with permission.)

selective progressive cell death caused by low level metabolic disturbance are blocked by NMDA antagonists *in vitro* or removal of cortical inputs *in vivo*.

## Strong and weak excitotoxic hypotheses

The fact that cell death resulting from metabolic disturbance can be blocked by glutamate antagonists suggests that metabolic toxicity and excitotoxic processes may work through a common pathway involving glutamate (and more specifically NMDA) receptors. As shown in Fig. 3.11, an impairment of cellular electron transport cascade results in a reduction of ATP production by mitochondria, which in turn leads to a deficit in the cellular levels of ATP necessary to maintain the membrane ion pumps regulating $Na^+$, $K^+$, and $Ca^{2+}$ balance. This failure produces a cascade of changes within the cell that disturbs the ionic balance across the cell membrane (Beal *et al.* 1993). For example, glutamate excitation depolarises the cell, which in the absence of an effective restoration of the membrane potential leads to prolonged opening of $Ca^{2+}$ channels, allowing calcium to build up within the cell and a failure

of its effective removal. In addition, prolonged depolarisation releases the protective voltage-dependent magnesium block of the glutamate receptor, increasing their responsiveness to endogenous levels of glutamate and increasing $Na^+$ and $Ca^{2+}$ influx. The accumulation of intracellular calcium itself leads to a cascade of additional intracellular changes in the production of proteases, phospholipases, and endonucleases that cause destructive intracellular damage (see Chapter 1), enhancing the glutamate-mediated cell death.

High levels of stimulation at glutamate receptors (either by potent agonists or abnormally high levels of glutamate itself) can cause cell death directly. The cell death induced by metabolic toxins involves many of the same excitotoxic processes, but these are recruited at normal rather than heightened levels of glutamate activation by a metabolic disturbance of the cell's endogenous capacity to autoregulate and maintain its normal ionic potential balance. The process whereby metabolic disturbance produces cell death through an indirect excitotoxic mechanism has been termed '*weak excitotoxicity*' to distinguish it from a primary process of cell death due directly to excess glutamate activation

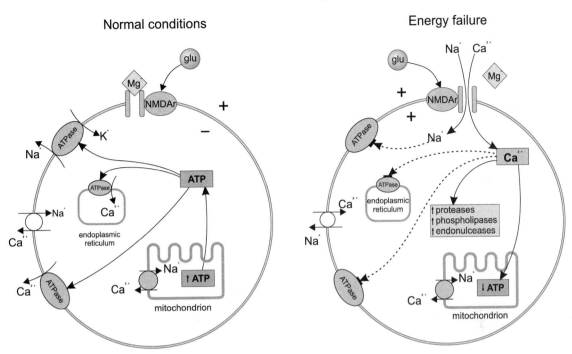

**Normal conditions**

**Energy failure**

**Fig. 3.11** Consequences of energy failure within nerve cells. (Redrawn from Beal *et al.* 1993.)

('*strong excitotoxicity*'). As we shall see, the indirect mechanisms involving compromise in cellular metabolism offer novel strategies for neuroprotection and repair.

## Oxidative stress

The brain has a high consumption of oxygen and is rich in oxidisable substances, such as unsaturated lipids and catecholamines. This environment has considerable potential for the formation of 'oxygen radicals', which in turn might contribute to the mediation of neurodegeneration in ischaemia and other conditions (Coyle and Puttfarcken 1993). *Oxidative stress* refers to the process whereby oxygen free radicals are toxic to cells.

### Nitric oxide

Nitric oxide is released in the anoxic brain via several mechanisms. Calcium entry into the neurone via NMDA channels, voltage gated channels, or release from internal stores will increase the activity of neuronal NO synthase, whose activity is controlled by calcium levels via calmodulin. NO production can be induced in

astrocytes through induction of the inducible NO synthase, and in microglia. That excessive levels of NO can be damaging in the CNS is shown by the neuroprotective effect of NO synthase inhibitors, and by the fact that animals with knockout of NO synthase are resistant to anoxic and excitotoxic damage. NO probably works via two mechanisms. The simpler mechanism is via reaction with reactive oxygen species to produce the highly toxic radical peroxynitrite. This probably only occurs when very high levels of NO are present in the CNS. NO in itself is only mildly toxic, but it reacts with the superoxide radical, $O_2^-$, to give peroxynitrite, $ONOO^-$. This is highly reactive in itself, has a long half life of 0.9 s, allowing it to diffuse over several cell diameters, and can break down to yield a highly reactive $OH^-$ radical (see Fig. 3.12). A combination of increased free radical and increased NO production together can therefore lead to widespread oxidation of lipids, proteins, and nucleic acids. At lower NO levels, the main effect may be on the mitochondria. NO has various effects on the mitochondrion, one of which is the inhibition of ATP production through inhibition of the enzyme cytochrome c. Low levels of ATP will slow down membrane pumps in neurones, leading to depolarisation and increased calcium entry via voltage-gated

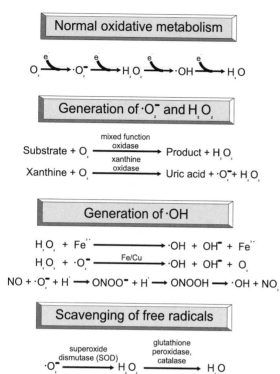

**Fig. 3.12** Free-radical reactions that may generate reactive oxygen species in the brain. (From Coyle and Puttfarcken 1993.)

channels. Low levels of ATP in astrocytes will reduce glutamate uptake. John Garthwaite and his colleagues were able to show a vicious cycle of neurodegeneration in a tissue culture model of striatal neurones and glia. He found that a short treatment with NMDA was insufficient to cause widespread necrosis, but initiated an apoptotic process that started after several hours, and continued over 24 h. This could be prevented by NO synthase inhibitors, NMDA blockers, or blockers of sodium channels. The interpretation is that the short pulse of NMDA started a cycle in which calcium entry triggered NO release, which affected neuronal and glial ATP production, leading to increased glutamate release and decreased uptake, leading to continuing NMDA receptor activation, thus continuing the cycle (Strijbos *et al.* 1996).

## Generation of free radicals

A free radical is any molecule that contains one or more unpaired electrons; they are mostly unstable and react freely with neighbouring molecules. The predominant free radical oxygen species affecting the brain are the superoxide anion $\cdot O_2^-$, hydrogen peroxide $H_2O_2$, and the hydroxyl radical $\cdot OH$ (see Fig. 3.12). These are formed in the normal process of mitochondrial aerobic energy respiration by the successive addition of electrons to $O_2$.

In addition to the production of free radical species during normal aerobic metabolism, toxic free radicals may originate from a number of other sources, both endogenous and exogenous (Ames *et al.* 1993). There are three major endogenous sources.

- *Infections.* Phagocytes release NO and other free radicals as a primary component of their defence in response to viral, bacterial, or parasitic infection.

- *Fatty acid metabolism.* Peroxisomes, the cellular organelles responsible for lipid degradation, produce $H_2O_2$ as a primary product, which is frequently incompletely degraded by catalase.

- *Toxins.* Cytochrome P450 enzymes provide one of the main endogenous defence mechanisms against a variety of naturally-occurring plant toxins but they can produce a variety of oxidant free radicals as by-products.

In addition, there are three main sources of exogenous free radicals that add to the endogenous production (Ames *et al.* 1993).

- Oxides of nitrogen in cigarette smoke increase oxidative activity and decrease levels of antioxidants in cells.

- Iron and copper salts (mainly derived from the diet) exacerbate the generation of highly toxic $\cdot OH^-$ radicals from $\cdot O_2^-$ and $H_2O_2$ (the Fenton reaction, see third panel, Fig. 3.12).

- Natural phenolic compounds in the diet (e.g. chlorogenic and caffeic acid) can generate oxidants via the redox cycle.

## Cellular defences against free radicals

Cells generate free radicals as by-products of both normal and aberrant cellular processing, but have also evolved a variety of mechanisms to scavenge and protect against such toxic damage.

- The enzyme *superoxide dismutase* (SOD) is specifically a scavenger of free $\cdot O_2^-$. SOD enzymes form the major defence system against excess $\bullet O_2^{\sim}$ formed in aerobic cells.

- The enzyme *glutathione peroxidase* metabolises glutathione and excess $H_2O_2$ to form glutathione disulphide and water.

- Similarly, *catalase* can also metabolise $H_2O_2$ to water in a number of body systems, although it has a less predominant role than glutathione peroxidase, and is found at only low levels in the brain.

- *Ferritin* and *transferrin* chelate free metal ions, in particular iron and copper, and reduce their capacity to promote toxic hydroxyl radical production.

- *NADPH: quinone reductase* reduces quinones to less toxic hydroquinones.

- *Vitamin E* is the most important endogenous lipid-soluble chain-breaking antioxidant.

- *Uric acid* has multiple effects on oxidative metabolism by tightly binding iron and copper, scavenging radicals, and inhibiting lipid peroxidation.

## Toxicity of free radicals

In excess, free radicals can be highly toxic to living cells. The exact mechanism of this toxicity is not certain. However, while $\bullet O_2^{\sim}$ can damage some biomolecules directly, under normal circumstances it rapidly becomes converted to $H_2O_2$ when in aqueous solution. It seems more likely that cellular damage occurs when $H_2O_2$ comes into contact with reduced forms of certain metal ions, such as iron or copper, which decompose the $H_2O_2$ into the exceptionally reactive and toxic hydroxyl radical $\bullet OH^-$. $\bullet OH^-$ reacts at great speed with almost every molecule found in living cells, leading among other things to strand breakage and base modification in DNA, to lipid peroxidation with gradual loss of membrane integrity, and eventually to cytotoxicity (Halliwell and Gutteridge 1985). In addition, free radicals may combine with nitric oxide, which is produced by neurones, astrocytes, and inflammatory cells in the damaged CNS to produce the highly toxic radical peroxynitrite.

Damage to DNA is through $\bullet OH^-$ modification of ribose phosphates and pyrimidine nucleosides and nucleotides, and reaction with the sugar phosphate backbone to break the DNA strands (Brawn and Fridovich 1981).

A second target of damage is proteins themselves (Stadtman 1986). $Fe^{2+}$ and $Cu^{2+}$ bind to cation-binding sites on proteins during redox cycling, and change amine groups into carbonyls when under attack from $\bullet O_2^{\sim}$ and $H_2O_2$. This leads to a complex range of changes in proteolysis and enzyme degradation. The pigment lipofuchsin, found in the ageing nervous system, is an end-product of the oxidative degradation of lipids, and is generally found in otherwise healthy cells that may be successfully dealing with intracellular oxygen radicals.

The toxicity of $\bullet O_2^{\sim}$ *in vivo* is dependent upon the concentration of available metal ion catalysts (Olanow and Arendash 1994). Thus, $O_2$ is itself relatively unreactive but will interact with metal ions to generate $\bullet O_2^{\sim}$. Similarly, $H_2O_2$ will decompose to the highly reactive hydroxyl ion $\bullet OH^-$ at a slow rate spontaneously, but this is markedly enhanced in the presence of free iron, $Fe^{2+}$. This potentiation is illustrated in an experiment by Liu *et al.* (1994). Injection of either $H_2O_2$ alone or iron alone into the CNS of rats had rather limited effects, but infusion of the two together induced a marked cellular degeneration.

Free radical induced cell death is by both necrotic and apoptotic processes. Their attack on lipids and proteins disrupts membrane ion gradients and produces rupture of the cell membranes, precipitating the essential processes of necrosis. However, an additional role for programmed cell death is also suggested by a variety of lines of evidence (Simonian and Coyle 1996); for example, that depletion of glutathione or SOD can induce apoptosis in cultured neurones, whereas antioxidant treatments (see below) can prevent the apoptotic death induced by tumour necrosis factor-$\alpha$ in cultured neuroblastoma cells.

As well as their direct effects on cell death, free radicals can also inhibit mitochondrial activity, promoting weak excitotoxicity, and their production is potentiated by rises in intracellular calcium. Consequently, excitotoxic, metabolic, free radical, and calcium-mediated mechanisms are not independent causes of cell death but interact in a 'cycle of neurodegeneration' (Fig. 3.13; Olanow and Arendash 1994).

One implication of this cycle of interactions is not only that a part of the cell death associated with free radical production may be compounded by excitotoxic and calcium-related mechanisms, but also that excitotoxically induced cell death may in part be alleviated by antioxidant treatments (Schulz *et al.* 1995) Thus, for example, NMDA-induced death of cerebellar cells in tissue culture has been shown to be associated with a rise in intracellular calcium and the formation of $\bullet O_2^{\sim}$, and the loss of cells was attenuated by antioxidant

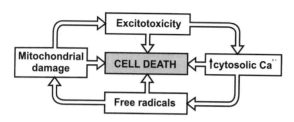

**Fig. 3.13** The cycle of neurodegeneration, involving a positive feedback of the influences of excitotoxicity, raised cytosolic calcium, free radical production and mitochondrial metabolic dysfunction on cell death in the nervous system. (Redrawn from Olanow and Arendash 1994.)

treatment with the free radical scavenger DMPO (Lafon-Cazal *et al.* 1993).

Protection by antioxidants is described in Chapter 7.

## *Metabolic mechanisms in types of CNS pathology*

### Free radicals in catecholamine systems and Parkinson's disease

The role of oxygen radicals in neurodegenerative conditions of the nervous system has been studied in most detail in Parkinson's disease, in part because of the apparent sensitivity to the forebrain catecholamine systems in general, and the dopaminergic substantia nigra in particular, to oxidative damage.

The normal metabolism of dopamine involves the generation of hydrogen peroxide both under enzymatic regulation by monoamine oxidase and by auto-oxidation. Although this is normally cleared by glutathione, it can interact with free iron to form highly toxic $\bullet OH^-$ (see Fig. 3.12). Dopamine is itself toxic in high concentrations. Thus, for example, direct injection of dopamine into the neostriatum causes substantial degeneration of striatal cells at the site of injection and an extensive degeneration of nigrostriatal nerve terminals in the vicinity (Hastings *et al.* 1996). Both the cellular and the terminal degeneration was substantially blocked by injections of ascorbic acid or glutathione, indicating that the toxic reaction was due to an oxidation process. The toxicity of dopamine is further exac-

erbated in the substantia nigra itself, where dopamine neurones (at least in humans and other primates) are pigmented with neuromelanin, which selectively binds iron. Consequently the substantia nigra exhibits particularly high levels of free iron, which may potentiate toxic free-radical production by these neurones. In a direct test of this hypothesis Sengstock *et al.* (1992) showed that local injection of ferric chloride ($FeCl_3$) produces a selective degeneration of the dopamine neurones in the substantia nigra of rats

These experimental observations have led naturally to the hypothesis that the pathophysiology of Parkinson's disease may be attributable to oxidative damage of the substantia nigra. Although the causative mechanisms remain elusive, support for this hypothesis is gained from observations of raised levels of iron, and reduced levels of glutathione and ferritin in the substantia nigra in post-mortem Parkinsonian brains (Simonian and Coyle 1996). Consequently, we should consider whether the onset or progression of the disease might be inhibited by antioxidants.

An experimental rationale for this approach has been provided by a number of lines of research indicating neuroprotective effects of various antioxidant strategies in experimental models. Thus, embryonic dopamine neurones do not readily thrive in culture or following transplantation in the brain, but their survival is promoted both *in vitro* and *in vivo* by treatment with antioxidant lazaroids or by blockade of glutathione (Frodl *et al.* 1994; Nakao *et al.* 1994). Moreover, the toxicity of the exogenous toxin MPTP (see Chapter 6) is substantially reduced in transgenic mice that overexpress superoxide dismutase (Przedborski *et al.* 1992).

These studies provided the basis for the DATATOP trial of antioxidant treatment in Parkinson's disease (Parkinson's Study Group 1993). This was a large, prospective, double-blind trial evaluating two treatments, the antioxidant $\alpha$-tocopherol (vitamin E) and a monoamine oxidase inhibitor deprenyl on the development of disorder in early Parkinson's disease patients. Although deprenyl did yield demonstrable benefit (see Chapters 6 and 7), in this study the antioxidant treatment was not effective.

## *Ischaemia*

### Ischaemic damage to the CNS

Ischaemia occurs when blood supply is cut off to the brain. This primary event combines several different toxic processes, including excitotoxicity, metabolic toxicity and oxidative stress, which converge to produce CNS degeneration following stroke.

Human patients may experience two main forms of CNS ischaemia: transient global ischaemia and focal prolonged ischaemia. Transient global ischaemia occurs when there is generalised circulatory failure, as in cardiac arrest. Focal ischaemia occurs when a circumscribed area of brain loses its blood supply, due to blockage or rupture of an artery, generally associated with stroke. Focal events may be associated with permanent blockage of the artery, or there may be reperfusion after the thrombosis is removed, whether occurring spontaneously or as a result to thrombolytic therapy.

## Animal models

In order to study ischaemia, several different models have been developed in experimental animals (Seta *et al.* 1992). Global ischaemia with reperfusion is achieved by completely interrupting the blood supply to the brain for a period of a few minutes. If the experimental interest lies in studying the acute cellular and molecular changes associated with total loss of blood perfusion to the brain, then this can be studied by analysis of tissue changes following decapitation (e.g. Lowry *et al.* 1964). However, if we are interested in the longer term dynamics of injury and recovery, then a variety of surgical approaches have been developed in rats and other rodents for reversible episodes of ischaemia to one or both hemispheres.

An early model involved occluding the common carotid artery (CCA) in gerbils. Since the circle of Willis is incomplete in gerbils, it is possible thereby to produce unilateral hemispheric infarction. However, this procedure is not very reliable, and has largely been replaced by two main methods of global ischaemia that can apply in other species such as rats also, the so called 2-vessel occlusion (2VO) and 4-vessel occlusion (4VO) methods. In the 2VO model, both CCA are again occluded, but since this still allows partial brain perfusion, additional stress is placed on the brain circulation by lowering blood pressure to approximately 50 mmHg. This lesion affects, in particular, those areas of the brain supplied by the middle cerebral artery, such as the lateral neocortex and striatum in rats, as well as other particularly vulnerable areas such as the hippocampus.

Finally, the 4VO method although surgically the most complex is the most reliable and allows controlled reversible ischaemia in the awake rat. In the first stage, the vertebral arteries are cauterised, and a loop of suture thread is placed around the two CCAs. Twenty-four hours later, the ends of the thread are drawn to seal the CCA. The extent of damage in the 4VO model is related to the duration of occlusion: 15 min will induce selective cell loss in the dorsal blade (field CA1) of the hippocampus, whereas after occlusion for 30 min or more, damage is more extensive, in particular in the neocortex and striatum (Pulsinelli *et al.* 1982).

The alternative is to induce ischaemia at a focal site in the brain, for which the two predominant approaches are to occlude the arterial supply to a particular region of the brain and to induce focal thrombotic lesions surgically, physically or chemically. The most widely used method involves occlusion of the middle cerebral artery (MCA) in rodents (see Fig. 3.14). The occlusion is, typically, made permanently by ligation or cauterisation of the artery under general anaesthesia; although recently a reversible method has been used, in which a thread is passed up the artery to block it, and then removed after the required period (Seta *et al.* 1992). Permanent MCA occlusion typically involves more extensive damage with widespread necrosis through the affected frontal and parietal neocortex and neostriatum than does transient global ischaemia, although the extent can depend on the degree of compensatory inflow and overlap from adjacent cerebral arterial systems.

A recent alternative is the development of photosensitive dyes with the capacity to induce local cerebral infarction (De Ryck 1990). Rose Bengal is a halogenated derivative of fluorescein, which on illumination yields single oxygen molecules that will cause endothelial cell damage and platelet aggregation when blood borne. The relatively non-invasive surgical method for inducing ischaemia is to inject Rose Bengal into the rat tail vein and then illuminate a circumscribed area of neocortex with a fibre optic white light or laser source, inducing a photothrombic lesion at the site of illumination. In rats, a high-intensity light source can penetrate the skull, offering the great flexibility of relatively non-invasive surgery, although a more precise and reproducible lesion is produced with removal of a circumscribed skull bone flap and direct illumination of the cortical surface.

## *Cell death in ischaemia*

The biology of the events following these experimental insults is rather different from one model to another. In addition, there are a number of *in vitro* models in which monolayer or slice cultures are exposed to anoxia,

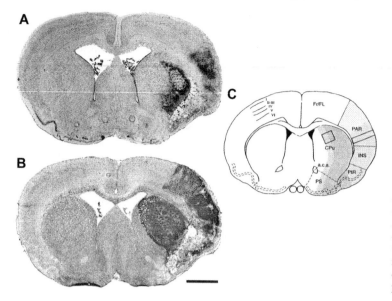

**Fig. 3.14** Focal ischaemia. Degeneration in the lateral neocortex and neostriatum in the rat brain following occlusion of the middle cerebral artery unilaterally. A Schematic outline, showing infarct and penumbral area as heavier and lighter shading. B Nissl cell body stain with cresyl violet. C Ox42 immunohistochemistry for increased microglia and macrophage activity. (Reproduced from Lehrmann *et al.* 1997, with permission.)

excitotoxic agents, or other toxins. The profusion of different models complicates any attempt to give a general view of the biology of anoxic damage, but there are several general mechanistic themes that run through the whole literature. Not surprisingly, the extent of tissue damage relates to the area of perfusion loss, the completeness of the reduction in blood flow, and the duration of the ischaemia. Certain areas are predictably affected in the different models, either because of their dependence on a particular cerebral artery (such as the lateral striatum and neocortex on the MCA), or because of the sensitivity of particular cells to anoxia (e.g. CA1 pyramidal neurones of the hippocampus).

Any form of injury to the CNS, whether it be due to mechanical trauma or anoxia, will, if it continues for long enough, damage some cells so badly that they will be disrupted and die rapidly. In focal ischaemia models this will lead to an area of necrosis at the centre of the lesion that is not rescuable. The disrupted cells release their contents, and some blood vessels are generally disrupted leading to further bleeding. There are no features of cell damage and death in this region that are peculiar to the CNS, and no potential therapy other than prevention of the insult that led to it. However, in the region surrounding the area of immediate cell death is a *penumbra* of tissue in which cell death takes time to develop (see Fig. 3.15). Within this zone, most cells do not die immediately but death may take 2 or 3 days to occur. Cell death here is not due to a rapid primary necrosis but is largely apoptotic (see Chapter 1), and due to a cascade of secondary changes induced by the initial

ischaemic event, and has the potential, with suitable intervention, to be preventable. Clearly there must be a gradation of anoxic damage from the centre of the lesion out into this penumbra, so the more central cells are more severely at risk than the more peripheral. In addition, some neurones fairly distant from the lesion, but whose axons pass through it or connect to it, may die in the days following anoxia due to events associated with axotomy and loss of trophic support rather than to the ischaemic event *per se* (see Chapter 2).

## Mechanisms of ischaemic neuronal death

Analysis of the events associated with ischaemic injury in the brain, suggests that excitotoxicity may contribute significantly to the mechanisms of delayed cell death in the penumbra, which has opened up over the last decade novel strategies for remediation. In particular, many of the mechanisms share the property of increasing intracellular calcium, and the large and often irreversible rise in intracellular calcium triggers many of the mechanisms that lead to cell death.

## Anoxia and vasoconstriction

A region of hypoxia exists around the central core of a stroke lesion, simply by reason of blood-vessel blockage. Thrombolytic treatment aimed at restarting blood flow will, to some degree, reperfuse such an area. In global ischaemia, restarting the circulation will lead to

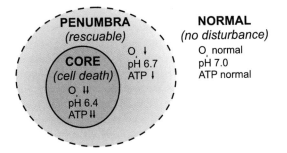

**Fig. 3.15** Core and penumbra surrounding a site of focal ischaemia in the brain. (From Choi 1990.)

reperfusion. However, there are still a number of mechanisms leading to vasoconstriction.

Damage to the endothelial cells lining blood vessels leads to the release of endothelins, which have also been found in some astrocytes and neurones. The tissue destruction caused by CNS damage will therefore release endothelin into the local circulation, leading to vasoconstriction.

Platelets release many active molecules when they are disrupted during the clotting process. Serotonin, ATP, and ADP are released in particularly large amounts. Serotonin is generally an active vasoconstrictor, while ADP and ATP may be active as vasodilators.

Activation of the arachidonic acid cascade occurs wherever there is tissue damage, and leads to the formation of many active compounds. Several prostaglandins, leukotriemes, and lipoxins are formed, some of which are vasoconstrictors, whilst others increase vascular permeability and activate macrophages and neutrophils (see below).

Many patients become hypotensive following CNS damage, leading to a general decrease in the perfusion of the brain, and exacerbating the poor blood flow surrounding the lesion.

## Oedema

Damaged CNS tissue becomes oedematous. At its worst, this can involve a general increase in intracerebral pressure, coning of the brainstem down the spinal canal and death due to pressure on, and disruption of, the vasomotor, respiratory, and other vital centres in the pons and medulla. However, local oedema can also reduce blood flow through the capillaries, leading to worsening of hypoxia. The oedema is both intracellular and extracellular. Intracellular oedema arises when the sodium–potassium exchange pump is slowed, sodium

enters the cell, the sodium gradient across the membrane diminishes, and water is then able to enter, attracted by the osmotic potential of the intracellular macromolecules. Extracellular oedema occurs when vascular permeability increases, either because of damage to the endothelial cells, or because vasoactive substances, such as bradykinin, are released by the cells of the CNS, or by invading neutrophils and macrophages. The blood–brain barrier is usually so tight that effectively no osmotically active molecules can enter the CNS except by active transport, so the influx of proteins and other molecules from the blood through the now leaky capillaries leads to a major change in the osmotic potential of the brain extracellular environment, and therefore water enters leading to extracellular oedema.

The precise changes in blood flow following stroke are not well documented in humans, and this will not occur until it is possible to submit patients with recent strokes to PET scanning. It may then transpire that some patients have persistent diminution of blood flow, while others have reactive hyperaemia. The treatment for these two conditions would obviously be very different.

## Formation of free radicals

Stroke can lead to the generation of free radicals by a number of mechanisms, which we have detailed above. The major causes are effects on mitochondria, by generation and metabolism of arachidonic acid, by generation of nitric oxide, by the effects of iron released from red blood cells, and by the recruitment of neutrophils and macrophages that release free radicals. We have already seen the variety of ways in which free radicals are an important cause of CNS damage. Moreover, antioxidant treatments including free-radical scavengers, iron chelators, nitric oxide synthase inhibitors, and neutrophil depletion are all neuroprotective under appropriate conditions in both whole animal and *in vitro* models of ischaemia.

## Neutrophils and macrophages

Following CNS trauma or stroke, neutrophils are seen adhering to the blood vessel walls in the surrounding tissue within minutes, and entering the tissue within 1 or 2 h (Heinel *et al.* 1994). Macrophages can enter from two sources. Where there is severe damage, vascular destruction, and increased capillary permeability, monocytes can enter the CNS from the blood. However, there are also resident macrophages in the CNS in the form of microglia, and these become activated, migrate towards the lesion, and divide. However, macrophages are not a major feature of the pathology of CNS lesions until after 24 h or so, but will then persist for weeks.

Neutrophils adhere to blood vessel walls initially due to upregulation of E- and P-selectin on the endothelial cell surface, which interact with the LeX lectin on the neutrophil surface. Passage through the endothelial wall depends on the neutrophil integrins MAC-1 and LFA-1 interacting with ICAM-1 and -2, and VCAM on the endothelial cells. These ligands are also upregulated on astrocytes following a variety of types of CNS damage (Matsuo *et al.* 1994). The attraction of neutrophils and their adhesion to endothelial cells is initiated by the secretion of chemokines by cytokines, such as TNFα and IL-1, and by various arachidonic acid derivatives. These factors will also initiate degranulation by the neutrophils, releasing many molecules, particularly proteolytic enzymes such as cathepsins, gelatinases, and elastases, which have the ability to damage the surrounding cells and extracellular matrix. In addition, neutrophils undergo a respiratory burst, leading to the production of highly toxic free radicals. Neutrophil depletion has been shown to significantly reduce the size of lesions in both stroke and head-injury models, so the damage done by these processes is significant.

After 24 h or so the major inflammatory cell type is the macrophage. Its recruitment from the circulation is by a similar mechanism to that of neutrophils, and involves selectins, the integrins LFA-1 or MAC-1 adhering to ICAM-1, and -2, and VCAM. On a larger time scale, macrophages can be recruited from the microglial population (see Chapter 2). These again are capable of free-radical generation by respiratory burst, and of releasing many proteolytic enzymes. In addition, macrophages produce many cytokines, particularly TNFα and interleukin 1, both of which may be responsible for mediating further cell death.

## Plasminogen activators and proteases

A surprising finding was made in 1995 by Tsirka and colleagues in Strickland's laboratory, when they looked at excitotocity in a mouse in which the gene for tissue plasminogen activator (tPA) had been knocked out. They found that when they injected kainate into the hippocampus of these mice there was almost no neuronal death, unless they replaced the tPA by injecting it directly. tPA is produced in the CNS primarily by microglia, and its main action is to convert the inactive plasminogen into the active proteolytic enzyme plasmin, which degrades extracellular matrix and surface mole-

cules. In a further set of experiments, the laboratory looked at the effects of excitotoxic injury with kainate on mice deficient in plasminogen, and these were also resistant to neuronal damage, as were wild-type mice treated with inhibitors of tPA or plasmin. Since the main source of tPA is microglial cells, the hypothesis is that these cells are centrally involved in the excitotoxic process. The direct evidence in favour of this comes from experiments, again by Tsirka, in which macrophage inhibitory factor (MIF) was used to damp down the microglial response when kainate was injected into the hippocampus: this prevented excitotoxicity. There are large numbers of proteases in the CNS, mostly in an inactive form, but these are mostly activated by plasmin, which cleaves off a group to produce an active protease, so tPA is at the start of a protease cascade, which will activate not just plasmin, but also a number of metalloproteinases. How might these various enzymes cause neuronal death? Direct injection of metalloproteinases into the CNS can cause neuronal death, so direct enzyme action is probably the mechanism. A possibility is that the enzymes degrade a vital extracellular matrix molecule such as laminin, whose absence or degradation products trigger neuronal death.

## Excitotoxicity and ischaemia

The link between excitotoxicity and ischaemia was first suggested from the observation that elevating extracellular magnesium, which reduces glutamate transmission, reduced the vulnerability of cultured hippocampal neurones to anoxia (Kass and Lipton 1982). This suggestion was quickly followed by the direct demonstration that extracellular levels of glutamate and aspartate are raised in the brain followed transient ischaemia (Fig. 3.16; Benveniste *et al.* 1984), that lesion of the glutamatergic projections within the hippocampus reduces the extent of cell loss induced by hypoxia (Onodera *et al.* 1986), and that pretreatment with NMDA antagonists such as 2-aminophosphonoheptanoic acid or CGS-19755 can protect against hippocampal degeneration associated with 30 min transient global ischaemia followed by reperfusion (Fig. 3.17; Boast *et al.* 1988; Simon *et al.* 1984).

The concept behind excitotoxicity is the excitotoxic cascade. The excitotoxic cascade starts to produce major and irreversible damage when astrocytes start to release their intracellular glutamate stores, which are much greater than those in neurones. Normally astrocytes remove glutamate from the extracellular environ-

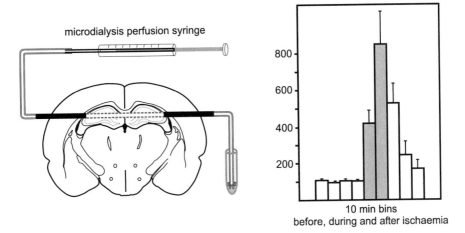

**Fig. 3.16** Changes in glutamate release measured by intracerebral microdialysis in the hippocampus induced by 10 min transient global ischaemia. (Redrawn from Benveniste *et al.* 1984.)

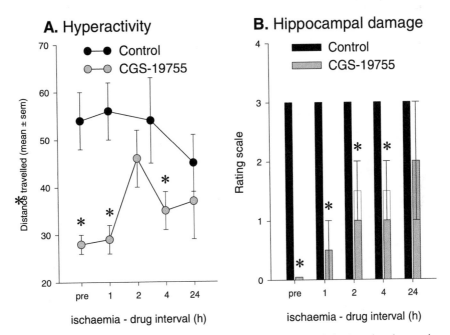

**Fig. 3.17** Treatment with the NMDA antagonist CGS-19755 can protect against behavioural and neurodegenerative consequences of ischaemia, even when given up to 4 hours after the insult. (Data from Boast *et al.* 1988.)

ment through an exchange pump, which exchanges two sodium ions and one glutamate for a potassium ion and a hydroxyl ion, the energy being provided by both sodium and potassium going down their concentration gradients, and sodium also going down a potential gradient. As the brain runs out of ATP, the transmembrane sodium and potassium concentration gradients are reduced, the membrane potential is diminished, and intracellular pH falls. All of these changes reduce the drive for the glutamate uptake pump, and eventually the changes are such that the pump goes into reverse. The reversal of the glutamate pump releases very large amounts of glutamate into the extracellular environment. This large amount of glutamate is sufficient to depolarise the CNS neurones to the extent that they fire action potentials, leading to more glutamate release, and to a vicious cycle of increasing depolarisation and increasing glutamate (see Szatkowski and Atwell 1994). NMDA receptors are fully occupied with glutamate, and the degree of depolarisation is sufficient to allow the NMDA channels to be open, increasing intracellular concentrations of $Ca^{2+}$, and long-lasting potentiation of NMDA-gated channels. This is the stage referred to by Choi as 'amplification' of the initial intracellular derangement. In direct parallel to the stages already outlined for primary excitotoxic injury (Fig. 3.8), these several processes induced by ischaemic injury converge on producing high levels of intracellular calcium, activation of degradative enzymes, and generation of toxic free radicals, which combine in a final phase of 'expression' of the injury to cause overt cell death.

Thus, anoxia or ischaemia do not predominantly involve unique mechanisms of cell death, but combine the major elements of excitotoxicity, calcium damage, metabolic disturbance, and free-radical production, amplifying the cycle of neurotoxicity outlined above (Fig. 3.13).

## Nitric oxide

NO synthase inhibitors are protective in models of ischaemia both *in vivo* and *in vitro,* and animals in which the NO synthase gene has been knocked out are also somewhat protected. As described earlier in this chapter, NO at high levels will combine with oxygen radicals to form the highly toxic peroxynitrite, and at lower levels will inhibit ATP production in mitochondria, yet further reducing neuronal and glial ATP levels.

The subject of neuroprotection is considered in Chapter 7.

# Further reading

Choi, D.W. (1990). Cerebral hypoxia: some new approaches and unanswered questions. *Journal of Neuroscience,* **10,** 2493–2501.

Choi, D.W. (1992). Excitotoxic cell death. *Journal of Neurobiology,* **23,** 1261–1276.

Meldrum, B. and Garthwaite, J. (1990) Excitatory amino acid neurotoxicity and neurodegenerative disease. *Trends in Pharmacological Sciences,* **11,** 379–387.

Simonian, N.A. and Coyle, J.T. (1996). Oxidative stress in neurodegenerative disease. *Annual Review of Pharmacology and Toxicology,* **36,** 83–106.

## Introduction

Although the CNS has conventionally been viewed as an immunologically privileged site, the importance of immunological responses in the pathogenesis of CNS disease has become increasingly apparent over the last few decades. Indeed, the concept of CNS isolation from the immune system is hard to reconcile with the favourable outcome of encephalitides commonly complicating some exanthemata, such as mumps, and with the brisk cerebrospinal fluid pleocytosis, which almost invariably accompanies brain infection; neither observation suggests that CNS invasion by infective agents proceeds unhindered by immune response. However, whilst *absolute* immune privilege can no longer be sustained, is has become clear that there are fundamental differences between the mechanisms of immunity in the CNS and those elsewhere in the body. In order to understand the part inflammation plays in both pathogenesis and repair, it is necessary to consider briefly both the principles of the systemic immune response and the blood–brain barrier, which protects nervous tissues from the systemic circulation.

## The immune response

A complex network of cells and soluble molecules is responsible for initiating, activating, targeting, co-ordinating, recalling, and regulating, the immune response. Despite the diversity of immune activities, and the vast range of cellular and humoral components of the immune response, the functions of the immune system may usefully be defined according to the biological activity expressed and the nature of the target. Thus, targets may either comprise foreign material (such as infectious microbes or transplanted cells) or host tissue (which may be normal as in autoimmune reactions, or abnormal as in neoplasms). This broad classification applies to most immune activities, and will be adopted in considering immune responses within the nervous system.

The conventional but perhaps oversimplified division into cellular and humoral immune responses remains a helpful way of classifying mechanisms of immune activity, but no longer may either immune reactions or autoimmune diseases be described as 'T cell' or 'B cell' mediated. These two arms of the immune response are wholly and inextricably interdependent. The basic elements of the immune response have been simplified and illustrated in Fig. 4.1.

## Elements of the immune response

The T cell is central to all elements of the immune reaction and T cell classification is detailed in Box 4.1 (p. 55). Recognition of antigen by T lymphocytes is responsible for initiating target-specific responses, and ultimately cytotoxic death of antigen-carrying cells. It is also responsible for modulation of the immune response, for example, by its suppresser actions; and for allowing activation of the B lymphocytes.

Antigenic stimulation of B lymphocytes results in secretion of circulating antibodies (immunoglobulins) by plasma cells. The combination of antibody with antigen may act to neutralise the antigen, recruit and activate macrophages, or bind and activate complement (a group of serum proteins that circulate in an inactive form and once activated result in the formation of vasoactive and chemotactic peptides, and terminal membrane attack complexes, which may injure or lyse target cells).

Cells of the macrophage/monocyte-lineage are represented in the CNS by the microglia. They have three key roles:

(1) initiation of immune responses by interacting with T cells;

(2) as effector cells, by phagocytosis of targets; and

(3) modulation of the immune response.

Antigen presentation is discussed below. Macrophages are able to attack their target by phagocytosis or

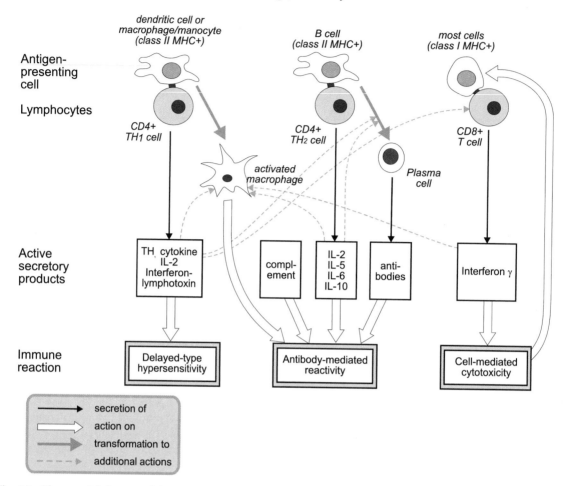

**Fig. 4.1** The essential elements of the immune response are presented according to the category of relevant antigen-presenting cell and class of immune response. The central role of the T cell is apparent in terms of enabling humoral responses, recruitment of other elements of the immune response, and regulation of the immune system. The main antigen-presenting cell of the CNS is the microglia (macrophage/monocyte lineage). Interactions between microglia and CD4+ TH1 cells stimulate the release of TH1 cytokines, which mediate delayed-type hypersensitivity. Similar interactions between antigen-presenting B cells and CD4+ TH2 cells, and other class I MHC+ cells and CD8+ T cells, are the primary interactions important in antibody-mediated and cell-mediated reactions, respectively. Complement and activated macrophages also contribute to the process of antibody-mediated reactivity, the latter by phagocytosis after opsination. Secretion of cell products (*black arrow*). Cell activation (*hatched arrow*). Cell or cytokine action (*white arrow*). Some interactions between the three main pathways are also shown in light grey.

by secretion of toxic substances, such as free oxygen radicals and tumour necrosis factor. Immune regulation is effected by secretion of proteins and peptides (macrokines), which influence other immune cells.

Presentation of antigen to the T cell as a complex with a molecule encoded by the major histocompatability complex (MHC) is necessary for T-lymphocyte activation. Class II MHC molecules (HLA-DR) are consitutively expressed only by *antigen-presenting cells* (APC), e.g. macrophages and dendritic cells. B cells may also function as antigen-presenting cells. Other cell types may be induced by lymphokines to express class II antigens and so can acquire a role in T-cell stimulation — such cells are known as *non-professional APC*. The complex of HLA-DR molecule and antigen must bind to the surface T cell antigen receptor (TCR), and even then, additional binding is required between a number of *accessory molecules* expressed by the APC and T cell (see Fig. 4.2). These include B7, and various intercellular adhesion molecules such as lymphocyte function

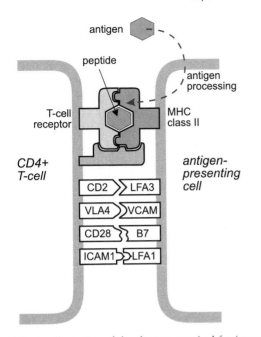

**Fig. 4.2** An illustration of the elements required for interaction between cells of the macrophage/monocyte line and T cells in delayed type hypersensitivity. Similar, although not identical, interactions take place between T cells and antigen-presenting cells to initiate antibody-mediated and cell-mediated cytotoxicity.

associated antigen 1 (LFA-1), and intercellular adhesion molecule 1 (ICAM 1). Engagement of HLA-DR antigen with TCR without additional accessory molecule interactions results in incomplete activation, T cell anergy, or possibly T cell apoptosis.

Antigen presentation by APC to T cells is a prerequisite for the development of the great majority of B cell (antibody) as well as cellular immune reactions, stressing the fundamental importance of T cells in the generation of immune responses. T lymphocytes play a key role in initiating and co-ordinating virtually every limb of the immune system, both through direct contact with other cells and by the secretion of numerous lymphokines, including interleukins and interferon $\gamma$.

## The blood–brain barrier

The blood–brain barrier (BBB) is the means by which differences in the constituents of the blood and the fluid bathing the brain can be maintained. The BBB arises from the way in which the endothelial lining of vessels penetrating the brain are constructed (see Fig. 4.3).

Whilst highly permeable to water and lipid-soluble molecules, the BBB prevents the free passage of solutes from the systemic circulation into the CNS. Essential nutrients, including glucose and certain amino acids,

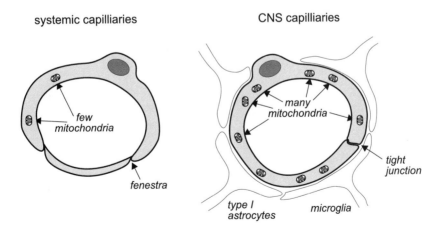

**Fig. 4.3** The essential differences between blood vessel structure in the periphery and the CNS are demonstrated. One major difference between the two is the presence of tight junctions between adjacent endothelial cells in CNS vessels, part of the machinery for limiting exchange between blood and tissue fluids. A continuous covering is provided by the extended foot processes, which were thought to be derived exclusively from type 1 astrocytes (Juhler and Neuwelt 1989), although it is now clear that a significant number of these processes are contributed by microglia. This covering is responsible for inducing endothelial cells to form this barrier between the systemic circulation and the CNS (Janzer and Raff 1987). Furthermore, CNS endothelial cells lack the vesicles that elsewhere effect transport of proteins into extravascular tissue, and also have many more mitochondria, presumably an indication of the reliance of specific transporter systems.

together with some ions, are transported by specific carrier mechanisms, but the majority of larger polar molecules, including proteins, cannot reach the abluminal surface.

The BBB normally excludes circulating immune effector molecules, such as immunoglobulin and complement, and most leucocytes, from extracellular fluid in the CNS. A similar barrier in the choroid plexus performs a parallel function, separating blood and cerebrospinal fluid (csf); this barrier is anatomically situated at the epithelial cell lining of the choroid plexus, not in the choroidal capillary endothelium.

BBB function may be disturbed by a variety of mechanisms, including infection and inflammation, neoplastic infiltration, circulating toxins, and malignant hypertension, often without physical disruption of the component cells or destruction of their tight junctions. Increases in BBB permeability are commonly reversible and often appear to be energy-dependent, neither observation being consistent with the simple concept of capillary leakage through a damaged cell lining. Rather, loss of BBB integrity is commonly the result of both increased vesicular transport across the endothelial cells and partial, but often transient, relaxation of endothelial tight junctions (for review see Bradbury 1979).

Impaired barrier function allows penetration into the CNS of circulating immune cells and molecules, exposing the brain to the complete canon of immune responses. It is generally accepted that activated T cells, regardless of their specificity, are able to penetrate the normal BBB, providing the CNS with a degree of immune surveillance. In experimental encephalomyelitis, lymphocytes infiltrate the CNS at a very early stage, when the BBB remains impermeable to horse-radish peroxidase (Simmons *et al.* 1987) and appears normal both structurally and functionally. Even systemic immune responses against antigens not expressed by neural tissue result in the appearance of activated T cells within the CNS (Hickey and Kimura 1987). T-cell blasts are able to secrete enzymes that degrade endothelial cell basement membranes; this presumably facilitates their passage through the BBB (Naparstek *et al.* 1984). There are also areas of the CNS where the BBB is constitutively incompetent — the hypothalamus, area postrema, periventricular areas, and spinal and cranial nerve roots (Bradbury 1979; Juhler and Neuwelt 1989). Thus traffic of activated T cells may occur through the CNS, providing the brain with a degree of immune surveillance but at the same time potentially exposing it to immune attack.

# The generation of CNS immune response

While the conventional dogma that the CNS is not routinely patrolled by lymphocytes is no longer tenable, this small volume of T-cell traffic would be unlikely to generate an immune response without encountering antigen-presenting cells or triggering BBB impairment, allowing other immune and inflammatory mediators to enter the CNS. In the normal CNS microglia, which are ultimately bone-marrow derived, are the major cell type constitutively expressing class II MHC molecules (Hayes *et al.* 1987). The interaction of T cells with microglia triggers the secretion of cytokines, which in turn amplifies microglial class II expression, and acts on local endothelia, impairing BBB function and recruiting further inflammatory and immunologically active cells (Hickey, and Kimura 1987).

Cytokines (such as interferon-$\gamma$) produced by T cell/microglia interactions may amplify the immune response further by causing the expression of class I and II MHC products on astrocytes and cerebral vascular endothelial cells, thus increasing the numbers of antigen-presenting cells. Neither of these cells normally express these molecules. Furthermore, astrocytes can express ICAM, and may also secrete interleukin 1, which is important in T-cell activation (Frohman *et al.* 1989). Thus, astrocytes and endothelial cells could have a central role in amplifying T-cell reactions and, since both are involved in maintaining normal BBB physiology, in augmenting BBB damage. It must be emphasised, however, that most results supporting this role derive from *in vitro* studies, with rather sparse supportive *in vivo* evidence.

# Autoimmune damage to the CNS

In general terms, autoimmune damage to the CNS may attack one or more basic elements: glial cells; neurones; or endothelial cells. Damage to each of these elements will be illustrated using selected disease examples.

## Glial damage

Two diseases produced by immune damage to glial elements of the CNS are acute disseminated encephalomyelitis, which as its name suggests is a monophasic illness, and multiple sclerosis, which is a chronic illness.

*Acute disseminated encephalomyelitis* (ADEM) is an

inflammatory demyelinating disease that is a rare complication of a number of infections, such as measles and vaccinations (Cohen and Lisak 1987). Characteristically it commences 1–3 weeks after the offending cause, with headache, fever, meningism, and impaired consciousness, accompanied by neurological symptoms referable to white matter disease affecting the cerebral and cerebellar hemispheres, brainstem tracts, spinal cord, and optic nerves. There is evidence of a brisk immune response with white cells in the CSF and oligoclonal bands; the latter are indicative of local immunoglobulin production and may only transiently be present, in contrast to more chronic forms of inflammatory demyelination.

Pathologically there are multifocal lesions comprising an intense perivascular infiltrate of lymphocytes and macrophages. In the more severe variant, acute haemorrhagic leukoencephalitis (AHLE), there are haemorrhagic changes, with fibrinoid necrosis of small veins. Demyelination is not seen initially in these hyperacute cases, and seems only to develop after several days. The difficulty in identifying persistent virus, and the histopathological similarity to experimental allergic encephalomyelitis (EAE), a well characterised T-cell mediated experimental autoimmune disease of the rodent CNS, suggest that ADEM, and indeed AHLE, represent a cell-mediated anti-myelin immune responses. A number of possible mechanisms have been proposed including changes in oligodendrocyte–myelin surface antigens induced by virus infection, induction of class II MHC by virus within the CNS, allowing antigen presentation, and cross-reactivity of viral and myelin antigens.

*Multiple sclerosis* is a relatively common chronic disease, characterised clinically by the classical relapsing-remitting course, each relapse representing an acute or subacute self-limiting episode of focal neurological disturbance. The pathological substrate for these episodes is the inflammatory demyelinating lesion, in which is found circumscribed perivascular oedema, and inflammation and demyelination. The inflammation, oedema, and demyelination all contribute to conduction block (Yule 1991). Imaging studies show, and histopathological studies have confirmed, that any part of the brain can be affected, but certain white matter tracts are particularly (and thus far inexplicably) susceptible (Fig. 4.4). This damage results in characteristic and recognisable clinical patterns — which, together with the relapsing course, result in a unique neurological picture. However, not all patients conform to this classical pattern, and a substantial variability

in the impact and severity of disease expression is found.

The cause of multiple sclerosis (MS) and related demyelinating diseases remains unknown. Both genetic and environmental factors contribute, but in both cases, the precise nature of the precipitant remains to be defined (reviewed in Scolding *et al.* 1994; Compston 1997). The high concordance rate in monozygotic twins, contrasting with the rate in dizygotes, offers powerful evidence that the genetic contribution is substantial and definite, and yet not absolute — environmental influences are implied by the 70% discordance in identical twins. Inheritance is polygenic, most models predicting that at least five or six genes are implicated (Compston 1997). Various groups have undertaken genome screens, and these have highlighted several areas of importance within the genome, excluding the possibility of any single gene making a major contribution to the development of multiple sclerosis. The identification of the important genes of influence is the next target. The nature of the environmental influence remains, however, to be identified. The most likely candidates are viral, the hypothesis being that the virus either has on its surface a protein that mimics myelin proteins, causes such a molecule to be expressed on the cells it infects, or causes infected cells to modify their cell surface so as to mimic a myelin molecule and initiate an immune response to it. Of the possible viruses, herpes-6 virus is one recent suspect.

Considerable effort has been expended in elucidating T-cell and B-cell reactivities in multiple sclerosis in attempts to identify a so-called 'multiple sclerosis antigen'. However, immune reactivities to numerous myelin antigens occur, often differing between patients with multiple sclerosis, or not differing from healthy controls, and these are clearly difficult to reconcile with pathological and other evidence supporting not just an immune pathogenesis but highly targeted damage to the oligodendrocyte-myelin unit. However, a coherent picture of the sequence of events culminating in demyelination is emerging that, while incomplete, can accommodate many of the complicated findings described above (Scolding *et al.* 1994). This is represented schematically in Fig. 4.5.

At the onset, T lymphocytes are activated in the periphery. The commonest suggestion is that this crucial immunological episode centres upon an antigen carried by infection — probably viral, and probably common, the (later) idiosyncratic cascade depending on the host gene complement rather than the organism. The responsible antigen may mimic an oligodendrocyte-myelin

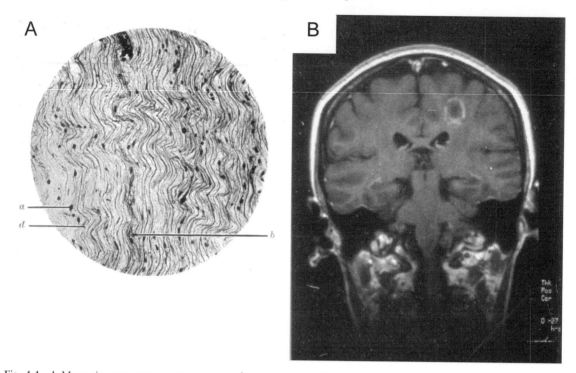

**Fig. 4.4** A Magnetic resonance spectroscopy scan from a patient suffering with MS. Areas of demyelination can be seen as hypodense regions (arrows), and the predilection for white matter is apparent. B Photomicrograph of a section through such a region of white matter tract damage, i.e. the so-called 'plaque' of MS. As can be seen from this section, axons are intact (arrows), but there is oligodendrocyte damage (arrow heads) so that the axon has lost it's myelin cover.

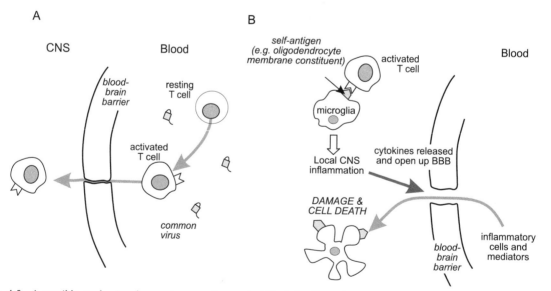

**Fig. 4.5** A possible mechanism for autoimmune damage in MS. A Small numbers of T cells are activated by a common viral antigen, and at some stage (possibly at a much later time), they pass across the blood–brain barrier (BBB), perhaps as part of a further non-specific reactivation of this response. B Once in the CNS, they cross react with the self-antigen presented by the macrophage/microglial cells and thus initiate an inflammatory response with BBB opening and the arrival of further elements of the immune cascade.

epitope. At a later stage — probably much later and perhaps as a consequence of non-specific reactivation of this immune response following viral infection or other events — a small number of these activated T cells, in common with other circulating activated T cells, traverse the blood–brain barrier (BBB). Within the perivascular brain parenchyma, they encounter the (unknown) target self-antigen presented to the T-cell receptor by perivascular macrophages and microglia. This interaction represents the initiating nidus of focal CNS inflammation, promoting local maintenance and propagation of the originally systemic immune response. Cytokine production upregulates expression of adhesion molecules on circulating lymphocytes and BBB endothelia, and directly increases the permeability of the barrier, causing increased binding and migration of inflammatory cells into brain parenchyma, together with an influx of humoral immune mediators, culminating in the formation of a perivascular hypercellular inflammatory infiltrate.

Oligodendrocyte and myelin damage is contingent upon this T-cell dependent event and probably involves several mechanisms. In the early phase, myelin function might be disturbed simply by the compressive effect of oedema. The restoration of blood–brain integrity might subsequently allow oligodendrocyte recovery and restitution of saltatory conduction through myelinated fibres. Animal models suggest that antibodies directed against oligodendrocyte-myelin surface components are important for targeting damage, activating complement and opsonising for macrophage/microglial attack. Others have proposed non-specific bystander damage by cytotoxic cytokines, enzymes, and oxygen radicals secreted by activated T cells and microglia, including TNF$\alpha$, lymphotoxin, nitric oxide, and myelin-degrading proteases; complement is also likely to be involved (Scolding *et al.* 1989). Ultimately, the damaged myelin sheath is engulfed and removed by microglia; astrocytes invade, hypertrophy, and proliferate, and the classical gliotic oligodendrocytopaenic demyelinated plaque is formed. It is clear that significant axon loss, particularly in chronic lesions, contributes to permanent disability in patients.

So far attempts to treat MS by immune manipulation have been largely disappointing (Hohlfeld 1997) (see Chapter 10). High-dose intravenous methyl prednisolone hastens recovery from acute relapses, but does not interfere with the long-term disease process. Of the conventional immune suppressants, azathioprine is probably the most useful, with a very small but statistically significant effect on progression of disability;

newer agents such as interferon-$\beta$, copolymer, and intravenous immunoglobulin may hold more promise (e.g. Paty *et al.* 1993), but the evidence that any has a substantial effect in slowing disease progression is scanty. Other treatments are under evaluation.

# Endothelial damage: vasculitis

Not surprisingly, when the autoimmune insult is directed against components of vessel walls, damage is frequently multisystem, and neurological involvement is an inconsistent feature of the many vasculitic conditions (Brick and Brick 1989; Heck and Phillips 1989; Kissel 1989; Serdaroglu *et al.* 1989). Since these conditions affect blood vessels, the result is usually CNS ischaemia, which may be focal, multifocal, or diffuse, and may affect any part of the brain. This explains the occurrence of almost any neurological symptom, sign, or syndrome (Sigal 1987; Moore 1994; Moore and Calabrese 1994). Thus, classification on clinical grounds has proven difficult, and insufficient is known to enable a useful classification based on aetiology or pathology. A number of systems have been proposed that depend variably on histological characteristics, such as the size of vessel involved and the presence or otherwise of granulomata; the clinical context and organ involved; and whether the disease is deemed to be primary or secondary. Primary vasculitic disorders include Wegener's granulomatosis, microscopic polyangiitis, and temporal arteritis, while vasculitis may alternatively be secondary to collagen vascular or rheumatologic disorders, malignancy (particularly myeloproliferative disease), drugs, or infections such as hepatitis B or C.

## Mechanisms of damage

The classical pathological change in vasculitis is that of an inflammatory infiltrate within the vascular wall associated with destructive changes, commonly described as fibrinoid necrosis. At present there is very limited understanding both of the initiating causes of vasculitis (in contrast to many autoimmune disorders, there does not even appear to be a class II MHC association upon which to build hypotheses of causation; see Zhang *et al.* 1995), and of the mechanisms of tissue damage. The exception to this general rule of aetiological ignorance is that group of vasculitides occurring in the context of infectious diseases, where, for example, direct bacterial invasion of the vascular wall causes the vasculitic process (see Chapter 5).

Of the two classical effector limbs of the immune system, cellular and humoral, the latter appears far more important in the development of the vasculitic process, although the constant qualification of this simplified approach to immune mechanisms — that humoral and cellular immunity are interdependent and cannot truly be divorced — again applies. Three principal pathways of vascular injury are commonly invoked (e.g. Jennette *et al.* 1994): direct antibody attack of the vasculature; immune complex mediated vasculitis; and ANCA-related vasculitis; all depend ultimately on antibodies. T cell dependent mechanisms are rather less commonly implicated in vasculitis, but will also be discussed

## Immune complex mediated vasculitis

Immune complex deposition in the wall of blood vessels triggers activation of the complement cascade and the consequent recruitment of polymorphs and macrophages, amplification of inflammation, and the generation of lytic and injurious membrane attack complexes. This sequence of events is widely quoted as a cause of the vasculitic process, although there are in fact rather few examples in which this has unequivocally demonstrated: hepatitis B and C associated vasculitis and Henoch Schnlein purpura amongst these.

## Direct antibody attack

Antibodies directed against endothelial cells have been reported in a variety of disorders, including MS, where a pathological role has been suggested, but by no means universally accepted. Studies of patients with vasculitic syndromes have also revealed the presence of anti-endothelial cell antibodies. Such antibodies have been shown to activate or to injure endothelial cells (Carvalho *et al.* 1996), although their lack of specificity, coupled with rather variable rates of detection, has left questions concerning their relevance. Medium- and large-vessel vasculitis (and therefore less often cerebral disease) are more frequently associated with anti-endothelial cell antibodies than small-vessel disease (Salojin 1996).

## Anti-neutrophil cytoplasmic antigen (ANCA)-related vasculitis

The description of antibodies directed against cytoplasmic antigens in polymorphonuclear cells in patients with systemic vasculitis represented a major advance in sero-

logical diagnosis of these disorders. Indirect immuno-fluorescence testing using ethanol-fixed neutrophils reveals two patterns of reactivity — cytoplasmic ('cANCA'), associated with Wegener's granulomatosis, and perinuclear, ('pANCA'), rather less specific, but commonly seen in microscopic polyangiitis and Churg–Strauss syndrome (and with glomerulonephritis). These fluorescence reactivities are associated with specificity for a neutrophil serine protease, proteinase 3, and myeloperoxidase respectively. Other antigen specificities continue to be described.

Despite the diagnostically useful specificity of these circulating antibodies, detailed histological studies of ANCA-related vasculitis often reveal little evidence of antibody-dependent tissue damage — neither immune complexes, complement components, nor immunoglobulins are readily identifiable — suggesting that the ANCAs may not play a direct role in tissue damage. One possibility is that ANCAs activate circulating mononuclear cells, stimulating an inflammatory cell attack on the vessel wall (Jennette *et al.* 1993). Ordinarily ANCA targets are cytoplasmic and thus inaccessible to antibodies, but tumour necrosis factor-$\alpha$ or interleukin 8 stimulate polymorphonucleocytes, and in this process PR-3 becomes detectable on the cell surface neutrophils (Csernok *et al.* 1994). ANCAs interacting with Fc-receptors cause degranulation with free radical production (Falk *et al.* 1990; Kallenberg *et al.* 1994).

PR3 and MPO, can also be identified in the lesions of, for example, Wegener's granulomatosis (Brouwer *et al.* 1994), where they may play a role in tissue damage. cANCA, specific to proteinase-3, inhibits inactivation of this enzyme, blocking the binding to it of the naturally occurring inhibitor $\alpha$1 antitrypsin (Dolman *et al.* 1993). Cytokines (including TNF$\alpha$, interferon-$\gamma$, and interleukins 1$\alpha$ and 1$\beta$) also induce endothelial cell PR-3 expression followed by its translocation to the cell surface (Mayet *et al.* 1993), re-emphasising the possibility of a direct effect of circulating ANCA antibodies on blood vessels might be mediated.

## Cell-mediated vasculitis

Interactions between adhesion molecules on endothelial cells, and circulating lymphocytes and other inflammatory cells clearly play a vital role in the development of inflammatory lesions (Springer 1994). The *selectins* are important in initiating the first adhesive contacts between leukocytes and endothelial cells, leading to the leucocytes rolling along vessel walls, while the *integrin* and *immunoglobulin gene superfamily* adhesion molecule groups mediate adhesion of leukocytes followed by penetration of the vascular endothelium. Various of these molecules are found in elevated concentrations in the serum, or are expressed on monocytes at higher levels in vasculitic syndromes (e.g. serum VCAM-1, ICAM-1, LFA-3, and monocyte expression of ICAM-1 and LFA-3 in Wegener's granulomatosis (Wang *et al.* 1993; Stegeman *et al.* 1994), reflecting vascular inflammation without illuminating the underlying reason. ICAM-1 and VCAM-1 are upregulated in hypertrophic endothelial cells within vasculitic lesions (Bradley *et al.* 1994).

Recent studies have clearly identified activated T cells and (putatively) antigen-presenting MHC class II positive dendritic cells in the lesions of microscopic polyartheritis nodosa (Cid *et al.* 1994) and Wegener's granulomatosis (Pall *et al.* 1994). Furthermore, in the latter disorder circulating T cells responsive to PR-3 have been demonstrated (Brouwer *et al.* 1994). MPO and PR3-directed T-cell responses are increasingly studied in systemic vasculitis (Griffiths 1996), and significant involvement of T cells seems more than likely.

In both primary CNS and peripheral nerve vasculitic lesions, the predominant infiltrate is CD4-positive and CD8-positive T lymphocytes and monocytes (Kissel *et al.* 1989; Gauthier *et al.* 1992; Cid *et al.* 1994; Parisi and Moore 1994). Eosinophils are rarely found to be prominent. B cells and plasma cells are also present, with giant cells of both Langerhans and foreign body type.

# Neural damage: paraneoplastic conditions

A number of clearly defined neurological syndromes occurring in the context of non-metastatic remote cancer are thought to be autoimmune in aetiology (Henson and Urich 1982; Arnason 1987; Anderson 1995). These may affect the peripheral nervous system — *paraneoplastic sensory peripheral neuropathy*, the *Eaton–Lambert myasthenic syndrome*, and *dermatomyositis* — or the CNS. Perhaps the most common of the latter is a *subacute cerebellar degeneration*. There is progressive ataxia, often presenting with vertigo; truncal ataxia is often marked, and the disorder commonly progresses to complete helplessness. *Opsoclonus-myoclonus* represents a second classical phenotype, while *limbic encephalitis*, with an amnesic presentation, may also be seen. These symptoms characteristically occur early in the course of the associated malignant

disease, frequently antedating tumour detection (by up to a year in some instances). Approximately 50% of reported cases have occurred in the context of bronchial small cell carcinoma, although the syndrome is also associated with cancers of the breast and ovary, and with lymphoma.

Subacute cerebellar degeneration is most commonly associated with small cell lung, ovarian, and uterine cancer. Encephalomyelitis, again most commonly associated with small cell lung cancer (Henson *et al.* 1965) may present as brainstem encephalitis with progressive vertigo, ophthalmoplegia, and nystagmus, and bulbar failure (Henson *et al.* 1965; Reddy *et al.* 1981; Dalmau *et al.* 1991) with or without more widespread features including pyramidal and extrapyramidal signs, ataxia, autonomic failure, and a sensory neuropathy. Myelitis may also occur (mostly in conjunction with signs of encephalitis) causing multifocal wasting and weakness, sometimes suggestive of amyotrophic lateral sclerosis. Limbic encephalitis, again usually associated with small cell lung cancer (Brierley *et al.* 1960) presents with a relatively selective subacutely progressive amnesic syndrome.

The principal pathological features associated with each of the above-described CNS syndromes are (anatomy apart) strikingly similar, with a few notable exceptions that will be described. The main changes are pronounced neuronal loss, with pyknotic changes, which would currently be interpreted as indicating apoptotic cell death; changes indicative of an inflammatory process, including perivascular lymphocytic cuffing with parenchymal infiltration by lymphocytes and macrophages, and the formation of microglial nodules; ubiquitous and relatively non-specific finding of astrogliosis. So, for example, in the paraneoplastic cerebellar degeneration these are the prominent changes in the cerebellar cortex (Brain 1965), where Purkinje cells are selectively lost. Similarly, dorsal root ganglion neurones are lost in paraneoplastic sensory neuropathy.

Pathologically, loss of Purkinje neurones is often accompanied by a lymphocytic inflammatory-cell infiltrate, and spinal fluid samples may exhibit a lymphocytosis, raised protein, and increased immunoglobulins, all consistent with an autoimmune process.

Further evidence for an immune pathogenesis lies in the demonstration, in many patients, of antibodies against neuronal cells that cross-react with antigens on tumour cells (see Kornguth 1989). Thus, in paraneoplastic cerebellar degeneration, antibodies directed against Purkinje cells are found, while in sensory neuropathy and limbic encephalitis, antibodies reacting less specifically with the majority of CNS and PNS neuronal populations are demonstrable. Similar cross-reacting antibodies have been found in patients with *paraneoplastic retinal degeneration* (see also Kornguth 1989); this is also associated with a range of tumours similar to the cerebellar syndrome, but here antibodies bind to photoreceptor antigens. The condition presents with bilateral visual failure progressing to complete blindness. Immunophenotypic analysis of the largely perivascular infiltrating inflammatory cells in paraneoplastic encephalomyelitis reveals a mixture of T and B lymphocytes (Graus *et al.* 1990; Szabo *et al.* 1991) and the presence of Hu-specific B lymphocytes in brain parenchyma of one patient. A direct role for these antibodies in mediating neuronal damage is yet to be proven, however.

The general pathogenetic model for paraneoplastic neurological disorders is that normal neural antigens come to represent the targets of immunological damage as innocent cross-reactive bystanders during the anti-tumour immune response. Antibody-mediated damage is at present thought to be more important than cellular responses. Disorders of the neuromuscular junction are very well described in this respect, and although they represent peripheral rather than central nervous system disease, their immunology represents a paradigm for the paraneoplastic CNS syndromes and is described below.

*Myasthaenia gravis* (MG) is a paraneoplastic syndrome that normally occurs outside the context of malignancy, although approximately 10% are associated with thymoma and are of paraneoplastic origin. Thymic tissue expresses the $\alpha$-subunit of the nicotinic acetylcholine receptor (Kornstein *et al.* 1995), and anti-acetylcholine receptor antibodies are developed in these patients. In this condition, it is clear that the antibody itself is the key cause of the disease. Thus passive transfer of immunoglobulins from patients with MG induces disease in rodents (Toyka *et al.* 1975), and there is a clinical response to removal of the tumour and to reducing the amount of circulating antibody by chemotherapy or plasmapheresis (Newsome-Davis *et al.* 1978).

Similarly, in at least a proportion of patients with a clearly paraneoplastic syndrome, the Lambert–Eaton myasthaenic syndrome (LEMS), antibodies directed against components of the neuromuscular junction have been identified. These impair calcium flux in the axon terminal *in vitro* (Roberts *et al.* 1985; Lennon *et al.* 1995), and therefore reduce acetylcholine release; they are probably directed against voltage-gated calcium channels (Leys *et al.* 1991; Lennon *et al.* 1995; Motomura *et al.* 1995). Small cell lung cancer is present

in 60% patients with LEMS (O'Neill *et al.* 1988), and the calcium channel proteins are expressed by both tumour and neurological target. Passive transfer of IgG from patients with LEMS into experimental animals induces the disorder, while immunosuppressive treatments again are symptomatically (and electrophysiologically) beneficial (Newsome-Davis *et al.* 1984).

A crucial difference between the CNS paraneoplastic disorders and paraneoplastic LEMS and myasthaenia gravis concerns the site of the relevant antigen: in the latter diseases, expression of the antigen on the cell surface allows antibodies easy access; in contrast, the antigens of proposed significance in CNS paraneoplasia are all intracellular, and on the wrong side of the blood–brain barrier. However, not all patients with proven cancer-associated disorders readily fitting into the above spectrum lack the 'appropriate' antibody; and, conversely, antibody-positive patients who lack either the correct tumour, or the required neurology, are well-described. Finally, there have been substantial difficulties in developing animal models of these diseases in that the autoimmune hypothesis remains to be proven.

Other possibilities must be considered. In paraneoplastic motor neurone disease, a possible opportunistic infectious aetiology has been suggested. The particular association with lymphoma offers immune paresis as a contribution to this suggestion; poliomyelitis represents an obvious example of viral disease of the anterior horn cell. A lower motor neurone disorder caused by a leukaemia retrovirus in mice has been described (Gardner 1991).

## Anti-Yo antibodies/anti-Purkinje cell cytoplasmic antibodies (APCA)

These antibodies are found in many patients with paraneoplastic cerebellar degeneration — almost invariably those with an underlying breast or gynaecological malignancy, significantly less often in those with small cell lung cancer (Greenlee 1983; Jaeckle *et al.* 1985; Anderson *et al.* 1988; Smith *et al.* 1988; Peterson *et al.* 1992). They are polyclonal IgG antibodies, commonly found in higher concentration in the csf than in serum, implying intrathecal synthesis or concentration (Furneaux *et al.* 1990).

A number of antigens for which anti-Yo/APCA are specific have been cloned, including PCD-AA, CDR62 and CDR3, which are all DNA-binding proteins that direct gene transcription, of the leucine-zipper family (Sakai *et al.* 1990; Fathallah-Shaykh *et al.* 1991). Others

**Table 4.1** Antibody specificities in paraneoplastic CNS disorders, indicating some of the antibodies associated with specific paraneoplastic syndromes

| Syndrome | Tumour | Antibody |
|---|---|---|
| Subacute cerebellar degeneration | Breast and ovary | Anti-Yo antibodies/anti-Purkinje cell cytoplasmic antibodies/APCA |
| Encephalomyelitis | Small cell lung cancer | Anti-Hu antibodies |
| Limbic encephalitis, subacute sensory neuronopathy; autonomic neuropathy | | Type 1 anti-neuronal nuclear antibodies/ANNA-1 |
| Opsoclonus/myoclonus syndrome | Breast | Anti-Ri antibodies/type 2 anti-neuronal nuclear antibodies/ANNA-2 |
| Cancer-associated retinopathy | Small cell lung cancer | Recoverin antibodies |
| Cancer-associated retinopathy | Melanoma | Anti-bipolar retinal cell antibodies |

---

## Box 4.1  T cell classification

As the T cell is so central to the immune response, it is worth elaborating further at this point. T lymphocytes may be divided into two groups: those expressing the antigen CD4, and those expressing CD8. Immature T cells are co-positive, and lose one or other as they mature. The majority of CD4+ve cells are responsible for the initiation of delayed type-hypersensitivity responses and for assisting B cells (hence the term *helper T cells* or $T_H$ *cells*), while CD8+ve T lymphocytes cells exhibit cytotoxic functions. They are able to recognise antigen when presented in conjunction with class I MHC molecules, which are expressed constitutively by most nucleated cell types, and bind to and lyse target cells by a variety of mechanisms. Contrary to initial suggestions, both CD4+ve and CD8+ve T lymphocytes can express suppresser function. *Suppresser T cells* provide a check on the activity of helper lymphocytes, and suppresser function is particularly important in immunological tolerance; its loss is thought to be central to the problem of autoimmune disease. Although the existence of suppresser activity is not in doubt, it has proved difficult to identify the functional sub-population and assign it a cluster-defined (CD) nomenclature using phenotypic markers.

T helper cells ($T_H$) may in turn be sub-divided into functional classes. $T_H$ cells are initially designated $T_H0$; they are long-lived, and their adhesion molecule profile commits them to circulation through blood and lymphatic organs, awaiting engagement and stimulation by professional APC. They thereupon differentiate into activated, effector cells secreting cytokines in a pattern that allows two polar types to be defined. $T_H1$ cells secrete pro-inflammatory cytokines, including tumour necrosis factor-b and interferon-g; $T_H2$ cells appear committed to promoting B-lymphocyte responses, producing cytokines important for B-cell activation and differentiation, including interleukin-4 (Il-4), Il-6, and Il-10.

Finally, a second type of T cell, the g/d T cell, has also been defined, so-named according to their usage of g- and d- chains — subunits of the TCR — in contrast to the majority of T lymphocytes (a/b-cells), which express TCRs comprising a- and b-chains. They also develop in the thymus and circulate, they express many of the same surface molecules as, and can secrete many cytokines in common with a/b-cells, and appear capable of generating immune responses and expressing cytotoxic effector function. However, their precise role and significance remains to be elucidated.

---

appear to have similar transcription-regulatory function, acting instead through zinc finger binding activity (Sato *et al.* 1991), while in yet other cases, antibodies to a protein (CDR34) abundantly expressed in cerebellar cortex and in breast and ovarian carcinoma, but of entirely unknown function, are found (Dropchko *et al.* 1987).

How, or indeed if, these antibodies interact *in vivo* with these antigens, and whether this interaction is responsible for Purkinje cell loss is unclear. Anti-

Yo/APCA antibodies do not bind in other areas of the CNS, while they are not detected in non-paraneoplastic cerebellar degenerations, arguing against their secondary generation triggered by (otherwise mediated) Purkinje cell damage. Anti-Yo/APCA antibody binding is, according to ultrastructural immunocytochemical studies, cytoplasmic rather than neuronal, which is clearly not readily reconcilable with a role in interfering with transcription. Purkinje cells exposed *in vivo* to specific (passively transferred) anti-Yo/APCA antibodies take up these (but not other) immunoglobulin molecules (Graus *et al.* 1991). Perplexingly, however, no cerebellar cell injury is apparent in these models — and there is indeed very little evidence from any immunological system that internalised antibody can cause cell damage. Active immunisation with recombinant (Yo) protein also fails to induce cerebellar disease, while passive transfer of Yo/APCA-specific lymphocytes into immune-deficient (SCID) mice similarly fails to replicate disease (Tanaka *et al.* 1995). The association between the presence of antibody and disease is summarised in Table 4.1.

### Anti-Hu antibodies/type 1 anti-neuronal nuclear antibodies (ANNA-1)

These antibodies are predominantly associated with paraneoplastic syndromes precipitated by small cell lung cancer, particularly the various encephalomyelitides and subacute sensory neuronopathy (Graus *et al.* 1985) — syndromes that may, of course, occur together. These are also polyclonal IgG antibodies and, in common with anti-Yo/APCA, appear to be synthesised within the CNS.

Ubiquitous staining of almost all neuronal nuclei by anti-Hu/ANNA-1 is described, not only throughout the brain and spinal cord, but also of sensory neurones of the dorsal root ganglia and of autonomic ganglia. A number of antigens have been identified using molecular cloning techniques: HuC, HuD, and Hel-N1 share sequence homology with each other and with a family of RNA-binding proteins thought to be important in post-transcriptional gene processing. Hel-N1 has been shown to bind to the mRNA molecules encoding the immediate early genes c-*fos* and c-*myc* and a number of growth factors including granulocyte-macrophage colony stimulating factor.

Small cell lung cancers almost invariably express anti-Hu/ANNA-1 antigen, particularly (and perhaps exclusively) HuD. Detectable expression occurs regardless of whether or not the tumour has triggered neurological paraneoplasia; one suggestion is that antibody production only occurs in those cases wherein the tumour co-expresses MHC class I antigens. B lymphocytes are prominent in the perivascular inflammatory infiltrates found in patients with paraneoplastic encephalomyelitis, while deposits of IgG are demonstrable within neurones. Complement-dependent and independent lysis of rodent cerebellar neurones by anti-Hu antibodies has been demonstrated. In parallel with those experiments concerning anti-Yo/APCA described above, attempts to develop animal models of anti-Hu/ANNA-1-related disease by injecting antibody have repeatedly failed (Dyck 1988; Rene *et al.* 1996).

### Cell-mediated immunity in paraneoplastic disorders

Paraneoplastic anti-neuronal antibodies have assumed an important diagnostic role of great practical help in investigating patients. There has properly persisted, however, some degree of scepticism concerning their potential pathogenetic contribution, and a small but significant body of evidence implicating the T cell has emerged.

In addition to B cells, macrophages and T lymphocytes are prominent in the lesions of paraneoplastic encephalomyelitis. CD4 and CD8-positive cells are present, but neither class I or class II MHC is detectable on the surface of neurones (Graus *et al.* 1990).

## Conclusions

The power of the immune system as a mediator of CNS damage has been illustrated by the disease processes described above. The involvement of inflammation as a final common pathway or as an adjunctive mechanism is apparent in a wide range of diseases (e.g. see Chapter 5 for infective agents), and as our understanding increases, many more diseases may be seen to have the immune response as a central damaging agent, as well as our major defence.

## *Further reading*

Scolding, N.J. (1999). *Immunological and Inflammatory Disorders of the Central Nervous System*. Heinemann Butterworths, London.

# 5 | Infection

## With Roger Barker and Steve Wharton

## Introduction

Infectious agents can cause a host of disorders within the nervous system, from fulminant bacterial meningitis to slow viral infections that underlie some neurodegenerative conditions. In this chapter the discussion will concentrate on the main pathogenic mechanisms of infective disorders rather than their neuropathological findings. These mechanisms involve direct invasion and damage by the infective organism, exotoxins, and the recruitment of an immune response that, whilst attempting to rid the body of the infection, can also damage the nervous system. Many, if not all, infections mediate their effect through a number of different mechanisms, one of which usually predominates. For clarity, these separate processes will be discussed individually with reference to specific disease examples.

Infective organisms usually enter the body either via breaches in the skin and mucosal membranes, or via the respiratory or gastrointestinal tract. Once inside the body the organism replicates and can then spread to other sites, including the nervous system (see Fig. 5.1), typically by way of the bloodstream (e.g. bacterial meningitis). However, infection can penetrate the CNS through a number of other routes, which include intracellular transport of the infective agent across the blood–brain barrier (BBB) by cells of the immune system itself (e.g. HTLV-1, JC virus, or HIV), or the retrograde transport of infective particles by neurones along their axons extending into the periphery (e.g. rabies). Once inside neural tissue the infection can start to mediate its pathogenic effect, which can be very selective both anatomically (e.g. HTLV-1 and thoracic spinal cord) as well as in terms of the cell type affected (e.g. oligodendrocytes in progressive multifocal encephalopathy, (PML)). This pathogenic effect typically takes the form either of direct damage and/or the generation of an immune response, although on occasions infecting organisms can mediate their neurological effects through the local or systemic release of a neurally active exotoxin (e.g. botulism, tetanus, and diphtheria).

The time from inoculation to disease presentation (latent period) varies between infections, ranging from hours in the case of some forms of bacterial meningitis (e.g. meningococcal meningitis) to years in the case of certain viral infections (e.g. HIV disease). Furthermore, the length of the latent period and the speed of disease progression are highly correlated, such that diseases with long latent periods tend to run a slower, more chronically progressive course. This, coupled to the mode of cellular damage induced by the invading organism, is a useful starting point for considering the infective disorders of the nervous system, and is schematically shown in Fig. 5.2.

The pathogenesis of CNS infection is not dissimilar to that seen at other sites within the body, although the CNS itself has unique properties both in terms of the immunogenicity of the cells within and its relationship to the afferent/efferent arms of the immune response. In this last respect, the immune response in the CNS is strongly influenced by its relative immunological privilege as a result of its very poorly developed lymphatic system and the presence of a blood–brain barrier (BBB). This latter structure isolates the CNS from circulating cells and antibodies, although some activated T cells are still able to cross it and effect immune surveillance in the non-diseased state (see also Chapter 4).

Neural tissue also represents a further difference from other cell types in that it is relatively non-immunogenic. Major histocompatability complex (MHC) expression, rather than being constitutive on most cells as elsewhere, is almost absent in the CNS, with MHC class I being restricted to endothelial cells, whilst MHC II expression is seen on a few microglial cells in the resting CNS. However, the situation is different in the disease state where the expression of MHC can be induced in astrocytes and microglia by pro-inflammatory cytokines released from activated T cells, so allowing for antigen presentation (Fabry et al. 1994; Neumann and Wekerle 1998) (see Fig. 5.3). Indeed the lack of constitutive MHC class I expression on neurones, may be of importance in allowing viruses to persistently infect neurones and escape immune elimination (Joly

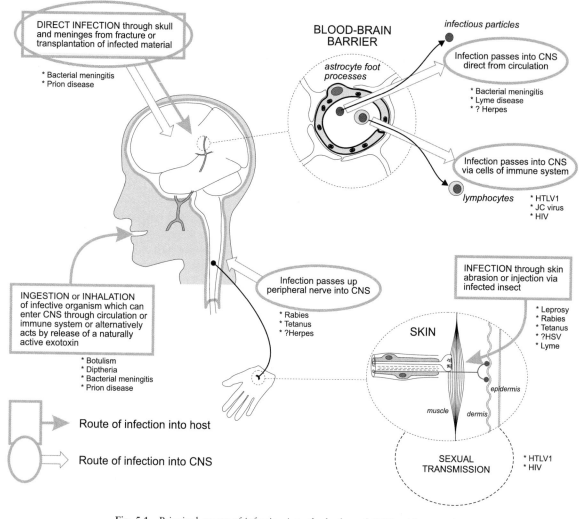

**Fig. 5.1**  Principal routes of infection into the body and CNS, with examples.

*et al.* 1991; Joly and Oldstone 1992) as abnormal MHC I expression on neurones in transgenic mice results in a more vigorous immune response. This improves the clearance of infective virus but results in greater damage with blood–brain barrier disruption (Rall *et al.* 1995).

This ability of an infective agent to induce immune-mediated damage within the CNS is not only a function of MHC expression but the age of the host at the time of inoculation (Ogata *et al.* 1991; Griffin *et al.* 1994; Oliver *et al.* 1997; Oliver and Fazakerley 1998). This is perhaps best illustrated with lymphocytic chori-omeningitis virus (LCMV) in mice. Intracerebral injection of adult mice with LCMV results in death from a

CD8+ T-cell mediated encephalitis, whilst in neonatal mice there is survival without an encephalitic illness. However, in some neonatal mice, the virus persists and depresses mRNA production, especially in the anterior pituitary, which can result in the development of a growth retardation syndrome (Oldstone *et al.* 1984; de la Torre 1992). Indeed, LCMV has similar effects on other cells including acetylcholine production in cultured neuroblastoma cells (Oldstone *et al.* 1977), as well as the *in vivo* expression of GAP-43 in the hippocampus, which in turn has been correlated to deficits in learning (de la Torre *et al.* 1996). Thus it is possible for cells of the CNS to support low-grade viral replication without structural effects but with functional

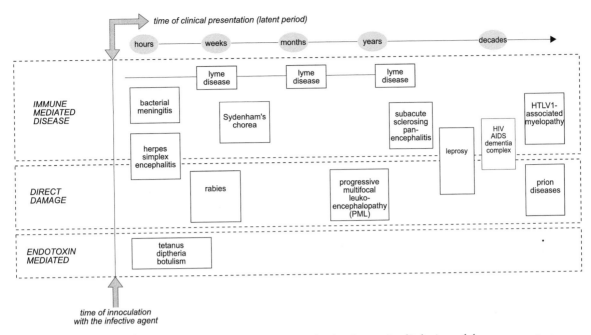

**Fig. 5.2** Schematic figure of latent period and primary mode of pathogenesis of infections of the nervous system.

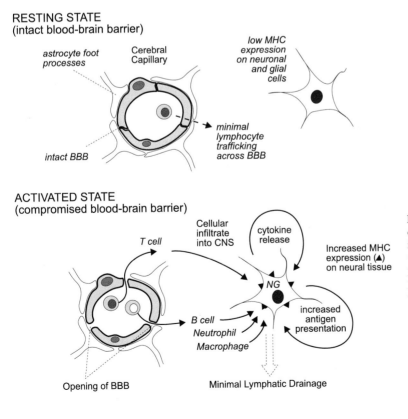

**Fig. 5.3** Schematic figure of the status of the immune system within the CNS in both the resting and activated states (for clarity some of the astrocytic foot processes have been omitted). CNS pathology leads to increased MHC expression on CNS glial cells, increased antigen presentation, and release of cytokines, as well as opening of the blood–brain barrier (BBB) and the passage of lymphocytes and, in some conditions, macrophages and neutrophils into the CNS parenchyma. NG, neuroglial cell.

impairments, and the extent to which this is part of the pathogenesis of infective disorders of the human brain remains to be determined (see, for example, Rabies below).

The pathogenic effects of an infection will therefore vary according to the state of the host, in terms of its age, MHC expression, BBB integrity, and immunological competence of the host, as well as the actual nature of that infective organism. Indeed there is often a fine balance between the immune system controlling disease due to the infectious agent and the avoidance of damage to the CNS as a result of that same immune response. This chapter will develop this theme and discuss infections of the CNS in terms of three major pathogenic mechanisms of damage: immune-mediated, direct toxicity, and exotoxin release. However, the linking of one infective organism to one pathogenic mechanism is somewhat artificial, and thus the chapter concludes with Lyme disease as an example of a disorder that employs many pathogenic mechanisms over varying lengths of time.

## Immune-mediated disease mechanisms

### Acute bacterially driven disorders: bacterial meningitis

Bacterial meningitis describes an inflammation of the pia, arachnoid, and the cerebrospinal fluid (csf) in the subarachnoid space in response to an infecting pyogenic organism. The whole neuraxis is bathed by csf and so is involved in the disease process, although the predominant pathological events are seen in supraspinal sites. These events are not so much the result of the infection *per se* but secondary to the inflammatory response it evokes. Thus, bacterial meningitis is a classical illustration of how a pathogenic organism can produce damage largely by way of the inflammatory response it generates.

The three organisms most commonly responsible for acute bacterial meningitis are *Neisseria meningitidis* (meningococcal meningitis), *Streptococcus pneumoniae*, and *Haemophilus influenzae* (see Table 5.1) — all of which colonise apparently healthy mucosal surfaces in the respiratory tract of normal subjects. The reason why these commensual organisms can cause meningitis is unknown, although their spread through the bloodstream with meningeal invasion seems to be a critical first step. However, exactly what triggers this invasion is not clear, although a number of possible factors have been postulated to be important including (Pfister and Scheld 1997):

- viral infection of the respiratory tract with impairment of mucosal defence mechanisms and passage of bacteria across the cribriform plate;

- BBB disruption by blood-borne bacterially-derived endotoxins;

- co-incident viral inflammation in the meninges, thus allowing infection to cross the BBB; and finally

- direct endothelial-bacterial interactions allowing bacteria to cross from the circulation into adjacent tissues.

Whilst the disease affects apparently 'normal' individuals in the majority of cases, there are, nevertheless, patients at particular risk of developing bacterial meningitis as a result of immune compromise. This includes patients with congenital agammaglobulineamia and those with more selective complement deficiencies, as well as acquired immunodeficiency states such as HIV.

The sequence of events that follows the bacterial invasion of the meningeal membranes and subarachnoid space is schematically summarised in Fig. 5.4, and discussed as such below.

### Stage 1

The bacteria on entering the subarachnoid spaces set up an inflammatory reaction of the meninges and structures lying within or adjacent to them. This acute inflamma-

**Table 5.1**  Common organisms causing bacterial meningitis

| Organism | Common age for infection | Other clinical features |
| --- | --- | --- |
| *Neisseria meningitis* | Children–young adults | Purpuric skin rash |
| *Streptococcus pneumoniae* | Infants and elderly | Pneumonia |
| *Haemophilus influenzae* | Infants and children | Middle-ear infection |

tory reaction is provoked by the bacteria and their toxins and leads to increased permeability of the local vessels with accompanying oedema, as is typical for infections in non-neural tissue.

During this period of acute inflammation there is migration of cells out from the vessels into the subarachnoid space. Neutrophils predominate at this stage and are probably brought in by chemoattractants produced by the meninges in response to the bacteria. These cells play an important role in the death and phagocytosis of the bacteria. Clinically during this early phase, patients complain of headache and examination reveals a stiff neck (so-called meningism) indicating early meningeal inflammation.

## Stage 2

The next phase of the inflammatory response (typically within 48–72 h) involves the rapid accumulation of the exudate into the subarachnoid space, which is heavy at certain sites such as the base of the brain (see Fig. 5.5A). At this latter site it may extend into the sheaths of cranial and spinal nerves, whereas more rostrally it may spread a short way into the perivascular spaces of the cortex. At this stage the inflammatory infiltrate starts to involve the adventitia (outer wall) of subarachnoid blood vessels with proliferation of cells in the intima (the inner lining). This early involvement of the vasculature reflects the fact that the adventitia of these vessels is actually an investment of the subarachnoid membrane, and is thus exposed early on to the invading organism.

Clinically, patients now start to develop confusion, stupor, and convulsions, which are likely to be due to the secondary toxic effects of the bacteria causing abnormalities of cerebral perfusion and cerebral oedema. Post-mortem studies during this acute phase of meningitis show few, if any, polymorphonuclear cell neutrophils infiltrating into cortical tissue (see Chapter 2), in striking contrast to the neutrophil infiltrate of the leptomeninges (see Fig. 5.5B). The underlying brain however, is oedematous, a change which may be marked.

## Stage 3

As the infection proceeds, the neutrophils in the subarachnoid exudate are replaced by lymphocytes, histocytes, and plasma cells, and there is a gradual increase in the exudation of blood proteins within this site, both

in the form of fibrinogen and antibodies produced by the plasma cells. Those remaining neutrophils continue to invade into the blood vessels with further intimal proliferation, which ultimately results in areas of focal vessel necrosis, subintimal fibrosis, and vessel occlusion causing ischaemic damage (see Fig. 5.5C; see stage 4). Veins are similarly affected and mural thrombi start to appear.

This process may also involve the perineurial sheaths of the cranial and spinal nerve roots, which become infiltrated by the inflammatory cells leading to ischaemic damage and thus focal nerve palsies typically the IIIrd, IVth, VIth, VIIth, and VIIIth cranial nerves. However, this type of damage has become uncommon since the advent of antibiotics.

## Stage 4

As the infection advances beyond the first week there are further vascular changes. Frank thrombosis of meningeal veins may occur causing further cerebral ischaemia with focal cerebral deficits, such as a hemiparesis and seizures. As the exudate increases and becomes more purulent, it may cause blockage of csf flow around the brainstem, which causes hydrocephalus.

At this more advanced stage, there is also proliferation of microglia and astrocytes in the outer layers of the cortex, which eventually spreads to involve all parts of it. The cause of this proliferation is not clear, but may be secondary to the diffusion of bacterial toxins or circulatory disturbances induced by the inflammatory infiltrate. These neuroglial elements in turn can modulate the ongoing immune response. In this respect, *in vitro* studies have shown that both microglia and astrocytes exposed to such bacterial toxins release cytokines such as interleukin 1 (IL-1) and tumour necrosis factor (TNF). For example, IL-1 initiates T-cell proliferation, whilst TNF stimulates IL-1 as well as activating neutrophils (see above). However the relevance of this to the *in vivo* situation is not clear.

Patients at this stage are comatose and even with appropriate antibiotic treatment, a significant number will die (Swartz 1984).

## Stage 5

If the patient survives stage 4, resolution occurs and the exudate organises into two layers: one adjacent to the pia and the other to the subarachnoid membrane.

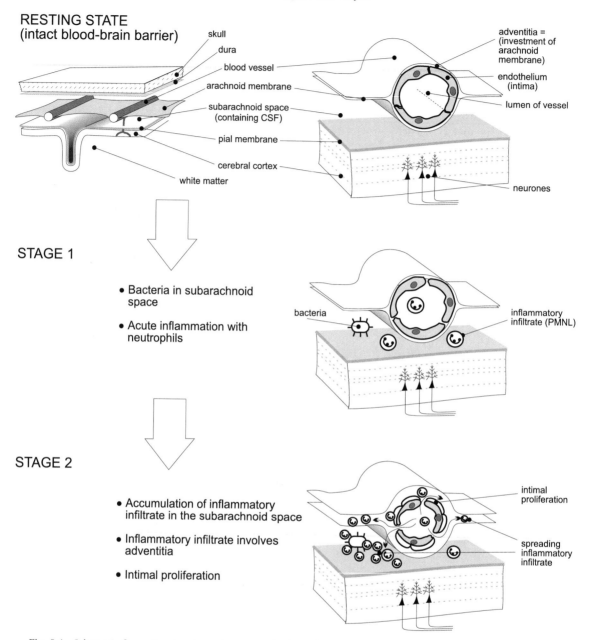

**RESTING STATE**
**(intact blood-brain barrier)**

skull
dura
blood vessel
arachnoid membrane
subarachnoid space
(containing CSF)
pial membrane
cerebral cortex
white matter

adventitia =
(investment of
arachnoid
membrane)
endothelium
(intima)
lumen of vessel
neurones

**STAGE 1**

- Bacteria in subarachnoid space
- Acute inflammation with neutrophils

bacteria
inflammatory
infiltrate (PMNL)

**STAGE 2**

- Accumulation of inflammatory infiltrate in the subarachnoid space
- Inflammatory infiltrate involves adventitia
- Intimal proliferation

intimal
proliferation
spreading
inflammatory
infiltrate

**Fig. 5.4** Schematic figure showing the various stages in the pathogenesis of bacterial meningitis (see text for details).

The fibrosis of the arachnoid membrane that characterises this stage of the process starts earlier in the course of the infection with fibroblast proliferation, although it is not until the second week that this fibrosis is conspicuous and may result in exudate loculation.

As the infection resolves, cells disappear in the order they appeared, although lymphocytes, macrophages, and plasma cells may be present in small numbers for several months. The extent of resolution depends on the stage at which the above inflammatory process is arrested. If this occurs early, there may be no lasting CNS damage, but at later stages when fibrosis is established, adhesions between the arachnoid and pia may contribute to the late sequelae of meningitis, such as

STAGE 3

- Subarachnoid exudate contains lymphocytes, histiocytes and plasma cells

- Increased protein exudation in subarachnoid space (fibrinogen and antibodies)

- Increased intimal proliferation and fibrosis

STAGE 4

- Vessel occlusion with ischaemic damage

- Changes within the cerebral cortex of astrocyte and microglia proliferation

STAGE 5

- Restoration, which can . be back to normal (see Resting state)

- Resolution can cause fibrosis of arachnoid membrane and pia with adhesions between the two causing hydrocephalus as a result of obstructing csF flow

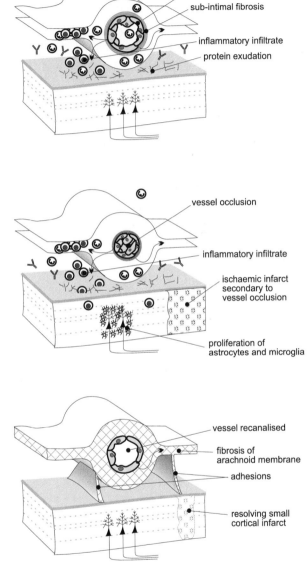

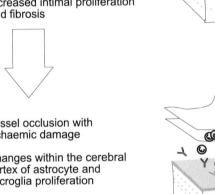

**Fig. 5.4** *Continued.*

chronic hydrocephalus, due to obstruction of the csf flow, and cranial nerve palsies.

Although the distribution of the pathogenic bacteria in this condition is largely limited to invasion of the meninges, it can be seen from the above description that there is the potential for damage outside this structure as a result of the immune response it generates. Therefore, the early treatment of this condition with antibiotics is critical, as any delay in clearance of the bacteria may result in long-term neurological sequelae secondary to the subsequent inflammatory damage.

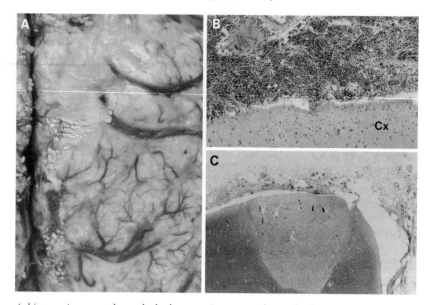

**Fig. 5.5** A Cream/white pus is present beneath the leptomeninges over the cerebral cortex. B An intense acute inflammatory cell infiltrate is present in the leptomeningeal space. Despite this, acute inflammatory cells do not infiltrate into the underlying cortex (Cx), ×75. C Low-power view showing an acute meningitis. A pale-shaped infarct, with its base at the cortical surface is seen secondary to inflammatory cell involvement of cortical arterioles, ×15.

## Acute virally driven disorders: herpes simplex encephalitis

The commonest form of acute encephalitis is herpes simplex encephalitis (HSVE), caused by the type 1 herpes simplex virus (HSVI). This encephalitis is a serious disorder which is still fatal in about 25% of treated cases (Whitley *et al.* 1986) and even in those who survive the acute illness, permanent neurological deficits are often seen consisting of an amnesic syndrome (secondary to bi-temporal lobe involvement) and seizures (Whitley 1990; Hokkanen and Launes 1997).

This virus responsible for HSVE is also the cause of common oral mucosal blisters known as 'cold sores', although interestingly reactivation of oral lesions rarely coincides with the encephalitic illness. However, HSVI is thought to initially gain access to the body via the oral mucosa or through abraded skin on the face, where it replicates, enters cutaneous sensory nerves, and then spreads axonally to reach the trigeminal ganglia where further replication may occur. Here it remains latent for years to be reactivated by stimuli such as intercurrent viral infections or UV light.

This ability of the herpes simplex virus to remain latent in sensory ganglia has attracted considerable interest, because although the virus is present there appears to be no replication or production of viral pro-

teins or peptides, in contrast to some other persistent viral states where there is low-grade viral replication. As a result, the virus is rendered invisible to the immune system; although it is not transcriptionally silent as an RNA species, the latency associated transcripts (LATs), may be detected by *in situ* hybridisation (Stevens *et al.* 1987; see Fig. 5.7B). However the functional effects of LATs currently remains unclear.

The fact that HSV remains latent raises the question as to whether the encephalitis it induces is secondary to reactivation of latent virus, or re-infection. In support of the former hypothesis is the observation that over half the patients with HSVE had identical strains of HSVI in the oral region and CNS (Whitley *et al.* 1982). If reactivation is thought to be the primary route of infection, then the virus should spread through the trigeminal nerve fibres innervating the leptomeninges of the anterior and middle fossae. Alternatively, it has been hypothesised that the virus gains access to the CNS via the nasal system and olfactory tracts. In favour of the trigeminal route is the fact that 40% of fatal HSVE cases have no olfactory pathway involvement at post-mortem, although the absence of virus in the meninges has led some authors to exclude a trigeminal nerve route of spread. Evidence in favour of the nasal route comes from the distribution of pathology in patients (Esiri 1982; see below) and the fact that the distribution of disease in the olfactory and limbic system structures of the central nervous system is replicated in animal models by intranasal inoculation (Anderson and Field 1983).

Controversy in HSVE is not only confined to the route of infection but extends to questions on why such a ubiquitous infection should cause an encephalitis in a tiny proportion of apparently healthy individuals — especially given the fact that three-quarters of these patients have antibodies to the virus at the onset of the illness. Indeed there is no clear evidence that the virus is particularly virulent in these cases, nor that there is any neuropathological difference between encephalitis due to primary infection or viral reactivation.

Pathologically, HSVE is characterised by bilateral, asymmetric damage of the temporal lobes (Fig. 5.6 and Fig. 5.7A), possibly because of the transneuronal spread of the virus along the anatomical pathways or, alternatively, due to specific tropism of the virus for these parts of the brain. Limbic system structures are particularly affected and, in addition to medial temporal lobe and orbitofrontal cortex, the insular and cingulate gyri are commonly involved. In these regions there is prominent oedema, necrosis, micro-

haemorrhages, perivascular and parenchymal infiltrates of activated T cells, macrophages, and granulocytes (see Fig. 5.7C) and meningeal inflammation is not an infrequent finding.

In early fatal cases intranuclear, eosinophilic inclusions (Cowdry type A inclusions, which are characteristic of HSV infection) are seen predominantly in oligodendrocytes, as well as neurones. In addition, viral antigen can be detected in these same cells by immunohistochemistry and viral particles by electron microscopy (see Fig. 5.7D). Additional evidence for direct viral cytopathogenicity comes from the finding that in animal models HSV infection is associated with the shutting-off of host macromolecular synthesis with both mRNA and protein being affected (Read and Frenkel 1983; Roizman and Sears 1990; Hardwicke and Sandri-Goldin 1994).

The virus can therefore be seen directly to infect and interfere with neuronal function, however in addition it recruits an immune response that may also be pathogenic. Chemokines, which attract and activate specific leukocyte subsets, are found to be high in the csf of patients with HSVE and show a specific profile of change over time, which is inversely correlated to the clinical state of the patient (Rosler *et al.* 1998). Furthermore, cell-mediated inflammatory processes may also play a role, as in animal models of HSVE, mononuclear CD4+ and CD8+ T cells are found in approximately equal numbers (Hudson *et al.* 1998). Moreover, these HSV-specific cytotoxic T cells were the predominant type found in temporal lobe tissue just prior to the onset of focal lesions in this same model, and were fully activated. Furthermore, antibody neutralisation of these specific cytotoxic cells removed their cytotoxicity, thus inhibiting neural damage implying that these cells direct the pathological insult. Interestingly such cells from the lymph nodes and spleen of these same mice failed to exhibit specific cytotoxic activity. Thus immune-mediated processes are critical to the pathogenesis of HSVE, as in bacterial meningitis, but in contrast cell death, as a result of direct viral infection, is also important.

## Chronic bacterially mediated disease: leprosy

Leprosy is the cause of the most common treatable neuropathy in the world. The causative organism *Mycobacterium lepra* (*M. leprae*) was identified by Hansen in 1873, and has several unique qualities — not least its fastidious growth requirements in animal models and the fact that it grows maximally at 27–30°C. The exact

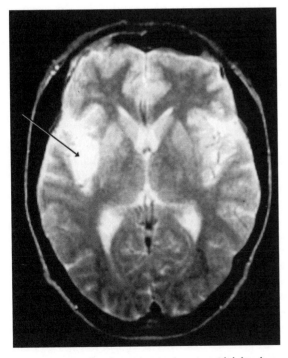

**Fig. 5.6** MRI showing asymmetric temporal lobe damage (*arrow*) in herpes encephalitis.

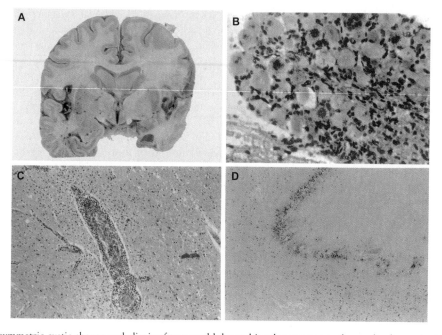

**Fig. 5.7** A Asymmetric cystic change and gliosis of temporal lobe and insular structures, the result of organised herpes simplex encephalitis, shows the characteristic distribution of damage in this condition. B Dorsal root ganglion of a mouse latently infected with herpes simplex virus type 1. *In situ* hybridisation, using a $^{35}$S-labelled riboprobe to latency associated transcripts, detects signal over the nuclei of a proportion of the neurones, ×300. C Histology from the temporal lobe of a case of herpes simplex encephalitis showing a perivascular lymphocytic cuff of inflammatory cells. Surrounding tissue similarly shows inflammatory cell infiltration which includes foamy macrophages, ×75. D Immunohistochemistry demonstrates abundant expression of herpes simplex virus in medial temporal lobe structures in a case of herpes simplex encephalitis. Expression is particularly strong in cells of the dentate gyrus, which runs in a band across the photograph, ×30.

mode of transmission is uncertain, although most probably occurs through abraded skin and/or nasal mucosa. However, once the bacillus has entered the host, it invades the peripheral nerve through binding to laminin-2 and then $\alpha$-dystroglycan (reviewed in Spear 1998), although there is a considerable delay from infection to clinical presentation (~3–5 years) and in some people no disease state is ever manifest.

The initial site of infection and replication is the endoneurium and Schwann cell of the cooler distal extremities and face (Miko *et al.* 1993). As one would expect, this infecting organism generates an immune response, and it is this that determines the clinical features of the disease (reviewed in: Ottenhoff 1994; Swift and Sabin 1996). A vigorous cell-mediated response produces tuberculoid leprosy, whilst a greatly reduced or absent response leads to lepromatous leprosy. However, in many cases an intermediate or mixed picture is seen, that is borderline or dimorphous leprosy. Furthermore, the nature of the disease may

change towards either a lepromatous or tuberculoid direction. These so-called reversal reactions are dependent on changes in the activity of host cell mediated responses.

Tuberculoid leprosy is characterised by a vigorous T-cell response with the production of high levels of IL-2 and interferon-$\gamma$ (i.e. Th1 response). This immune response checks bacterial proliferation and so dissemination, so that few bacteria are present although *M. leprae* antigen is still detectable. Thus, these patients have localised disease in which there are tuberculoid granuloma with epitheloid cells and lymphocytes surrounding neurovascular elements and extending up to the epidermis. This inflammatory reaction, whilst halting the spread of the disease, causes local damage to the skin and nerves, so that characteristically the patients have small hypopigmented, anaesthetic (somatic nerve involvement) areas of skin that are dry (autonomic nerve involvement).

In contrast, in lepromatous leprosy there is wide-

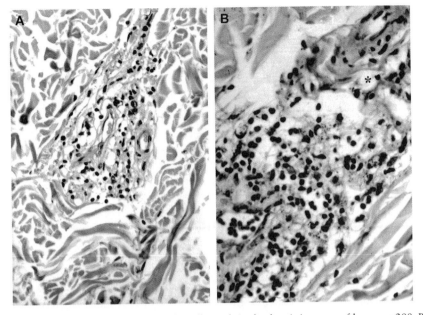

**Fig. 5.8** A An infiltrate of foamy macrophages around small vessels in the dermis in a case of leprosy, ×200. B Wade–Fite stain demonstrates elongated *Mycobacterium leprae* organisms within the foamy cells (*), ×450.

spread dissemination of the bacilli with very little in the way of a T-cell inflammatory response, and that which is generated is more of the Th2 type with relatively high levels of IL-4 and IL-10 (Sieling *et al.* 1993). As a result, the organisms proliferate in cool areas such as the skin, the upper respiratory tract, ears, testes, and eye, and cause local thickening due to the unchecked bacillary multiplication within macrophages, Schwann cells, and fibroblasts. Oedema and fibrosis of the endoneurium also occur, possibly due to fibroblast activation mediated by cytokines released from macrophages. Damage to the perineurium further damages the function of the blood–nerve barrier. In the early stages there is minimal peripheral nerve damage, in contrast to tuberculoid leprosy, but as the disease progresses, an evolving centripetal neuropathy develops with the cooler distal areas being affected first. Superimposed on this is an additional involvement of the main nerve trunks, which in combination with the loss of the more superficial sensory nerves, results in a severe disabling sensorimotor neuropathy.

Thus leprosy represents a classic example in which the immune responsiveness of the individual to an invading bacillus determines the clinical phenotype of the disease.

# Chronic bacterially mediated disease: Sydenham's chorea

Some infections, whilst not directly infecting the CNS, can produce effects through remote immunological mechanisms, similar to those seen in paraneoplastic conditions (see Chapter 4). A good example of such a condition is Sydenham's chorea, where choreic movements, muscle hypotonia, and psychological disturbance occurs some weeks after a streptococcal infection (Swedo *et al.* 1993). It is usually self-limiting, although a number of cases of more persistent neurological deficit have been described, which characteristically have radiological lesions within the basal ganglia (Emery and Vieco 1997).

Previously this condition was associated with numerous types of streptococcal infection, but nowadays it is most frequently associated with acute rheumatic fever (Cardoso *et al.* 1997). The mechanism is thought to be antibody mediated, against epitopes within basal ganglia structures. Anti-neural antibodies have been isolated in cases of Sydenham's chorea and may represent cross-reactivity with elements of group A streptococcal membranes, although the pathogenic nature of these antibodies has not been unequivocally demonstrated (Bronze *et al.* 1993). In addition, host factors have also been shown to be important in those patients developing Sydenham's chorea. For example, the B lymphocyte antigen D8/17 is preferentially expressed in the vast majority of patients with rheumatic fever and thus may represent a susceptibility trait (Murphy *et al.* 1997). Interestingly this trait appears to be shared with children developing Tourette's syndrome and childhood obsessive compulsive disorder. Thus, these conditions may have a common pathogenic mechanism (Murphy *et al.* 1997).

## Chronic virally driven immune disorder: human T-cell lymphotropic virus type 1 (HTLV-1) associated myelopathy

The human T-cell lymphotropic virus type 1 (HTLV-1) was isolated in 1980 and initially associated with a certain form of adult T-cell leukaemia (Poiesz *et al.* 1980). However, it soon became apparent that it was also responsible for certain forms of tropical spastic paraparesis, a condition in which a slowly progressive weakness of both legs (paraparesis) develops in adult life (Gessain *et al.* 1985). Tropical spastic paraparesis has therefore become known as HTLV-1 associated myelopathy (HAM). The disease targets the thoracic spinal cord of young women in the Caribbean, Japan, and Africa, and to a lesser extent South America and Australasia. Transmission is primarily through sexual intercourse, although contaminated blood products along with breast-feeding have also been identified as routes of infection.

The disease is characterised by a selectivity for the thoracic spinal cord, although it can involve peripheral nerve, muscle and even supraspinal sites (Montgomery *et al.* 1964; Mora *et al.* 1988; Izumo *et al.* 1989). Neuropathologically, HTLV-1 induces demyelination and axonal loss with an associated proliferation of capillaries and perivascular infiltration of lymphocytes and macrophages, which in time leads to gliosis (Cruikshank *et al.* 1989). It seems likely that the virus causes CNS damage through its ability to induce an immune reaction rather than by any direct toxicity. This is further supported by the presence of oligoclonal bands to HTLV-1 in the csf of affected patients (Cruikshank *et al.* 1989).

HTLV-1 is a type C retrovirus that has a specific tropism for the CD4+ T lymphocyte. In the associated adult T-cell leukaemia, it is thought that this viral infec-

tion is the first event in a 2–3 step leukemogenesis process (Höllsberg and Hafler 1993). In the case of HAM, it is unclear how the viral infection of CD4+ lymphocytes causes demyelination within the spinal cord, although two main theories are proposed (reviewed in: Höllsberg and Hafler 1993, 1995; see Fig. 5.9):

The *autoimmune model* proposes that HTLV-1 activates, through either infection or T–T cell interactions, specific T cells that have been primed to recognise antigens on glial cells presented with MHC class I or II antigens. These activated autoreactive lymphocytes can then migrate into the CNS where they recognise target antigen presented on these glial cells. This antigen may in fact be a processed part of the HTLV-1 virus, as the infected CD4+ cells are capable of passing the virus to the glial cells (see below), alternatively it may represent processed myelin antigens. The activated lymphocytes on recognising the presented antigen, secrete cytokines that in turn recruit a full inflammatory response and tissue destruction. However, the specificity of the disease in terms of CNS antigens and anatomical site is not explained by this theory.

The *cytotoxic model*, on the other hand, proposes that the disease is caused by a direct CD8+ mediated cytolytic attack against HTLV-1 infected cells. This may solely involve the CD4+ lymphocytes, in which case CNS damage is as a result of a 'bystander' effect. Alternatively, the infected CD4+ lymphocytes may pass on infection to the glial cells, which then become the target for the cytolytic CD8+ lymphocyte. Although some recent evidence has favoured this model by the demonstration of HTLV-1 mRNA within astrocytes in affected patients (Lehky *et al.* 1995), the number of infected cells is low and has not been reported by others (Hara *et al.* 1994).

Whilst both theories remain a possibility, neither can explain the following peculiarities of this disorder.

- The vast majority of HTLV-1 seropositive individuals remain asymptomatic throughout their life. The percentage doing so varies with geographical location, which implies that this may relate to HLA haplotype.

- Co-infection with HIV-1 increases the expression of neurological disease in HTLV-1 infected individuals, possibly by increasing the viral burden as a result of increased HTLV-1 replication (Berger *et al.* 1991, 1997).

- No immunosuppressive therapy has ever been shown to be consistently effective. This may reflect the fact that by the time of clinical presentation, the

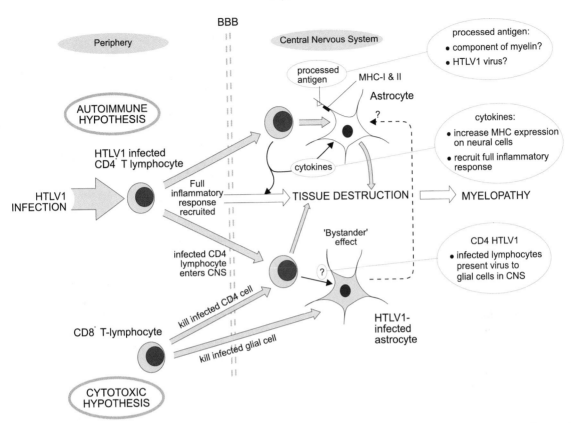

**Fig. 5.9** Possible mechanisms for the pathogenesis of HTLV1-associated myelopathy. The two major hypotheses illustrated in the figure are described in detail in the text.

majority of the damage has already taken place in a fashion analogous to secondary progressive multiple sclerosis, where the suppression of inflammation does not prevent the secondary progression that reflects axonal loss (Edwards *et al.* 1999).

- The selectivity of the disease process for the thoracic spinal cord.

However HAM is a clear example of a virally driven immune mediated CNS disorder.

## Chronic virally driven immune disorder: AIDS dementia complex

HIV is a retrovirus (like HTLV-1) that has a selective tropism for CD4+ T helper lymphocytes, which it infects and kills. As a consequence, HIV predisposes infected individuals to a number of opportunistic infections (e.g. PML), although in addition it can directly cause CNS damage. This direct viral damage produces cognitive

and motor dysfunction, which, whilst producing subtle changes early on in the course of the disease, culminates in the AIDS dementia complex (or HIV-1-associated cognitive/motor complex — reviewed in: Lipton and Gendelman 1995; Lipton 1997).

Within the CNS, HIV-1 selectively infects macrophages or microglial cells through the CD4 cellular receptor with the most characteristic histological feature being multinucleate giant cells (of macrophage/ microglial lineage: CD68 positive; see Fig. 5.10B) containing HIV nucleic acid and protein. These latter cells may act as a reservoir for the virus, although there is some evidence that astrocytes may also carry latent infection (Takahashi *et al.* 1996). However, the pathological substrate of the AIDS dementia complex is a combination of neuronal loss and white matter damage associated with gliosis (Everall *et al.* 1993; Esiri and Kennedy 1997; Scaravilli and Harrison 1997). Neurones themselves do not appear to be infected, so the mechanism of their loss must be indirect, secondary to the neuroglial cell infection (Fig. 5.10).

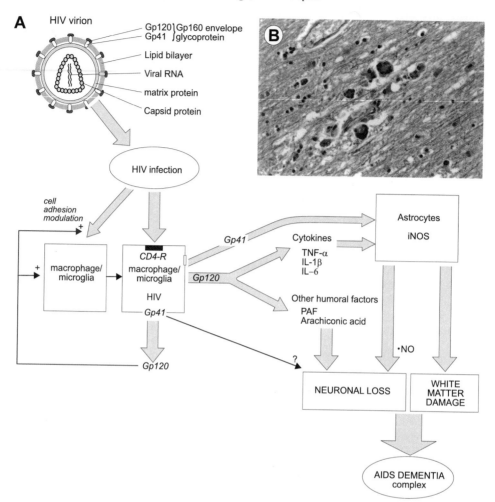

**Fig. 5.10** A Possible steps in the pathogenesis of the AIDS dementia complex. B Multinucleate giant cells in the white matter from a case of HIV encephalopathy. ×300. iNOS, inducible nitric oxide synthase; NO, nitric oxide; PAF, platelet activating factor

The mechanism underlying this indirect neuronal damage may be the release of toxic factors, either locally or through the recruitment of an immune response. For example, large numbers of cytokines are present in the csf of such patients, including arachidonic acid, nitric oxide, IL-1, and TNF (Adamson *et al.* 1996; Johnson *et al.* 1996). However most attention has been focused on the gp 120 component of the HIV envelope glycoprotein, as it has been shown to cause neuronal injury through macrophage and astrocyte activation in both rodent and human cultures. This may be via an excitotoxic mechanism, as gp120 has been shown to stimulate microglia to produce a number of factors, some of which inhibit glutamate uptake by astrocytes. In addi-

tion, gp 120 has been shown to affect the expression of intercellular adhesion molecules, which may be important in facilitating the entry of HIV-1 infected macrophages into the nervous system, which allows the disease process to proceed (reviewed in Lipton 1997).

Although gp 120 has always been thought to be the main mediator of neurotoxicity, the remaining membrane bound gp41 component of the envelope gp160 glycoprotein has recently been shown to have a possible role in the neuropathogenesis of the AIDS dementia complex. The increased expression of this protein in AIDS brains coincides with the expression of inducible nitric oxide synthase (iNOS), which in culture is associated with neuronal death. Also in culture the upregulation of iNOS in astrocytes by cytokines released from HIV-infected macrophages has been shown to be important in the disease process (reviewed in: Lipton and Gendelman 1995; Adamson *et al.* 1996).

Finally, the HIV regulatory protein Tat in experimental situations has been shown to be neurotoxic, although the relevance of this to the neuropathogenesis of the AIDS dementia complex is not known (Weeks *et al.* 1995).

Overall, HIV infection causes a primary neurological disorder characterised by cognitive and motor decline secondary to progressive neuronal loss and gliosis within the CNS. The neuronal death may be through apoptotic or excitotoxic mechanisms, which are activated through the interaction of components of HIV with microglia and astrocytes. Certainly the neuronal loss is secondary to the expression of diffusible factors from both these cell types, rather than direct viral infection of the neurones themselves, although the exact role for each of these factors is currently unresolved.

## Chronic virally driven immune disorder: subacute sclerosing panencephalitis (SSPE)

In the 1960s an association was recognised between a rare syndrome seen in children and teenagers with previous measles (a paramyxovirus) infection (Tellez and Harter 1966). This syndrome was characterised by subacute progressive behavioural abnormalities, mental deterioration, and limb jerking (Risk and Haddad 1979; Prabhakar and Alexander 1995). The link between this syndrome and the measles infection was established by:

- the demonstration of paramyxovirus-like tubular filaments in brain biopsies from these patients (Bouteille *et al.* 1965; Tellez and Harter 1966);

- elevated levels of measles antibodies in the sera (Connolly *et al.* 1967);

- the presence of measles antigen in the brain (Connolly *et al.* 1967);

- the demonstration of measles viral replication in co-cultures of infective brain tissue with permissive HELA cells (Horta-Barbosa *et al.* 1969; Payne *et al.* 1969).

Nevertheless it is unclear why only a small proportion of children with previous measles exposure developed SSPE. The most likely explanation is an interaction between a slightly altered infective agent and a host with an immunological predisposition. Furthermore, why such an infection many years previously should cause this progressive, eventually fatal illness is unknown, although certain trigger factors have been suggested, such as an intercurrent illness, vaccination, and exposure to sick animals.

SSPE and the measles virus are identical except for some minor, but possibly crucial, differences. These changes may occur with years of passage in the body, or the SSPE virus may be a natural mutant of the measles virus. A frequent, but not consistent difference, between the measles and SSPE virus is the absence of M protein (Hall and Choppin 1979; Hall *et al.* 1979) — a protein with a major role in replication. A series of animal experiments have demonstrated the importance of the virus and the immune response it generates, in particular such work has shown that the:

- disappearance of the M protein coincides with the disappearance of the infectivity and the development of cell associated infection (Johnson *et al.* 1981);

- chronic subclinical infection occurs only in weaning animals; and

- the presence of measles antibody is necessary for persistent infection.

It is therefore presumed that small amounts of virus persist within the MHC negative neural cells of the CNS, which not only allows the viral genome to go undetected but also permits the spread of the virus from cell to cell. The failure of cytotoxic T cells to recognise the virally infected neural cells (Dhib-Jhalbut *et al.* 1989) allows for its persistence in the CNS, but the low level of antigenic stimulation it generates will nevertheless allow the viral specific antibodies distinctive of SSPE to develop, although the relevance of these to the pathogenesis of SSPE is unclear (Johnson 1984). Histologically, biopsies or post-mortem brains demonstrate antibody, complement, and immunoglobulins, within CNS blood vessel walls (reviewed in: Prabhakar and Alexander 1995), although SSPE can occur in conditions such as hypogammaglobulinaemia. Overall, the clinical picture, histology, and immunological markers of SSPE suggest that the disease is associated with inflammation and demyelination and that it is primarily an immune-mediated disorder driven by a persistent intracellular viral infection.

## *Direct damage from infective organism*

### Rabies: an infection targeted at neurones

Rabies is a zoonotic disease that is endemic in many parts of the world and still causes a large numbers of fatalities every year; estimated at over 34 000 deaths in 1994. The rabies virus and four genotypes of rabies-related viruses form part of the *Lyssavirus* genus of the RNA viral family, Rhabdoviridae. All reside in different animal hosts and are spread to humans through bites from infected animals, usually dogs. The rabies virus is inoculated into humans through the bite and replicates locally before spreading up the peripheral nerves to invade the CNS (see Fig. 5.11). This period between the time of the bite and the CNS invasion allows for prevention of the disease by wound cleaning and post-exposure immunisation. In the absence of such measures, the risk of developing rabies is between 35 and 70%, and once developed the disease is universally fatal.

The virus can enter the body through a number of routes (e.g. inhalation of infected nasal secretions in caves containing rabid bats), although the commonest mode of infection is through a rabid dog bite (see Fig. 5.11). The local replication of the virus typically takes place in the muscle, although if the bite is deep the virus may be directly injected into peripheral nerves. In this latter case, the incubation period from bite to neurological dysfunction is shorter, especially if the bite is located close to the brain (e.g. shoulder). This local replication provokes some irritation at the wound site, but there are few systemic features of infection as there is typically no viraemia in rabies. The virus then gains access to the peripheral nerve possibly through the acetylcholine receptors at the neuromuscular junction (Tsiang 1993). It is then transported retrogradely up the axon towards the cell body, typically of the motor neurone (see Fig. 5.11). Once inside the CNS, the virus rapidly replicates and spreads trans-synaptically, and it is at this time that the neurological manifestations of dumb and furious rabies become apparent (see Table 5.2). These different clinical phenotypes reflect the preferential localisation of the virus to the spinal cord in dumb rabies, and the brainstem and limbic systems in furious rabies (Warrell and Warrell 1996). In time the virus actually spreads outside the CNS through efferent autonomic nerves, so that it can be found in a number of different organs and tissues (Wunner and Dietzschold 1987).

The virus does not induce an immune response until symptoms develop, which suggests that it either evades or suppresses the immune response. Indeed recent evidence suggests that the known effect of rabies virus on suppressing cytotoxic T-cell responses and Natural Killer (NK) cell activity may be mediated via a CNS action through the hypothalamo-pituitary-adrenal axis (reviewed in: Hemachudha and Phuapradit 1997). This in turn may have some effect on the clinical manifestations of rabies, in that patients with intact cell-mediated immunity are more likely to manifest furious rabies and die more quickly (Hemachuda 1994). However, whilst the form of the clinical expression of rabies may be influenced by the immune response it generates, this is not a necessary part of its pathogenesis. The inflammatory reactions seen in the early stages of this disease are usually scant and when they are present, do not correlate with clinical symptoms. It is therefore likely that the virus directly interacts with neurones and by so-doing causes them to dysfunction and eventually die — a process that can be arrested if a sufficient antibody response can be generated. This is the aim of the post-exposure immunisation procedure mentioned above.

The mechanism by which the virus induces neuronal dysfunction and death is not known, but altered neurotransmitter functions, as well as nitric oxide (NO) induced cell death, have been implicated. For example,

**Table 5.2**  Features of furious and dumb rabies

|  | Furious rabies | Dumb rabies |
|---|---|---|
| % cases | 70–80% | 20–30% |
| Mean incubation period | 7 days | 13 days |
| Main site of pathology | Midbrain/medulla | Spinal cord |
| Clinical features | Hydrophobia with muscle spasms<br>Heightened arousal to stimuli<br>Brainstem signs<br>Autonomic disturbances | Flaccid paralysis in bitten limb that spreads<br>Urinary incontinence<br>hydrophobia is RARE |

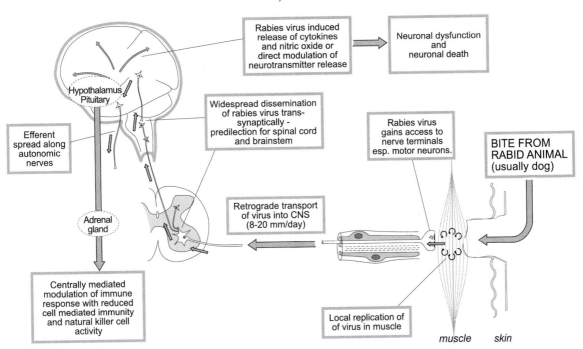

**Fig. 5.11** Steps in the pathogenesis of rabies, showing the route by which the rabies virus can reach the CNS and cause central damage, followed by peripheral spread along autonomic nerves.

rabies has been shown to affect the binding capacity of acetylcholine receptors in rat brain and opiate receptors in cell lines (Tsiang *et al.* 1982; Koshel and Munzel 1984) and this may affect neuronal function in an analogous fashion to LCMV infection in mice (see above). Ultimately though cell death does occur and the rabies virus has been shown to induce neuronal apoptosis in some experimental animals (Jackson and Park 1998).

Rabies is therefore a disorder in which the virus directly invades the neuronal cells of the nervous system and by so doing causes dysfunction and death with the CNS. The mechanism by which this is achieved is not known. The importance of the immune response to rabies is more in terms of protecting the individual from the disease and its clinical expression (dumb versus furious), than its pathogenesis. In other words the immune response is secondary to the pathogenic effects of viral invasion and is thus not the main player in the evolution of this neurological disorder.

## Progressive multifocal leukoencephalopathy (PML): a viral infection of glia

PML is an opportunistic demyelinating infection of the CNS caused by the JC virus and was originally described as a rare complication in chronic lymphocytic leukaemia and Hodgkin's disease (Aström *et al.* 1958). Nowadays it is most commonly associated with HIV disease where it accounts for 4% of all deaths among patients with AIDS (Berger *et al.* 1998), although the introduction of highly active antiretroviral therapy has improved the prognosis of PML in this condition (Clifford *et al.* 1999).

The JC virus is a papovavirus that is found in most people, where it is non-pathogenic; however, in the immunocompromised state the virus is able to infect and directly destroy oligodendrocytes. Indeed the presence of the virus in the blood correlates with the degree of immunosuppression, although not necessarily with the development of PML (Koralnik *et al.* 1999). PML therefore presents as an evolving subcortical disorder with a predisposition for the posterior white matter of the cerebral hemispheres (see Fig. 5.12A), and as such the patients often have cognitive dysfunction, visual impairment, and speech disturbance; although weakness and gait abnormalities are not uncommon (Berger *et al.* 1998). There is no effective treatment and the median survival is around 6 months from the first clinical signs.

The host and viral factors leading to the development of PML are not well known (Greenlee 1998). Over 70%

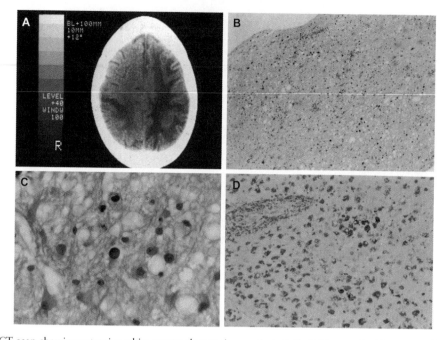

**Fig. 5.12** A CT scan showing extensive white matter changes in a patient PML. B Biopsy of white matter showing vacuolation, gliosis, and enlarged oligodendroglial nuclei in a case of progressive multifocal leucoencephalopathy, ×75. C High-power view of white matter from a case of progressive multifocal leucoencephalopathy. An enlarged oligodendroglial nucleus is present in the centre of the field, surrounded by gliotic cells and occasional foamy macrophages, ×450. D Immunohistochemistry to CD68 demonstrates numerous macrophages in the white matter in a case of PML. A light perivascular lymphocytic infiltrate is present in the *top left-hand corner*, ×250.

of the normal population have antibodies to the JC virus, which can persist in B lymphocytes as well as the kidney. Indeed the virus can even be detected in the brain in the absence of PML, although it is unclear in these situations whether it is in the neuroglial cells or circulating B lymphocytes. Consequently it is not known whether the invasion of the brain by the JC virus in PML is through infected B lymphocytes or reactivation of latent infection in glial cells (Gallia *et al.* 1997). Certainly the virus has a predilection for glial cells, oligodendrocytes more than astrocytes, and enters the cell via a limited number of cell surface receptors (Liu *et al.* 1998). The mechanism by which the virus ultimately kills the infected cell is not known (reviewed in: Weber and Major 1997) but it may be significant that the HIV 1 nuclear protein, Tat, is capable of increasing the transcriptional activation of the JC viral genome in these cells (Chowdhury *et al.* 1993). It is of further interest that, by analogy with SV40, JC virus also produces a T antigen that binds to p53 and the retinoblastoma protein, causing p53 stabilisation and accumulation (Ariza *et al.* 1996) as well as affecting the expression of host cyclins and Ki-67 (Ariza *et al.* 1998).

PML is therefore an example of a disease in which a virus is directly lytic to cells in the nervous system, in this case oligodendrocytes. As a result the condition is characterised by a progressive and fatal demyelination of subcortical white matter.

# Exotoxin-induced neurological damage

## Tetanus, botulism, and diphtheria

A number of infectious organisms produce an effect on the nervous system by releasing an exotoxin that interferes with normal neuronal function. These organisms, and the effects of their exotoxins, are summarised in Table 5.3 (reviewed in: Critchley 1991; McDonald and Kocen 1991; Trucksis 1995).

In these diseases neither the infective organism itself, nor the immune response it generates, are responsible for the neurological disorder. In both botulism and diphtheria, the toxin primarily acts locally; whereas in tetanus the main effect of the toxin is to be found

**Table 5.3** Main features of exotoxin induced neurological disease

| Organism | Action of exotoxin | Clinical features |
|---|---|---|
| *Clostridium tetani* | Inhibits transmitter release at inhibitory central synapses | Rigidity and muscle spasms with autonomic instability |
| *Corynebacterium diphtheriae* | Inhibits protein synthesis or kills cells | Paralysis of bulbar muscle with loss of pupillary accommodation. A delayed demyelinating polyneuropathy can develop. |
| *Clostridium botulinum* | Prevents release of acetylcholine at autonomic ganglia and neuromuscular junction | Paralysis and autonomic failure |

within the CNS; as a result of its retrograde transport (see Fig. 5.13).

## Complex polyphasic infections

### Lyme disease

Lyme disease is an infectious disorder caused by the spirochaete *Borrelia burgdorferi* and transmitted by *Ixodes* ticks. It is a disease that affects many different organ systems and although the first description of the skin rash characteristic of this condition was described in 1909, it was not until 1922 that first account of neuroborreliosis was reported (Garin 1922). The disease, however, takes its name from a small town on the eastern bank of the Connecticut river following the investigation of an outbreak of juvenile rheumatoid arthritis in the late 1970s (Steere *et al.* 1977).

Lyme disease, like other spirochetal infections (e.g. syphilis, relapsing fever), occurs in distinct stages and encompasses the range of pathogenic mechanisms discussed in this chapter. However, the relative roles of these different mechanisms during different phases of the illness are not understood. Lyme disease thus serves as an example of a polyphasic illness due to a single infective organism, with each phase possibly having different pathological mechanisms underlying it.

The recognised phases of Lyme disease are acute localised (stage I) followed by a disseminated stage which is divided into early (stage II) and late (stage III). In the disseminated phase a number of organ systems are preferentially affected including the heart, joints, and nervous system. This latter involvement, termed neuroborreliosis, is seen in about 10–40% of patients with Lyme disease and can occur at any time during the disseminated phase. It involves both the peripheral and central nervous systems, although the clinical presentation tends to be different in the late, as opposed to the early, disseminated stage.

The clinical features characteristic of each of these phases are given below(reviewed in: Agger *et al.* 1991; Pfister *et al.* 1994; Garcia-Monco and Benach 1995; Haas 1998).

### Stage I: acute localised disease

Stage I occurs within days and weeks of inoculation with the organism and is characterised by a distinct rash that is often centred on the tick bite itself (erythema chronicum migrans). The rash often develops in the context of a non-specific systemic illness characterised by malaise, fatigue, headache, fever, myalgia, arthralgia, and lymphadenopathy, all of which implies that Borrelia disseminates early in its clinical course (see below). However, at this stage of the illness there is no clinically overt involvement of the nervous system.

### Stage II: early disseminated disease

From the neurological point of view, stage II includes the classic triad of lymphocytic inflammation of the meninges, cranial nerve palsies, and painful inflammation of both the nerve at its site of exit from the CNS as well as in the periphery (polyradiculoneuropathy). Each of these presentations can occur alone or in combination, and is seen weeks to months after the initial bite. Examination of CSF at this stage reveals a lymphocytic pleocytosis with both CD4+ T lymphocytes as well as plasma cells, the latter accounting for the presence of oligoclonal bands within the CSF to Borrelia. Pathologically, nerve biopsies at this stage reveal a lymphocytic vasculitis with an infiltration of the vasa nervorum by lymphocytes and plasma cells but without evidence of vessel wall necrosis. The patient usually recovers with

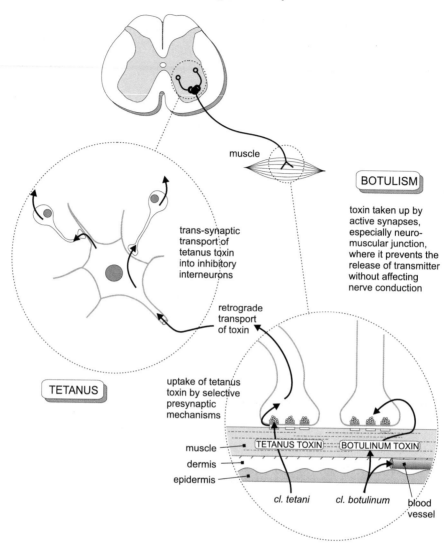

**Fig. 5.13** The mechanism by which the toxins produced by *Clostridium tetani* and *Clostridium botulinum* produce neurological dysfunction.

appropriate antibiotic therapy, although 20% are left with some sequelae.

## Stage III: late disseminated disease

Stage III occurs months to years after the initial tick bite and again affects both the peripheral and central nervous systems. In the PNS, the patient develops a polyradiculoneuropathy, which on biopsy is similar to that seen in stage II of the disease. In the CNS the patient can develop anything from a mild encephalopathy to a chronic encephalomyelitis, the latter presenting as a

spastic paraparesis, ataxia, cranial nerve palsies, bladder dysfunction, and cognitive impairment. These patients pathologically have a mild gliosis with focal demyelination and a perivascular infiltration mainly by CD4+ lymphocytes. Many of these patients are left with sequelae, even when treated with antibiotics, as a result of the advanced state of the pathological process and the fact that the primary process is immune rather than infectively mediated.

The pathogenesis of Lyme disease is complex and understanding has been hampered by the lack of suitable animal models, although recently murine and primate models have been developed (see for example: Coyle *et al.* 1995; England *et al.* 1997). However, the heterogeneity of the strains of *Borrelia burgdorferi*, even within one tick, coupled to the variable (possibly genetically derived) host response, makes it extremely difficult to be precise about the relative roles of the pathogenic mechanism during each phase of the illness. It is generally accepted that a number of different pathogenic mechanisms are seen in chronic infection with *Borrelia*.

On entering the body, *Borrelia* has to invade into the CNS and this it does early on, perhaps within the first few days to weeks. Certainly in experimental models using mice, *Borrelia* has been seen to cross the BBB within 8 days following intraperitoneal injection (Pachner and Itano 1990). This is probably through a specific mechanism of adhesion and penetration across the endothelium of the CNS blood vessels. Once inside the CNS the spirochete is thought, from *in vitro* studies, to be able selectively to adhere to astrocytes, oligodendrocytes, and possibly neurones, whilst in the PNS the process involves Schwann cells (Garcia Monco *et al.* 1989; Thomas *et al.* 1994). Once bound, the spirochaete can then damage the cells through a number of mechanisms:

- Direct damage (e.g. Baig *et al.* 1991; Oksi *et al.* 1996).

- *Borrelia* infection promotes an inflammatory response with the elaboration of pro-inflammatory mediators, such as interleukin-6 (Habicht *et al.* 1991), although the ability of the organism to induce a CD4+ lymphocyte Th1 response has been linked to chronic infection (Coyle 1995). The inflammatory response so evoked then mediates the cellular damage.

- In the late stages of the disease, damage can occur in the absence of persistent organisms by the recruitment of autoreactive responses. Antibodies to myelin components, as well as flagellin in neurones, have been reported (Garcia-Monco *et al.* 1988; Martin *et al.* 1988b), along with T-cell clones directed to similar antigens (Martin *et al.* 1988; Baig *et al.* 1991)

- *Borrelia* invades vessels and by so doing induces a lymphocytic vasculitis both within the CNS and PNS. This therefore means that some of the damage it induces is secondary to ischaemia consequent to vessel narrowing and occlusion (Oksi *et al.* 1996; Garcia-Monco and Benach 1995).

However, the exact role of each of these mechanisms to the different phases of Lyme disease is not known, but does help explain the protean manifestations of this disorder and its failure on occasions to respond to antibiotic therapy.

# Unconventional infections

## Spongiform encephalopathies

Unconventional infectious agents, which may contain no nucleic acid (prions), are thought to be responsible for the transmissible or inherited spongiform encephalopathies, kuru, Creutzfeldt–Jacob disease, Gerstmann–Straussler syndrome, and familial fatal insomnia (reviewed in: Collinge and Palmer 1997). Although the agents have conventionally been thought to provoke no immune response, and to cause non-inflammatory neural degeneration, the involvement of microglia has recently been demonstrated, and an immunological component to the propagation of disease processes has been suggested. These mechanisms are discussed further in Chapter 6.

# Conclusion

In this chapter a number of infections of the nervous system have been presented in terms of the pathogenic mechanisms they employ. The vast majority of these infections use a number of different pathological mechanisms to produce their damage, and their division by mode of action must be seen as a gross simplification. However, the important point that this approach makes is that the mechanisms involved in producing damage in CNS infection, and the consequent outcome, are due to the interaction of the target cell, the infective agent, and the immune response. Whilst the latter is desirable to clear infectious agents and protect the central nervous system from infection, the powerful mechanisms elicited by an immune response may themselves cause considerable damage in the special environment of the central nervous system, with its compliment of irreplaceable cells.

A large number of disorders that can affect the nervous system indirectly have not been discussed (e.g. encephalopathies with atypical pneumonias or cerebral malaria) for reasons of clarity and brevity. However, many of these disorders have ill-understood pathogenic mechanisms, although it is probable that they produce their effects through the pathways detailed in this chapter.

## Further reading

Shaker, R.A., Newman, P.K., and Poser, C.M. (ed.) (1996). *Tropical Neurology*. WB Saunders Co. Ltd, London.

*Neurodegenerative disease*

*With Harry Baker*

## Amyloid and tau pathology in Alzheimer's disease

### Alzheimer's disease, plaques, and tangles

Most dementias are associated with a widespread pattern of atrophy in the forebrain, which is most apparent as a reduction in the weight of the brain measured post-mortem. As the brain undergoes loss of cells, there is a thinning of the neocortex, and an associated flattening of the sulci on the surface of the brain and the ventricles in its depths.

Dementia can come about through a number of different causes. In a series of studies in the 1950s and 1960s, Sir Martin Roth and his colleagues at the University of Newcastle undertook a systematic evaluation of the nature of the post-mortem pathology in a large series of patients dying (both with and without dementia) in a psychogeriatric hospital. These studies highlighted the fact that the cognitive disturbances of senile dementia can be associated with a number of distinct patterns of neuropathology, associated with different causes and disease processes (Tomlinson *et al.* 1970).

The commonest form of cellular neuropathology in silver-stained sections of affected brains is the appearance of abnormal extracellular and intracellular deposits, the senile plaques and neurofibrillary tangles, respectively (see Fig. 6.1). This distinctive pattern of pathology was first described at the turn of the twentieth century by Alois Alzheimer (1907). Although that first report was based on just two patients dying with dementia at a 'presenile' age, the description applies also to the predominant form of dementia in the elderly (i.e. senile dementia), and so his name has come to be associated with this distinctive pattern of cellular pathology (and the disease process that is inferred) at whatever age it develops.

The precise cellular pathology of Alzheimer's disease can only be analysed properly post-mortem. Although Alzheimer's disease can be anticipated in the demented patient on the basis of the particular pattern of psy-chopathology, disease progression, and data from brain scans, final diagnosis in life is still not unequivocally possible. Consequently, such patients are most properly diagnosed as dementia of the Alzheimer type (DAT) whilst still alive.

The second commonest form of pathology in dementia is a spongiform appearance of the brain associated with multiple small and recurrent infarcts of the microvascular systems of the brain, so called multi-infarct dementia (MID).

In the Newcastle studies, the third commonest profile was a mixture of both the abnormal plaque and tangle deposits combined with multi-infarct vacuolation, as well as a number of rarer or distinctive forms that did not fall into any of these categories. Some of the rarer forms of dementia are believed also to be due to other idiopathic disease processes, such as Pick's, which is associated with globular intracellular deposits in cortical neurones, or a form of dementia associated with Parkinson's disease in which the Lewy body deposits that decorate substantia nigra neurones in typical

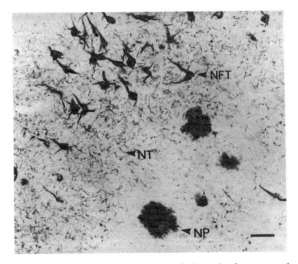

**Fig. 6.1** The cardinal neuropathological features of Alzheimer's disease seen in silver stained sections of neocortex: intracellular neurofibrillary tangles (NFT), extracellular senile neuritic plaques (NP), and neuropil threads (NT).

parkinsonism are also found to affect cortical neurones widely (q.v.). In some cases, dementia may be precipitated by traumatic injury (such as the 'dementia pugilistica' syndrome of boxers). In yet other cases dementia may be caused by explicit toxic processes, such as intoxication with aluminium salts, in particular after prolonged exposure, whether in an industrial context (miners) or by iatrogenic origin (as in dialysis dementia, suffered by long-term kidney patients who were exposed to abnormal levels of aluminium in the course of treatment in early dialysis machines) (for review see: Dunnett and Barth 1991).

It is most plausible to interpret the common patterns of cognitive impairment that characterise dementia, whether occurring at a senile or a presenile age, as due to a generalised and widespread disturbance in the integrity of the brain, in particular in the higher cognitive centres of the neocortex. Conversely, widespread disturbance of cortical function can come about through a variety of cellular and molecular processes, and it is necessary to study the individual diseases if there is to be any understanding of the neuropathological process itself. Analysis of the structure and development of the senile plaques and neurofibrillary tangles in Alzheimer's disease in particular has, over the last decade, begun to reveal the cellular and molecular basis of the commonest neurodegenerative processes in dementia.

## Senile plaques and the Aβ amyloid protein

Senile plaques are made of a relatively soluble and inert protein known as amyloid. Amyloid is a histological description of proteinaceous deposits, seen in a number of conditions within the CNS and elsewhere. It is identified in classical histology by a distinctive pattern of birefringence when viewed under phase contrast optics, and it can be stained by a number of classical dyes such as Congo red or thioflavin-S. Classical neuropathology has described the typical growth of small amyloid deposits into mature plaques with an amyloid core surrounded by a tangle of neurites, best visualised in silver-stained sections, which were believed to comprise degenerating nerve terminals. In a number of forms of dementia, amyloid deposits are also seen in blood vessels and this, rather than the brain neuropil, is the predominant site of pathology in a number of rare inherited dementias such as familial Dutch congoangiopathy.

The amyloid protein was finally isolated and its structure determined in 1984 by Glenner and Wong, who isolated and sequenced a 41 amino acid peptide ('β-

peptide') from blood vessel walls. Soon after, Masters and colleagues isolated and sequenced a similar 42-amino acid peptide (the A4 protein) from Alzheimer brain. The common molecule is now known by the consensus title of the Aβ amyloid protein. It has no clear structural homology with any other polypeptide and its precise normal function remains unclear.

The gene for the amyloid protein was identified by Kang and colleagues in 1987. The gene is located on chromosome 21 and encodes a 695 amino acid precursor protein (APP, see Fig. 6.2). APP is of neuronal origin and its structure suggests that it is a membrane-bound molecule with a large extracellular and small intracellular domains. The Aβ amyloid peptide is a short fragment of this much longer precursor protein from which it is derived by an enzymatic cleavage. Since one end of the Aβ fragment is embedded within the cell membrane, the cleavage site is not accessible to enzymes in intact cells. Rather, in the intact cell, the extracellular portion of APP is cleaved within the middle of the Aβ sequence by normal protease digestion. However, it has been hypothesised that under pathological conditions, breakdown of the cell membrane exposes the C terminal end of the Aβ amyloid protein to enzymatic cleavage, resulting in deposition of Aβ fibrils that aggregate at the core of plaques, precipitate degeneration in adjacent neurites, which in turn expose more APP molecules to abnormal cleavage, leading to a cascade of neuritic degeneration and further amyloid deposition in a positive feed-back loop (Beyreuther 1993).

Several lines of evidence support a critical role for the Aβ amyloid protein as a primary cause of degeneration. First, individuals with three copies (trisomy) of chromosome 21 develop Down syndrome. With improving health care services, Down syndrome cases are now living into mature adulthood, and this has revealed dementia as an inevitable consequence of the chromosomal abnormality. Although dementia develops in Down syndrome at 40–50 years of age (i.e. several decades earlier than typical senile dementia), the neuropathological pattern of plaques and tangles is indistinguishable from classic Alzheimer's disease. This provides an opportunity to study the early development of the Alzheimer-like pathology because, whereas we cannot determine which individuals in a general population will develop Alzheimer's disease, we know that every adult with Down syndrome will develop the same pathology within a circumscribed age range. David Mann has systematically analysed the time course for appearance of different signs and markers of disease and has identified amyloid deposition as the first clear sign

## Amyloid precursor protein (APP₆₉₅)

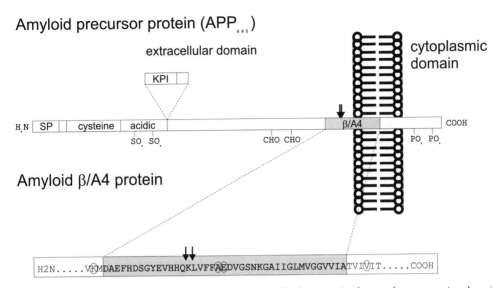

**Fig. 6.2** Structure of the amyloid precursor protein and the amyloid Aβ protein in the membrane-spanning domain. Sites of reported amino acid mutation are *ringed*. The normal cleavage site is indicated by *double arrows*, whereas the 42 amino acid Aβ protein is the deposited after abnormal cleavage. (Kang *et al.* 1987.)

of impending pathology, occurring some 20–30 years earlier than overt cellular degeneration (Mann *et al.* 1992). The association with Down syndrome provided the critical clue for Kang and colleagues to focus their search on chromosome 21 in first identifying the APP gene.

A second strand of evidence implicating the Aβ protein as a primary component of the disease process comes from studies of familial Alzheimer's disease. Although it accounts for no more than 5% of cases, there are a number of rare pedigrees in which Alzheimer's disease runs as an autosomal dominant trait with early onset (typically in the 30s or 40s) within families. Linkage studies first identified a number of markers closely associated with a disease locus on the long arm of chromosome 21, which turns out to be the obligate region for Down syndrome and is where the APP gene is located. More recently, specific APP mutations have been identified in several pedigrees of familial Alzheimer's disease, a theme that we shall develop in the next section of this chapter.

A third line of evidence relates to the direct toxicity of the Aβ protein on nerve cells *in vivo* and *in vitro*. In 1990, Yankner *et al.* first reported that the Aβ protein can be both neurotrophic for, and neurotoxic to, neurones grown in culture. Thus, when administered in low concentrations to undifferentiated embryonic hippocampal neurones, there was significant enhancement

in neuronal cell survival over the first 1–3 days in comparison to control cultures. By contrast, when administered at a higher concentration, and to mature neurones, Aβ treatment induces a marked retraction of both dendrites and axons followed by cell death. In the following year, Kowall and colleagues reported that the Aβ protein is also toxic when applied to mature neurones *in vivo*. They found that direct injections of the protein into the neocortex of rats produced profound neurodegenerative changes in cortical neurones, and subsequent studies confirmed generalised neurotoxicity following injections into the neocortex also in monkeys.

However, the specificity of these effects has been a matter of dispute. For example, control injections in the cortex also invariably produce some necrotic damage at the site of injection. Podlisny *et al.* (1992) replicated the general neuronal damage following amyloid injection into the cortex of monkeys, but could find no evidence for induction of the specific plaque or tangle pathology of the human disease.

Perhaps the clearest evidence that amyloid deposition can provide the critical event in development of an Alzheimer-like pathology comes from experiments using transgenic mice. The first attempts to obtain overexpression of the amyloid precursor protein in transgenic mice were rather disappointing in producing limited and equivocal patterns of pathology and behavioural deficits that lacked specificity. However, Dora Games

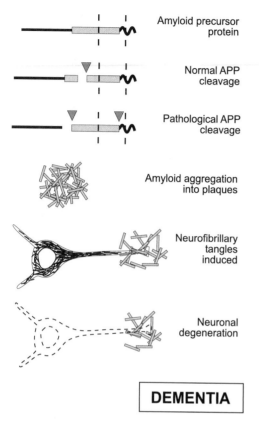

Amyloid precursor protein

Normal APP cleavage

Pathological APP cleavage

Amyloid aggregation into plaques

Neurofibrillary tangles induced

Neuronal degeneration

**DEMENTIA**

**Fig. 6.3** Hypothesised mechanisms of neurodegeneration attributable to abnormal processing of the amyloid precursor protein (APP; after Beyreuther 1993).

and colleagues have been successful in producing much clearer results by insertion into transgenic mice of the human APP gene containing the valine–phenylalanine mutation at residue 717, which is associated with one of the variants of familial Alzheimer's from Sweden. This mutant human gene was placed under the control of a neurone specific promoter (the 'Athena' mouse; Games *et al.* 1995). No pathology was obvious up to 6 months of age, but thereafter the mice developed a pattern of extracellular pathology involving β/A4 deposits in the hippocampus, cerebellum, and neocortex, and formation of numerous plaque-like structures that stained for thioflavin-S, and had an amyloid core surrounded by a tangle of dystrophic neurites. The histochemical features of the plaques was thus very similar to the critical human pathology. By contrast the brains were relatively devoid of abnormal tau deposits or neurofibrillary pathology. At the time of writing, the behavioural characterisation of this transgenic strain has not been reported.

Consequently, a variety of lines of evidence points to a critical involvement of the β-APP in the pathogenesis of Alzheimer's disease. However, up to this point, the role of intracellular neurofibrillary tangles and their constituent microtubule-associated tau protein has not been emphasised. There are cogent reasons to believe that this second aspect of the critical Alzheimer's disease neuropathology may also contribute to the pathogenic disease process and the development of dementia.

## Neurofibrillary tangles and the tau protein

Neurofibrillary tangles are the second major neuropathological feature of affected areas of the brain in Alzheimer's disease. In classical silver stains, neurofibrillary tangles are distinguishable as dense tangles of neurofilaments located intracellularly, particularly in the large pyramidal neurones of the neocortex and the hippocampus. As neurones degenerate in the disease, insoluble 'ghost' tangles of neurofibrils remain in the neuropil, as tombstones of the lost cells. Like the senile plaques, neurofibrillary tangles are not unique to Alzheimer's disease but are found in a number of other progressive neurodegenerative conditions.

Before the advent of modern molecular techniques, analysis of the role of different components of the neuropathology to disease pathogenesis centred on evaluating the relationship between post-mortem pathology and dementia in life. First, Sir Martin Roth and colleagues in Newcastle, and subsequently Wilcock and Esiri in Oxford, undertook systematic correlations between mental test scores in life and different components of the subsequent pathology. Many of these studies indicated that the degree of functional deficit correlated closer with the density of neurofibrillary tangles than it did with plaque formation (Wilcock *et al.* 1982). Moreover, many normal elderly people dying without signs of dementia exhibited a substantial accumulation of plaques, whereas neurofibrillary tangles were only exhibited above very low levels in cases of dementia. These observations have led a number of authors to consider that neurofibrillary tangle formation is critical for the expression of Alzheimer's dementia, whether or not it represents the cardinal neuropathological event in the disease process.

Perhaps a more fruitful approach is to consider the development of the disease as involving interactions between intracellular and extracellular events. Braak and Braak (1991) have provided the most systematic analyses of the development of the disease in terms of both amyloid deposits and silver-tained sections of neurofibrillary pathology (see Fig. 6.4). They highlight the variability of the distribution of senile plaque formation from individual to individual and conclude that amyloid deposition itself cannot provide a systematic basis for classification of disease progression. By contrast, the neuropil threads associated with nerve terminals and neurofibrillary tangles in the cell bodies have a rather selective involvement of particular cell types and architectonic areas, that allows a more consistent, predictable, and precise mapping of the course of the disease. The earliest appearance of neurofibrillary pathology appears to develop in the entorhinal cortex (Fig. 6.4). From there, neurodegeneration subsequently spreads into the hippocampus and thence into

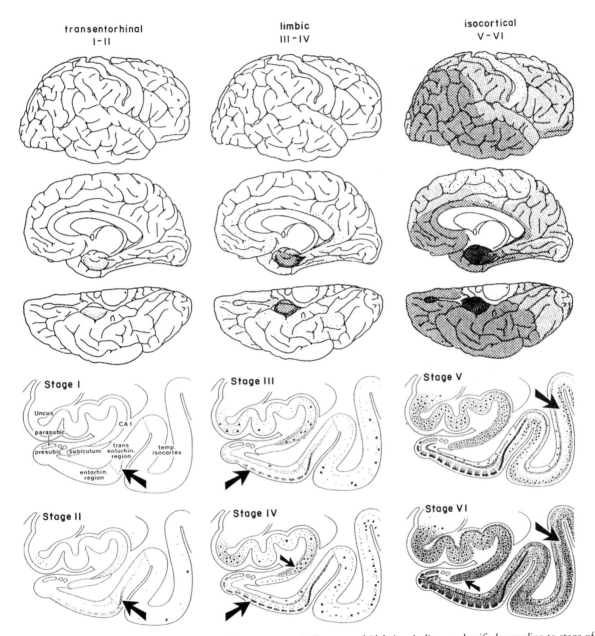

**Fig. 6.4** Distribution of neurofibrillary pathology in neo- and allocortex of Alzheimer's disease, classified according to stage of the disease. (From Braak and Braak 1991.)

association areas of neocortex. Only in advanced disease do sensory and motor areas of neocortex become implicated.

The specific pattern of the spread of the disease maps closely to the anatomical connections of the neo- and allocortex. This was highlighted by Pearson and colleagues (1985) in a study of the detailed location and clustering of amyloid and tangle pathology in different areas of neocortex. Neurofibrillary tangles were located predominantly in clusters in the layer 5 pyramidal neurones, and to a lesser extent in the layer 3 neurones. However, the layer 5 and layer 3 clusters are in register. Senile plaques were more widely distributed in all cortical layers and did not show the same tendency for clustering. From a combination of the laminar distribution and the pathological involvement of different areas of neocortex, they proposed that the pathology occurs in areas that are interconnected anatomically and that the disease process spreads along connecting fibres. Thus from an initial focus in the olfactory, limbic, and entorhinal parts of the temporal lobe, the disease spreads as a cascade of retrograde degeneration via afferent pathways to that area, both from the hippocampus and from corticocortical areas, first to affect limbic, then association, and only finally the primary sensory and motor areas of the neocortex. However, if this hypothesis is correct it is necessary to understand the molecular basis of the disease before it is possible to identify the mechanisms of trans-synaptic spread.

Identification of the structural constituents of the neurofibrillary tangle has been technically complex. The neurofibrils are relatively insoluble, which means that they persist even after the cell has died, but which makes their isolation for chemical analysis extremely difficult. Crowther and Wischik (1985) identified at the ultrastructural level that the neurofibrils that constitute intracellular tangles have a distinctive paired helical twist. These paired helical filaments vary in width from 8 to 20 nm with a regular period of about 80 nm. The filaments can be stained with anti-tau antibodies, in particular, when the fuzzy coat of the paired helical filaments is removed by protease treatments to reveal the pronase-resistant core.

Tau is a phosphoprotein that has long been known to have a potent influence on the ability of microtubules to polymerise. When microtubules bind tau they become more stable. Thus, tau is a natural candidate for involvement in the abnormal accumulation of neurofibrillary tangles. The tau molecule has been sequenced and identified as the core protein in the formation of paired helical filaments (Goedert *et al.* 1988). Six different

isoforms are produced from a single gene through alternative splicing of the mRNA (Fig. 6.5). Each isoform of tau carries three or four 31–32 amino acid tandem repeats close to the carboxyl terminus of the protein, which constitute microtubule-binding domains. The second distinguishing feature of the different isoforms is the presence of 0–2 29 amino acid inserts at the amino terminal of the peptide. In the immature brain, only the short form with three tandem repeats is expressed, but expression is developmentally regulated such that all six forms are seen in adults. It has now been shown that paired helical filaments, like those purified from Alzheimer's disease tangles, can be artificially produced from bacterially expressed tau, which provides strong evidence that tau is the primary, if not the only, essential component necessary to form paired helical filaments. Whether tau is broken down normally or aggregates to form paired helical filament is believed to be dependent upon the level of phosphorylation of the molecule. In the normal adult brain, tau is only phosphorylated at a few of the 17 available sites, whereas in the diseased brain tau is hyperphosphorylated for reasons that are not yet identified. Nevertheless, hyperphosphorylation of tau impedes its ability to bind to microtubules and precedes its aggregation into paired helical filaments.

The abnormal assembly of tau may be regulated by sulphated glycosaminoglycans (GAGs), such as heparin or heparan sulphate. Goedert *et al.* (1996) found that in the presence of GAGs the capacity of non-phosphorylated tau to bind to microtubules was inhibited, and the tau molecules would self-aggregate into paired

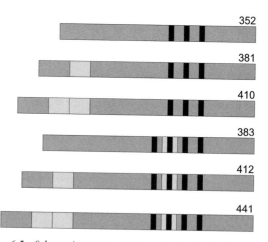

**Fig. 6.5** Schematic representation of the six isoforms of human brain tau. Numbers indicate the amino acid length of each isoform. (Redrawn from Goedert 1993.)

helical filaments. Moreover, heparan sulphate and hyperphosphorylated tau coexist in neurones in the Alzheimer's disease brain, suggesting that this may be a key factor in the formation of neurofibrillary pathology in Alzheimer's disease.

## The Baptists versus the Tauists

The relative roles of β-APP and tau proteins as either initial trigger or the primary components in the neuropathological cascade of Alzheimer's disease remain unresolved. There are strong advocates for the importance of each process, characterised by Beyreuther and Masters, as the Baptist versus the Tauist camps.

Amyloid deposits are not unique in Alzheimer's disease (AD); they are found in a wide variety of diseases and neurodegenerative conditions, and are also observed in normal ageing and in elderly animals of some large species (such as bears, dogs, and monkeys). Nevertheless, amyloid deposits are particularly marked in the human disease, and do appear to correlate to some extent with the extent of dementia. On the one hand this could be taken as suggesting that AD is an extreme stage of the normal ageing process — we will all die of dementia if we live long enough. This seems unlikely in the light of cases of familial AD inherited as a result of identified mutations in the APP gene. On the other hand it is argued that amyloid pathology cannot be the sole determinant of AD, and tau almost certainly plays a major role in the cascade of neuropathological development.

## Genetics of Alzheimer's disease (AD) and other dementias

### Familial AD

Following the identification of linkage of familial AD to chromosome 21 and the subsequent sequencing of the amyloid precursor protein, it was natural to seek to identify variations or mutations in this gene in the familial cases. This strategy has been successful in identifying a number of distinct mutations in APP that result in familial inheritance of the disease. The first of these was found by Alison Goate and her colleagues in 1991. Detailed mapping of the APP gene in affected members of one pedigree identified a mutation of valine to isoleucine at residue 717, just adjacent to the intramembrane Aβ cleavage site. Subsequent studies have identified several other mutations in other cases of familial

AD, not always at the same precise site, but always close to the transmembrane Aβ protein segment of APP when associated with chromosome 21. This suggests that in the early onset families, the disease develops at an early stage due to a rapid formation of Aβ protein by abnormal cleavage following a mutation-induced block of the normal pathway for processing of amyloid and its precursor protein.

It remains unclear, however, what might trigger a similar process in normal sporadic cases of AD. Critically, several other mutation sites have now been identified in other pedigrees of familial AD.

## Apo E

The chromosome 21 mutations are typically associated with early onset disease. For example, affected cases in the linkage study of an extensive Belgian pedigree by van Broeckhoven *et al.* (1987) had a mean age of onset of 35 years. By contrast, there are other pedigrees in which the age of onset is much later, typically in the 60s and 70s. Genetic linkage studies in these late onset families suggested a second susceptibility locus on chromosome 19. Location of the gene for the apolipoprotein E (ApoE) close to this linkage site, along with the findings that ApoE binds to Aβ amyloid protein and occurs in senile plaques, together suggested a potential role for this peptide in the disease process.

There are three common isoforms of the ApoE gene in humans, designated ε2, ε3, and ε4. Following initial observations by Saunders *et al.* (1993) and Corder *et al.* (1993) there have now been many studies indicating that the relative frequency of these genes differ in Alzheimer's disease (Table 6.1). Patients exhibit a raised incidence of the ε4 allele in comparison to unaffected individuals (from 15% to 40%) suggesting that carrying this allele increases susceptibility to the disease, and far lower than normal incidence of the ε2 allele (from 10% to 2%), which may therefore indicate a protective influence (Roses 1996). Moreover, the presence of ε4/ε4 homozygosity not only further raises the risk but lowers the age of onset, whereas the age of onset is further raised in the rare cases of disease in an individual carrying the ε2 allele.

The mechanism by which different isoforms of the ApoE protein influence the disease process is not entirely clear (for review see: St George-Hislop *et al.* 1998). *In vitro*, ApoE-ε4 binds to the Aβ amyloid protein more avidly than does ApoE-ε3, suggesting a role in the production, metabolism, or clearance of Aβ in plaque formation. Conversely, ApoE-ε4 binds less

**Table 6.1** Incidence of ApoE alleles in normal and Alzheimer's disease (AD)

| ApoE allele: | ε2 | ε3 | ε4 |
|---|---|---|---|
| Normal Caucasian | 10% | 75% | 15% |
| AD | 2% | 58% | 40% |

well to tau than do the ε2 and ε3 isoforms. This may suggest that ApoE has a role in sequestering free tau protein, thereby reducing the ability of tau molecules to bind with each other, become hyperphosphorylated, and accumulate as PHF tangles.

## Presenilins

A third set of polymorphic markers associated with AD have been identified on chromosome 14, in this case linked more commonly with earlier onset disease, and pinpointed as involving the presenilin 1 gene, encoding a 50 kDa peptide that is strongly conserved across species, and is expressed in intracellular membranes associated with the endoplasmic reticulum and perinuclear envelope. It has variously been considered to play a role in protein and membrane trafficking, and the regulation of signal transduction and apoptosis (St George-Hislop *et al.* 1998).

The role of presenilin 1 in AD is suggested by the identification of a large number of different mutations in over 35 different family pedigrees at the last count (St George-Hislop *et al.*1998) — which is considerably higher than the incidence of familial disease attributable to chromosome 21-based mutations in the amyloid precursor protein. However, these molecules may interact at the protein level. It appears that at least one effect of presenilin mutation is to alter the processing and enzymatic cleavage of amyloid precursor protein to favour production of the most toxic 42 and 43-amino acid long forms of the β/A4 protein. Thus, for example, transgenic mice that overexpress mutant forms of presenilin 1 exhibit higher brain concentrations of long forms of the β/A4 protein but little change in the short form (Duff *et al.* 1996), and more recently it has been seen that in a line of APP transgenic mice that exhibit Alzheimer-like pathology, breeding of the double presenilin-APP mutation reduces the age of onset and exacerbates the severity of neuropathology (Holcomb *et al.* 1998).

## Chromosome 17 and tauopathies

The fourth set of genes involved in the development of dementia are suggested by a number of familial demen-

tias linked to chromosome 17 (Spillantini *et al.* 1998). These cases were first identified in several instances of late-onset dementia running strongly in a number of families in which AD was excluded by the absence of a major incidence of amyloid plaques. The pattern of dementia is essentially frontal in type with additional parkinsonian features, but there was also an absence of Pick's and Lewy bodies, which excluded neuropathologically other established diseases with similar symptoms such as Pick's and Parkinson's. Conversely, incidence of dementia is closely linked to a marker on chromosome 17q21–22 in these families, and further neuropathological analysis indicated atrophy in the frontal and temporal neocortex and basal ganglia, and a high incidence of tau-rich neurofibrillary tangles in both neurones and glia in affected areas of the brain.

The common clinical and neuropathological features of the disease suggest a distinct disease that has been designated frontotemporal dementia with parkinsonism linked to chromosome 17 (FTDP-17; Foster *et al.* 1997), characterised neuropathologically by abnormal accumulation of tau ('tauopathy') as filamentous deposits forming intracytoplasmic tangles, which are ultrastructurally similar to those seen in AD, but which differ both in their topographic distribution and in their occurrence in glia as well as neurones. Clinical symptoms reflect the distinctive distribution of cellular pathology, involving both cognitive aspects, such as disinhibition, apathy, and personal neglect, characteristic of frontal impairment, and motor disturbances including bradykinesia, rigidity, and postural instability characteristic of basal ganglia disease. However, apart from linkage to particular chromosomal markers, the genetic basis for this disease, in particular identification of the specific genes implicated, is yet to be determined.

# Degeneration due to environmental toxins: Parkinson's disease

## The role of nigrostriatal dopamine

The loss of pigmentation in the substantia nigra and loss of the large neurones of the pars compacta was first recognised as a primary neuropathological feature of Parkinson's disease by Tretiakoff in 1919, and anticholinergic drugs were introduced as clinically effective on empirical grounds in the 1950s. However, the fundamental role of neurodegeneration of dopamine neurones in this disorder was not recognised until the early 1960s.

The critical observations that underlay our contemporary understanding of the functional pathology of Parkinson's disease came from Carlsson's (1959, 1987) studies into the pharmacology of central catecholamine systems. Carlsson found that injections of either the catecholamine depleting drug, reserpine, or the catecholamine synthesis inhibitor, α-methyl tyrosine, induced an immobility syndrome in rats and rabbits that was remarkably similar to the akinesia of human Parkinson's disease. Although the role of noradrenaline as a neurotransmitter was known at that time, a similar role for dopamine had not been established, Nevertheless, Carlsson hypothesised that loss of dopamine was critical; first, because the functional deficits correlated better with biochemical assays of dopamine depletion than of noradrenaline depletion, and second, because dopamine was concentrated in the basal ganglia, which had long been known to be implicated in motor function, whereas noradrenaline was localised in more cortical forebrain areas more associated with higher associative functions.

The second critical set of observations by Carlsson was that both reserpine and α-methyl tyrosine induced akinesia in animals could be reversed by treatment with the dopamine precursor L-DOPA (Fig. 6.6). As a

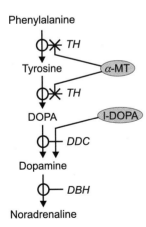

**Fig. 6.6** Synthetic pathway of dopamine. The amino acids phenylalanine and tyrosine are taken up from the blood, and converted in dopamine neurones via L-DOPA to dopamine under the control of the enzymes tyrosine hydroxylase (TH) and dopa-decarboxylase (DDC). Noradrenaline neurones contain the additional enzyme dopamine-β-hydroxylase that regulates conversion of dopamine to noradrenaline. The enzyme TH is blocked by the drug α-methyl tyrosine (α-MT), but can be bypassed by L-DOPA.

replacement therapy, L-DOPA bypasses the critical stage of precursor synthesis regulated by tyrosine hydroxylase that is blocked by α-methyl tyrosine, and has the advantage over dopamine that it will cross the blood–brain barrier and so can be administered peripherally.

Together, these observations led Carlsson (1959) to two speculative hypotheses.

1. From the similarities of the pharmacologically-induced syndrome in animals, he proposed that human Parkinson's disease is due to a deficiency in forebrain dopamine in the basal ganglia.

2. He proposed that, if Parkinson's disease is indeed due to dopamine depletion, then it may be alleviated by treatment with the precursor drug, L-DOPA.

These two hypotheses were first tested in patients by Oleh Hornykiewicz.

First, in 1960, Ehringer and Hornykiewicz measured dopamine and noradrenaline in the brains of Parkinson's disease patients post-mortem, and found a marked decline in dopamine in the caudate nucleus, putamen, and substantia nigra. From this they inferred that Parkinson's disease involved degeneration of a dopaminergic projection from the striatum to the substantia nigra. Almost right. These studies preceded, but were closely followed by, the introduction of the catecholamine fluorescence histochemical technique that allowed Dahlström and Fuxe (1964) to provide the first detailed anatomical mapping of forebrain dopamine systems, which demonstrated that the critical dopamine pathway that degenerated in Parkinson's disease projected from the substantia nigra to the striatum rather than *vice versa*.

Second, in the following year, Birkmayer and Hornykiewicz (1961) published the first trial of L-DOPA as a dopamine substitution therapy in Parkinson's disease patients. Even though effective against the patients' akinesia and rigidity, L-DOPA was not at first considered very useful, because it induced marked peripheral, especially cardiovascular, side-effects. However, the peripheral effects can be blocked by combining L-DOPA with a dopa-decarboxylase inhibitor that does not cross the blood–brain barrier (such as carbi-DOPA). This combination drug treatment then permits conversion of L-DOPA to active dopamine only in the CNS, where the inhibitor does not penetrate. The fist large-scale trials of L-DOPA with carbi-DOPA were conducted with remarkable effect in 1967 by Cotzias *et al.*, and since then L-DOPA therapy has been the cornerstone in the clinical management of Parkinson's disease.

## Incidence of Parkinson's disease

The causes of Parkinson's disease are not known but there are a variety of indications that, in contrast to clearly genetic causes of degeneration, such as seen in Huntington's or familial AD, it may be due to some form of externally-derived toxic process. It has been known for many years that a number of specific environmental toxins can cause Parkinson's disease-like symptoms. For example, a distinctive neurological disease with marked parkinsonian movement disorder has been described among workers in manganese mines and after carbon disulphide poisoning. However, in each of these two disorders, the primary degeneration is in striatal neurones and the striatal output pathways. Consequently in, seeking to understand the basis of selective nigral cell death in idiopathic Parkinson's disease, we must be careful to distinguish it from degeneration in other components of the basal ganglia circuitry that can have similar clinical consequences. Apart from the characteristic clinical picture, there are two main guides to identifying true parkinsonian syndromes. First, fluorodopa PET scans will identify a selective loss of dopaminergic neurones in the substantia nigra and their terminals in the striatum, whereas other structures of the basal ganglia are unaffected in PET and MRI. Second, true Parkinson's disease is responsive to L-DOPA therapy to replace lost dopamine, at least at early and middle stages of the disease, before the drug effects lead to switching between on and off stages, and the dyskinetic side-effects of L-DOPA become intolerable. In the last analysis, however, idiopathic Parkinson's disease can only be finally confirmed based on post-mortem evidence of the selective and specific Lewy body pathology and loss of dopaminergic neurones in the substantia nigra.

Even in the normal brain, there is a steady loss of dopaminergic neurones with age, the rate of loss being around 5% per decade. This means that even a normal person, if they live long enough, will lose around 50% of their dopaminergic neurones, which is the threshold for the onset of parkinsonian symptoms. However, in patients with idiopathic Parkinson's disease, the rate of cell loss is greatly accelerated to around 45% per decade. This implies that there must be a long-term ongoing neurotoxic process. However, it is also possible to acquire parkinsonism by the sudden loss of large numbers of dopaminergic neurones, as may occur following head injury, viral infection, or due to the action of toxic chemicals such as MPTP (see later) (reviewed in: Dunnett and Björklund 1999).

If we look at the world-wide incidence, Parkinson's disease occurs in all developed countries at approximately similar levels, although pockets of higher incidence are found, e.g. in Swedish populations in Finland. From a historical perspective, it has often been remarked that descriptions of the characteristic movement disorder of Parkinson's disease only appear in the medical literature from around the time of the industrial revolution, although a Parkinson-like syndrome may have been described earlier by Leonardo da Vinci. Moreover, the incidence world-wide is higher in industrialised than in non-industrialised societies. These observations give credence to the suggestion that chemical pollutants or some other toxic feature of industrial processes may be a contributory factor in the disease.

## Epidemiology of Parkinson's disease

To address these issues, Barbeau and colleagues (1987) undertook a series of detailed epidemiological studies of the incidence of Parkinson's disease in the Province of Québec in Canada. This turns out to be a unique population for this purpose: there is a full range of industrial and agriculture activities; the peoples are located in everything from large cities to remote farmsteads, and yet, as a result of the unique language situation (a French speaking population embedded in an otherwise predominantly English and Spanish speaking continent), there are rather low levels of migration into and out of the province.

The incidence of the disease was not completely homogeneous. First, the background levels of incidence varied depending on the agricultural communities, with a higher incidence in the areas associated with market gardening than with the growth of corn and other large-scale grain crops. Importantly, within towns and villages, the incidence was higher in those areas in which the water supplies were collected from the drainage from market gardening land than from the corn belt areas (see Fig. 6.7). There tends to be a much higher use of fertilisers and pesticides in the former type of agriculture. Second, pockets of still higher incidence of disease were identified in communities associated with lumber and paper mills, which are also associated with a variety of industrial chemicals.

Since then, many other epidemiological studies have yielded similar results (Koller *et al.* 1990; Butterfield *et al.* 1993; Chaturvedi *et al.* 1995). Together these suggest

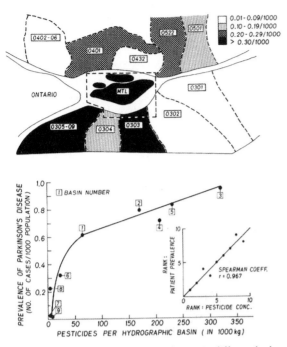

**Fig. 6.7** Prevalence of Parkinson's disease in different hydrographic sub-basins of southern Québec province. There is a clear correlation between the observed prevalence and the use of pesticides during the year 1992. (From Barbeau *et al.* 1987.)

that the increased incidence of idiopathic Parkinson's disease is due to neurotoxicity from agrochemicals or other industrial chemicals and waste products. Although many candidates have been suggested, none have yet been specifically implicated.

## MPTP in humans

In 1979 Davis *et al.* first reported the apparently spontaneous occurrence in New York of a parkinsonian-like disorder of sudden onset in a 20-year old drug abuser, but they were unable to trace the source of the disorder. Several years later, Bill Langston encountered several more cases, also of rapid onset in young adult drug addicts (Langston *et al.* 1983), and he successfully traced the cause of this new neurological disease to a contaminant of a designer drug that was circulating in San Francisco at the time. This remarkable chance discovery, although devastating for the individual addicts, has revolutionised the study and treatment of Parkinson's disease.

The critical substance is 1-methyl-4-phenyl-1,2,3,6-tetrahydropyridine, usually abbreviated to MPTP. Although not itself a drug of abuse, it is a by-product

generated in the synthesis of the heroin substitute, meperidine. When self-administered, only two or three doses were necessary for the drug users to develop full parkinsonian symptoms, and become 'frozen addicts'. It is not just a similarity of symptoms. The patients appear to have fully developed Parkinson's disease, albeit at an abnormally young age. They were initially responsive to L-DOPA, and PET scans revealed the typical Parkinson's pattern involving a marked loss of fluorodopa signal in the basal ganglia. However, in comparison to the very slow progression of the disorder in the idiopathic disease, many of the affected addicts only benefited from the L-DOPA therapy for a short time and rapidly progressed to an intolerance of drug treatment and marked side-effects, including the profound dyskinesias and on-off cycles typical of advanced disease (Langston and Ballard 1983). This does not necessarily indicate a fundamental difference between idiopathic and MPTP-induced parkinsonism in the neuropathological changes but rather reflects the introduction of drug treatment at a very late stage to a patient in whom the degeneration is already advanced: the description in the drug patients is similar to the brief respite followed by relapse due to intolerance of the drugs in the post-encephalitic parkinsonian patients described by Oliver Sacks in his book (and the film) *Awakenings* (1973).

## MPTP in monkeys

The critical proof that MPTP is the culprit comes from the experimental induction of an identical syndrome when the purified drug is administered to experimental animals. In 1983, Burns and colleagues first reported that MPTP injected i.p. into rhesus monkeys produced an identical syndrome of profound parkinsonian L-DOPA responsive akinesia. Moreover, the motor symptoms correlated well with pathological changes in the brain, in particular with a marked degeneration of the dopaminergic neurones of the substantia nigra and loss of dopamine in the striatum, an effect soon confirmed in the squirrel monkey by Langston and colleagues (1984).

The MPTP-treated monkey provides the closest animal model to human Parkinson's disease and so is widely used to assess new strategies for neuroprotection (e.g. GDNF) or repair (e.g. nigral transplants). The model has the clear advantage that the toxin can be given peripherally and still target the nigrostriatal dopamine system. The major experimental problem with this approach, however, is that the animals are severely debilitated and require intensive long-term nursing care for their survival. Bankiewicz and colleagues (1986) therefore introduced a unilateral lesion model by injection of the toxin into the ascending carotid artery. This retained the advantages of peripheral administration (and so avoiding the need for more complex neurosurgery) but leaves the nigrostriatal system intact on one side to maintain all vital functions to keep the animals in good health. The unilateral lesioned animals then exhibit parkinsonian motor impairment and neglect on the contralateral side of the body, as measured by simple tests of turning, postural bias, and use of the contralateral limbs or hands for retrieving food, play objects, or grooming.

## MPTP in rats and mice

Much of the basic neurochemistry to identify mechanisms of neurotoxicity and protection from MPTP has been developed not in the primate but in rodent models. It turns out that MPTP is not itself the active compound. Rather, MPTP is metabolised extraneuronally by monoamine oxidase to the meperidine ion MPP+ (Fig. 6.8). MPP+ is taken up selectively into catecholamine neurones via the active dopamine and noradrenaline uptake channels, and then is further metabolised intraneuronally to form a number of highly toxic free radicals, which are the active constituents of neurotoxicity (see Chapter 3).

Whereas mice show a similar susceptibility to MPTP as do primates, remarkably rats are almost totally resistant to the toxin. This is because the conversion of MPTP to MPP+ is subserved by the B but not the A form of monoamine oxidase. Rat MAO is almost exclusively of the A form, whereas mice and monkeys (like humans)

use both MAO-A and MAO-B. Rats are therefore insensitive to MPTP because they are unable to convert MPTP to the active isomer. Nevertheless, if this stage is bypassed, rats do show full behavioural and pathological response when injected with the active metabolite, MPP+. Conversely, since absence of MAO-B blocks the metabolism and thereby inhibits the toxicity of MPTP, this suggests that selective inhibition of MAO-B might be neuroprotective in animals that use both forms of MAO. This hypothesis turns out to be well founded. Administration of the selective B-type MAOI, deprenyl ('Selegiline') was found to be effective in blocking both the nigral degeneration and the development of parkinsonian-like symptoms in both mice and monkeys following MPTP administration.

## DATATOP trial

Although no exogenous toxin has been identified to account for most forms of idiopathic Parkinson's disease, MPTP is structurally similar to the pesticide Paraquat, and is of the class of compounds, the pyridines, that are trace compounds in many industrial processes. Consequently, it was proposed that deprenyl may provide neuroprotection against other environmental toxins, if they operate by a similar mechanism to MPTP. This led to a large multicentre trial, known as DATATOP (Deprenyl and tocopherol antioxidant treatment of parkinsonism), using a fully randomised, double-blind design to evaluate the effects of deprenyl and the antioxidant, tocopherol (vitamin E), on the progression of newly diagnosed Parkinson's disease (The Parkinson's Study Group 1993). Although tocopherol was found to have little effect, deprenyl was found apparently to slow the progression of the disease, and to extend the time that patients could continue in work, and until death. However, MAOIs such as deprenyl may not work through a neuroprotective mechanisms but may instead have a direct dopamine-enchancing effect on symptoms. More worryingly, there is accumulating evidence that early introduction of deprenyl treatment may shorten the useful period that L-DOPA is effective, and trigger side-effects at an earlier stage.

Following the appearance of the DATATOP trial report, deprenyl was routinely used for a period as an adjunctive therapy in all newly diagnosed cases of Parkinson's disease. However, the doubt cast over its ability to slow disease progression, worries about acceleration of side-effects, and more recent specific concern about possible cardiotoxicity have severely curtailed its recent use.

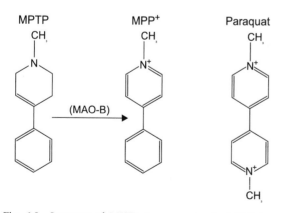

Fig. 6.8 Structure of MPTP, its conversion by MAO-A to MPP+, and structural similarity of MPP+ to the herbicide Paraquat.

# *Lewy bodies in Parkinson's disease and dementia*

## The Lewy body in Parkinson's disease

Lewy bodies are a pathological spherical inclusion seen in cells of the substantia nigra and elsewhere when sections from the parkinsonian brain are stained with the classical haematoxylin and eosin (H&E) method. They have a characteristic spheroid shape with a dense eosinophilic core surrounded by a lighter halo in the cytoplasm of cells, predominantly neurones. In the electron microscope, the dense core of tightly compacted electron dense material is surrounded by radiating filaments (Fig. 6.9). Lewy bodies also stain strongly with antibodies against ubiquitin, and stain to a variable degree with different neurofilament antibodies.

When he first described these inclusions, Lewy (1914) reported on their appearance in the nucleus basalis of Meynert, the hypothalamus, and the vagal motor nucleus. It was Tretiakoff (1919) who first noted the occurrence of Lewy bodies in the substantia nigra in Parkinson's disease, and who emphasised the relationship between nigral pathology and the rigidity and tremor of the disease. Although a variety of other sites (such as the locus coeruleus and nucleus basalis) are known also frequently to display Lewy bodies in post-mortem Parkinson's disease brain, it is their occurrence in the substantia nigra that is now considered to be a defining neuropathological feature of the idiopathic form of the disease, over and above the dopamine deficiency that arises from degeneration of the affected cells.

Until recently, the structure of Lewy bodies has remained opaque. However, recent developments in the genetics of Parkinson's disease have thrown a surprising new light on the classical pathology.

## Familial Parkinson's disease (PD), α-synuclein and Lewy bodies

Except for rare families with clearly-inherited disease, idiopathic PD has traditionally been considered not to involve a strong genetic component. Thus, for example, twin studies by Calne and colleagues (1987) suggested that when this relatively common disease occurred in two or more members of a family, the onset was more closely matched by date rather than by the age of the affected members, suggesting the impact of a common environmental factor rather than inherited genes.

However, as in AD, there are a few family pedigrees in which a parkinsonian-like disease appears to be an autosomal dominant inherited disorder. Linkage with markers on chromosome 4 in one large Italian family recently led to the identification of a mutation in the α-synuclein gene associated with the PD phenotype in this and several other families with familial parkinsonism (Polymeropoulos *et al.* 1997).

The functions of α-synuclein are currently unknown. It was first identified in electric fish, and subsequently

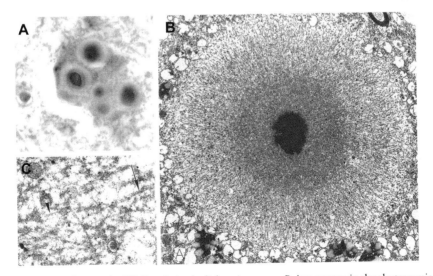

**Fig. 6.9** Lewy bodies. A Visualisation by H&E stain in the light microscope. B Appearance in the electron microscope, ×6000. (Reproduced from Forno 1996.)

characterised in a variety of species including zebra fish, rat, mouse, and humans. The protein is expressed at high levels in the brain where it is largely concentrated in presynaptic nerve terminals. Moreover, Polymeropoulos *et al.* (1997) highlighted the fact that the distribution of α-synuclein as studied in the rat brain (Maroteaux, and Scheller 1991) overlaps closely with the occurrence of Lewy bodies in the PD brain. These associations led Spillantini and colleagues (1997) to analyse Lewy bodies immunohistochemically, revealing that α-synuclein (in its normal rather than mutated form) is a major component of both the core and peripheral halo of the Lewy body, both in idiopathic PD and in other dementing diseases which show Lewy body pathology.

## Lewy body dementias

The human form of α-synuclein was first identified because of its cross-reactivity to certain tau antibodies and it has an anatomical appearance indistinguishable from the non-Aβ form of amyloid found in the AD brain. That this same molecule comprises the structural core of the PD Lewy body suggests a potential overlap in the underlying mechanisms of disease (Dunnett and Bjorklund).

Lewy bodies are concentrated in the substantia nigra of PD but may also occur in other cortical and subcortical sites in the parkinsonian brain, as well as occurring in other diseases, in particular with features of dementia. To this point we have treated Parkinson's and Alzheimer's as quite distinct diseases, involving very different symptoms, different types of pathology, and different regions of the brain. And yet PD can involve cognitive as well as motor impairments, Lewy bodies may appear in the cortex as well as the midbrain, and the Lewy body pathology involves molecular constituents that interact with amyloid and tau. Conversely,

Lewy bodies and other Parkinson-like features are frequently seen in many cases of Alzheimer's (Ditter, and Mirra 1987). The incidence of overlapping features is far higher than could be explained by co-occurrence of two independent disease processes. Rather, from these observations has grown the concept of a spectrum of Lewy body disease (Kosaka *et al.* 1984), including an intermediate condition known as diffuse Lewy body disease (DLBD) characterised by widespread and particularly cortical Lewy bodies, resulting in dementia (Fig. 6.10). In DLBD there is a lack of extensive plaques and tangles that distinguish it from AD, and a predominance of cortical pathology and dementia that distinguish it from PD, where the Lewy bodies predominate in the brainstem.

This distinction highlights our lack of understanding of the cognitive impairments seen in PD. Whereas there is a consensus that the motor dysfunctions reflect pathology of the substantia nigra and consequent disturbance of dopaminergic regulation of the basal ganglia, it remains ambiguous whether the more cognitive components involve the same ascending dopamine projections to basal ganglia and/or association cortex, Lewy body pathology in other subcortical (e.g. NBM) and/or cortical areas, or coexisting pathology of another type, such as AD.

## *Metabolic disturbance of neuronal integrity in trinucleotide repeat diseases*

### Huntington's disease

Huntington's disease is an inherited neurodegenerative disease involving a complex pattern of motor, cognitive,

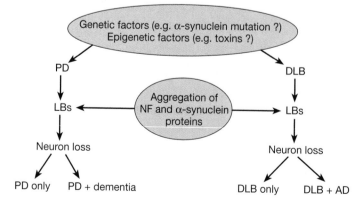

**Fig. 6.10** The spectrum of Lewy body disease. (Based on Trojanowski and Lee 1998.)

and psychiatric impairments. The disease is characterised by a progressive degeneration first and foremost of the neostriatum. As the disease progresses, the caudate nucleus is the first area to degenerate, then other nuclei of the basal ganglia including the putamen and globus pallidus, and then major areas that project into and out of the basal ganglia including the neocortex and substantia nigra.

The main symptoms of the disease can be well understood in terms of the primary loss of the striatum and its input and output connections. Thus, striatal lesions in animals also produce motor and cognitive impairments, although it is more difficult to evaluate psychiatric disturbance in experimental rats. The cognitive impairments are distinct from those seen in AD. Although both Alzheimer's and Huntington's disease both induce forms of dementia, the deficits in the former are particularly of new learning and memory, functions that are typically associated with the temporal lobe and hippocampus. By contrast, the dementia of Huntington's disease involves disturbances in thinking, planning, and decision-making that are more characteristic of frontal cortex function and show some similarity to those seen after frontal lobe damage. Consequently the motor cognitive and psychiatric disturbances of Huntington's disease are typical of disruption of corticostriatal circuits, whether studied in animals or man.

At the cellular level, the GABAergic medium spiny neurones of the striatum are the first to degenerate in Huntington's disease. These are by far the commonest type of neurones in the striatum (about 85% of the total); they receive the cortical, thalamic, and dopamine inputs and they give rise to the main striatal output projection to targets in the globus pallidus and substantia nigra. By contrast, the medium and large interneurones of the striatum that use somatostatin, neuropeptide Y, and acetylcholine as their transmitters appear to be relatively spared in the early stages of the disease.

The first animal models of Huntington's disease were based on excitotoxic lesions, using first kainic acid, and subsequently ibotenic and quinolinic acids. As outlined in Chapter 1, these toxins not only create selective damage of striatal neurones while sparing axons of passage, but under appropriate conditions of dose and concentration they can reproduce the selective profile of toxicity seen in the human disease involving preferential degeneration of medium spiny projection neurones and relative sparing of striatal interneurones. This was at first taken to indicate an excitotoxic mechanism of cell death in the human disease. However, it was soon recognised that the most selective excitotoxin quinolinic acid occurs naturally and is a component in the kynurate pathway, suggesting that the toxicity may be related to a disturbance in cellular energy metabolism. This in turn led to the identification of a variety of metabolic toxins, such as 3-nitroproprionic acid and malonate, as perhaps even more accurate models of the disease in animals, and suggesting that the selective striatal degeneration is related to a fundamental metabolic disturbance (see Chapter 3).

Nevertheless, in spite of these leads from relatively good animal models for reproducing the neuropathology and psychopathology of the human disease, they fail to explain why the striatum is selectively targeted. Thus, for example, peripheral administration of 3-nitropropionic acid results in widespread down-regulation of succinate dehydrogenase activity throughout the brain, but selective toxicity in just the striatal neurones. Why? Some clues may be provided by recent advances in understanding the molecular genetics of the human disease.

## Molecular genetics of Huntington's disease

The familial pattern of Huntington's disease is one of relatively pure autosomal dominant inheritance. The risk of an affected parent passing on the gene to his or her children is 50% for each child. Nevertheless, there are certain strange features of the classical inheritance pattern. Although the disease typically affects sufferers in middle age, once they have had children and have passed on the affected gene, the age of onset tends to be younger and younger in successive generations if the gene is inherited from the father but to remain stable if inherited from the mother. It proved extremely difficult to account for this effect, known as 'paternal anticipation', in terms of classical Mendelian genetics.

The search for the Huntington's disease gene was extremely protracted. Indeed it required over ten years of hard study by many groups between the first discovery of linkage markers on chromosome 4 and the isolation and sequencing of the gene (Huntington's Disease Collaborative Research Group 1993). The gene was prosaically named IT15 (for 'interesting transcript no. 15') and codes for a novel protein, given the more relevant designation, 'huntingtin'.

The nature of the gene defect in Huntington's disease turned out to be an example of a novel form of mutation: it is not a change or deletion of essential bases/amino acids, but rather an expansion of a CAG repeat sequence in the gene, encoding a polyglutamine ('poly

Q') expansion in the protein. In the normal individual, both copies of the IT15 gene typically have strings of 10–20 CAG repeats, whereas in Huntington's disease the repeat is typically >40. Indeed, the transition from normal to affected is quite sharp, with 35 copies or less consistently associated with no disease, and 39 copies or more consistently associated with the full disease state. There is a modest inverse correlation between the number of repeats and the age of disease onset, but this is nowhere near as strong as that suggested by the very tight affected/not affected cut-off.

The normal functions of huntingtin within the cell are not known, let alone why an abnormal repeat length results in striatal disease. Max Perutz (1994) has suggested that the expanded repeat length may reflect a profound conformational change in the tertiary structure of the protein that changes the protein function. This hypothesis can account for the sharp transition between a normal and disease-related repeat length, but not why the striatum is its target. Huntingtin is expressed ubiquitously not only throughout the brain but widely in peripheral tissues also. However, in the search for its normal function, a number of other proteins have recently been identified, which appear to interact selectively with huntingtin. Of these, the 'huntingtin-associated protein' HAP1 has a heterogeneous distribution in the brain, being at its lowest concentration first and foremost in the striatum and then in association cortex, globus pallidus, and thalamus, which are the areas most affected in the disease. This led Page *et al.* (1998) to propose that HAP1 and related interacting proteins may exert a neutralising action on huntingtin, so that the striatal selectivity of the disease may reflect a local failure in the neuroprotective activity of these proteins, in particular when confronted with an enhanced toxicity from the huntingtin protein itself.

Several groups have now made transgenic mice that overexpress either full-length copies or fragments of the human huntingtin gene containing the expanded CAG repeat (Burright *et al.* 1997; Reddy *et al.* 1999). Whereas several of these mice exhibit a marked neuronal phenotype, the degeneration is not selectively striatal — indeed it has proved hard to identify any extensive overt neurodegeneration in some mice that are markedly affected neurologically (Mangiarini *et al.* 1996).

The more interesting development from the transgenic mice has been the identification of an intracellular pathology (Davies *et al.* 1997). When stained with antibodies against huntingtin, many neurones throughout the transgenic (but not normal) mouse brain show small dense accumulations of protein that at the EM level are seen to comprise dense filamentous inclusions within the cell nucleus. The same 'intranuclear inclusions' are also stained with ubiquitin antibodies, a widely used antibody for identifying degenerating neurones in a variety of dementing diseases. Following this observation in the transgenic mouse brain, DiFiglia and colleagues (1997) quickly confirmed that similar intranuclear occlusions occur in Huntington's disease in humans, although again the pathology appears to be more widespread rather than exclusively concentrated within striatal neurones. How fragments of the huntingtin protein come to accumulate as filamentous deposits within the cell nucleus is at present completely unknown: indeed, it remains ambiguous whether the deposits reflect an abnormal process of nuclear accumulation in the disease, or whether they reflect the breakdown of a normal scavenging process is completely unknown. Nevertheless, the phenomenon offers the first real handle on the search for understanding the neuropathological process at the heart of Huntington's disease.

## Other trinucleotide repeat diseases

Huntington's disease is just one of a series of trinucleotide repeat diseases that have been identified by the new developments in molecular genetics (see Table 6.2). Although they are mostly extremely rare and are associated with expansions in quite different genes, they all have several remarkable features in common (Paulson and Fishbeck 1996).

- They all involve repeats of C- and G-rich triplets of bases, and in all cases disease results from an abnormal expansion, rather than mutation, in the number of repeats seen in the normal gene.

- The critical number of repeats for transition to a disease phenotype is similar at around 40–50 triplets in all cases.

- In each case inheritance is autosomal dominant or X-chromosome linked.

- Disease severity can vary in each disease, but is typically more severe and with earlier onset, the greater the repeat expansion.

- Expanded trinucleotide repeat lengths are unstable when transmitted from parent to child. Expansions are more common than retractions between generations, resulting in the phenomenon of 'anticipation', i.e. the tendency to increase repeat length, increasing severity and reducing age of onset in successive

**Table 6.2**  Key features of the trinucleotide repeat diseases

| Disease | | Phenotype | Repeat | Normal | Disease | Gene Product |
|---|---|---|---|---|---|---|
| Huntington's disease | HD | Cognitive, motor and emotional disturbance | CAG | 11–34 | 36–121 | huntingtin |
| Spinal and bulbar muscular atrophy | SBMA | Neuromuscular weakness, atrophy and fasciculation | CAG | 11–34 | 40–62 | androgen receptor |
| Fragile X type A | FraxA | Inherited mental retardation with dysmorphic features | CGG | 6–52 | 60–>2000 | RNA-binding protein |
| Fragile X type E | FraxE | Milder retardation | GCC | 6–25 | >200 | ? |
| Myotonic dystrophy | | Progressive weakness and myotonia | CTG | 5–37 | 50–>2000 | myotonin protein kinase |
| Spinocerebellar atrophy 1 | SCA1 | Ataxia, ophthalmoparesis, and muscle weakness | CAG | 6–39 | 41–81 | ataxin 1 |
| Dentorubral-pallido-luysian atrophy | DRPLA | Ataxia, dementia, myoclonus, choreathetosis, and epilepsy | CAG | 7–25 | 49–88 | atrophin |
| Machado-Joseph disease | MJD | Spinocerebellar degeneration | CAG | 11–36 | 68–79 | MJD 1 gene product |

generations. By contrast, normal repeat lengths tend to stability between generations.

- Parental effects are also common — for example, the anticipation effects are predominantly paternal in Huntington's and other neurological diseases, whereas maternal inheritance is associated with more severe disorder in myotonic dystrophy and fragile X syndromes.

In spite of these similarities, a number of authors have divided the trinucleotide repeat disorders into two subgroups (Paulson and Fishbeck 1996):

The *type I disorders* comprise the five diseases with expanded repeats of the CAG triplet of bases, coding for glutamine. These all result in neurological disorders (HD, SBMA, SCA1, DRPLA, MJD, see Table 6.2), they all have moderate instability of the CAG repeat between generations, the repeats are all transcribed into proteins, and they all target specific populations of neurones in the CNS. The patterns of inheritance and neuronal targeting in each case suggest that even though the normal functions of the affected proteins are not yet fully understood and are likely to differ considerably in each case, the expanded repeat confers a toxic gain of an abnormal function to the affected proteins, rather than the loss of a normal one.

The *type II disorders* comprise the three diseases with expanded GCC, CGG, or CTG triplets. In these diseases, it appears that the expanded repeat results in an altered expression of the gene rather than a change of function of the resulting protein, resulting in abnormalities in the development of multiple brain and neuro-

muscular systems. These diseases are also characterised by much greater repeat instability and the occurrence of some very large expansions.

In their theoretical review, Paulson and Fishbeck (1996) propose three alternative hypotheses for how an expanded trinucleotide repeat might lead to neurodegeneration and disease.

1. *Transregulation model.* In the first model, the expanded repeat might alter the protein's binding with other proteins with which it interacts, thereby changing the strength of the influence of the resultant complex on normal cell metabolism. A series of interacting proteins are now being identified, such as the huntingtin-associated and huntingtin-interacting proteins that interact with huntingtin, although the function of these molecular interactions remains to be elucidated (Page *et al.* 1998).

2. *Protein aggregation model.* In the second model the expanded polyglutamine segments of the protein exert an abnormal influence of their own, not restricted to interactions with a limited set of interacting proteins. For example, Perutz (1994) has proposed that an expanded polyglutamine tract may yield abnormal folding of the molecule and may tend to form a highly attractive polar zipper structure increasing the tendency of the molecule to aggregate both with itself and with other proteins with similar repeats.

3. *Transglutaminase model.* In the third model, Green (1993) has proposed that glutamine expansions

beyond approximately 30 amino acids in length become unusually avid substrates for transglutaminase activity, resulting in increased cross-linking with other proteins that are toxic to all cells. However, by virtue of their longevity, neurones would be particularly susceptible to the toxic effects of the accumulation of such cross-linked complexes over time.

As described in the preceding section, the recent identification of the neuronal intranuclear inclusions in Huntington's disease strongly argues in favour of the second of these models. Moreover, transgenic mice with expanded repeats of the SCA and DRPLA genes have recently also been seen to produce similar neuronal intranuclear inclusions, suggesting that this may be the common mechanism of cellular pathology associated with the expanded polyglutamine tract rather than the individual proteins within which they are included, which may instead influence the target population of cells that are most affected to yield the particular disease.

## Prion diseases

Prion diseases, also referred to as transmissible spongiform encephalopathies, are fatal neurodegenerative diseases of humans and animals whose pathogenesis involves the abnormal metabolism of *prion protein* (PrP). The normal cellular form of prion protein (PrP$^C$)[1], found in brain and some other organs, is a 33–35 kDa glycoprotein encoded by a single copy gene on chromosome 20 in humans, and on homologous chromosomes in other species (e.g. chromosome 2 in mice). In the scientific literature the human gene is referred to as PRNP and the mouse gene as Prn-p, but for ease of discussion the gene in all species will be called the PrP gene. The PrP gene is highly conserved across many species, suggesting an essential function, but 'knock-out' mice, in which the gene has been ablated, appear to develop into healthy adults with few indications of abnormality (Büeler *et al.* 1992; Manson *et al.* 1994). Although the function of PrP$^C$ is unknown, it has been suggested that it might act as a cell surface receptor. *In vitro*, PrP$^C$ is soluble in non-denaturing detergents and is degraded by treatment with the proteolytic enzyme, proteinase K.

In cases of prion diseases, a proteinase K resistant form (PrP$^{SC}$)[2] accumulates in affected brain tissue. Although the amount of PrP$^{SC}$ found in the brains of mice or hamsters infected with scrapie (the endemic prion disease of sheep) is ten-fold higher than the amount of PrP$^C$ found in uninfected mouse or hamster brains, there is no difference in the level or distribution of prion protein mRNA. Thus it appears that the production of prion protein is not increased during disease pathogenesis; rather, there is a reduction in the turnover of the protein. In the presence of detergent, *in vitro*, PrP$^{SC}$ tends to aggregate to form amyloid fibrils, known as scrapie-associated fibrils (SAFs). In some cases of prion disease, amyloid deposits in the form of plaques are found in the brain and these contain PrP$^{SC}$. When affected tissue is digested with proteinase K, a 27–30 kDa fragment (PrP27–30), which derives from PrP$^{SC}$, can be detected. The difference between PrP$^C$ and PrP$^{SC}$ probably results from a post-translational modification of PrP$^C$ leading to a conformational change in which the $\alpha$-helical content is decreased and the $\beta$-pleated sheet content is increased (for review see: Prusiner 1996a,b, 1997a). What sets these diseases apart from other neurodegenerative diseases, however, is their experimental transmissibility. Animals injected intracerebrally with brain tissue from an affected individual (human or animal) will usually develop prion disease after a prolonged incubation period of many months and, sometimes, years.

### Human prion diseases

The human prion diseases include Creutzfeldt–Jakob disease (CJD), Gerstmann-Sträussler–Scheinker disease (GSS), Fatal Familial Insomnia (FFI), Atypical Prion Disease (APD), and kuru. Individual cases of prion disease can be classified as *familial, acquired* or *sporadic. Familial* cases occur in an autosomal dominant pattern within pedigrees. They have been described in terms of their clinical and neuropathological features, as shown in Table 6.3.

*Acquired* cases are those where prion disease is known to have been contracted through contact with tissue (usually brain or near-brain tissue, such as cornea or dura mater) from other cases of prion disease. About 100 cases of *iatrogenic* CJD have occurred in Western

---

[1] PrP$^C$ denotes the normal cellular form of prion protein. PrP denotes protease-resistant protein.

[2] PrPSC denotes the abnormal, disease-associated form of prion protein. The superscript reflects the fact that this form was first identified in scrapie-affected animals, although the term is used when describing the protein in all the animal and human diseases.

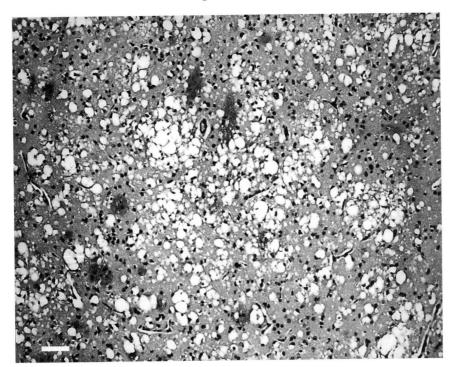

**Fig 6.11**   Spongiform change in the cortex of a patient with sporadic CJD. Bar = 25 μm (Quote source.)

cultures as a result of contamination during surgical procedures or among those treated with human pituitary-derived hormones (Brown 1996), and between 1995 and the end of 1999, some 48 people in Britain had died from a new variant form of Creutzfeldt-Jakob disease (nvCJD), which has been linked to the epidemic of bovine spongiform encephalopathy (BSE) — see below. *Kuru*, an epidemic prion disease, spread among the tribal people of Papua-New Guinea as a result of endocannibalism and claimed the lives of several thousand between the mid-1940s and the mid-1960s (Alpers 1987).

*Sporadic* cases of prion disease are those in which there is no evidence of a contaminating event, no family history of prion disease, and no disease-related PrP gene mutation. They comprise ~85% CJD cases but extremely few cases of GSS or APD. Cases of sporadic CJD usually present with cognitive impairment that may or may not be accompanied by cerebellar dysfunction, visual failure, and pyramidal and extra-pyramidal signs, depending on which brain areas are most seriously affected. The mean age at onset is about 60 years and the median duration of illness is about 4–5 months (de Silva 1996). The new variant form of CJD was identi-

fied in 1996 because the clinical presentation differed subtly from that of sporadic CJD. These patients usually present with behavioural changes (the early cases were often referred to psychiatrists rather than to neurologists) and become ataxic with amnesia and dementia developing later. The age at onset is much lower than that described for sporadic CJD and the duration of illness is longer, but confirmation of nvCJD depends on the neuropathological picture, which differs substantially from that seen in sporadic CJD. Striking, and very consistent between cases, is the occurrence of numerous PrP-plaques throughout the cerebrum and cerebellum. These plaques resemble those seen in the brains of kuru victims (kuru-plaques) but, additionally, are surrounded by a zone of spongiform vacuolation. This particular type of 'florid' plaque has become pathognomic for nvCJD. (Prp-plaques are seen in ~25% of cases of sporadic CJD and ~75% of cases of kuru; diffuse PrP-deposits and large multicentric PrP-plaques are seen in GSS, and plaques may be seen in the cerebellum and spinal cord of patients with iatrogenic CJD associated with growth hormone treatment.)

Apart from kuru and the iatrogenic cases, there is no evidence of transmission of prion disease between

**Table 6.3**   Familial prion diseases

*Inherited Creutzfeldt-Jakob disease (CJD)*
Rapidly progressive dementia (< 2 years duration), movement disorder (myoclonus), characteristic EEG. Neuropathological examination reveals widespread spongiform encephalopathy (SE), astrocytic hyperplasia and, in 10–15% cases, PrP-positive amyloid plaque deposition.

*Gerstmann-Sträussler-Scheinker syndrome (GSS)*
A more slowly progressive dementia and/or cerebellar ataxia with 2–15 year duration. Neuropathological examination reveals severe PrP-positive amyloid plaque deposition and, sometimes, SE.

*Atypical Prion Disease (APD)*
There are a number of cases in which neither the clinical nor the neuropathological features of CJD or GSS are present but where a diagnosis of prion dementia is warranted because there is a fatal neurological condition plus biochemical evidence of PrP$^{SC}$ accumulation and/or a mutation in the PrP gene not found in the normal population.

*Fatal Familial Insomnia (FFI)*
Cases present with progressive dysautonomia and profound insomnia. Later signs include dysarthria, ataxia, myoclonus, and pyramidal signs. Duration of illness is about 15 months. Neuropathological findings include severe neuronal loss in thalamus, atrophy of inferior olives, and variable amount of SE in cortex.

**Table 6.4**   Sufficient criteria for a diagnosis of prion disease

Spongiform encephalopathy which must be distinguished from the spongy changes sometimes seen in other neurodegenerative diseases.
Transmission of spongiform encephalopathy to animals by intracerebral injection of brain material.
Detection of PrP$^{SC}$ by immunodetection methods (for example, Western blotting).
In situ PrP staining with appropriate antibodies after brief digestion with proteolytic enzymes.
Preparation of scrapie-associated fibrils (SAFs) from brain and subsequent visualisation by electron microscopy and / or by staining with anti-PrP antibody.
Some fatal neurological illness plus mutations within the PrP gene which are not found in the normal population.

humans by normal social or sexual contact, and no evidence of maternal transmission from affected mother to offspring either *in utero* or in the post-natal period. Of the more than 1000 children born after the ban on cannibalism to women who were suffering from kuru, or who were incubating kuru, none has developed kuru. And at least three children have been born to women in the terminal stages of CJD; none has developed disease.

## Animal prion diseases

*Scrapie* is probably the only truly endemic animal prion disease. It affects sheep and occurs in many parts of the world. It is still widely believed that scrapie is maintained in the sheep population by lateral and maternal transmission, though the evidence for this is unconvincing and has been challenged (Ridley and Baker 1995). Although scrapie is widespread in British flocks, some breeds seem to be resistant to the disease, and within sheep breeds, susceptibility or resistance to scrapie is determined by PrP genotype. It is also reported in goats. Other animal prion diseases, including spongi-

form encephalopathy of cat, kudu, nyala, and mink, and the best known, BSE of cattle, are all believed to be acquired by contamination, probably through eating scrapie- or BSE-affected meat, or meat- and bone-meal food additives. About 170 000 cattle died from BSE during the epidemic in Britain between 1986 and 1997, and a further 700 000 infected cattle were slaughtered for food (Anderson *et al.* 1996).

## Diagnosis of prion disease

When scrapie, CJD, and GSS were shown to be experimentally transmissible to animals after a long incubation period they became known as 'slow viral diseases' and experimental transmissibility became the diagnostic criterion. However, transmissibility is an inadequate tool for diagnosis since attempts to transmit disease are frequently unsuccessful because of the 'species-barrier'. Primary transmission of prion disease from a human with CJD or a sheep with scrapie to an animal of another species (e.g. a rodent) may be difficult to achieve. It may be necessary to inject many animals to ensure that a few develop disease. However, once disease has been established in the second species, subsequent passage of disease to another animal of that species is usually much easier, with shorter incubation times. This species-barrier depends on the ease with which the infecting PrP$^{SC}$ interacts with the host PrP$^{C}$ (see below). While there is no one feature that is *necessary* for diagnosis, there are several features that are *sufficient*, although in individual cases the information is often absent for technical or logistical reasons. The sufficient criteria are shown in Table 6.4.

# Genetics of prion disease

The first prion disease-linked mutation in the PrP gene was found in a large British family in which GSS is inherited, and involves a cytosine to thymine change at codon 102, leading to a proline to leucine substitution in the prion protein (Hsiao *et al.* 1989). Since then a further 20 or so disease-linked mutations have been found in the PrP gene. While some are point mutations, others are insertions of extra repeats of the octapeptide repeat sequence found in the normal PrP gene (Poulter *et al.* 1992). Between codons 51 and 91 there is an octapeptide sequence that is repeated five times with minor variation; in a British pedigree with dominantly inherited atypical prion disease, affected members carry an extra six octapeptide repeats. A few of the mutations linked to prion disease are listed in Table 6.5. The linkage of prion disease to mutations in the PrP gene argues persuasively that in these inherited cases the disease is *caused* by the mutation. It is also clear that in at least some of these inherited cases the disease is experimentally transmissible.

Although there is quite wide variability in phenotype between these mutations, and within families with a specific mutation, it is possible to generalise to a certain extent. So, for example, codon 200 (glutamine to lysine) mutation cases tend to be of short duration and to have a CJD-like presentation, while codon 102 (proline to leucine) and 117 (alanine to valine) mutation cases are more likely to have a long duration with amyloid plaques (proteinaceous deposits within the brain parenchyma, consisting largely of PrP$^{SC}$) and to have a younger age at onset, i.e. a GSS-like picture (Collinge *et al.* 1992). Cases with insertion mutations tend to be atypical, of long duration, and of variable age at onset. The codon 178 (aspartic acid to asparagine) mutation cases are very interesting. Several North European families with this mutation present with fairly typical CJD, and disease has been experimentally transmitted from these cases (Goldfarb *et al.* 1992a). In a number of Italian families, however, individuals carrying the codon 178 mutation develop 'fatal familial insomnia'. Although this condition presents as a severe insomnia, there is progressive autonomic breakdown, ataxia, and pyramidal signs. Neuropathologically, there is marked neuronal loss in thalamus and cerebral atrophy, but usually little or no spongiform encephalopathy (Medori *et al.* 1992).

In addition to the disease-related mutations, there is a common polymorphism in the PrP gene. In Caucasians, codon 129 encodes methionine (M) or valine (V) with allele frequencies 0.68 : 0.32, respectively. In Japanese, the valine substitution is rare and it has been reported that in the tribal people of Papua-New Guinea the methionine is rare, suggesting wide ethnic variation.

Early reports suggested that the different phenotypic expression of the codon 178 mutation may be determined by the codon 129 polymorphism. It was found that when the codon 178 mutation is in an allele encoding methionine at codon 129, the clinical presentation is fatal familial insomnia, whereas if the mutation is in

**Table 6.5** Some PrP gene mutations in prion disease

| Codon* | Changes | Comments |
|---|---|---|
| 51–91 | Octapeptide repeats: | |
| | 5 | Normal |
| | 7 | CJD-like illness |
| | 10 | Dementia, cerebellar ataxia. Age at onset 31–45; duration 5–15 years. Spongiform change. |
| | 11 | Linked to APD. Attempts to transmit disease to monkeys have not been successful |
| | 12–14 | Various clinical presentations, some with spongiform change. |
| 102 | Proline–Leucine | GSS |
| 117 | Alanine–Valine | GSS |
| 178 | Aspartic acid–Asparagine | CJD or FFI depending on codon 129 (see text). |
| 198 | Phenylalanine–Serine | Variant GSS; has features of Alzheimer pathology as well as PrP plaques. |
| 200 | Glutamic acid–Lysine | Most common inherited CJD. |

* There are, in addition, a number of other mutations at codons 108, 208, 210, and 217 that have been identified either in single cases or single families. Two Japanese patients with subacute dementia and myoclonus were found to have a valine to isoleucine substitution at codon 180. Neuropathological examination revealed the characteristic CJD 'triad' of spongiform change, neuronal loss, and astrocytosis. One of these patients was also found to have a methionine to arginine substitution at codon 232 on the other allele, and this mutation has also been found in other Japanese patients. As investigators become more aware of the many different clinical presentations of prion disease, the number of mutations linked to prion disease is increasing.

an allele encoding valine at codon 129, the presentation is of typical CJD (Goldfarb *et al.* 1992b). However, in an Australian family carrying the codon 178 mutation in a Met[129] allele, affected individuals present with fatal familial insomnia, CJD, or a cerebellar ataxia-like illness, suggesting that the genotype/phenotype association is not so tight as was originally thought (Mclean *et al.* 1997).

## Pathogenesis of prion disease

The experimental transmission of scrapie in the 1930s, and kuru and CJD in the 1960s, led to the search for a transmissible agent variously called a virus, a 'virino', or a defective retrovirus. No such agent has been identified, however, and the only macromolecule known to be associated with transmissibility or 'infectivity' is PrP[SC]. Even after it was confirmed that some dominantly inherited forms of human prion disease were experimentally transmissible (Baker *et al.* 1985), the question remained of whether the PrP gene mutations confer susceptibility to an exogenous causative agent or whether they are sufficient in themselves to cause disease. This question may have been answered by a series of experiments in which transgenic mice were created containing multiple copies of a PrP gene with a codon 101 (proline to leucine) mutation, homologous to the human codon 102 mutation known to be linked to GSS. At approximately 180 days of age these mice *spontaneously* developed neurological disease and spongiform encephalopathy (SE), and it has subsequently been shown that this genetically caused disease is experimentally transmissible to normal animals (Hsiao *et al.* 1992; Prusiner 1997b). However, in other experiments with mice carrying only a single copy of the codon 101 mutant gene, none of the animals developed disease (Manson 1996). Interestingly, older mice carrying multiple copies of normal mouse, hamster, or sheep PrP genes developed truncal ataxia, hind limb paralysis and tremors, associated with necrotising myopathy involving skeletal muscle, a demyelinating polyneuropathy, and, in some cases, focal spongiform degeneration of the grey matter. In these animals, however, no protease-resistant PrP[SC] was detectable (Westaway *et al.* 1994; Prusiner 1997b).

An increasingly influential hypothesis, which attempts to explain the familial, acquired, and sporadic occurrence of prion diseases, as well as experimental transmissibility and the lack of direct evidence for a causative virus, was first proposed by Prusiner (1982), who was awarded the 1997 Nobel Prize in Physiology or Medi-

cine. Prusiner coined the name prion protein (from *pro*teinaceous *in*fectious) and suggested that the transmissible agent of the spongiform encephalopathies probably consisted solely of prion protein. He argued that during the disease process, PrP[SC] acts as a template for the conversion of more PrP[C] to PrP[SC], and that this process can continue even if the PrP[SC] is transferred to the brain of another host. When affected brain tissue containing PrP[SC] is injected into the brain of a new host, it combines with the new host's PrP[C] and catalyses its conversion to the abnormal form. Since the newly accumulated abnormal form is host-coded, there is no immune response. Experimental transmission within species is more readily achieved than between species (the so-called species-barrier) and this probably reflects the ease with which the PrP[SC] derived from one species can act as a template for the conversion of the normal protein from another species. This appears to depend, amongst other things, on the sequence homology between different PrP[C] structures and many experiments have demonstrated that the species-barrier between hamsters and mice can be abolished by introducing hamster PrP genes into the mice. These experiments have shown that the infecting hamster PrP[SC] converts the hamster PrP[C] produced by the hamster PrP transgenes in the mice into hamster PrP[SC] (for review see Westaway 1996).

It is not clear why PrP[C] should undergo such a conversion in the first place but it may be related to processes that mediate senescence. It is proposed that this conversion is a rare stochastic event in the normal population, leading to sporadic CJD (which occurs with an annual incidence of 1–2 per million of the population world-wide), while in individuals who carry specific PrP gene mutations the probability of the change being initiated approaches unity by later middle age. In these genetic cases the efficiency with which PrP[SC] will 'recruit' PrP[C] may depend on the sequence homology between the proteins produced by the two PrP alleles. Some evidence for this idea has been provided by two recent findings. Within each pedigree, the disease-related mutation will be carried on either a M[129] or a V[129] allele and it has been shown that in a large pedigree with an insert consisting of six extra octapeptide repeats carried in a M[129] allele, age at death is later in those who are heterozygous at this codon (M[129], V[129]) than in those who are homozygous (M[129], M[129]). Age at onset may also be later and illness duration longer in heterozygotes (Baker *et al.* 1991). A similar finding has been reported in a large Indiana kindred with the codon 198 mutation (Dlouhy *et al.* 1992). Evidence for an

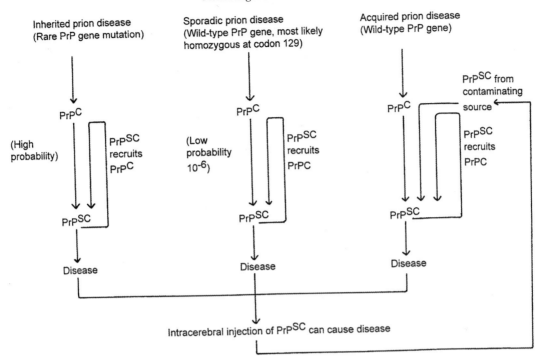

**Fig. 6.12** Scheme illustrating the relationship between the normal and abnormal forms of prion protein and possible pathogenesis of prion disease.

interaction between the prion protein products of each allele was provided by the observation that of 22 confirmed cases of sporadic CJD, 21 were homozygous at codon 129, while only 1 was heterozygous. The difference in homozygosity between the CJD group (95.5%) and a large control group (49%) is highly significant (Palmer *et al.* 1991). This finding has been confirmed in other studies (Laplanche *et al.* 1994; Windl *et al.* 1996).

A major problem for the protein-only hypothesis has been the existence of multiple strains of agent, which are capable of changing or 'mutating' as they are passaged through mice of different PrP genotypes. This has been interpreted as evidence that the transmissible agent must contain an informational molecule, capable of mutation, and probably a nucleic acid (Bruce *et al.* 1992). These authors claim that there are at least 20 strains of the scrapie agent, but others have argued that there are probably no more than two or three (Ridley and Baker 1996). Strain types are defined by the pattern of pathology and the incubation times they produce when inoculated into a panel of mice of different PrP genotypes. When brain tissue from cattle with BSE, or from kudu, nyala, and cats with SE, was injected into

the panel of mice they all produced the same pattern of incubation periods and distribution of pathology, suggesting they contained a single strain of agent. This was presumed to be the BSE agent. When brain tissue from several new variant CJD cases also produced the same incubation times and pathology this was taken as direct evidence that nvCJD is linked to BSE (Bruce *et al.* 1997).

It remains the case, however, that no agent-specific nucleic acid has been identified and many scientists have proposed that strain-specific information may be encoded or encrypted within the tertiary structure or conformation of PrP$^{SC}$ and that this information can be conserved when PrP$^{SC}$ converts PrP$^{C}$ from the same species into PrP$^{SC}$ (e.g. see Prusiner 1991; Ridley and Baker 1997). Evidence for this proposition has come from the elegant experiments carried out by Caughey and colleagues, in which they demonstrate that strain characteristics can be preserved during the conversion of PrP$^{C}$ to PrP$^{SC}$ in a cell-free system, in the absence of nucleic acid (Kocisko *et al.* 1994; Bessen *et al.* 1995). The mechanism by which PrP$^{SC}$ converts PrP$^{C}$ to more PrP$^{SC}$ remains unknown and is the subject of most of the research into the prion diseases, but it is already suspected that another protein molecule is involved (Telling *et al.* 1995). It is also likely that any therapeutic approach to the prion diseases will target this mechanism (Prusiner 1997a).

The increasing appreciation of the importance of the amyloidogenic nature of prion protein (Prusiner *et al.* 1983) has highlighted several important similarities between the prion diseases and other neurodegenerative diseases that involve amyloid production, the most prevalent of which is AD. One of the key neuropathological features of AD is the widespread occurrence of plaques containing degenerating neuritic elements and deposits of A$\beta$ protein. Both AD and human prion disease occur in sporadic, familial, and acquired forms. In both diseases, sporadic cases have a mean later age at onset than familial cases, and familial cases are associated with mutations in the genes, which make, or are involved in processing, the protein that accumulates as an amyloid. AD is found in families that carry one of several mutations in the APP gene on chromosome 21, or in genes whose products modulate the processing of APP (see above). Familial prion disease is seen in families that carry one of several mutations in the PrP gene. Acquired cases of CJD result from accidental contamination with PrP$^{SC}$. Acquired AD (together with other neurological damage) results from head trauma, particularly repeated head trauma, such as that seen in professional boxers. Metabolic perturbations cause an increase in APP production, which results in the production of A$\beta$. The link between prion disease and AD is brought even closer in the 'Indiana Pedigree' of GSS. In addition to plaques composed of PrP, the brains of these patients contain many neurones bearing 'neurofibrillary tangles', deposits of yet another amyloid (tau protein, which is characteristic of AD, and in older affected members of this pedigree the PrP-plaques in the brain are surrounded by 'haloes' of the A$\beta$ protein found in AD (Ghetti *et al.* 1995). Until the techniques of immunohistochemistry became available, the brains of patients from the 'Indiana Pedigree' were indistinguishable from those of patients with AD (Ghetti *et al.* 1989). That prion disease might initiate the deposition of ß-amyloid, especially in fairly elderly patients, is perhaps not too surprising since the deposition of ß-amyloid in normal ageing, and in response to neurotrauma, suggests that it may be a natural response of the elderly brain to any sort of damage.

Prion disease and AD differ radically in that prion disease is experimentally and accidentally transmissible, whereas AD is not (although the majority of familial forms of human prion disease, especially those of long duration with the deposition of many PrP-plaques, have not been transmitted experimentally). The process of corruption of molecules is, nonetheless, a common theme occurring in both types of disease. In artificial conditions, the precursor molecule of A$\beta$ protein, or synthesised portions of that precursor molecule, are biochemically unstable and may rapidly and unpredictably form A$\beta$ fibrils. PrP$^{sc}$ forms PrP-amyloid on extraction from brain, and does so spontaneously within the brain to form amyloid plaques in a proportion (but, importantly, not all) cases of prion disease. Artificially synthesised portions of PrP will also spontaneously polymerise in a test tube. A$\beta$-amyloid and PrP$^{sc}$ are both made up structurally of 'ß-pleated sheet' formations.

Just as in some cases of familial prion disease it has been possible to show that the protein product of both copies of the PrP gene enter into the disease process, so too in 'hereditary cerebral haemorrhage with amyloidosis, Dutch type', which is caused by a mutation within the APP gene and which is characterised by the accumulation of $\beta$-amyloid in the brain, is there evidence that the A$\beta$ protein is produced from both the abnormal and the normal APP molecules (Gajdusek 1994). This suggests that the A$\beta$, or a pathological pre-amyloid molecule, is recruiting or corrupting normal molecules in a manner that bears some similarities to the crucial pathological process of prion disease. Furthermore, small numbers of A$\beta$ plaques have been found in the brains of middle-aged monkeys injected with human AD brain tissue, but not in those injected with other sorts of brain tissue, nor in age-matched controls (Baker *et al.* 1994).

# Common mechanisms of neurodegeneration in CNS disease

## Intracellular inclusions

From the analysis of pathology in Huntington's disease and related expanded trinucleotide repeat diseases, the formation of neuronal intranuclear inclusions that are toxic to neurones suggested a common mechanism of neurodegenerative insult. By contrast, the specific proteins that include the polyglutamine expansion will determine the particular nuclear targets and the pattern of clinical disorder that are affected in each particular disease.

Recently this principle has been expanded to apply

more generally to a broad range of neurodegenerative diseases of adulthood as reviewed in this chapter. Thus, AD appears to be attributable to the intraneuronal accumulation of aggregates of tau to form neurofibrillary tangles and/or the extraneuronal accumulation of A$\beta$-amyloid to form senile plaques, throughout the brain but in particular in the higher level association centres of the neocortex and limbic system. PD involves the intracytoplasmic development of Lewy bodies from the aggregation of normal and mutant forms of $\alpha$-synuclein, in particular in the substantia nigra, but involving other basal forebrain nuclei as well. Lewy body formation in other centres, such as the neocortex, presumably by an accumulation of $\alpha$-synuclein also, yields other distinctive patterns of dementia. Prion diseases result in accumulation and transformation of normal to abnormal conformations of the PrP that self-aggregate to generate toxic complexes leading to vacuolar degeneration.

All of these diseases involve an abnormal deposition of a normally occurring protein that may suggest a common mechanism of toxicity (Lansbury 1998). In each case, the particular proteins produce distinctive pathological formations and affect different populations of neurones to form distinctive profiles of neurological symptoms. However, there may be a common pathogenic mechanism at heart whereby under certain conditions particular proteins (tau, amyloid, PrP, $\alpha$-synuclein, huntingtin) can become transformed into a form that will self-aggregate and be deposited. These aggregates not only form toxic complexes in cells but can additionally act as a seed for the for the further transformation of other normal proteins into the self-aggregating form. Thus the initial transformation, once it starts, results in a positive-feedback process involving aggregation of toxic complexes, followed by the recruitment and transformation of other normal molecules into the toxic cascade. Thus, Lansbury proposes that a wide range of chronic brain diseases, including AD, PD, prion disease, and the trinucleotide repeat diseases including HD and SCA, may all involve a similar pathological process in which protein polymerisation is endogenously seeded to produce intracellular or extracellular aggregates that are toxic to neurones, resulting in neuronal cell death and consequent neurodegenerative disease.

Although very recent at the time of writing, this hypothesis opens completely new avenues for therapy, making the seed the therapeutic target, and opening the way for new prophylactic, as opposed to symptomatic, treatments.

# Further reading

Markesbury, W.R. (ed.) (1998). *Neuropathology of Dementing Disorders*. Arnold, London.

Harper, P.S. (1996). *Huntington's Disease*. (2$^{nd}$ edn). W.B. Saunders, London.

Huber, S.J. and Cummings, J.L. (1992). *Parkinson's Disease: Neurobehavioural Aspects*. Oxford University Press, New York.

# Section II
## Damage limitation

# 7 | *Neuroprotection*

The introductory chapters of this volume introduced the primary mechanisms of cell death in the nervous system. Excitoxic damage, metabolic imbalance, oxidative stress, and calcium influx are each capable of inducing cell death by both necrotic and apoptotic mechanisms. If these various mechanisms contribute, separately and together, to neurodegeneration, then a rational strategy for treatment must be to search for ways of blocking the individual components of the cascade that leads to death. The last decade has seen active development of pharmaceutical strategies targeted at each major component of this cascade.

## *Calcium antagonists*

One of the major events in the cycle of excitotoxicity and cell death is the influx of calcium, and the consequent imbalance of intracellular homeostasis leading to cell death. This is particularly true in stroke, where calcium imbalance has been seen to provide an important component in the development and spread of the penumbral damage (see: Chapter 3; Morley *et al.* 1994). Consequently, pharmacological inhibition of calcium influx has provided a major target for neuroprotection, in particular against ischaemic injury. Since calcium influx triggers both apoptotic and necrotic processes of cell death, strategies to inhibit toxic rise in intracellular calcium levels, either by blocking its influx or by promoting binding and export, may be neuroprotective against both classes of mechanism. Calcium enters cells in ischaemic brain largely via glutamate-gated and voltage-gated channels. The NMDA channel opens in response to a combination of glutamate and cellular depolarisation, admitting calcium directly into the cell. Since ischaemic neurones are both depolarised and exposed to high levels of glutamate, NMDA channels have been a major focus of efforts to achieve neuroprotection. Of the other glutamate-activated channels, those kainate receptors that include the GluR4 subunit, also permit the passage of calcium. The other major route by which calcium can enter depolarised neurones

is via voltage-gated calcium channels, which will tend to be open in ischaemic neurones that are depolarised both by changes in the ionic composition of their intracellular and extracellular fluid, and by the action of glutamate.

## Anti-excitotoxic treatments

The first and earliest treatments for neuroprotection were targeted against excitotoxic damage of cells. If endogenous release of glutamate from excitatory nerve terminals can trigger cell death by overstimulation of their post-synaptic targets, then perhaps a receptor antagonist may be able to ameliorate the major deleterious effects of excess glutamate. We saw in Chapter 3 that calcium influx through the NMDA receptor in particular has been implicated in excitotoxic cell death, and the NMDA antagonist MK-801 was the first major antagonist to be explored for neuroprotective capacity.

## MK-801

The first demonstrations of the neuroprotective actions of the NMDA antagonist MK-801 came from tissue-culture models, in which neuronal death was induced either by applying glutamate directly, or in which anoxia and glucose withdrawal were used to trigger neuronal death. MK-801 (dizocilpine) blocks the toxicity of exogenously applied glutamate or glutamate agonists. Thus, for example, when cerebellar granule cells in culture are deprived of glucose for 40 min, they become sensitive to (and are killed by) micromolar concentrations of glutamate. This toxicity was completely blocked in the presence of 20 nM MK-801 (Lysko *et al.* 1989). By contrast, antagonists with selectivity for other classes of glutamate receptor are without effect.

The protective effects of MK-801 against exogenous excitotoxicity also work *in vivo*. Foster and colleagues (1988) injected four different excitatory amino acids — NMDA, quinolinic acid, kainic acid, or AMPA — stereotaxically into the neostriatum to induce 60–80% loss of striatal neurones, as measured by assays for the

GABA synthesising enzyme GAD (as an index of loss of the medium spiny striatal neurones) and of the ACh synthesising enzyme ChAT (as a marker for the giant cholinergic neurones of the striatum). Different groups of animals were either pretreated with peripheral injections of MK-801 prior to the lesion, or given the injections from 1 to 24 h after the lesion. As shown in Fig. 7.1, not only did pretreatment with MK-801 provide almost total protection against the toxicity induced by quinolinic acid or NMDA, but the effects were apparent even when the drug was administered up to 5 h after lesion. The receptor specificity of neuroprotection was apparent in the fact that whilst fully effective against excitatory amino acids acting at the NMDA receptor (quinolinic acid and NMDA itself), it was completely ineffective when toxicity was induced by excitatory amino acids acting at the other two main classes of glutamate receptor (kainic acid and AMPA).

## Other NMDA antagonists and neuroprotection in ischaemia

Given the primary importance of NMDA-receptor mediated processes in the generation of damage in the anoxic/ischaemic brain (see Chapter 3), it is not surprising that NMDA antagonists are also potent neuroprotective agents against stroke in experimental animals. This was first demonstrated for transient global ischaemia using the antagonist 2-aminophosphonoheptanoic acid, in the study by Simons *et al.* (1984). A similar strategy can also be neuroprotective in focal ischaemia. For example, George *et al.* (1988) administered injections of the NMDA antagonist, dextromorphan, to rabbits 1 h prior to occlusion of the medial

cerebral artery and demonstrated protection of cortical and striatal neurones that would otherwise degenerate. Such results have been widely replicated in many subsequent studies using a wide range of NMDA antagonists and in a wide variety of ischaemic models

Of particular interest is the fact that such drugs can work when administered during a period following the ischaemic episode, as well as in the situation of experimental pretreatment. For example, Boast *et al.* (1988) treated gerbils with two different competitive NMDA antagonists, *cis*-4-(phosphonomethyl)-2-piperidine carboxylic acid (CGS-19755) and 4-(3-phosphonopropyl)-2-piperazine carboxylic acid (CPP) prior to, or at various times following, transient global ischaemia. Motor activity was measured 1 and 4 days after treatment, following which the animals were perfused and the brains analysed for hippocampal damage on a five-point scale of pathology. CGS-19755 turned out to be the more neuroprotective compound. As shown in Fig. 7.2, CGS-19755 significantly reduced the gerbils' hyperactivity and the extent of hippocampal damage when administered 1 and 4 h after the occlusion. Small effects were even apparent when given after a 24-h delay.

The neuroprotective effects of NMDA antagonists, even when given several hours after onset of the ischaemic episode, suggests that the processes leading to cell death continue for some time, and opens up distinct opportunities for therapeutic intervention prior to the stage of irreversible damage. Certainly many neurones are killed rapidly by the initial influx of calcium after anoxia but other neurones die hours or days later, and it is presumably this latter population that are rescued by NMDA blockers administered after the anoxia has been relieved. When the circulation is restored, gluta-

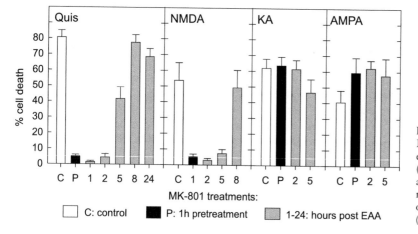

Fig. 7.1 The NMDA antagonist MK-801 blocks cell death induced by excitatory amino acid agonists (quisqualic acid or NMDA itself) that act primarily at the NMDA glutamate receptor, but not toxins acting at other (Kainic acid, AMPA) receptors. (Redrawn from Foster *et al.* 1988.)

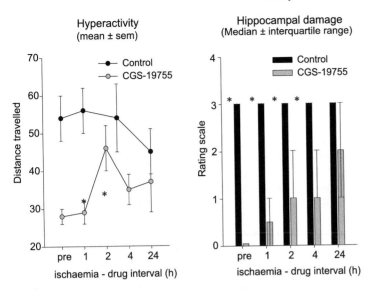

**Fig. 7.2** Treatment with the NMDA antagonist CGS-19755 can protect against behavioural and neurodegenerative consequences of ischaemia, even when given up to 4 h after the insult. (Data from Boast *et al*. 1988.)

mate levels, intracellular calcium levels, and membrane potentials and mitochondrial potentials rapidly return to normal levels. Yet NMDA blockade after this time will still reduce the subsequent degree of neuronal death. The implication is that calcium entering the cell after the period of explicit anoxia is also damaging. It is possible that some of the mechanisms responsible for potentiation of transmission may greatly increase calcium entry through NMDA channels following the massive depolarisation that occurs during anoxia. Thus, normal brain activity will lead to massive calcium entry through these greatly potentiated synapses, leading to neuronal damage. Raised arachidonic acid levels, increased protein kinase C activity, and increased production of NMDA channels may all contribute to this potentiation.

## Blockers of voltage-gated calcium channels

The term 'calcium-channel antagonist' is usually taken to apply to blocking $Ca^{2+}$ through specific voltage-gated calcium channels. A variety of different channel subtypes has been identified on the basis of pharmacological properties, of which the P, N, Q, and R channels are of particular relevance in the central nervous system (Hunter 1997). The other major routes of calcium influx, described in this chapter and elsewhere, are the glutamate-gated NMDA channels and kainate channels, which include the GluR4 subunit.

In the light of the clear association of excitotoxicity with calcium influx, early *in vitro* studies focused on the ability of broadly acting calcium-channel antagonists, such as nifedipine and nimodipine, to block cell death induced by application of excitotoxic amino acids on cultured neurones, with mixed success (Hunter 1997). These mixed results may be due to the fact that excitotoxicity itself involves a convergence of different processes, only some of which are responsive to treatment with calcium antagonists. Thus, for example, cortical and cerebellar cell cultures respond to NMDA agonists or low oxygen by exhibiting both an acute swelling mediated by influx of $Na^+$, $Cl^-$, and water (which is blocked by reducing extracellular levels of calcium), and a delayed response that correlates with uptake of radioactive $^{45}Ca$ (Goldberg and Choi 1993). It is only this delayed component that may be blocked by nifedipine or nimodipine (Madden *et al*. 1990; Weiss *et al*. 1990). More recently, these broadly acting calcium-channel antagonists, have been supplemented by compounds that are more selective at individual calcium-channel subtypes, and as yet the preliminary studies on their individual profiles of selective uptake blockade have not yet been complemented by detailed analysis of their neuroprotective capacities (Hunter 1997).

Perhaps contrary to expectation, further progress has been achieved *in vivo*. Thus, for example, calcium-channel antagonists can block the degeneration associated with excitotoxic lesions. Luiten *et al*. (1995) gave nimodipine mixed in the normal lab food over 2 weeks before inducing excitotoxic lesions of the basal forebrain cholinergic system by injection of NMDA unilaterally into the basal forebrain of rats. As shown in Fig. 7.3, nimodipine induced a partial, but significant

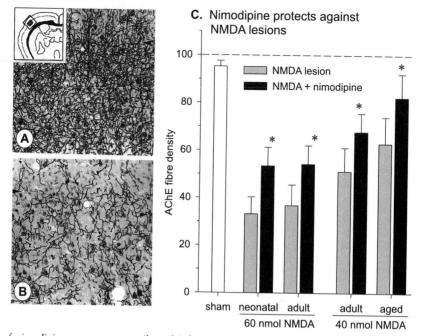

**Fig. 7.3** Effects of nimodipine treatment on unilateral infusions of NMDA into young and adult (60-nmole dose), and into adult and aged (40-nmole dose) rats. The loss of cortical innervation was quantified microscopically by counting AChE-positive fibres crossing a grid, in the cortex on the intact (A) and lesioned (B) sides. For analysis (C) the extent of innervation on the lesion side was expressed as a percentage ± s.d. of the intact contralateral side. Nimodipine was seen to provide a similar degree of protection at both doses of NMDA and at all ages. As an additional control, sham injections of saline induced minimal effect. (Data from Luiten *et al.* 1995.)

reduction in the loss of cholinergic fibres in the neocortex ipsilateral to the lesions, and the neuroprotective effect was apparent both at different lesion doses and at different ages from birth to old age.

Although this result appears relatively clear, there have been rather few direct *in vivo* studies of the effects of calcium-channel antagonism of excitotoxicity. By contrast, research in this area has concentrated on neuroprotection in models of ischaemia and, as reviewed by Hunter (1997), the results have been rather variable. Thus, whereas some studies using first generation calcium-channel antagonists have reported clear-cut neuroprotection against experimental ischaemia, there have been recurrent difficulties with failure to replicate. Hunter concludes that the differences between studies and the difficulties in observing consistent effects are not just due to wide variations in species (mice, rats, gerbils) and ischaemia models (focal lesions, most typically middle-cerebral artery occlusion, versus global ischaemia induced by bilateral carotid artery occlusion), and the use of a wide range of compounds with very different doses and routes of administration. The experimental studies are further confounded by the sys-

temic hypotension induced by many of these compounds, having indirect effects on cellular toxicity by changes in hypo- and hyperperfusion of affected areas, following treatment of the insult.

A clearer experimental picture may result from studies of recent generations of more specific calcium-channel antagonists, such as SB-201823, SB-206284, and SNX-111, which can inhibit calcium uptake via antagonism of specific calcium channels without additional effects on blood pressure and heart rate, at doses that are effectively neuroprotective *in vivo*. Moreover, such compounds have been used not just to demonstrate reduction in infarct volumes histologically (Bailey *et al.* 1995; Barone *et al.* 1995), but also to alleviate neurological and sensorimotor measures of deficit (Benham *et al.* 1993; Barone *et al.* 1995).

There have been a number of clinical trials in recent years of calcium-channel antagonists for stroke and other forms of cerebral vascular damage, although with little consistent success. However, the results of these trials, at least in stroke, have generally been disappointing (Wahlgren 1997) and the only application currently licensed is for the use of nimodipine in subarachnoid haemorrhage. However, as the contribution of different calcium-channel subtypes in the regulation of intracellular calcium balance becomes elucidated, and their different roles in ischaemia and other forms of neurodegeneration become clarified, it is likely that improved applications will develop based on new compounds with more selective profiles of action and lesser side-effects than was achieved with the first generation, which have proved more promising in theory than in practice.

## Free-radical scavengers and antioxidants

Oxidative stress to a cell, and the consequent extent of actual damage, is the result of a net imbalance between the generation and leakage of oxidant free radicals on the one hand and the capacity of the normal cellular metabolism and antioxidant scavenging machinery to remove any excess. Consequently, since normal metabolism continually creates free radicals, neurotoxicity and degeneration may be due as much to a degradation of the cells scavenging capacity as to an increase in endogenous or exogenous free radical load. Similarly, we may seek neuroprotective therapies by a combination of strategies designed to reduce free-radical production or exposure, and ones designed to enhance the antioxidant and scavenging capacity of cells.

A variety of strategies for neuroprotection based on reducing oxidative stress have been found to be effective, at the cellular level, and some of these have already shown promising results for application in clinical disease.

The first and most obvious strategy is the administration of free-radical scavenging agents. Scavengers react directly with the free radicals to neutralise their toxic actions on other oxidant species or biological molecules, as well as to inhibit chain reactions such as those involved in lipid peroxidation.

The cell's own defences include the generation of free-radical scavengers, notably the water soluble *ascorbic acid* (vitamin C) and the lipophilic α-*tocopherol* (vitamin E). Glutathione, as well as playing a role in the enzymatic metabolism of $H_2O_2$, also has the capacity in its reduced state to scavenge singlet oxygen and •OH⁻. A large number of naturally occurring antioxidant molecules are derived from the diet, in particular in fruits, which may be a major factor in the demonstrated relationship between diet and susceptibility to a wide range of neurodegenerative diseases (Ames *et al.* 1993).

A number of synthetic exogenous spin-trap agents with antioxidant activity are also available. For example, α-phenyl-*tert*-butyl-nitrone (PBN) reacts with oxygen radicals to form nitroxide radicals that are stable and hence non-toxic. PBN will therefore scavenge free radicals, it readily crosses the blood–brain barrier after peripheral administration, and has been shown to be protective in a variety of pathological situations (Novelli *et al.* 1985; Sen and Phillis 1993).

Other free-radical scavengers can inhibit lipid peroxidation. Within this class of compounds are the non-glucocorticoid steroids known as *lazaroids*, which are a novel class of 21-aminosteroids. Lazaroids appear to interact physically with membrane lipids, confine lipid radicals close to their site of production, and prevent radical diffusion through the cell membranes (Jacobsen *et al.* 1990; Hall 1997). The most widely studied of these compounds is tirilazad (or U-74006F), which has been found to be neuroprotective in a variety of pre-clinical neuroprotection models of ischaemia, and is the furthest advanced for application in clinical trails. Thus, for example, Park and Hall (1994) performed a systematic dose–response analysis of the degree of neuroprotection provided by tirilazad in a permanent unilateral middle-cerebral artery occlusion model in rats. Rats were given tirilazad at several different doses, by either the intravenous or intraperitoneal routes, and administered from 15 min to 6 h after the occlusion. Neurological function was rated on the following day prior to sacrifice and analysis of the degree of striatal and cortical degeneration. At the higher doses, and when administered soon after injury, tirilazad reduced the size of the cerebral infarct by 25–33%, and significantly reduced the scores on the test of neurological deficit. Subsequent studies using electron paramagnetic resonance imaging in gerbils suggests that the protection provided by tirilazad (as well as by hypothermia-induced neuroprotection) is mediated specifically by a reduction in the oxygen-based free-radical burden rather than on other components of the cellular response to ischaemic injury (Zhao *et al.* 1996).

Nevertheless, when a variety of global and focal ischaemia models are compared in different species, the results are not always consistent. As reviewed by Hall (1997), in general tirilazad is more effective for protection of cortical degeneration after focal ischaemia models than of the highly sensitive CA1 cells of the hippocampus after brief global ischaemia. Following the initial focus on stroke, subsequent studies have reported that tirilazad and other 21-aminiosteroids can be neuroprotective against other forms of acute neurological damage also, including spinal cord injury, fluid percussion or concussion head injury, subarachnoid haemorrhage, experimental allergic encephalitis (a model of human multiple sclerosis), and motor neurone degeneration (Hall 1997).

On the basis of these and many similar studies, tirilazad has now been subjected to phase II and phase III trials as a neuroprotective treatment for stroke in humans (Hall 1997). There have been two large double-blind multicentre trials, in Europe and North America, respectively (Peters *et al.* 1996; Scott *et al.* 1996), In both series, patients were treated over 3 days with 6 mg/kg/day tirilazad, commencing within 6h of the stroke episode. Although the drug treatment itself was well tolerated, no significant benefit was found for tirilazad in either study, either in terms of improvements in the neurological disability, or of measures of activities of daily living. Conversely, tirilazad has been found to provide beneficial protection in a trial restricted to subarachnoid haemorrhage (SAH; Kassell *et al.* 1996). In this study, involving a multinational collaboration between European, Australian, and New Zealand centres, alternative doses of tirilazad (0.6, 2, or 6 mg/kg/day) were compared, administered over 8–10 days starting within 48h of the SAH. In this study, the highest dose produced significant reductions in mortality after 3 months, and significant improvements in functional indices. Notably, there were clear sex differences, with male subjects benefiting more than females in achieving a beneficial outcome (see Fig. 7.4).

Lazaroids have also been shown to reduce cell degen-

eration following spinal cord and brain trauma in experimental animals (Braughler *et al.* 1989).

A second potential strategy for antioxidant therapy is to prevent the generation of toxic free radicals by promoting the action of the cellular enzymes superoxide dismutase, glutathione peroxidase, and catalase, responsible for limiting toxic free-radical generation. The potential efficacy of such a strategy is demonstrated in transgenic mice that overexpress several-fold the human Cu/Zn superoxide dismutase gene (Epstein *et al.* 1989). These mice exhibit an enhanced protection against traumatic, hypothermic, and ischaemic injury of the CNS.

*N-acetyl cysteine* (NAC) is a potent antioxidant and prevents apoptotic death of neuronal cells in a variety of *in vitro* systems (Ferrari *et al.* 1995). NAC appears to affect oxidative stress at several levels of action. It has a direct capacity to reduce reactive oxygen species (Aruoma *et al.* 1989). Moreover, it increases intracellular levels of glutathione and so increases the substrate for peroxidation of $H_2O_2$ (Meister 1988). In addition, it may directly interfere with apoptotic mechanisms of cell death by inhibiting DNA synthesis and regulation of the cell cycle (Ferrari *et al.* 1995).

Other mechanisms of free radical production in excitotoxic cell death include activation of calpain I and the conversion of xanthine dehydrogenase to form xanthine oxidase with the consequent generation of superoxide radicals. Calcium-induced activation of the phospholipase A2 and initiation of the arachidonic acid cascade can also result in the generation of reactive oxygen molecules during the metabolism of prostaglandins, leukotrienes and thromboxanes via the cycloxygenase

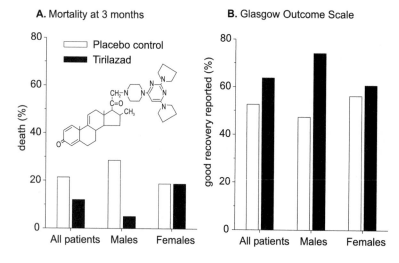

**Fig. 7.4**  Clinical trial of tirilazad in subarachnoid haemorrhage.: A Mortality as measured by percentage of deaths over the 3 month trial. B Functional outcome as measured by the widely used Glasgow coma rating scale. (Data from Kassell *et al.* 1996, as presented by Hall 1997.)

and lipoxygenase pathways, and release of iron from extravasated and clotted blood. Iron is a catalytic generator of hydroxyl radical and the initiating agent of injurious lipid-peroxidative reactions.

## Promotion of cellular metabolic efficiency

Along with generation of excitotoxic amino acids and free radicals, a third interacting component in the cycle of toxicity (as outlined in Chapter 3) is the impairment of mitochondrial energy production, whether in response to excitotoxic or other changes in cellular calcium, or as a primary target of metabolic toxins such as malonate, aminooxyacetic acid, 3-nitroproprionic acid, or MPP+. Consequently, a third strategy to neuroprotection is to seek strategies that enhance mitochondrial function. The most widely used pharmaceutical for this purpose is coenzyme $Q_{10}$, one of the substrates for mitochondrial electron transport (Fig. 7.5A). In animal experiments, coenzyme $Q_{10}$ can be administered in the food, and at doses of 200 mg/kg/day will provide substantial protection of striatal neurones in rats lesioned with local injections of the metabolic toxins aminooxyacetic acid (Brouillet *et al.* 1994) or

malonate (Fig. 7.5B; Schulz *et al.* 1996), and of striatal dopamine terminals when mice are lesioned by peripheral injections of MPTP (Schulz *et al.* 1995).

Neuroprotection at these different levels may be additive. Thus, Schulz *et al.* (1995, 1996) have employed the strategy of comparing inhibitors of glutamate release (such as lamotrigine or BW-1003C87), glutamate receptor antagonists (e.g. memantine), enhancers of mitochondrial function (e.g. coenzyme $Q_{10}$ or nicotinamide), and free-radical scavengers (such as the spin-trap agent, n-tert-butyl-$\alpha$-(2-sulfophenyl)-nitrone, S-PBN), singly and in combination (see Fig. 7.5).

Since the striatal cell death in Huntington's disease is believed to be related to an impairment in mitochondrial energy production similar to that induced by malonate (see Chapter 6; Browne *et al.* 1999), there is therefore now considerable interest on whether a similar strategy may work in patients. Initial safety studies indicate the good tolerability of both coenzyme $Q_{10}$, and another free-radical scavenger, OPC-14117 (Feigin *et al.* 1996; Shoulson *et al.* 1998), as well as of the glutamate NMDA receptor antagonist (Kieburtz *et al.* 1996a), in small groups of patients, but although suggestive these trials were too small to demonstrate efficacy. However, on the basis of these safety trials, a large multicentre clinical trial of neuroprotection in patients at early

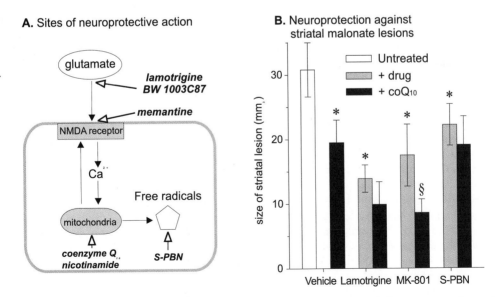

**Fig. 7.5** Dietary supplement with the mitochondrial electron transport substrate, coenzyme $Q_{10}$, protects against malonate toxicity. A Site of action of coenzyme $Q_{10}$ and other agents that can also offer neuroprotective action. B Coenzyme $Q_{10}$, protects against malonate toxicity following intrastriatal administration of this metabolic toxin. It can also enhance the actions of other neuroprotective agents, such as the NMDA antagonist, MK-801. *, p<0.01 in comparison to vehicle; §, p<0.05 of combined treatment in comparison to MK-801 alone. (Redrawn from Schulz *et al.* 1996.)

stages of the disease is now underway. The patients are now all recruited for this CARE-HD (Coenzyme Q$_{10}$ and remacemide evaluation in Huntington's disease) trial, but it will be another 2 years before the efficacy of these treatments, singly or in combination, will be known (Kieburtz 1999).

## Anti-apoptotic treatment

As described in Chapter 1, the apoptotic cascade is regulated by a cascade of genes and associated proteins of the ced-3/ICE family, now known as the 'caspases'. Inhibition of individual caspases and other apoptosis regulatory genes, such as bcl-2, may therefore provide a means to protect neurones against apoptotic death triggered by upstream changes, e.g. via excitotoxicity or calcium influx. Caspase inhibitors have now been shown to protect against apoptotic cell death in a wide variety of *in vitro* systems, as well as a growing number of *in vivo* models of neurological disease.

First, a variety of caspase inhibitors will protect against injury induced by acute experimental toxins. Thus, for example, intrastriatal injections of the caspase inhibitor zVAD-fmk protects striatal neurones from degeneration induced by intracerebral injections of malonate (Schulz *et al.* 1998). Moreover treatment of embryonic dopamine neurones *in vitro* with YVAD will enhance their survival following transplantation into the dopamine-deplete host brain (Schierle *et al.* 1999).

More naturally occurring insults occur in axotomy and ischaemia, and alternative caspase inhibitors are equally effective here. Thus, for example, de Bilbao and Dubois-Dauphin (1996) transected the facial nerve in developing mice to induce retrograde degeneration of facial motor neurones in the brainstem. Application of the ICE caspase inhibitor, YVAD-cho, reduced apoptotic cell death in the facial nucleus as evidenced by a 32% decline in TUNEL-labelled cells in the treated mice. Similarly, degeneration of retinal ganglion cells induced by ischaemia resulting from transiently raised intraocular pressure, and demonstrated to be due to an apoptotic mechanism by TUNEL staining, is substantially reduced when the rats are treated with a variety of caspase inhibitors, including TVAD and YVAD (Lam *et al.* 1999). YVAD will also induce increased sprouting and axon regeneration in retinal ganglion cells following axotomy (Lucius and Sievers 1997).

Caspase inhibitors can also protect against the slow neuronal death induced by ischaemia. Thus, Himi and colleagues (1998) used the general irreversible caspase inhibitor zDCB substantially to reduce the slow death of CA1 neurones in the hippocampus over 4–8 days after transient bilateral carotid artery occlusion in the gerbil. Again, to be effective, intracerebral delivery was required, given in three injections directly into the hippocampus, 0 12 and 24 h after the insult. Not only was the treatment effective in atrophy and pyknotic staining of hippocampal neurones at 4 days, and overt loss of neurones at 8 days after the insult (Fig. 7.6A), but it also substantially alleviated the animals' deficits in both step-down and step-through versions of the passive avoidance test of one-trial learning (Fig. 7.6B).

One recent result of particular interest is the demonstration that inhibition of caspase-1 can protect against the development of abnormal pathology and neurological phenotype in a transgenic model of Huntington's disease (Ona *et al.* 1999). The R6/2 strain of mice that overexpress exon 1 of the huntingtin gene, including an expanded CAG trinucleotide repeat, was described in Chapter 6. This mouse exhibits a progressive brain atrophy, the development of neuronal intranuclear inclusions, and a neurological phenotype involving a broad range of developing motor impairments before a precipitous weight loss and death at around 13–17 weeks of age (Mangiarini *et al.* 1996; Davies *et al.* 1997; Carter *et al.* 1999). The Ona *et al.* (1999) study provided three distinct findings. First, raised levels of caspase-1 were observed in both HD brain and the brains of R6/2 mice, suggesting an apoptotic component in cellular pathology. Second, HD mice were cross-bred with caspase-1 knockout mice, and it was found that in the caspase-deficient brain, the HD mice showed later development of neuronal inclusions and astrocytic pathology, dramatically reduced deficits on a rotarod test of motor co-ordination, and a delayed weight loss and increased longevity of the mice (Fig. 7.7A). Third, R6/2 mice were treated by intracerebral infusion of the caspase 1 inhibitor, ZVAD-fmk, and it was found that again the mice improved rotarod performance and delayed mortality (Fig. 7.7B). Together these data not only corroborate a clear role for apoptotic mechanisms in cell death, but also suggest that it may be possible to develop anti-apoptotic therapies, not only to treat acute insults but also to protect against slow progressive degeneration in neurological disease.

## Anti-inflammatory treatment

One of the mechanisms implicated in neuronal cell death after stroke and head injury is inflammation. In

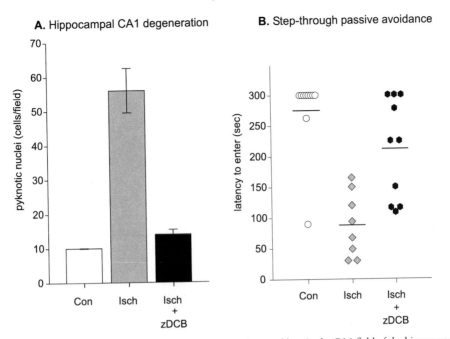

**Fig. 7.6** The caspase inhibitor zDCB protects against ischaemia. A Neuronal loss in the CA1 field of the hippocampus. B Latency to re-enter the chamber in which the animal had received foot-shock 24 h earlier in the step-through passive avoidance test. (Data from Himi *et al.* 1998.)

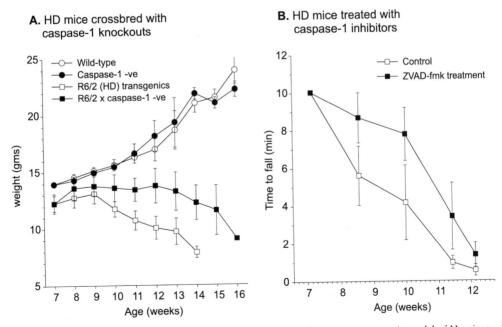

**Fig. 7.7** Caspase-1 inhibition blocks progression of the neurological progression in a transgenic model of Huntington's disease (HD). A Cross-breeding HD transgenic mice with caspase-1 knockouts mice indicates that the caspase-1 double negative reduces weight loss and premature death in the HD mice. B Direct intracerebral injections of the caspase inhibitor zVAD reduces motor deficits on a rotarod test in HD transgenic mice. (Data from Ona *et al.* 1999.)

the complex series of events that lead to the production of toxic molecules by inflammatory processes, there are many potential points for intervention. Successful treatments in experimental ischaemia models have been:

- blockade of adhesion molecules responsible for neutrophil recruitment, particularly with antibodies to ICAM-1;

- neutrophil depletion prior to the ischaemic insult;

- prevention of the effects of the inflammatory mediator IL-1, using specific inhibitors or antibodies;

- deletion of the gene for interferon regulatory factor 1, a transcription factor involved in the co-ordination of the expression of inflammation-related genes;

- inhibitors of the enzyme cyclooxygenase-2, which produces superoxide and toxic prostanoids.

Of these treatments, anti-ICAM-1 antibodies have reached clinical trial, but like other treatments that have shown promise in animal models, no effect was seen in human stroke patients.

## Experience of neuroprotective therapies in human patients

The sad fact is that although many treatments, as outlined in this chapter, have shown considerable efficacy in animal models of focal and general ischaemia, and in head-injury models, none of those tested in stroke or head injury in human patients have been proven to have a consistently beneficial effect. Other than lysis of thrombus that is blocking blood vessels with infusion of tissue plasminogen activator or urokinase, there is no approved neuroprotective treatment that can be given to patients in the immediate aftermath of a stroke or head injury. Considering the enormous investment of effort and money in the development of neuroprotective treatments, it is depressing to have to write that the treatment of acute insults to the CNS is still largely bed-rest and symptomatic therapy, followed by physio-therapy in the aftermath. Since so many treatments have shown such promise in animal models, how can it be that all have failed in therapeutic trials? There are various possibilities:

1. *Fundamental differences between animal models and humans.* The human and rodent brain are dis-

similar in many respects. A major difference is one of size. The primary theoretical focus of neuroprotective treatments is to preserve the neurones in the penumbra region, which are affected by the insult but not immediately killed. In rodents, the size of the penumbra is well-established, at around 0.5 cm, which represents a large proportion of the rat cortex. In humans, the existence of a penumbra has not been directly proven. Moreover, there is no particular reason to expect the penumbra to increase in size with increasing brain size. Preserving neurones in a 0.5-cm penumbra in humans would preserve only a small part of the cortex, and have little functional impact, while a penumbra of the same size in rodents represents a much greater proportion of the brain, and therefore should have more influence on functional outcome. There are also differences in the collateral circulations in humans and rodents, which may effect the response to ischaemia.

2. *Concentrations of drugs.* Some neuroprotective drugs have psychomimetic, cardiovascular, and other side-effects, which limit the dose that can be given to patients. In addition, it is likely that the drugs do not reach even these concentrations in ischaemic areas of the brain. Some drugs may, therefore, have seemed ineffective due to inadequate dosage.

3. *Timing of administration.* Some of the neuroprotective drugs have proven to be effective even when given to animals some time after the ischaemic insult. However, the effectiveness is almost always greatest if the drug is given at the time of, or before, ischaemia, with declining effectiveness thereafter. In human patients it is usually not clear when the ischaemia started, only when they first complained of symptoms. Drugs may, therefore, often have been given too late.

4. *Design of trials.* Stroke in human patients may affect many different parts of the CNS, and produce lesions of widely varying size. The outcome of a stroke or head injury is rather unpredictable at the time of admission, and there is therefore enormous variability in the disability that patients will eventually experience. Given this variability of outcome, only a drug with very major effects could be expected to show efficacy. On the other hand, animal models have been refined to give very repeatable lesions and infarcts, so that drug effects are more readily seen.

Given these difficulties, it may not be surprising that it has so far been impossible to prove efficacy in the many drugs that have reached phase III trials. It is possible that some of the drugs that have failed were effective, but not sufficiently so to show statistically significant effects in the trials that have been performed. The future must lie not only in new compounds, but also in designing trials in which the patient's neurological damage is more closely standardised using MRI and PET imaging, and in which the variability of outcome is therefore reduced.

## Neuroprotection in Parkinson's disease

Since the neurodegenerative process in PD is likely to involve a cascade of inter-related events — oxidative stress, mitochondrial dysfunction, excitotoxicity with excess formation of •NO and $O_2^-$, and inflammatory changes, leading to both apoptotic and necrotic cell death (see Chapter 6; Dunnett and Björklund 1999) — strategies directed towards reducing the oxidative stress on dopamine neurones have been a major target for study. Since the dopamine neurones are likely to be dysfunctional for a period — perhaps for years — before they are irreversibly damaged, both neurotrophic and anti-apoptotic agents may be used to prevent delayed cell death and/or restore function.

As outlined above, there are two basic strategies to reduce oxidative stress: the reduction of free radical formation, and the enhancement of free radical scavenging mechanisms; although in practice these often overlap. The different points of intervention can be identified if we consider the two basic pathways by which dopamine and other products of cellular processing are metabolised and neutralised (see Fig. 7.8; Dunnett and Björklund 1999). Enzymatic oxidation of dopamine by monoamine oxidase produces hydrogen peroxide (1), which under normal circumstances in intact neurones is converted by glutathione peroxidase to water (2). However, in the presence of excess iron, dopamine can also generate the highly toxic hydroxyl ion by the

Fenton reaction (3). Excess dopamine can also be auto-oxidised to generate superoxide (4), which may be neutralised by the enzyme superoxide dismutase (5) but which in the presence of high levels of nitric oxide also generates further toxic hydroxyl ions (6). The toxic consequences of excess free radical production will be reduced to the extent that we can promote processing down pathways generating the normal, rather than the highly toxic, end-products (see Fig. 7.8). To this end, a variety of metabolic and pharmacological strategies are under investigation

The neutralisation of hydrogen peroxide holds a key point of convergence in the ability of the cells to handle free radicals, and so a first strategy must be to seek its detoxification by shifting the balance from pathway (3) to (2), enhancing peroxidation and limiting the availability of free iron to catalyse the Fenton reaction.

*Promoting glutathione peroxidase activity.* One side of this balance is by promoting effective peroxidation, increasing activity of the enzyme glutathione peroxidase or increasing levels of the glutathione substrate. Thus, for example, addition of glutathione peroxidase to the medium can enhance the survival of dopamine cells in culture, in particular under high concentrations of oxygen (Fig. 7.9; Colton *et al.* 1995). This same study found an even greater effect by treatment with N-acetyl cysteine (NAC), a precursor of glutathione that has antioxidant properties by increasing the substrate for neutralisation of hydrogen peroxide by endogenous glutathione peroxidase. Moreover, NAC almost completely blocks the toxicity of dopamine when applied to cultured rat forebrain neurones (Hoyt *et al.* 1997).

*Inhibiting iron.* The other side of this equation is to reduce the metabolism of hydrogen peroxide by inhibiting the Fenton reaction (pathway (3) in Fig. 7.8). This reaction involves the transformation of $Fe^{3+}$ to $Fe^{2+}$ in the formation of the highly toxic hydroxyl ion, to which the neurones of the substantia nigra may be particularly susceptible by virtue of their high iron content associated with neuromelanin granules. Indeed, there is a higher level of interaction between iron and melanised dopamine neurones in the parkinsonian than in the control substantia nigra. This has led to the suggestion that iron chelators, such as deferoxamine, which inhibit lipid peroxidation, may be neuroprotective in Parkinson's disease (Ben-Shachar *et al.* 1992; Olanow 1997).

The alternative pathway for generation of the highly toxic hydroxyl ion is by conversion of excess superoxide arising from auto-oxidation of dopamine. Again, there are two outcomes: superoxide may be neutralised by

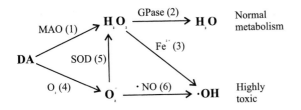

**Fig. 7.8** Role of dopamine and its metabolites in free radical formation (see text for details). (From Dunnett and Björklund 1999.)

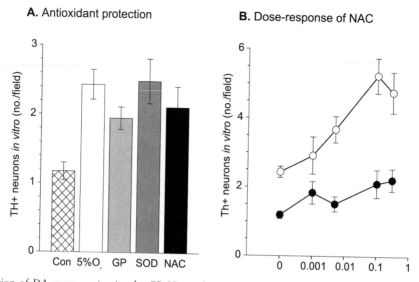

**Fig. 7.9** Protection of DA neurones *in vitro* by GP, N-acetyl cysteine (NAC), and superoxide dismutase (SOD). (Data from Colton *et al.* 1995.)

superoxide dismutase (pathway (5) in Fig. 7.8), or it may combine with •NO to form peroxynitrite, which then decomposes to form the highly toxic •OH hydroxyl radical (pathway (6) in Fig. 7.8; Jenner 1998). Consequently, we may expect effective neuroprotection to result if we can switch the balance towards the former pathway by promoting superoxide dismutase (SOD) activity and /or inhibiting the peroxynitrite reaction.

*Promoting SOD activity.* If we can increase SOD activity, then this might enhance the metabolism of superoxide down non-toxic pathways. A number of strategies have been attempted to increase SOD activity *in vivo*. First, transgenic mice have been generated that overexpress human Cu/Zn SOD. Nigral cells derived from transgenic embryos show improved survival *in vitro* under suboptimal culture conditions, and these same cells survive transplantation better than grafts derived from control mice (Nakao *et al.* 1995). Moreover, whereas intraventricular injections of 6-OHDA in normal mice result in both shrinkage and loss of dopaminergic cells in the substantia nigra, along with massive loss of dopaminergic terminals and atrophy in the striatum, all of these neurodegenerative effects of the toxin were largely abolished when 6-OHDA was injected similarly into transgenic mice (Asanuma *et al.* 1998).

Whereas the studies in transgenic mice provide proof of principle, it is more difficult to upregulate SOD activity pharmacologically. However, one strategy that may

prove effective is by using viruses to transfer the SOD gene into the cells that require protection. The technology for *ex vivo* and *in vivo* gene transfer is described fully in a later chapter (Chapter 26). Barkats *et al.* (1996) used adenoviral vectors to insert the human SOD gene into rat striatal neurones in culture. The infected cells expressed the SOD gene for at least 48 h, and they were totally resistant to glutamate excitotoxicity at a dose that killed over 50% of uninfected cells.

*Inhibiting NO formation.* Formation of •NO, the essential substrate for the peroxynitrite reaction, is regulated by the enzyme nitric oxide synthase (NOS), and formation of peroxynitrite may therefore be blocked if NOS activity is inhibited. Thus, transgenic mice with knock-out of the gene for neuronal NOS, show markedly reduced death of dopaminergic neurones in response to injections of the pyridinium ion MPTP (Przedborski *et al.* 1996). Moreover, in rats, the selective NOS inhibitor 7-nitroindazole (7-NI) and the non-selective inhibitor l-NAME have both been seen to block hydroxyl ion formation and reduce toxicity in rats treated with the pyridinium ion MPP+ or 6-OHDA (Jenner 1998). Thus, for example, Hantraye and colleagues have examined the efficacy of 7-NI to alleviate the MPTP-induced parkinsonism in baboons. As shown in Fig. 7.10, the 7-NI pretreatment entirely blocked the loss of striatal dopamine, which is induced by MPTP in control monkeys, and in parallel reversed not only the

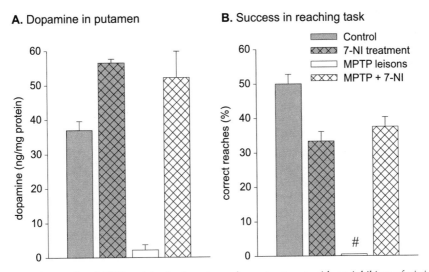

**Fig. 7.10** Neuroprotection against MPTP toxicity in the primate by pretreatment with an inhibitor of nitric oxide synthase (NOS). In four groups of baboons, two groups received subacute injections of MPTP. One control group and one MPTP treated group also received twice daily injections of the NOS inhibitor, 7-nitroindazole, starting the day before treatment. A 7-NI protects against MPTP-induced loss of dopamine from the putamen. B 7-NI pretreatment alleviated the MPTP-induced deficit in a barrier reaching task. (Data from Hantraye *et al.* 1996.)

animals' hypokinesia but also the lesion induced deficits in a complex barrier reaching motor task.

*Other antioxidants.* Vitamin E has long been considered to have general antioxidant properties. In particular, the biologically active component of vitamin E, α-tocopherol (Halliwell and Gutteridge 1985), can attenuate the effects of lipid peroxidation by trapping free radicals. This provided the foundation for one arm of a major clinical trial of neuroprotection in Parkinson's disease — the 'DATATOP' study (see Chapter 6). The other arm involved treatment with the monoamine oxidase B inhibitor, deprenyl, which blocks conversion of MPTP to MPP+ and dramatically limits its toxicity in experimental primates. Therefore, the trial asked whether deprenyl, tocopherol, or both together, could slow the progression of the disease when given long-term, starting early in the disease prior to the stage where severity of disability required initiation of L-DOPA therapy. An interim report 3 years into the study found that the deprenyl treatment produced a highly significant slowing of the disease progression and that fewer treated patients have given up work, irrespective of whether or not they also received tocopherol (Parkinson's Study Group 1993). However, subsequent studies failed to confirm the dramatic nature of the benefit of deprenyl in the initial report and suggested significant side-effects of the deprenyl treatment (Le Witt 1994; Lees 1995). Indeed, since deprenyl can itself have direct symptomatic effects, a neuroprotective mechanism of any beneficial action is further thrown into doubt (Dunnett and Björklund 1999). Notwithstanding the focus on the monoamine oxidase inhibition, there was no demonstrable neuroprotective effects of the antioxidant arm of the trial using tocopherol.

## Summary

Cell death in the nervous system can be induced by a variety of mechanisms: excitotoxicity, metabolic compromise, free radical toxicity and oxidative stress, and raised intracellular calcium, which can all, singly and in combination, induce cells to die by an active apoptotic process. Effective neuroprotection can be provided by antagonising each of these mechanisms using a variety of molecular and pharmaceutical strategies — blocking release or receptor activation of excitatory amino acids; scavenging free radicals; promoting mitochondrial energy production; mopping up excess calcium — as well as by inhibitors of the downstream apoptotic cascade itself. Each strategy can prove effective under appropriate precipitating conditions, and there are examples where each is currently under investigation for clinical application in conditions as diverse as stroke, trauma, and particular neurodegenerative diseases.

Nevertheless, most clinical neuroprotection pro-grammes to date have not proved dramatically effective. It is now necessary to recognise the diverse range of mechanisms that can apply and feed back on each other, which implies that future strategies must not only attempt to characterise in detail the particular mecha-nisms of cell death that apply in any particular disease condition, but also develop effective combinations of neuroprotective therapy that block the cycle and cascade of interacting processes that converge on cell death. In addition, given the numbers of potential pre-cipitating conditions in any particular context, it is likely that considerable advances are still to be made in particular in inhibition of the final common pathway of cell death, i.e. inhibitors of the apoptotic cascade itself.

## Further reading

Green, A.R. and Cross, A.J. (1997). *Neuroprotective Agents and Cerebral Ischaemia*. Academic Press, San Diego.
Dimagl, U., Iadecola, C., and Moskowitz, M.A. (1999) Patho-biology and ischaemic stroke: an integrated view. *Trends in Neuroscience*, **22**, 391–397.

# 8 | Steroids

## By Joe Herbert

The adrenal cortex secretes a wide range of steroids. Nearly all attention has been focused on the role in brain damage of cortisol (or corticosterone, its counterpart in some species). Only recently have the powerful effects on neural function of other adrenal-derived steroids been recognised.

## Control of cortisol levels

The secretion of cortisol (or corticosterone — the following applies to both) is highly labile. There are marked diurnal variations: highest levels coincide with the start of activity, irrespective of when that occurs (e.g. in the early morning in humans, but at the start of the night in rats and other nocturnal species) (Krieger *et al.* 1971). Since the response of corticoid-sensitive tissues (such as the brain) is a function of their exposure to hormone across time, the shape of the diurnal rhythm is important. So, therefore, is the time at which blood or other samples are taken for assay. Stress, a general term encompassing a variety of states of unusual demand, reliably raises cortisol levels (Munck *et al.* 1984). Though cortisol is by no means the only hormone to react to stress, it does respond to a remarkably wide range of both physical and psychological events (Herbert 1987). Persistent stress-induced hypercortisolaemia will, therefore, result in exposure of tissues to higher levels of steroid; it may also result in loss of the diurnal rhythm, and thus the period of relatively low exposure. This may be equally important: there is evidence (mainly from other steroids such as oestrogen) that intermittent low tissue levels are a significant physiological event and important for the restoration of receptor levels.

### Entry of cortisol into the brain

Blood levels of cortisol are much higher than in the brain — or, more accurately, in the cerebrospinal fluid (csf), which is presumed to reflect levels in the brain extracellular fluid. The blood of most species (including humans) contains a protein, corticoid-binding globulin (CBG), that binds cortisol with relatively high affinity ($K_D \cong 20\,nM$), though with limited capacity (Westphal 1970). Serum albumin also binds corticoids, but with much lower affinity (though with greater capacity). Levels of bound and free cortisol are maintained in dynamic equilibrium, represented by the total amount of corticoid, and the amount of CBG occupied:

$$C + CBG \; [\leftrightarrow] \; CBG\text{-}C \qquad (8.1)$$

Under basal conditions, about 5% of total cortisol is in the free form. This is the amount that can pass across the blood–brain barrier into the brain (Baxter, and Tyrrell 1987). As blood levels begin to increase, the same relative proportion will remain free, so that the absolute amount of cortisol available to the brain rises steadily but proportionately. However, as soon as the binding capacity of CBG is exceeded, any additional cortisol will stay in the free condition, so that amounts passing into the brain rapidly and disproportionately increase (Herbert and Martinesz 1982). Thus, during states of acute or persistent hypercortisolaemia, the amount to which the brain is exposed cannot be determined solely from measuring total cortisol concentrations in the blood, but only by some estimate of the 'free' fraction.

Once it enters the brain, levels of cortisol are regulated by clearance from the cerebral compartment. Though information is limited, it seems that this is much slower from the brain than from the blood (Herbert 1989). So increased levels in the blood (or changes in the diurnal cortisol rhythm) will have disproportionate (magnified) effects on concentrations in the brain.

### Corticoid macromolecular receptors

Once within the brain, corticoids act on cytoplasmic receptors (De Kloet 1991; Funder 1992). These are proteins that are probably bound to heat-shock protein (hsp90) in the unactivated state. Corticoids bind to a specific region near the C-terminus, thereby dissociating the receptor from hsp90, and causing it to translocate to the nucleus. Here it dimerises, and binds to a consensus palindromic sequence on the genome (the glu-cocorticoid regulatory element — GRE) to act as a tran-scription regulator (Carlstedt-Duke *et al.* 1988). A considerable number of genes have GREs associated with their promoters. The brain contains at least two classes of receptors: 'mineralocorticoid' receptors (type 1 receptors or MR) have high affinity ($K_D \cong 0.5$ nM) for both mineralocorticoids, such as aldosterone, and glu-cocorticoids, such as cortisol or corticosterone (Herman *et al.* 1989). So-called glucocorticoid receptors (type 2 receptors or GR) have (paradoxically) lower affinity for glucocorticoids ($K_D \cong 5$ nM) and an even lower one for aldosterone. In some tissues, type 1 receptors may respond preferentially to mineralocorticoids because they contain an enzyme (11-$\beta$OH steroid dehydroge-nase) that converts cortisol to cortisone (which does not bind to MR) or a protein (similar to CBG) that sequesters glucocorticoid. An important point is that some synthetic glucocorticoids (e.g. dexamethasone) have a preferential affinity for GR, unlike the major naturally-occurring ones.

The relative affinities of GR and MR for glucocorti-coids means that under 'basal' conditions — particularly during the circadian trough — it seems likely that less than 20% of GRs are occupied. However, when brain levels of glucocorticoids are elevated (e.g. during stress, when the binding capacity of CBG may be exceeded) GRs will become more fully occupied. There may, there-fore, be a neuronal response, represented by GR, that is relatively specific for hypercortisolaemic conditions. GRs are found widely distributed in the brain, unlike the more restricted MRs.

## Experimental evidence for a role for corticoids in brain damage

Experimental and clinical evidence shows that high levels of cortisol or corticosterone can both induce brain damage and accentuate contemporary neurotoxic processes (Sapolsky 1992). Experimental studies have focused on the hippocampus, long known to contain high concentrations of both MR and GR. Giving pro-longed corticosterone to rats increases the age-related rate at which pyramidal neurones are lost. Chronic stress does likewise. Neonatal handling, which reduces subsequent stress responses, delays hippocampal degen-eration (Meaney *et al.* 1988). Corticoids also potentiate neurodegeneration induced by such agents as anoxia, glutamate analogues such as kainic acid, or cholinergic agents (adrenalectomy offers partial protection)

(Hortnagl *et al.* 1993). Similar effects are reported for cultured hippocampal neurones (Tombaugh *et al.* 1992). Prolonged exposure to high levels of circulating corticosterone in rats have been seen to increase the age-related rate at which hippocampal pyramidal neurones are lost (Sapolsky 1996; Sapolsky *et al.* 1985), and to induce atrophy of apical dendrites (Magarinos and McEwen 1995).

## Mechanisms of corticoid-induced brain damage

There are a number of ways in which increased corti-coids could enhance brain damage. It is not entirely clear why the hippocampus is so vulnerable to damage from toxic, ischaemic, or metabolic agents, though this has been related to its content of corticoid receptors and its ability to modify its structure and function (i.e. it's 'plas-ticity'; McEwen 1994). Detailed studies suggest that there are several distinct corticoid-dependent mecha-nisms that are additive in their effects. The re-uptake of glutamate by glial cells, which reduces perineuronal con-centrations, may be impaired by corticoids. As outlined in Chapter 3, glutamate analogues, such as NMDA, can damage neurones by increasing intracellular $Ca^{2+}$ levels and by generation of reactive oxygen species, and both of these effects are accentuated by corticoids (Chou *et al.* 1994; McIntosh and Sapolsky 1996).

Intact animals subjected to stress show increased levels of extracellular glutamate (Moghaddam 1993). Situations that result in increased corticoid levels may thus predispose to brain injury, either by a direct action or by potentiating other pathological processes. Since aged rats seem to have higher basal levels of corticos-terone (and show more prolonged hypercortisolaemic responses to stress), this may increase their vulnerabil-ity to brain damage. However, corticoids alter many other processes and genes, many of which could be implicated in brain damage or resistance to injury; these include regulating levels of neurotrophic molecules, such as FGF-2, NT3, NGF, and BDNF (Chao and McEwen 1994; Smith *et al.* 1995a; Mocchetti *et al.* 1996), as well as those implicated in apoptosis, such as bcl-2 (McCullers and Herman 1998). It is not at present clear whether one or more of these elements are pri-marily responsible either for the sensitivity of the hip-pocampus to the damaging effects of corticoids, or for the process whereby corticoids induce or enhance brain damage. Moreover, different mechanisms may be more prominent in specified circumstances.

## Neurogenesis in the hippocampus

The hippocampus has one extraordinary feature, which may well have a bearing on its vulnerability to damage and its sensitivity to steroids. Unlike other areas of the brain, active neurogenesis occurs in the dentate gyrus well into adult life (see Chapter 25). This, first described over 30 years ago by Altman and Das (1965), seems — like many other significant findings — to have been largely ignored until recently. Now, however, it is recognised that neurogenesis of both neurones and glia occurs in adulthood, not only in rats but also in monkeys and humans (Eriksson *et al.* 1998; Kornack and Rakic 1999). Furthermore, this process seems to be modulated both by NMDA receptors and glucocorticoids (Gould *et al.* 1991a,b; Cameron and Gould 1994). Stress (and age) reduces hippocampal neurogenesis (Fuchs and Flugge 1998). Conversely, adrenalectomy stimulates it (Montaron *et al.* 1999). Whether or how newly-formed neurones actually become part of the adult hippocampus, and what contribution they make to its function, is still unclear. However, if they are functional, neurogenesis offers an important avenue through which stress, the ageing process, and adrenal steroids can influence part of the brain known to be important for episodic and spatial memory, and which shows both environmental and age-related degeneration.

## Clinical evidence

Humans do not show a clear overall age-related change in either cortisol or CBG, although there are individual differences in the way that blood levels alter with age, and cortisol in the csf may increase in older people (Swaab *et al.* 1994; Guazzo *et al.* 1996). This has been related to age-dependent deficits in cognitive function (explicit memory and attention span) and reduced hippocampal volume (Lupien *et al.* 1994, 1998). There is also clinical evidence that corticoids may potentiate brain damage. Hypercortisolaemia is common after strokes (Olsson *et al.* 1992). There is a negative relation between post-infarct cortisol levels and both survival and functional recovery (Murros *et al.* 1993). The evening levels may be particularly significant; this is the time when cortisol is otherwise at its lowest. Thus the absence of this relatively cortisol-free interval may be important.

Depressive illness is associated with hypercortisolaemia in about 50% of cases, in both adults and adolescents, and may be one factor impeding recovery (Dolan *et al.* 1985; Goodyer *et al.* 1998). A high proportion of those with raised corticoids (e.g. Cushing's syndrome) are clinically depressed (Jeffcoate *et al.* 1979), and this mood disorder resolves when adrenal hypersecretion is corrected (Starkman *et al.* 1981). Giving glucocorticoids (e.g. prednisone) can induce mood disorders, predominantly depression (Lewis and Smith 1983). This suggests that raised corticoids may impair brain function in ways additional to actually inducing structural damage, though whether the two sets of effects are related is unknown. The longer term consequences of persistent hypercortisolaemia, such as that observed in some cases of depression, is also not known.

Resistance to the negative-feedback effects of dexamethasone may occur following stroke (Olsson *et al.* 1992). This is also seen in other conditions, notably major depressive disorder. Post-infarct depression has been linked to stroke-induced hypercortisolaemia (Åström *et al.* 1993). Since hyperglycaemia is also detrimental to recovery from stroke, there is debate over whether increased cortisol may contribute to this condition (O'Neill *et al.* 1988). If so, this might be one precipitating cause of the detrimental effects of cortisol on neural recovery. However, the experimental evidence clearly points to the possibility of a more direct adjunctive role for corticoids, though they may also interfere with glucose transport into neurones.

# *Neurosteroids*

Nearly all attention has been focused on cortisol. However, there is a second class of adrenal steroids, known for many years to endocrinologists, but only recently becoming of interest to neuroscientists. These are the so-called 'neurosteroids'.

Corticoids are formed from cholesterol, which is first metabolised to pregnenolone. At this point, biosynthesis can take two paths (Fig. 8.1). One leads to corticoids such as cortisol, corticosterone, and aldosterone (all C-21 steroids). The other leads to dehydroepiandrosterone (DHEA), a C-19 steroid, and thence to a series of compounds such as androstenedione (a weak androgen). DHEA is sulphated (mainly in the liver) to DHEAS (Labrie *et al.* 1994). So the blood contains both DHEA and DHEAS. DHEAS shows two remarkable properties. First, its concentration in the blood is about 10 times that of cortisol (itself one of the most abundant steroids). DHEA levels are about one-tenth those of cortisol. The second is that levels of DHEAS (and DHEA) decline steadily and profoundly with age (at about

10–20% per decade) (Barrett-Connor and Khaw 1990; Orentreich *et al.* 1992). DHEA levels also decline during certain illnesses, including major depression (Goodyer *et al.* 1996).

There is increasing interest in the possibility that the brain can make pregnenolone and (perhaps) DHEA from cholesterol, and thus that there may be local sources of these neuroactive compounds within the CNS (Akwa *et al.* 1991; Doostzadeh *et al.* 1997). Whether or not the adult brain can make DHEA is still debated.

## Effects on membrane-bound receptors

Neurosteroids have been shown to have a direct action on membrane-dependent events in the brain, such as the synaptic actions of GABA and glutamate (Majewska 1992). Both pregnenolone (sulphate) (P(S)) and DHEA(S) act as GABA antagonists, blocking $GABA_A$-stimulated chloride channels and inhibiting agonist (e.g. muscimol) and benzodiazepine binding. Conversely, these steroids potentiate the actions of glutamate (or its agonists), increasing depolarisation and

$Ca^{2+}$ entry. Only micromolar concentrations of steroid (e.g. $\cong 100\,\mu M$ or less) are needed, and the effects are seen *in vitro* only in the presence of GABA or glutamate (i.e. a true synergism; Majewska *et al.* 1988; Irwin *et al.* 1992). *In vivo*, DHEA and pregnenolone can depolarise neurones in the septum and pre-optic area (Carette and Poulain 1984), perhaps by accentuating endogenous glutamate or inhibiting GABA. However, these neuroactive steroids can also alter gene expression in the brain, a second (and more classical) mechanism of action (Rupprecht 1997).

An intriguing finding, in many ways comparable to the relation between glutamate and GABA, is that some of the later products of steroid biosynthesis have the opposite effect on membrane-bound receptors. For example, ring A-reduced metabolites of progesterone, DHEA, or cortisol (pregnenolone, androsterone, tetrahydrocortisol) potentiate $GABA_A$ activity (Harrison *et al.* 1987; Morrow *et al.* 1987; Lan *et al.* 1991). These compounds, however, are not major constituents of the blood, though they may be formed in peripheral tissues (including the brain).

## Anti-glucocorticoid actions of DHEA

As well as a direct role in neuromodulation, neurosteroids may have another, significant, role in brain damage. There is evidence that DHEA(S) can act as a potent anti-glucocorticoid. For example, it antagonises the immunosuppressant and lympholytic actions of cortisol (May *et al.* 1990; Blauer *et al.* 1991). Thus, circumstances in which DHEA(S) is lowered (e.g. during illness or as part of the ageing process), may result in relative increases in unopposed cortisol, and hence the neurotoxic effects described above.

## Entry into the brain: the effect of conjugation

Like any other steroid, the entry of DHEA(S) and P(S) from blood into the brain depends on their hydrophobicity. For the free steroids (DHEA), levels in csf are about 5% of those in plasma (i.e. comparable to cortisol). However, conjugation increases hydrophilicity. Penetration of DHEAS is, consequently, only about 0.2% that of blood levels (Guazzo *et al.* 1996). Bearing in mind the very high blood levels of DHEAS, this is an important consideration; the brain, may be (partially) protected against DHEAS. However, there is the suggestion that pregnenolone may be made in the brain itself (Corpechot *et al.* 1983). The enzymes required for cholesterol metabolism have been isolated from the

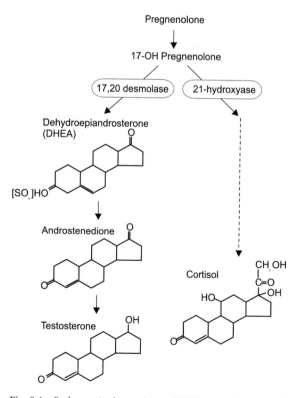

**Fig. 8.1** Pathways in the synthesis of C-21 corticoids (cortisol, corticosterone, and aldosterone) and C-19 neurosteroids (dehydroepiandrosterone, DHEA) from cholesterol.

brain, and levels in the rat brain have been reported to exceed those in the blood (Corpechot *et al.* 1993; Mellon and Deschepper 1993). If these findings are substantiated, a role for pregnenolone (and, perhaps, other neuromodulatory steroids) in brain damage or repair is further suggested by the enzyme (a cytochrome $P_{450}$) being abundant in astrocytes.

## Neurosteroids and brain damage

There is accumulating evidence that these neurosteroids may themselves contribute to brain damage or to the resilience of the brain to such damage. Pregnenolone may exacerbate NMDA-induced degeneration of hippocampal neurones (Weaver *et al.* 1998), but DHEA (and its sulphate, DHEAS) seem to be neuroprotective. DHEA and DHEAS can protect the hippocampus against the neurotoxic effects of both glutamate analogues and corticoids (Fig. 8.2; Kimonides *et al.* 1998; Mao and Barger 1998). Whether DHEA is the active agent, or whether locally-produced metabolites such as 7α-OH-DHEA (Akwa *et al.* 1992; Rose *et al.* 1997) will prove to be more potent, awaits further work.

The immediate early gene, *c-Jun*, in particular has been implicated in the response of neurones to injury, as part of both degenerative and restorative processes. Recently, a Jun kinase, SAPK/JNK, has been reported to phosphorylate *c-Jun* in striatal neuronal cultures following glutamate treatment (Schwarzschild *et al.* 1997). Immunohistochemical studies on the nuclear translocation of a range of stress activated protein kinases in hippocampal cultures showed that DHEA attenuated the activation of one, SAPK3, by corticosterone (Kimonides *et al.* 1999).

If DHEA (or its various metabolites) do prove to have significant brain-protective actions, then this clearly has considerable significance in the light of the marked (but individually variable) age-related decreases in the blood (and csf) levels of this group of steroids (Guazzo *et al.* 1996).

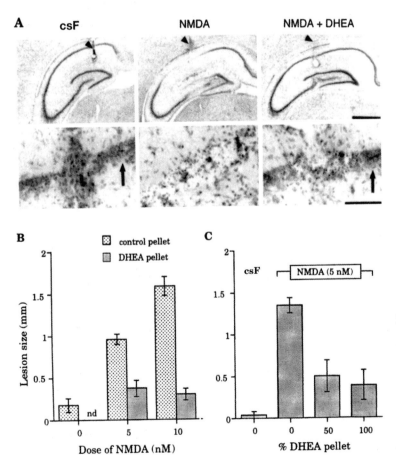

**Fig. 8.2** Subcutaneous administration of the neurosteroid DHEA protects hippocampal pyramidal neurones from NMDA-induced excitotoxicity. A Nissl-stained sections illustrating control, lesion, and DHEA treated hippocampus. B Lesion size measured as length of CA1 pyramidal layer indicating cell loss. C Half-dose of DHEA is as effective as the full dose: one pellet = 100 nM DHEA. (From Kimonides *et al.* 1998, with permission.)

## DHEA in some other neurological conditions

Reports of an association between DHEA and other age-related neurological conditions, such as Alzheimer's, have been variable and are not conclusive. An early finding that Alzheimer's patients had lower levels of DHEA than age-matched controls has not been confirmed (Schneider *et al.* 1992). Whether or not there is such an association is hardly relevant to the putative role of DHEA in such conditions. Since DHEA decreases so dramatically with age, it may act as a trigger or permissive factor allowing the expression of other (e.g. genetic) vulnerability factors, leading to the development of Alzheimer's (or other age-related conditions, such as Huntington's disease). Whilst individual variations in the age-related decline in DHEA may thus play a role, this may be obscured by equally individual differences in the operation of other, adjunctive, factors (e.g. specific genotypes, environmental factors such as preceding depressive illness, etc.). In other words, the DHEA threshold at which the brain becomes vulnerable to age-related disease may itself vary. This would not be apparent from simple between-group comparisons, but negative results from such studies would not invalidate this general proposition.

It is clear that the interactions between cortisol and other adrenal steroids in the context of the increased vulnerability of the brain to insult in the aged, or recovery from ischaemic or neurotoxic damage, has still to be adequately assessed. The large effects described above suggest that this would be a valuable exercise, and might open new avenues of therapy.

## *Oestrogens and brain damage*

Though the adrenal is only a minor source of oestrogens, these steroids (largely from the gonads) interact with glucocorticoids, and have themselves been shown to possess significant brain-protective actions. Oestradiol protects dentate neurones against the neurotoxic actions of systemic kainic acid (Azcoitia *et al.* 1998). Oestrogen also has a generally stimulating action on the growth and sprouting of neurones. For example, it increases dendritic spine synapses on hippocampal CA1 pyramidal cells (Woolley 1998), and encourages sprout-ing following entorhinal cortex lesions, perhaps through an action on apolipoprotein E (Stone *et al.* 1998). The mechanisms for these effects are still under investigation, but it is known that oestrogen can increase (and ovariectomy decrease) levels of growth factors, such as NGF and BDNF (Singh *et al.* 1995).

Oestrogen levels decline in women quite dramatically at the menopause, which thus represents the start of a prolonged period of relative or absolute oestrogen deficiency. However, increasing numbers of women now take steroid supplements (or 'HRT') that include oestrogens during the post-menopausal years, largely because of reported beneficial effects on bone density and heart disease. Several reports now suggest that such women also lessen their risk of developing Alzheimer's disease (Paganini-Hill and Henderson 1996; Tang *et al.* 1996), which, in untreated women, is about twice the age-adjusted rate in men. Oestrogen-treated elderly women had better cognitive function (short-term memory) than controls (Carlson and Sherwin 1998) and similar findings have been reported in transsexual males receiving oestrogen therapy (Miles *et al.* 1998).

There are complex interactions between oestrogen and corticoids, which are yet to be fully defined before the relative contributions of these two types of steroid are understood. An example is the effect that oestrogen has on blood levels of CBG — it increases it. This will reduce the proportion of 'free' cortisol and hence the entry of corticoids into the brain. Whether or not this is a significant factor in the neuroprotective actions of oestrogens is unknown, but the question needs clarification.

## *Conclusion*

The steroidal environment of the brain is a complex matter, but enough is now known to make it evident that changes in this environment, for whatever reason, can have highly significant effects on the onset, course, and risk of brain damage.

## *Further reading*

Sapolsky, R.M. (1992). *Stress, the Aging Brain, and the Mechanisms of Neuron Death*. MIT Press, Cambridge Mass. USA.

# 9 | Trophic factors

The original concept of the neurotrophins was that their function was restricted to development, where they were involved in determining which neurones survived into adulthood, and which axonal processes connected to particular targets (see Chapter 1). The developing nervous system produces about twice as many neurones as will survive into adulthood, and then at the end of development, around the time of birth in mammals, there is a short period termed the 'period of ontogenetic cell death' during which about half the neurones die. Trophic factors have a well-characterised role in the control of this process. The first trophic factor to be characterised was nerve growth factor (NGF): Rita Levi-Montalcini and Stanley Cohen received a Nobel prize for their pioneering work in the identification of this molecule (Levi-Montalcini 1987). Subsequently, many other neuronal trophic factors have been discovered, many of them mentioned later in this chapter and elsewhere in the book, but NGF has provided the prototype for all that followed.

During development, NGF acts to keep many sensory and all sympathetic neurones alive during the period of ontogenetic cell death. Thus, if developing embryos are deprived of NGF (which can be done by giving NGF antibodies to the mother or by making NGF genetic knockouts), then many of the sensory and all the sympathetic neurones die before birth (Pearson *et al.* 1983). The source of NGF in the embryo, which normally keeps these neurones alive, is mainly the target tissues innervated by the sympathetic and sensory neurones. Thus axons that have made successful connections to a target organ will receive plentiful NGF, and this will keep their neurones alive, while axons that have not made large connections will die back and their neurones will die.

The actions of NGF on developing neurones were demonstrated beautifully by Bob Campenot in an elegant tissue culture chamber system, now known as the Campenot chamber (Campenot 1981, 1982). As shown in Fig. 9.1, a Campenot chamber divides a tissue culture dish into three compartments, but the walls of the chamber that divide the dish are attached to the

axon growth surface with soft grease, which growing axons can penetrate. Therefore, axons can grow between the compartments, but molecules dissolved in the medium cannot diffuse. This arrangement made it possible to test for the effects of NGF on cell body and axonal survival when it was applied to different parts of the neurone. As shown in the diagram, NGF applied to any part of a neurone will promote survival. Thus, NGF available only at the end of the axon, which would

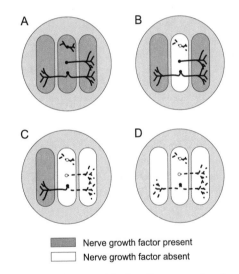

Fig. 9.1 Experiments with the Campenot chamber. The diagram shows a tissue culture dish seen from above, with a divider that separates it into three compartments, sealed to the dish with grease, which allows axons to grow between chambers but prevents exchange of dissolved molecules. Three sensory or sympathetic neurones are in the central chamber. A NGF is present in all chambers, and all three neurones and their processes survive. B NGF is withdrawn from the centre chamber, and the top neurone, which now has no access to NGF, dies. However, the other two neurones have access to NGF in the side-chambers from their axons, and they survive. C NGF is now withdrawn from the entre and right-hand chambers. Both the neurones, which have no access to NGF, die. However, the bottom neurone has access to NGF via the left-hand well and survives, but its right-hand process receives no NGF and dies. D All the NGF is withdrawn, and all the neurones die.

be the target area *in vivo,* is sufficient to maintain the neurone alive. NGF also has an effect on the survival of neuronal processes, and a process that does not have access to NGF will die back (Fig. 9.1), although the neurone itself may survive if it has contact with NGF from elsewhere. Therefore NGF, which has been the model for all the trophic factors, has effects on the survival of both whole neurones and neuronal processes.

Early experiments suggested that this clearly defined role for NGF, and therefore by implication for other trophic factors, might end after development, with the neurones becoming insensitive to the presence or absence of trophic factor. This view particularly grew out of experiments in which pregnant females were given NGF-neutralising antibodies in order to examine the effects of NGF withdrawal on the foetus. The foetus would grow up with few sensory and no sympathetic neurones, while the mother appeared unaffected. However, this interpretation begged the question of why trophic factors and their receptors are so widely expressed in the adult central and peripheral nervous systems. Could they simply be residual leftovers from development, or do they in fact play a part in adult neuronal and glial function? As detailed in this chapter and elsewhere in this book, we now know that trophic factors have many different roles in the adult CNS and PNS, on neuronal survival and plasticity, and on glial cells, both in normal brain function and in degenerative and regenerative responses to injury. In this chapter we will examine their ability to promote neuronal survival following adverse events such as axotomy, anoxia and neurotoxicity.

## Distribution of neurotrophins and neurotrophin receptors in the CNS

A huge number of molecules with neurotrophic effects have now been identified. The major factors and their superordinate families are summarised in Table 9.1, although it is beyond the scope of this book to give a detailed account of all of them. However, a few main families of trophic molecules account for most of the functional effects on neuroplasticity and regeneration that have been described to date.

The first major family of centrally acting growth factors are those neurotrophins related in structure to NGF. This family consists of NGF, BDNF, NT-3, and NT-4/5. These in turn bind to three main neurotrophin

**Table 9.1** The main families of neurotrophic factor and some of their members

A NEUROTROPHINS
(Factors of the prototypic NGF family)
Nerve growth factor (NGF)
Brain-derived neurotrophic factor (BDNF)
Neurotrophin-3 (NT3)
Neurotrophin-4/5 (NT4/5)
Neurotrophin-6 (NT6)

B NEUROPOIETIC FACTORS
(Factors with a predominant neuronal action, but can also effect blood cells)
Ciliary neurotrophic factor (CNTF)
Cholinergic differentiation factor (CDF)
Leukaemia inhibitory factor (LIF)

C HAEMOPOIETIC FACTORS
(Factors with a primary action in blood cell production, but also affect neurones)
Platelet derived growth factor (PDGF)
Interleukins (IL-1, -2, -6, -11)
Other lymphokines

D GROWTH FACTORS
(Other neurotrophic factors of the CNS)
Epidermal growth factor (EGF)
Fibroblast growth factor (FGF-1–5)
Glial cell line-derived neurotrophic factor (GDNF)
Neurturin, Persephin
Insulin
Insulin-like growth factors (IGF-I, -II)
Transforming growth factor (TGF$\alpha$, $\beta$)
Tumour necrosis factor (TNF$\alpha$, $\beta$)

E NEUROPEPTIDES
(Peptides identified in the PNS, subsequently found to have central neurotrophic actions)
ACTH
Calcitonin gene related peptide (CGRP)
Cholecystokinin (CCK)
Neuropeptide Y
Neurotensin
Substance P, and other tachykinins
Vasoactive intestinal polypeptide (VIP)
Vasopressin

Based on: Schwartz 1992; Baird 1993; Patterson and Nawa 1993.

receptors: trkA, trkB, and trkC; trkA binding to NGF, trkB to BDNF, NT-4 and NT-3, and trkC to NT-3. In addition, there is the low-affinity NGF receptor, p75, which is from a completely different receptor family to the trks, and which binds NGF and BDNF (Lindsay 1994). TrkA has a rather limited distribution in the CNS, being found on some neuronal types, particularly cholinergic neurones, while trkB and trkC are widely distributed throughout the nervous system, being found on most CNS neurones. TrkB also exists in a truncated form, which lacks the tyrosine kinase domain that is responsible for signalling, and this is the predominant form in the adult CNS, found on glial cells and neurones, although there is little in the embryo. The function of the truncated receptor is not yet well understood; it could be a way of restricting the spread of BDNF, of concentrating it at the cell surface, or of removing it by internalisation linked to the receptor (Valenzuela *et al.* 1993). NGF, NT-3, and BDNF are also widely expressed in the CNS, and at particularly high levels in the hippocampus.

Also widely expressed in the CNS is the receptor for CNTF, another molecule with neurotrophic properties. CNTF itself, however, is found in Schwann cells in peripheral nerves, with almost undetectable levels in the normal CNS, although it is produced by astrocytes after CNS injury (Sendtner *et al.* 1992; Ip and Yancopoulos 1996; Oyesiku *et al.* 1997).

FGF-2 is similar, in that the receptors are widely distributed on neurones and glial cells, and upregulated on glial cells after injury. FGFs are also widely produced, mainly by astrocytes, and promote survival and proliferation of most populations of neurones in the developing CNS. Along with EGF, FGF-2 has been of particular importance in promoting the division and proliferation of CNS-derived precursor/stem cells, which may provide an important renewable source of cells for transplantation (see Chapter 25).

Two further major families of trophic factors with more circumscribed actions in the nervous system are those related to TGF$\beta$, and the GDNF family that includes GDNF itself, neurturin, and persephin. GDNF, neurturin, and persephin are fairly widely expressed in the CNS, with GDNF and neurturin being largely of neuronal origin, while persephin is also in glia. The receptors (GFR$\alpha$1, GFR$\alpha$2, RET) are expressed on those neurones, such as the dopaminergic neurones of the substantia nigra, which respond to the trophic factors (Golden *et al.* 1998; Jaszai *et al.* 1998). Specific interest in GDNF arises from the fact that this molecule appears to be the most potent yet identified for promoting survival and growth of dopamine neurones both *in vitro* and *in vivo*, with obvious clinical applications (see below).

## Neurotrophins and the damaged nervous system

The role of trophic factors in modifying the neuronal death response to various types of insult has been examined in many areas of the nervous system. We will concentrate on the several model systems that have been investigated in most detail, and which demonstrate the main principles: peripheral nerve damage, amyotrophic lateral sclerosis, optic nerve damage, axotomy and neurotoxic lesions in the nigrostriatal pathway, damage to the cholinergic basal forebrain innervation of the cortex, and protection of the neurones of the striatum.

### Peripheral nervous damage

Damage to peripheral nerves affects the axons of motor sensory and sympathetic neurones. These neurones generally survive axotomy and, as described in Chapter 11, they mount a vigorous regenerative response. However, if the axotomy is close to the cell body, neuronal death is much greater. For instance, injuries in which the shoulder is dragged downwards may exert a great deal of force on the nerves of the brachial plexus, and this may result in avulsion of ventral and dorsal roots from the spinal cord. Motor neurone axons are damaged very close to the cell body, and this leads to immediate death of some neurones, and the atrophy or delayed death of others.

There has been a great deal of interest in the part that trophic factors may play in maintaining the damaged neurones alive after axotomy, and in whether application of trophic factors can improve neuronal survival and enhance the regenerative response. After axotomy, neurones projecting into the periphery will lose contact with their targets, and therefore will no longer receive target-derived trophic factors. However, they continue to receive trophic support from cells in the peripheral nerve. Schwann cells in the peripheral nervous system after nerve damage are capable of making NGF, BDNF and NT-3, although production in undamaged nerves is low or absent, and CNTF is made by myelinating Schwann cells and released after nerve damage, but it is down-regulated in the degenerating nerve (Lindholm *et al.* 1987; Meyer *et al.* 1992; Sendtner *et al.* 1992). If a peripheral nerve is damaged, however, production of NGF, BDNF, and some other cytokines, increases rapidly, and CNTF, which is present at high levels in Schwann cells, is released. Sensory axons almost all carry trk receptors, with the small nociceptive and temperature-sensitive neurones carrying trkA and, therefore, being supported by NGF; the large proprioceptive fibres carrying trkC and, therefore, being supported by NT-3; and fine touch and vibration-sensitive fibres carrying trkB and being supported by BDNF. There is also a population that is supported by GDNF.

Sympathetic axons are supported by NGF, while motor neurones have been shown to be supported *in vitro* by a wide range of trophic factors, including CNTF, BDNF, FGF-5, GDNF, and others. To some extent, axotomised neurones are protected by trophic factors within the animal. Thus, adult myelinating Schwann cells contain large amounts of CNTF, and it can be shown that CNTF released at the time of axotomy has a protective effect on motor neurones (Sendtner *et al.* 1997), although CNTF is soon down-regulated in the Schwann cells that have lost contact with axons, and there is upregulation of trkB and of BDNF production in motor neurones after axotomy, which will provide autocrine trophic support (Kobayashi *et al.* 1996).

Given the presence of the receptors, we may wonder whether the complementary trophic factors could help rescue neurones from axotomy-induced death. These studies have mainly focused on the motor neurones. However, there is a considerable amount of data on neurotransmitter plasticity in sympathetic neurones after axotomy (see also Chapter 11).

- Motor neurones vary in their susceptibility to death after axotomy depending on the age at which the axons are damaged, and the position of axotomy.

- Damage to a peripheral nerve in newborn animals up to the age of 10 days leads to extensive motor neuronal death, but damage in adults does not. Sciatic nerve crush in rats before post-natal day 10 leads to 65% death of motor neurones, while crush after day 10 leads to hardly any cell death (Li *et al.* 1994).

- Damage to a peripheral nerve in adulthood leads to little motor neurone cell death, but root avulsion causes 70% loss.

- Motor neurones in adults after axotomy lose much of their choline acetyltransferase enzyme, while in newborns the surviving axotomised neurones continue to express the enzyme (Kou *et al.* 1995).

The two main experimental models for studying regeneration of motor axons through the peripheral nerve environment involve damage (by cut or crush) to the sciatic nerve and to the facial nerve. A major advantage of the facial-nerve model is that the facial-nerve motor nucleus in rodents is anatomically distinct, and contains a readily counted and predictable number of motor neurones.

Trophic factors can protect against motor neurone

death after axotomy in both newborn and adult animals. In most studies the factors have been applied topically to the site of damage through an infusion pump or via a pad of gel foam. Of the many factors that have been applied, the three most effective have been BDNF, GDNF, and CNTF, each of which can rescue around half of the neurones that would normally die (Fig. 9.2; Sendtner *et al.* 1990; Li *et al.* 1995). The fact that addition of small quantities of these factors are effective indicates that the amounts available from within the animal are insufficient to keep all the neurones alive. BDNF is also able to maintain the levels of choline acetyltransferase in the axotomised neurones (Fernandes *et al.* 1998).

Peripheral nerve damage in newborn humans is a significant clinical issue, since root avulsion in the brachial plexus area can occur as a result of birth trauma. The ability of trophic factors to protect at this age is therefore important. The trophic factors that are effective are basically the same as in adulthood, with IGF, BDNF, and NT-3 being the most effective factors, and CNTF slightly less so (Li *et al.* 1994).

## Motor neurone disease

Another condition in which motor neurones die is motor neurone disease, also known as amyotrophic lateral sclerosis (ALS) or, in the USA, Lou Gehrig's disease. This is the most common neurodegenerative disease affecting neurones that project into the peripheral nervous system. In this condition there is a steady and unrelenting loss of motor neurones in the spinal cord over a period of usually less than 10 years. The disease results in progressive weakness and eventually death, usually following loss of function in the muscles that subserve swallowing, regurgitation, and breathing. In view of the findings (above) that motor neurones can be rescued from axotomy-induced death by the appropriate trophic factors, there has been a great deal of interest in trying to rescue motor neurones in motor neurone disease with trophic factors, and thereby to develop a treatment for this presently untreatable disease.

The development and testing of neurotrophic treatments against spinal motor neurone degeneration has been made much easier by the development of relevant transgenic animal models. Some inherited forms of ALS have been found to be associated with mutations in the gene for superoxide dismutase (SOD) (Deng *et al.* 1993; Rosen *et al.* 1993). From this observation, the most widely used transgenic model for motor neurone disease

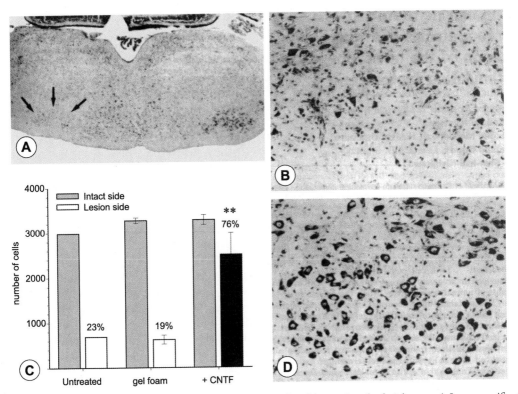

**Fig. 9.2** CNTF protects facial motor neurones against axotomy, induced by cutting the facial nerve. A Low magnification of the facial nuclei in the brainstem; the nucleus on the *left* has been axotomised, leading to death of most neurones. B, D High magnification of axotomised facial nucleus in animals treated with vehicle or gel foam soaked in 5 μg CNTF, respectively. CNTF protects the majority of neurones that are lost following axotomy. C Cell counts of surviving large motor neurones in the facial nucleus contralateral (intact side) and ipsilateral (lesion side) to axotomy. (From Sendtner *et al.* 1990.)

has similarly been the generation of mice that express a variety of mutant forms of the superoxide dismutase gene. These animals develop a syndrome similar to motor neurone disease, in which motor neurones die over a period of weeks (Wong *et al.* 1995). Various trophic factors have been applied. The two most active molecules in these models, as might be predicted from the axotomy experiments, are BDNF and CNTF. Individually they slow motor neurone degeneration in the mouse mutants, and they also behave synergistically (Sendtner *et al.* 1992; Lindsay 1994). IGF also has an effect in transgenic models, although the effect is less than with BDNF or CNTF (Dore *et al.* 1997). GDNF has been shown to preserve motor neurones but, surprisingly, it did not appear to prevent axonal degeneration (Sagot *et al.* 1996).

A major issue during these experiments has been the route of administration of the trophic factors. A theoretical attraction of motor neurone disease, as the first condition in which to attempt neuroprotection with

trophic factors, is that the factors do not have to cross the blood–brain barrier in order to reach the target neurones. Trophic factor injected in muscle can be transported retrogradely in the axons of the motor neurones, and many of the initial successful animal trials were therefore done with intramuscular injections. However, the other consequence of giving trophic factors by intramuscular injection is that they enter the systemic circulation and are distributed throughout the body. Treatment with recombinant human CNTF underwent a phase II–III trial, given by subcutaneous injection three times per week over 9 months, but the high doses of CNTF were not tolerated well, causing anorexia, weight loss, and coughs (and in extreme cases causing patients to become cachectic), which was not offset by the treatment producing any significant clinical benefit in progress of the disease (Lotz *et al.* 1996).

Potential side-effects also make it impractical to deliver BDNF by peripheral injection. Alternative routes of administration have therefore been tried. Both BDNF and CNTF are effective in animal models if given intrathecally, so that the highest concentrations are delivered to the spinal cord itself. One method of delivering trophic factors that has been developed is to genetically engineer cells to secrete trophic factor, then encase these cells in a semi-permeable capsule and implant it next to the spinal cord (Sagot *et al.* 1995). This approach has led to protection in animal models. A trial of CNTF in human motor neurone disease patients, delivered in this way directly to the CSF bathing the cord, has been carried out. The CNTF-secreting cells increased trophic factor levels in the CSF to the nanogram range, at which level there would be a detectable survival effect *in vitro*, but although there were no side-effects from the treatment, there was no detectable slowing of the disease progression (Aebischer *et al.* 1996). Also under trial at present is BDNF delivered by intrathecal infusion. Encapsulation of engineered cell lines for transplantation is developed in more detail in a later chapter (Chapter 26).

While CNTF and BDNF are the most effective trophic factors on motor neurone survival *in vitro*, their systemic side-effects limit their use. Another trophic factor with widespread trophic effects in the nervous system, IGF-I, does not produce such adverse systemic effects. IGF-I is an effective survival-promoting factor for motor neurones *in vitro*, and also protects in axotomy and in animal models of motor neurone disease. The growth factor was therefore tried out in human trials in motor neurone disease patients in Europe and in the USA, the IGF-I being delivered by subcutaneous injection for up to 9 months. The North American patients showed a clear slowing of the disease process, but the results in the European patients were less clear (Yuen and Mobley 1996; Doré *et al.* 1997). IGF-I is currently the only trophic factor licensed for clinical use in motor neurone disease.

## Retinal ganglion cells

The retina has its embryological origins in the central nervous system, and its cellular makeup is of CNS type. The anatomical arrangement of the eye, physically separated from the brain by the optic nerve and contained within a separate structure, makes it uniquely convenient for conducting analytical experiments on aspects of CNS neuroprotection and repair. In terms of injury response, retinal ganglion cells are like other CNS neurones in that they can be killed by axotomy, the percentage of cell death increasing as the axotomy is moved closer to the back of the eye. When Alan Harvey and

his collaborators looked at the timing of cell death in the retina by looking for pyknotic nuclei, they found that there was a phase of cell death that occurred almost immediately after axotomy, within 4 h, and a later phase that began at 24 h. Cell death is complete by 7 days (Cui, and Harvey 1995). The factors that have been shown to protect the ganglion cells include:

- trophic factors BDNF, CNTF, GDNF, NT-3, NT-4/5;

- inhibitors of protein synthesis;

- protease inhibitors;

- free-radical scavengers;

- NO synthase inhibitors;

On the other hand, NGF, which can be produced by microglial cells, has been shown in the developing eye to be toxic to retinal ganglion cells via the p75 receptor (Frade and Barde 1998). The various survival factors may protect against different phases of axotomy-induced cell death. Antioxidants by themselves were found to be effective only at the earliest stages, and do not have any effect on long-term survival, whereas BDNF and CNTF inhibit cell death at all stages. However, even the most effective of the trophic factors, BDNF, only has a rather temporary effect on increasing ganglion-cell survival, and repeated injections do not lead to permanent neuroprotection. Matthias Bahr and his colleagues wondered whether this was because BDNF can also trigger toxic effects by upregulating the production of free radicals. They therefore coupled BDNF treatment with inhibitors of free-radical effects (see Chapter 7), and found greatly increased long-term neuroprotection. One free radical that has been shown to be upregulated in neurones by BDNF is nitric oxide, through upregulation of the neuronal nitric oxide synthase gene, and this has been shown to produce toxic effects in neurones. Bahr and his colleagues, therefore, coupled BDNF treatment with an inhibitor of nitric oxide production, and again showed greatly increased long-term survival of retinal ganglion cells after axotomy (Klocker *et al.* 1998). BDNF also has effects that might be expected to increase the ability of ganglion-cell axons to regenerate, although BDNF by itself does not promote regeneration. Thus BDNF treatment reduces the die-back of axons from the site of an optic nerve injury, and also promotes the upregulation of GAP-43 (Weibel *et al.* 1995; Fournier *et al.* 1997).

## The nigro-striatal pathway

One of the major and common neurodegenerative diseases affecting humans is Parkinson's disease. This results from the death of the dopaminergic neurones of the substantia nigra. As described in Chapter 6, these dopaminergic neurones are lost even in normal humans at a slow rate such that anyone who lives into their 90s can expect to have some degree of parkinsonism. However, in some people the rate of loss of the neurones is increased, or there is some event such as head injury, exposure to a neurotoxin, or a viral disease that triggers increased loss. There are probably several causes of Parkinson's disease, which in itself makes the development of animal models problematic, and there is no model that reproduces the slow steady loss of dopaminergic neurones seen in most forms of the human disease. However, there are three main animal models that are used to assess neuroprotective strategies.

1. Mechanical axotomy of the nigro-striatal tract. Around 85% of dopaminergic neurones die over a period of up to 10 weeks following axotomy close to the substantia nigra, while there is less death if axons are cut nearer to the striatum.

2. Injection of the toxin 6-hydroxydopamine (6-OHDA) into the striatum or the nigro-striatal tract (see Chapter 6). Injection into the nigro-striatal tract leads to an almost 100% loss of dopaminergic neurones within 10 days, while injection of the toxin into the striatum leads to removal of the striatal dopaminergic innervation, and a slower and smaller loss of dopaminergic neurones.

3. Treatment with MPTP (See Chapter 6). MPTP is converted to its active metabolite MPP+, which is an inhibitor of mitochondrial complex 1, and probably works by inducing free-radical production in the dopaminergic neurones, and therefore an acute form of the free radical related loss of neurones that probably occurs in human Parkinson's disease. Cell loss is slower than with 6-hyroxydopamine, and dose related. The compound is given systemically or by injection into the carotid artery to target one hemisphere of the brain.

In order to try to develop treatments that might slow the death of the neurones, several trophic factors have been applied to substantia nigra neurones, both *in vitro* and following *in vivo* challenge, by axotomy or neurotoxins. Nigral dopamine neurones do not survive particularly well in culture, due at least in part to their sensitivity to oxidative stress (see Chapters 3 and 7), and *in vitro* experiments indicate that these neurones are responsive to a wide range of factors. Thus, CNTF, FGF-2, BDNF, NT-3, NT-4/5, TGFβ, GDNF, neurturin, and persephin, all have some ability to rescue the neurones in various types of experiment.

The first *in vivo* protection was achieved with BDNF, which also has powerful survival effects on dopaminergic neurones in tissue culture, and the neurones carry the trkB receptor. BDNF has been delivered to the substantia nigra by direct injection, by implanting cells that have been genetically engineered to secrete it, and by injecting into the brain an adenovirus that infects cells in the brain and increases their synthesis of BDNF. These treatments have been able to reduce the death of dopaminergic neurones in the substantia nigra following administration of both MPTP and 6-OHDA (Frim *et al.* 1994; Yoshimoto *et al.* 1995). The ability of BDNF to protect against axotomy-induced cell death is less clear. When given into the ventricles, BDNF did not protect, but in other experiments BDNF injected very close to the substantia nigra was protective (Knüsel *et al.* 1992; Hagg 1998). BDNF diffuses very poorly in the adult CNS, probably because it adheres to the large number of truncated trkB receptors that are present, so it may be that ventricular injections did not deliver a sufficient dose.

While BDNF clearly has neuroprotective effects, a more recently discovered family of trophic factors, GDNF, neurturin, and persephin, are more effective. The first family member to be discovered was GDNF, and this has potent protective effects against axotomy, 6-OHDA, and MPTP-induced neuronal death in the substantia nigra, whether delivered by adenoviral transfection of intrinsic brain cells or by direct injection into the brain (Beck *et al.* 1995, Tomac *et al.* 1995, Gash *et al.* 1996, Choi-Lundberg *et al.* 1997). GDNF injections appear to be effective both in protecting nigral neurones and rescuing striatal dopamine terminals, dependent upon the site of injection in the nigra or the striatum (Fig. 9.3; Beck *et al.* 1995; Tomac *et al.* 1995; Gash *et al.* 1996; Choi-Lundberg *et al.* 1997; Rosenblad *et al.* 1997; Lapchak *et al.* 1997a), and are associated with functional neuroprotection on a range of behavioural tests, including rotation, locomotor activity, and stepping (Fig. 9.3; Tomac *et al.* 1995, Shults *et al.* 1996, Rosenblad *et al.* 1997). To take just one example, Rosenblad and colleagues (1997) used terminal injections of 6-OHDA into the striatum to provide a slow and partial degeneration of nigral neurones, followed by

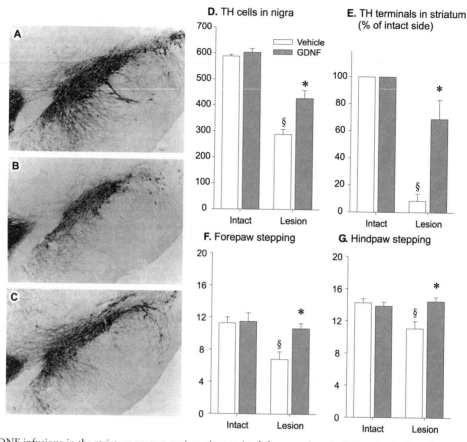

**Fig. 9.3** GDNF infusions in the striatum protect against nigro-striatal degeneration. A–C Tyrosine hydroxylase (TH) immuno-histochemistry of substantia nigra to visualise dopamine neurones in the intact nigra (A), after partial 6-OHDA lesion (B), and after treatment with GDNF (C). D–F Histograms of quantification of loss and protection of nigral TH+ cells (D), loss and protection of striatal TH+ terminals (E) and deficits and recovery of stepping, on the contralateral side-lesioned and GDNF-treated rats. Significant differences: *, from intact side, § from lesion only p<0.05. (Redrawn from Rosenblad *et al*. 1997.)

10 repeated injections of 5 μg GDNF into the striatum every other day over 3 weeks, from 4 to 7 weeks after the lesion. The animals then underwent a series of tests of motor function prior to perfusion and post-mortem analysis of nigral cell survival and density of striatal terminals. As shown in Fig. 9.3, not only did the GDNF injections reduce the slow degeneration of TH+ nigral neurones, but the injections were also associated with a dramatic increase in the density of dopamine terminals in the striatum, and an amelioration of the deficits in stepping with the contralateral fore- and hindpaws.

Subsequently, two more trophic factors from the GDNF family have been identified: neurturin and persephin. Neurturin protects in 6-OHDA and axotomy models, while persephin has so far only been proven in 6-OHDA lesioned rats (Horger *et al*. 1998; Milbrandt *et al*. 1998; Tseng *et al*. 1998). However, the expectation is that these factors will have much the same effects as GDNF.

In addition to protecting dopaminergic neurones against death, it was noticed that GDNF given to animals that had received a lesion some time previously, and in which the degree of Parkinsonism was stable, would produce considerable improvements in function. In primates there were improvements in the three main Parkinsonian deficits: bradykinesia, rigidity, and postural instability. Moreover, these changes last for up to a month after a single intracerebral dose, and repeated doses at monthly intervals can produce a long-term improvement. The biochemical correlate of this effect is an increase in the size of the dopaminergic neurones in the substantia nigra, in their production of dopamine, and in levels of the key synthetic enzyme tyrosine hydroxylase (Gash *et al.* 1998). The trophic factors of the GDNF family, therefore, have two beneficial effects: to promote survival of the neurones that would otherwise die; and to increase the function of those that survive.

A preliminary clinical trial in one patient with Parkinson's disease has recently been reported by Kordower and colleagues (1999). This patient received monthly i.c.v. injections of GDNF. The patient continued to show worsening parkinsonian symptoms over the trial period of 1 year, with an unacceptable range of side-effects, including nausea, loss of appetite, tingling, hallucinations, depression, and what is discreetly described as 'inappropriate sexual conduct'. A concurrent study in monkeys showed that it was likely that the GDNF administered via a similar intraventricular route of delivery would not actually reach the substantia nigra or deep levels of either caudate nucleus or putamen.

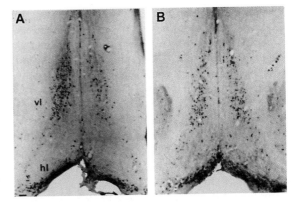

**Fig. 9.4** NGF infusions rescue axotomised septal cholinergic neurones. A Septum, in which approximately 60% of the cholinergic neurones of the vertical limb (vl) on the right side are lost after unilateral transection of their axons in the fimbria. Neurones of the horizontal limb (hl) do not project via the fimbria and so are unaffected. B Following central injection of NGF there is an almost complete rescue of the axotomised neurones. (From Montero and Hefti 1988.)

## The cholinergic basal-forebrain neurones

While few CNS neurones express the NGF receptor trkA, it is present at high levels on the cholinergic basal forebrain neurones. These are of particular interest, since many of them die in Alzheimer's disease and the consequent reduction in cholinergic innervation of the cortex and hippocampus is probably responsible for part of the cognitive deficit associated with the condition (see Chapter 6). In experimental animals a similar deficit can be caused by cutting the fimbria-fornix, through which the axons of these neurones pass. Following axotomy, some of the cholinergic neurones die and the rest atrophy. Local administration of NGF infused into the ventricles or into the septum is effective in reversing this effect. NGF diffuses sufficiently far in the rodent brain to be able to reach the cholinergic neurones and their axons. The result was a substantial rescue of the axotomised neurones and a reduction in their atrophy (Fig. 9.4; Hefti 1986; Williams *et al.* 1986). Even in normal rats, NGF infusion leads to an increase in choline acetyltransferase in these neurones. Again, the biggest practical difficulty with this model is how to deliver the NGF, which does not cross the blood–brain barrier, chronically into the CNS. The first studies implanted cannulae into the brain ventricles through which local infusions of NGF could be administered daily (Hefti 1986; Williams *et al.* 1986; Kromer 1987). This model system was used to evaluate implantation of cells engineered to secrete NGF in one of the

first attempts at *ex vivo* gene therapy (see Chapter 26; Rosenberg *et al.* 1988).

Whereas Alzheimer's disease involves a variety of neuropathological hallmarks and degeneration in wide areas of the brain, the degeneration of central cholinergic systems has been considered one important component (Coyle *et al.* 1983). Experimental lesions of forebrain cholinergic systems in the rat, and aged rats both exhibit cognitive impairments that have been taken to mimic key features of human dementia. Although the validity of this as a good model of dementia is not uncontroversial (see Dunnett *et al.* 1991), infusion of NGF both into aged rats and into rats with basal-forebrain lesions has been seen to improve aspects of cognitive performance, in particular in water-maze tests of spatial navigation (Williams *et al.* 1986; Chen and Gage 1995). The basal-forebrain neurones have trkB and trkC on their surface, as well as trkA, and both BDNF and NT-3 have been shown to have similar effects to NGF (Knüsel *et al.* 1992).

On the basis of these observations, preliminary trials of infusing NGF into the brains of humans with early Alzheimer's disease have been carried out. Moreover, Alzheimer's disease affects many neurones other than those in the basal forebrain, particularly ascending systems that provide a diffuse innervation of the cortex and hippocampus, and also intrinsic cortical and hippocampal neurones, and most of these do not have the trkA receptor. Hefti (1983) first proposed that Alzheimer's disease might actually be caused by a loss of NGF. Although this hypothesis has not been sustained, it may nevertheless be that cholinergic neuroprotection or the enhancement of residual cholinergic function may provide a functional benefit in patients. With this hypothesis in mind, Seiger and colleagues have undertaken preliminary clinical observations of the central administration of NGF infusion of three patients with Alzheimer's disease (Fig. 9.5; Seiger *et al.* 1993; Jonhagen *et al.* 1998). A total of 0.55 mg to 6.6 ng of NGF was administered by continuous infusion into the lateral ventricles for up to 3 months, and then the patients were evaluated on an extensive battery of neuropsychological, physiological, and scanning tests. Although a few of the neuropsychology tests showed modest change, and slow-wave cortical activity was reduced, no significant cognitive improvement was demonstrated (Jonhagen *et al.* 1998). Moreover, the infusions did result in negative side-effects including back pain and weight loss. Consequently, as in the other growth factors described above, further improvements in dosing and delivery are required before any clear therapeutic benefit can be assured. Moreover, many of the cholinergic neurones also carry trkB and trkC receptors, and respond to BDNF and NT-3 in culture. Consequently, a treatment based on a combination of factors may have theoretical advantages, and produce fewer

side-effects associated with high doses, over one based solely on NGF.

## Lesions of the striatum

A final model system that has been heavily investigated for neurotrophic protection has been the striatum, in animal models of Huntington's disease. Using a variety of excitotoxic and metabolic toxin lesions to model the human disease, striatal neurones can be rescued by co-infusion of a number of different neurotrophic molecules, including NGF, BDNF, NT-4/5, $\beta$FGF, TGF$\alpha$, CNTF, and GDNF (Frim *et al.* 1993; Anderson *et al.* 1996a; Emerich *et al.* 1996, 1997; Pérez-Navarro *et al.* 1996). Again, to take but one example, Anderson *et al.* (1996a) implanted stainless steel cannulae into the lateral ventricle of rats, and connected these to subcutaneous 'Alzet' mini-pumps that could deliver one of several trophic factors — 0.9 mg/mg NGF, 1 mg/ml BDNF, 1 mg/ml NT-3, or 0.78 mg/ml CNTF — which were then infused at a rate of 0.5 $\mu$l/h over 2 weeks. Three days after implanting the cannulae, the rats received unilateral striatal lesions made by local injection of 1 $\mu$l of 0.05 M quinolinic acid into the striatum. A little over 1 week later, all animals were killed for post-mortem analysis of the lesions. Animals with lesions alone consistently produced extensive loss of medium-sized projection neurones of the striatum (Fig. 9.6B), which was not alleviated by treatment with NGF, BDNF, or NT-3. By contrast, rats treated with CNTF showed a substantial sparing of striatal neurones in the area of the toxin infusion (Fig. 9.6C). Quantitative counts of the numbers of striatal neurones, ipsilateral and contralateral to the lesions, indicated 69 ± 17 % of the neurones surviving in the CNTF-treated rats as compared with a >70% loss in the striatum of rats treated with quinolinic acid alone (or indeed following treatment with any of the ineffective factors).

As in the other models, a key issue here has been delivery of the trophic molecules, and in addition to direct infusion, good progress has been made in the development of engineered cells for transplantation both directly into the striatum (Frim *et al.* 1993) and after encapsulation (Emerich *et al.* 1996, 1997). A discussion of this new technology is developed further in Chapter 26.

On the basis of such experimental studies, clinical trials of CNTF administration are presently underway in Huntington's disease, although no results of safety or efficacy are yet reported.

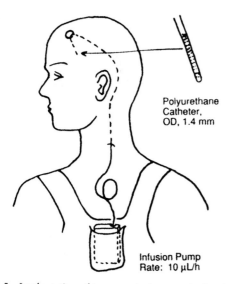

**Polyurethane Catheter, OD, 1.4 mm**

**Infusion Pump Rate: 10 µL/h**

**Fig. 9.5**  Implantation of intraventricular cannula for chronic delivery of NGF in the first trial on an Alzheimer's disease patient. (Reproduced from Seiger *et al.* 1993.)

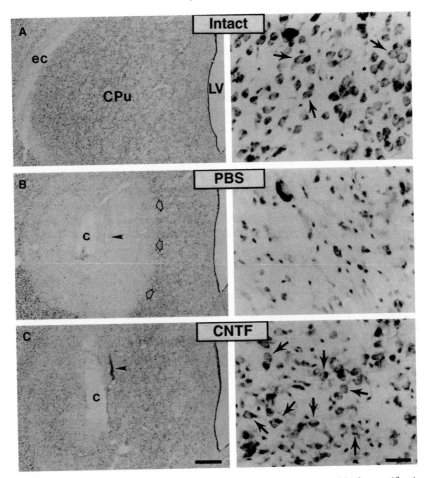

**Fig. 9.6** CNTF protects against quinolinic acid lesions of the neostriatum. A Low- and high-magnification images of intact striatum containing predominantly medium-sized neurones in the striatum. B Quinolinic acid induces massive neuronal loss in animals treated with additional injections of PBS vehicle. C Cell loss after a similar quinolinic acid lesion is markedly reduced in animals treated with 2 week infusion of CNTF. Abbreviations: c, cannula tip, i.e. the site of the PBS or CNTF infusion; CPu, caudate-putamen; ec, external capsule. Arrow head, site of the quinolinic acid injection; open arrows in B, borders of the area of cell loss in the lesion area; arrows, healthy neurones at higher magnification within the same area in intact (A) and CNTF infused (C) cases. Nissl stain. Scale bars: left = 0.5 mm, right = 30 $\mu$m. (Reproduced from Anderson *et al.* 1996a.)

## Use of trophic factors for neuroprotection

From the above, it is clear that some trophic factors are able to rescue damaged neurones in the adult nervous system. As such, these or related molecules may have a place in the treatment of a variety of acute and chronic conditions. However, there are significant problems in their use. The first is that the trophic factors are all large proteins, and therefore cannot be given by mouth. Even when given systemically, the proteins will not cross the

blood–brain barrier unless it is damaged. This is one of the reasons why motor neurone disease is an attractive prospect from the therapeutic point of view, since trophic factor given intramuscularly is effective on motor neurones. However, the problem is that the actions of trophic factors are not restricted to the CNS, neither are they restricted to promoting neuronal survival. Both CNTF and BDNF, when given intramuscularly to patients with motor neurone disease, cause unacceptable side-effects, and NGF has important peripheral influences on pain. These experiences lead to the conclusion that trophic factors must be administered to the place where they are needed in the CNS. Trials of CNTF and BDNF by intrathecal delivery for motor neurone disease are therefore in progress or completed, and further trials of NGF in Alzheimer's disease and CNTF in Huntington's disease are initiated. However, within the CNS the actions of the neurotrophic molecules are not just in the promotion of neuronal survival. There are important actions on neuronal plasticity, glial function, and other basic CNS processes. Delivery of trophic factors into the ventricles in high dose will affect large areas of the brain, and may therefore cause unacceptable effects. It may be that the use of intracerebral GDNF in Parkinson's disease will be restricted because of this. However, another important issue when delivering trophic factors into the CNS is their pharmacodynamics. Some factors, such as GDNF, spread for some distance after local injection, but BDNF remains almost completely localised to the site of injection, probably because of the large numbers of truncated trkB receptors in the adult CNS, which bind the molecule and internalise it. Increasingly, therefore, it looks as if the trophic factors may need to be delivered rather precisely to the neurones where they are needed to prevent degeneration. However, intraparenchymal infusion in humans will always be a difficult therapeutic option. Other possibilities, such as delivery via transfection of local cells with retrovirus or implantation of cells that secrete trophic factor, may turn out to be the best options in the long term (see Chapter 26). One situation in which trophic factor delivery is relatively easy is in the damaged peripheral nervous system, where surgical intervention is normally undertaken at which time implantation of a device to infuse trophic factors is not difficult. As an alternative approcah to the problems of delivery, trophic factor therapy will also be greatly facilitated by the development of small molecule trophic factor receptor agonists, and by agents that act on the downstream signalling pathways. These are currently highly active areas of pharmaceutical research.

# Further reading

Lindsay, R.M. (1996). Role of neurotrophins and trk receptors in the development and maintenance of sensory neurones: an overview. *Phil. Trans. Roy. Soc. Lond. B*, **351**, 365–373.

Yuen, E.C. and Mobley, W.C. (1996). Therapeutic potential of neurotrophic factors for neurological disorders. *Annals of Neurology*, 346–355.

# 10 | *Control of inflammation*

The nervous system is affected by inflammatory processes in many diseases. In general, these are diseases in which the primary pathological process is thought to be autoimmunity. The commonest and most serious of these conditions for the CNS is multiple sclerosis, which affects around 100 in every 100 000 of the population. However, the CNS is not infrequently involved in other autoimmune conditions, such as systemic lupus erythaematosis, the paraneoplastic diseases, and vasculitis. The CNS involvement in these various conditions is described in Chapter 5.

While inflammatory diseases affecting the CNS can produce a huge range of symptoms, depending on the exact nature of the disease process (see Table 10.1), the range of therapeutic options in these conditions is rather limited. Almost all the available treatments depend on some form of suppression of immunological function. These have been explored to the greatest extent in the treatment of multiple sclerosis, so the present account will focus on this disease, and we will mention other inflammatory conditions under the headings of the various types of available therapies.

**Table 10.1** Immunological conditions that affect the nervous system

| |
|---|
| **CNS** |
| Multiple sclerosis |
| Rheumatoid arthritis |
| Sjögren's syndrome |
| Systemic sclerosis |
| Mixed connective tissue disease |
| Systemic lupus erythematosus |
| Seronegative arthritides (ankylosing spondylitis, Reiter's disease, psoriasis) |
| Paraneoplastic disorders |
| Cerebral vasculitis, (including giant cell arteritis and Takayasu's disease, Behçet's disease, Vogt-Koyanagi-Harada syndrome) |
| Inflammatory bowel disease (ulcerative colitis, Crohn's disease, Whipple's disease, coeliac disease) |
| **PNS** |
| Guillain–Barré disease |
| Paraneoplastic disorders |

## Corticosteroids

The mainstay of immunosuppressive treatment in almost all the autoimmune diseases is the corticosteroids. These have multiple immunosuppressive actions, through effects on blood vessels, inflammatory cells, and inflammatory mediators. The major actions are:-

- decreased activity of T helper cells, and reduced proliferation of T cells, mainly due to decreased IL-2 production;

- reduced recruitment of leucocytes to areas of inflammation;

- reduced production of toxic free radicals by neutrophils and macrophages;

- decreased production of leukotrienes and prostanoids

- decreased production of cytokines by lymphocytes and other leukocytes;

- reduction in the concentration of complement components in plasma.

In multiple sclerosis, corticosteroid treatments offer faster recovery from relapses, possibly because they improve the function of the blood–brain barrier (Milligan *et al.* 1987). However, there is no evidence that they slow progression of the disease if given in the long term. Steroids are, therefore, given during the relapse phases of multiple sclerosis, but are withdrawn when maximal recovery has been achieved.

Steroids are also the mainstay of treatment for the complications of rheumatoid arthritis, Sjögren's syndrome, and systemic lupus erythematosus. High-dose intravenous steroids are given for acute exacerbation, and an oral maintenance dose for long-term disease control. Treatment of cerebral vasculitides also relies on high doses of corticosteroids as the mainstay, to which other agents are added.

## Azathioprine

Azathioprine is widely used as an immunosuppressant, often in combination with corticosteroids. The drug is metabolised to mercaptopurine, which in turn is converted to ribonucleotides. These abnormal molecules can be incorporated into DNA, affecting cell division, and can inhibit normal purine synthesis. The drug is cytotoxic to all dividing cells, but the lymphocytes are particularly susceptible, leading to depression of the induction phase of the immune response.

In multiple sclerosis a meta-analysis of trials of long-term azathioprine has shown an effect on disease progression and relapse rate (Yudkin *et al.* 1991). Azathioprine is frequently used as an adjunct to steroids in the major multi-system autoimmune diseases, such as systemic lupus erythematosus, where it is used to maintain remission, and to allow a lower dose of steroids to be given.

## Cyclophosphamide

Cyclophosphamide is an alkylating agent that affects all cells, but has a particularly strong effect on lymphocytes. The main targets for alkylation are adenine and guanine, which are particularly vulnerable in unpaired DNA during replication. Dividing cells are affected during S phase, then become blocked during $G_1$ and undergo cell death. It affects the clonal proliferative phase of the immune response, and reduces both antibody and cell-mediated immune reactions.

In multiple sclerosis, cyclophosphamide has been reported in one trial to stabilise the disease when used in combination with corticotrophin, but in another there was no slowing of the disease from a combination of cyclophosphamide and prednisone. The drug has substantial toxic side-effects, so it is not used for treatment of multiple sclerosis.

In the autoimmune diseases, such as systemic lupus erythematosus, cyclophosphamide is usually reserved for severe and steroid-resistant exacerbations, but it has also been used successfully for maintenance in the form of weekly, low doses. Cyclophosphamide is also used with steroids in cerebral vasculitis.

## Cyclosporin

Cyclosporin is a fungal cyclic peptide with powerful immunosuppressive effects on lymphocyte proliferation, affecting both cell-mediated and antibody-mediated immune responses. The drug binds to cyclophilin in the cell and the complex inhibits calcineurin, and thus interferes with the signalling pathway from activation of the T-cell receptor.

In multiple sclerosis, cyclosporine has a modest effect on slowing the progression of the disease, but only at the risk of unacceptable cardiovascular and renal side-effects (Faulds *et al.* 1993). However, the fact that the drug has some effect in multiple sclerosis provides some evidence for the involvement of CD4+ve T cells in the disease.

## Intravenous immunoglobulin

Immunoglobulins derived from normal human plasma can be used as replacement therapy in patients with immune deficiency. However, they have also been used in autoimmune conditions, on the assumption that normal levels of normal immunoglobulins will help control the immune system.

In multiple sclerosis, one study has shown a 38% reduction in relapse rate and a slowing of disease progression in patients treated with intravenous immunoglobulins (Achiron *et al.* 1998). This treatment is also reported to prevent the exacerbation of the disease that can occur after childbirth. In large-vessel cerebral vasculitis, immunoglobulins have achieved partial remission in around half the patients treated.

## Plasma exchange

On the assumption that factors such as immunoglobulins and other immune mediators are involved in the pathology of autoimmune disease, a treatment that has been developed is plasma exchange, in which the patients' plasma is separated from blood cells, then the cells and fresh normal plasma returned to the patient, and the patients' own plasma is then discarded.

This treatment has been reported to be effective in individual cases of multiple sclerosis, but a large trial in Canada failed to show significant benefit.

Plasma exchange is reported to be helpful in severe

encephalopathy and stroke due to systemic lupus erythematosus.

## *Interferon-α and interferon-β*

The interferons are cytokines produced by cells in response to viral infection, or in response to other cytokines, such as IL-1, IL-2, and TNFα. They have several actions, which include the inhibition of viral replication by interaction with signalling pathways and destabilisation of mRNA to inhibit protein production. They also induce MHC class 1 expression, which makes cells more susceptible to lysis by CD8+ve T cells, activates NK cells, and prevents IFN-γ induced upregulation of class II MHC.

Interferons have been given in multiple sclerosis on the theoretical basis that viral infection might be a root cause of the disease, and that viral infections may lead to relapses. Various forms of IFN-β have been the subject of four large trials. All of these showed a roughly 30% reduction in the relapse rate of the disease, although in only two of the trials was there an effect on the accumulation of long term disability (Duquette *et al.* 1995). IFN-α has also been the subject of a trial, and may have a similar effect to IFN-β.

## *Co-polymer-1 (glatirimer acetate)*

Co-polymer-1 is a random co-polymer of alanine glutamic acid, lysine, and tyrosine. It was originally produced to simulate the activity of myelin-basic protein in the induction of experimental allergic encephalomyelitis (EAE), and the amino acids are present in the same proportions. Surprisingly, the co-polymer-1 suppressed EAE, and is also able to induce a form of immune regulation that moderates activity against other myelin antigens.

Co-polymer-1 has been the subject of a large, multicentre trial in multiple sclerosis, and a 30% reduction in relapse rate was reported, as well as an improvement in disability, although little or no effect on the progression of disability (Johnson *et al.* 1998).

## *Monoclonal antibodies against leukocytes*

Treatment with cyclophosphamide and azathioprine is undertaken in autoimmune disease in order to kill rapidly dividing lymphocytes. However, the specificity of the drugs is low, since they kill all dividing cells, and side-effects are therefore numerous. Attempts have been made to target leukocyte populations directly, using monoclonal antibodies. Two antibodies have been tried: anti-CD4, which affects the CD4+ve lymphocytes; and Campath-1H, which affects lymphocytes and monocytes. Anti-CD4 leads to a large reduction in the CD4+ve lymphocyte population for over 1 month, while Campath-1H causes a rapid lymphopaenia which lasts for up to 1 year. However, aggressive immunodepletion is not without side-effects.

Both of these monoclonal antibodies have been tried in multiple sclerosis. Anti-CD4 had no quantifiable effect in a trial involving 21 patients (van Oosten *et al.* 1997). Campath-1H has been tried in only seven patients to date. After a single administration, the rate of appearance of new lesions, as assessed by gadolinium enhanced MRI, was suppressed for about 6 months, and the condition stabilised for up to 1 year (Moreau *et al.* 1994). The effects of anti-leukocyte antibodies in other autoimmune diseases are somewhat controversial. Anti-CD4 is reported in some case studies to be helpful in systemic lupus erythematosus and in some forms of vasculitis, but ineffective in rheumatoid arthritis. Campath-1H has been reported to have some beneficial effects in rheumatoid arthritis.

## *Anti-coagulation*

In patients with stroke due to cerebral vasculitis and systemic lupus erythematosus, anti-coagulation with warfarin and aspirin is used to prevent recurrence.

## *Further reading*

Scolding, N.J. (1999). *Immunological and Inflammatory Disorders of the Central Nervous System.* Heinemann Butterworths, London.

# Section III
## Intrinsic mechanisms of recovery

# *Peripheral nerve regeneration*

If we consider the animal kingdom as a whole, successful axon regeneration is the norm rather than the exception. Invertebrates and vertebrates up to the primitive amphibians can regenerate axons and reform accurate connections in both peripheral and central nervous systems. By contrast, in mammals, damage to the nervous system is generally considered to lead to permanent paralysis. However, there is an important exception. Mammals have retained the ability to regenerate axons in the peripheral nervous system (PNS) and, if properly treated, can regain much of the function that is lost after peripheral nerve damage. Not only do the axons regenerate in the periphery, but they restore functional motor connections with muscles, and functional sensory connections with the skin. Nevertheless, peripheral nerve repair is seldom perfect, due both to problems of axon guidance and to other factors that can limit regeneration. There are, therefore, several problems that need to be solved before a regenerated peripheral nerve can completely restore normal function.

In some respects, peripheral nerve regeneration can serve as a model for successful regeneration in the brain and spinal cord. The differences in axon regeneration between the peripheral and the central nervous systems of mammals are profound, but by working out the factors that lead to successful regeneration in the periphery, we hope to delineate the conditions for successful regeneration and thereby to discover the limiting factors that lead to abortive regeneration in the central nervous system (CNS).

## *The environment in which regeneration occurs in the PNS*

When a peripheral nerve is cut or crushed, the axons distal to the damage are disconnected from their cell bodies and start to degenerate (see Chapter 2). As the axons degenerate, the Schwann cell processes, which surround the axons as myelin, also degenerate, although the Schwann cells themselves do not die because they are maintained by several autocrine trophic factors (Jessen and Mirsky 1999). The degenerating axonal and myelin debris is removed over a period of 1–2 weeks, largely by macrophages that migrate into the degenerating nerve from the bloodstream, and also to some extent by the Schwann cells themselves. The Schwann cells are stimulated to divide, and they also secrete various growth factors, including the neurotrophins NGF and BDNF. Growth factor secretion is under the control of several stimuli, including cytokines (particularly interleukin 1) secreted by the invading macrophages (Meyer *et al.* 1992). There are also changes to the Schwann cell surface membrane on which cell surface adhesion molecules, such as L1, N-CAM, and N-cadherin, are increased, low-affinity nerve growth factor receptor (p75) appears, and the Schwann cell extracellular matrix changes, with increases in tenascin and several proteoglycans. Which of these changes is necessary for regeneration to occur is discussed later.

Each axon–Schwann cell unit in an undamaged peripheral nerve is surrounded by a basal lamina sheath, composed of molecules such as collagen, laminin, and fibronectin. Except where it is mechanically disrupted, this sheath remains intact in the degenerated nerve. The Schwann cells of the damaged nerve are, therefore, contained within these tubes of basal lamina. Each tube represents the course of a degenerated axon, and is continuous all the way from the lesion site to the place where the axon terminated. Within each tube the Schwann cells have divided sufficiently to provide a continuous column of end-to-end cells, the whole basal lamina/Schwann cell cylinder being called the band of Büngner (see Fig. 11.1).

The cellular events that happen at the site of nerve damage itself depend on the nature of the injury. At one extreme is a major disruption of the nerve, such as is caused for instance by a gunshot wound. Here the nerve may be cut through, and a substantial length of it so badly damaged that all the Schwann cells will die, leaving just a strip of fibrotic tissue. At the other extreme is a localised crush injury, which may be sufficient to kill the axons but may leave their basal lamina sheaths intact. If the nerve has been cut right through, no regeneration can occur unless the continuity of the Schwann cells is restored by surgically rejoining the proximal and distal nerve stumps. The combination of injury and repair causes a considerable amount of fibroblastic scarring, due to local proliferation of the perineurial and endoneurial fibroblasts. If the repair is badly performed, with residual tension pulling the nerve ends apart, scarring may extend right across the repair and act as a barrier to regeneration. However, if the nerve is merely crushed, there may be sufficient damage to kill the axons and Schwann cells, but the basal lamina sheaths enclosing them survive and remain as a continuous structure joining the axons proximal to the damage and the band of Büngner distal to it. This, then is the environment in which axon regeneration will occur: columns of Schwann that have lost their myelin, changed their cell surface, and started to secrete trophic molecules, encased in a basal lamina sheath, with perineurial fibroblasts interspersed.

## *Axonal regeneration*

### Processes within the axons and neurones

Many structural and biochemical changes and ion fluxes occur in neuronal cell bodies in response to axotomy, and have been described earlier (Chapter 2). The first structural responses to axotomy occur at the site of damage itself, in the axon stump proximal to the lesion. Usually, within an hour of injury, the cut end of the axon seals off, and there is formation of a growth cone-like structure. This occurs long before any molecules could have been transported from the site of damage back to the cell body or from the cell body to the site of damage. Axons must, therefore, have an intrinsic capacity to form a motile growth cone without the production of new molecules. However, within a day or so — the time depending on how far from the cell body the axon was cut — major changes in gene expression and protein production occur within the cell body, and new proteins are transported to the axon tip. Some of these proteins are building-blocks needed for regenerating a new axon, such as tubulin. There are six separate tubulin genes in the rat. Of these, one (T$\alpha$1) is the main tubulin gene expressed during axonal growth in embryonic neurones; and it is this same gene that is turned on again during regeneration.

The pattern of expression of other cytoskeletal proteins in neurones regenerating their axons also in general recapitulates the pattern seen during development, with little production of neurofilament protein, and increased synthesis of tubulin. On the other hand, the pattern of expression of microtubule-associated proteins, which probably play an important role in controlling the polymerisation of tubulin in the region of the growth cone and its stability in the axon, does not revert to the embryonic pattern but remains like the adult. One particular molecule that has attracted much study is the growth associated protein, GAP-43. This protein is localised to the inside surface of growth cones, and was originally identified because its expression is upregulated, sometimes up to 1000 times in neurones with regenerating axons, but not in neurones whose axons are failing to regenerate. All regenerating axons in the PNS contain GAP-43 (see Box 12.1), which is upregulated rapidly after the axon is cut — even if the cut is made a considerable distance from the cell body. As explained in Chapter 2 (see Fig. 2.3), there is also a good correlation between GAP-43 expression and the variations in the vigour of axon regeneration between different parts of the PNS. The clearest example of this is seen in the regeneration of the central and peripheral branches of sensory axons. The dorsal roots are part of the PNS, since they contain Schwann cells and fibroblasts rather than oligodendrocytes and astrocytes, yet axons crushed in the roots regenerate slowly and poorly, and they also contain little GAP-43; there is much less GAP-43 expression in the dorsal root ganglia after dorsal root crushes than after peripheral nerve crushes (see Chapter 2). However, if the peripheral nerve is crushed several days before a dorsal root crush, GAP-43 is already increased by the time of the dorsal root crush, and there is much more axon regeneration. GAP-43 is present on the inside of the growth cone, interacts with various kinases, and probably plays an important role in the communication between the growth cone and its surroundings (Chong *et al.* 1994; Aigner *et al.* 1995). The possible roles of these molecules in permitting central axonal regeneration are discussed in the next chapter.

### Interactions between regenerating axons and their environment

Regenerating axons are always found associated with the bands of Büngner, rather than with the many fibroblastic perineurial cells that are interspersed between them. A cross-section of a regenerating nerve reveals that the axons grow in between the basal lamina sheath and the Schwann cell membrane, so that half of the growth cone membrane is in contact with Schwann cell membrane, and half in contact with basal lamina (Fig 11.1). The cell–cell interactions that result in regeneration must, therefore, be between these three elements: growth cone, Schwann cell, and basal lamina.

Which cellular and molecular interactions are important for axonal regeneration?. First, it is important to know whether it is the Schwann cell plasma membrane or the basal lamina sheath which contains the molecules that are essential for regeneration. Two experiments

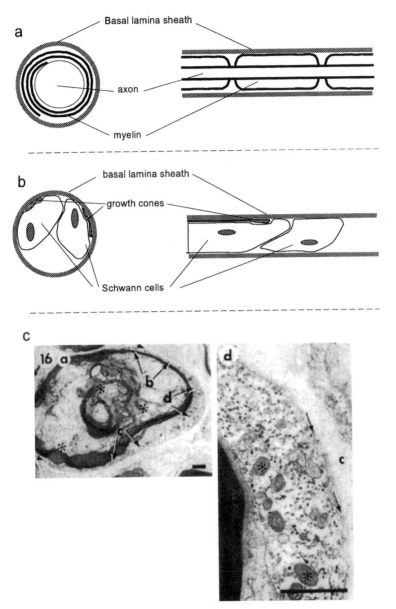

**Fig. 11.1** Axon regeneration in peripheral nerve. a) Arrangement of axon, Schwann cell, and basal lamina sheath in a normal nerve. b) Arrangement in a regenerating nerve. The basal lamina sheath remains, and Schwann cells have divided to fill it and form a band of Büngner. Axon growth cones are seen in between the Schwann cell and the basal lamina sheath. c (*Left*) electron micrograph of a growth cone regenerating in a peripheral nerve, showing a degenerating myelinated axon, with a large growth cone (*arrows* d) growing alongside it. (*Right*) area of the same photograph at higher magnification, showing the growth cone in the region marked d on the left-hand picture, which is in contact with Schwann cell membrane on its left side, basal lamina (*arrows*) on the right. (Micrographs from Scherer and Easter 1984.)

that address this question rely on grafting tissue containing basal lamina, but no Schwann cells, between the proximal and distal stump of a cut nerve. One such tissue is a section of peripheral nerve that has been frozen and unfrozen, while another is a preparation of muscle extracellular matrix from which the cellular material has been removed. Axons regenerate through both these substrates, but only when accompanied by Schwann cells that have migrated into the acellular graft from the proximal or distal stump. Moreover, if Schwann cell migration into frozen nerve grafts is prevented by applying a mitotic inhibitor to the preparation, then there is no axonal regeneration. Clearly, in these experiments, basal lamina by itself cannot support axonal regeneration — Schwann cells are also required (Hall 1986; Feneley *et al.* 1991).

Macrophages enter the degenerating peripheral nerve in quantity, and are responsible for removing axonal and myelin debris. They also secrete a variety of cytokines, which promote Schwann cell division, increasing the number of Schwann cells available for the axons to interact with. Macrophage-produced interleukin 1 also causes the Schwann cells to produce nerve growth factor, whose possible importance is discussed below.

After nerve damage, Schwann cells undergo many changes to their cell surface and in the molecules that they secrete. How important are these changes to the process of regeneration? The importance of macrophage invasion, and the various changes to Schwann cells that occur in degeneration, to the process of regeneration is shown by an inbred mouse strain, the Ola mouse, in which normal Wallerian degeneration is defective. As described in Chapter 2, cutting a peripheral nerve in this mouse does not lead to the normal rapid degeneration of nerve fibres and macrophage invasion. Instead the nerve distal to the cut continues to look almost normal for many days (see Fig. 2.1). Into this almost normal-looking distal stump, a few regenerating axons can penetrate. However, regeneration of both sensory and motor axons is greatly reduced in both speed and number. The changes initiated during degeneration are, therefore, essential for effective regeneration. The Ola mouse does not tell us, however, which of these changes are important, since both macrophage recruitment and Schwann cell changes are absent. It is not possible, therefore, to say whether the Schwann cell changes are initiated by macrophage invasion. The primary defect in the Ola mouse is probably in the axons, which are unable to undergo the active autolysis that is the basis of degeneration. But from the point of view of under-

standing what factors stimulate regeneration, the mouse shows that the changes in Schwann cells, which result from them losing contact with axons and from their interactions with macrophages, are very important in making them a suitable substrate for regenerating axons (Perry and Brown 1992).

## Molecular interactions necessary for regeneration

The regenerating axons interact with their environment through a variety of molecules, which are on the surface of axons and Schwann cells, in the extracellular matrix, and surrounding the axons as soluble secreted molecules.

In order to exert tension on the growing axons and make progress, growth cones must be able to adhere to the surfaces around them. This is done through the interaction of adhesion molecules on the growth cone surface with molecules on neighbouring cells, and through the interaction of substrate adhesion molecules with ligands in the extracellular matrix. On the surface of Schwann cells are two main adhesion molecules: L1 and N-cadherin. By growing axons over Schwann cells *in vitro* in the presence of antibodies that block the binding site of these molecules, John Bixby (working in the Reichardt laboratory) was able to assess whether they are necessary for axon–Schwann cell interaction (Bixby *et al.* 1988). Antibodies to both L1 and N-cadherin reduced axon elongation on Schwann cells, L1 antibodies to a greater extent than N-cadherin antibodies. When antibodies to both molecules were applied, growth was inhibited to a greater extent but still not prevented. Only when antibodies to integrins (the receptors on the axonal surface for extracellular matrix molecules, such as laminin) were applied as well, was axonal growth blocked. We can conclude, therefore, that L1, N-cadherin, and extracellular matrix, all promote axon regeneration over Schwann cells. L1 and N-cadherin via homophilic interactions with the same molecules on the axonal surface, and matrix molecules via binding to integrins. It may be important that levels of L1 are greatly increased on both axons and Schwann cells in regenerating nerve, as are levels of N-CAM, another homophilically binding adhesion molecule, which may also play a part in axon-glial interactions. In a different form of *in vitro* peripheral nerve regeneration assay, however, laminin was the critical component: frozen sections of peripheral nerve can be laid flat and used as a tissue culture surface, and on such a surface an antibody to laminin–heparan sulphate proteoglycan complex was able to completely prevent growth (Sandrock and Matthew 1987). This last result, however, should be interpreted in the light of the *in vivo* experiments detailed above, which show that Schwann cells must be present for regeneration to occur.

Schwann cells separated from axonal contact and stimulated by macrophages secrete NGF, BDNF, and several other growth factors. There is now a considerable body of evidence that suggests that these trophic factors increase the ability of neurones to survive the trauma of axotomy (see Chapter 2). Trophic factors also have an important action in stimulating axons to regenerate. While it has been appreciated for many years that NGF is essential for the survival of sensory and sympathetic neurones during development, it was assumed that it had little function in adults because its withdrawal from adults does not cause any immediate neuronal death. However Eugene Johnson and his co-workers showed that when the action of NGF in adult animals is blocked with an antiserum, peripheral neurones are less able than normal to survive axotomy (Yip *et al.* 1984). In addition, it has been shown that many trophic factors increase the ability of adult sensory neurones to regenerate their axons *in vitro*. *In vivo*, NGF-blocking antibody reduces sensory axon regeneration, and added NGF enhances nerve repair. Other soluble molecules are also important. IGF-1 can enhance peripheral nerve regeneration, as can CNTF. Trophic-factor release in the damaged nerve is almost certainly a key factor in helping axotomised neurones to survive, and in promoting regeneration of their axons. In addition, trophic events around the cell bodies in peripheral ganglia are important. Inflammation around the sensory neurones, which causes the release of many cytokines, also enhances sensory regeneration. In the CNS, Schwann cells and fibroblasts have been grafted into lesions in attempts to provide axons with a permissive environment in which to regenerate, and here too when the grafted cells have been engineered to secrete a variety of trophic factors, axon growth into the grafts is greatly enhanced.

## Inhibition of axon regeneration by scar tissue in the nerve

Not all axons are successful at regenerating across nerve injuries, but instead they grow into the fibroblastic scar tissue that forms at sites of nerve damage, then they are unable to grow further, and develop a swollen club ending. Apart from causing the failure of axons to regenerate, neuromatous regions of scar tissue can become extremely sensitive to light touch, and lead to agonising pain. The greater the physical damage to a nerve, the more scar tissue is formed, and the fewer axons can regenerate. Thus nerves that are traumatised over long distances by contusion or by stretch injuries, will have scarring over the whole length of the injury, and axons will not regenerate through these regions unless the damaged region is surgically excised and the gap bridged by an autologous nerve graft. Severe scarring may also be brought about by surgical nerve repairs in which tension has had to be exerted on the nerve ends to bring them together; under these circumstances it is more successful to use a nerve graft to bridge the gap between nerve ends, rather than dragging them together with tension.

Since scar tissue is so effective at preventing axon regeneration in peripheral nerves, the question arises as to why. We have already seen in the chapter on regeneration of CNS axons that fibroblasts can be a successful material for promoting the regeneration of CNS axons, and sensory axons grow fairly well on fibroblasts *in vitro*. The reasons are probably two-fold. One reason is probably that fibroblasts do not normally secrete trophic factors, so axons trying to grow through scar tissue receive no trophic support. The other reason is that peripheral nerve fibroblasts produce large amounts of the highly inhibitory proteoglycan NG2.

## Bridge grafts for nerve repair

After severe nerve damage there may be a gap between the proximal and distal stump of the nerve. If the nerve ends are pulled together under tension, an impenetrable scar will form and regeneration will fail. In order to allow axons to grow across these gaps it is necessary to provide some sort of bridge material. Considerable success has been achieved with cable grafts of nerve removed from elsewhere in the patient. The standard graft site is the sural nerve, which can be removed with little long-term loss of sensation. As long as the grafts are inserted so as to minimise scar formation at the suture lines, this can be a very successful technique. However, in severely injured patients it may not be possible to obtain enough graft material. For these cases, there has been interest in developing alternative forms of bridge material. The most successful of these materials have been collagen-based tubes, into which the ends of the nerves can be inserted, and a basal lamina material derived from muscle. Axon growth into these grafts depends on the migration of Schwann cells.

## Re-innervation of target structures by regenerating axons

When regenerating peripheral nerve axons reach appropriate targets they are able to re-innervate them, and it is this that makes the whole process functionally useful. Moreover there is an important level of specificity in the connections made by the axons, which is also essential to the restoration of function. Regenerating motor axons reconnect to muscles, and regenerating sensory axons reconnect to sensory structures. This implies that there are molecular recognition processes that allow regenerating axons to recognise appropriate targets. The molecular interactions that might underlie this behaviour are discussed below.

As first noted by Ramon y Cajal, (Cajal 1928) the majority of regenerated connections within muscles contact the muscle fibres at the exact site of the old muscle end-plate; even the pattern of axon branching within the end-plate often reproduces the previous pattern. This indicates that previous innervation leaves behind some molecular imprint, which can be recognised by the regrowing axon.

What is the molecular nature of the imprints left behind by degenerating axons at the muscle end-plate? The molecules must be associated with the end-plate basal lamina because, as Glicksman and Sanes showed in 1983 {Glicksman and Sanes 1983}, regenerating axons will find the old denervated synaptic sites, even when the muscle fibres inside their basal lamina sheaths are caused to degenerate, so that only the ghost of the muscle in the shape of its basal lamina sheath is left behind (Fig. 11.2). The old synaptic regions on these sheaths are still recognisable from their distinctive anatomy, and it is to these regions that axonal ingrowth is directed.

A candidate molecule for this role is agrin, which is found at the end-plate, is secreted there by both motor nerves and muscle, and is at least partly responsible for making acetylcholine receptors cluster under the terminal. This molecule can act as a stop signal for axons growing in tissue culture (Fig. 11.3). Another relevant molecule is a type of laminin, s-laminin, which is only found in synaptic junctions. This molecule also acts as a stop signal for motor axon growth *in vitro* and a transgenic mouse, which lacks functional s-laminin, has abnormal neuromuscular junctions. Also important in guiding axons back towards the end-plate, and in sprouting at the end-plate itself, are the specialised Schwann cells whose processes envelope it (Campagna *et al.* 1995; Sanes *et al.* 1995; Son *et al.* 1996). A combination of these factors probably allows the regenerating axons to recognise the old end-plate regions. However, the axons first have to be guided to somewhere near this region of the muscle, and for this they rely on the pathway formed by the degenerated nerve and its bands of Büngner.

In one important respect the reformed innervation differs from the original. In normal muscle, as a result of the removal of polyneuronal innervation late in development, each muscle fibre receives input from only one axon. Early in regeneration, polyneuronal innervation of muscle is found again, with several axons making contact with each muscle fibre at the end-plate. A new process of withdrawal of polyneuronal innervation now occurs, which generally results yet again in each muscle fibre being singly innervated. As in development, this process is delayed by blockade of electrical activity in the nerve fibres, and so to some extent it is likely to be a recapitulation of the developmental event. However, there may be many fewer axons innervating the muscles than normal because only a proportion of axons may regenerate, and each nerve fibre may therefore end up innervating many more muscle fibres than in undamaged innervation, leading to much larger motor units.

Sensory re-innervation is less clear-cut. Some sensory end-organs, such as Pacinian corpuscles, may degenerate after denervation and are therefore only available for re-innervation if it occurs rapidly, but nevertheless they attract regenerating axons, as do muscle spindles. However, many regenerated nerve endings in the skin are not associated with particular sensory organs, but are simple branched nerve endings ramifying in the skin, rather different to those that existed before the nerve was damaged (Zelena and Zacharova 1997).

## Specificity of connections

Regenerating PNS axons exhibit considerable specificity in making their connections. Motor axons reconnect to muscle, and sensory axons remake sensory endings. However, there is another level of specificity at which the regenerating axons are much less successful. In order

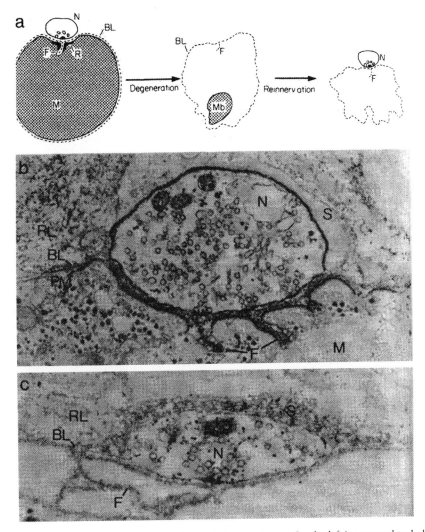

**Fig. 11.2** Re-innervation of previous end-plate sites. a Steps of the experiment. On the *left* is a normal end-plate. In the *centre* the axon has been cut, and the muscle damaged to make it degenerate, leaving behind the sheath and the synaptic fold. On the *right* the nerve has grown back to terminate on the old synaptic site, marked by the fold. b Normal end-plate with synaptic folds. c Nerve fibre reconnecting with the old synaptic site on the basal lamina sheath which is empty of muscle. (From Covault and Sanes 1985.) (N = nerve ending, S = Schwann cell, M = muscle, BL = Basal lamina, F = junctional told.)

for the reformed connections to function as well as the originals, particular motor neurone pools must reconnect to specific muscles, and particular sensory neurones must reconnect to specific areas of skin, or other specific sensory organs. A simple sensory map of the skin of a patient who has had a peripheral nerve repair will reveal that there are many positional errors made by regenerating axons. Thus a pinprick to the skin on one place may be perceived by the patient elsewhere on the skin. Equally, muscle connections are somewhat mixed

up, which results in a weak and clumsy limb, since an attempt to activate a particular muscle may lead to unintended contraction of other muscles, some of which may antagonise the intended movement. Some of the misguidance of regenerating axons may be a consequence of the anatomy of a degenerated nerve, with the bands of Büngner marking out the path of degenerated axons. It is very rare for regenerating axons to cross from one band of Büngner to another, since this would involve them penetrating the basal lamina wall of the band and

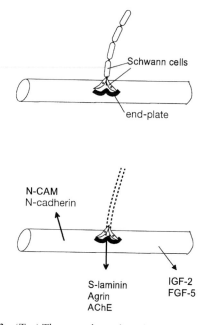

**Fig. 11.3** (*Top*) The normal muscle and end-plate before denervation. (*Bottom*) After denervation the muscle upregulates several adhesion molecules and growth factors. The end-plate region contains several molecules with the potential to attract regenerating axons. (Redrawn from Hall and Sanes 1993.)

growing into a neighbouring band. If a nerve is sectioned longitudinally, all the axons can be seen to be tracking down a single Schwann cell tube. However, as illustrated in Fig. 11.4, if the nerve has been disrupted at the site of injury so that basal lamina tubes are broken, there is often random and tangled growth in this region, so that axons are unlikely to get back to the correct band of Büngner, while other axons may fail to regenerate past the injury site at all, ending up in the fibroblastic scar tissue, which proliferates at the injury site where they form swollen club endings. Once in the wrong band of Büngner, axons are not able to correct their mistake, and will be carried down the path of the band of Büngner to wherever it leads. On the other hand, if the nerve is crushed rather than cut, the basal lamina sheaths may survive in continuity. This has important functional implications, because it means that a regenerating axon will never lose contact with its original basal lamina sheath, and it will therefore be led down the band of Büngner that resulted from the degeneration of that very axon. Since the band of Büngner follows the course of the cut axon, the regenerating axon, in following that band, must regenerate to the same target area that the parent axon originally innervated.

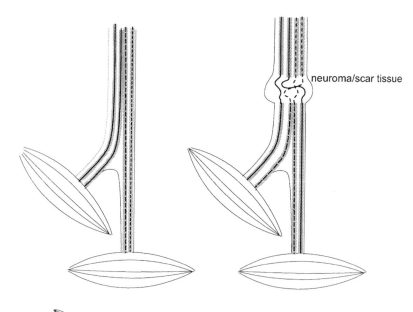

muscle

axons to right hand muscle

axons to left hand muscle

Band of Büngner, Schwann cell sheath

**Fig. 11.4** The mechanism by which axons get guided to the wrong target in regeneration. At the repair site axons may grow onto the wrong band of Büngner, and thus be guided to the wrong target.

Opinions vary as to whether regenerating axons in peripheral nerves exhibit any positional specificity of regeneration, or whether they are railroaded to a particular target from the moment that they join a particular band of Büngner. Thomas Brushart and colleagues have shown that axons regenerating in the rat sciatic nerve show specificity in that motor axons grow preferentially down a motor branch. The mechanism behind this specificity may be the expression of the HNK-1 carbohydrate epitope by Schwann cells in the motor branches of the peripheral nerve (Martini *et al.* 1994). It is also the case that many experiments that demonstrate a degree of specificity are ones in which the axons are forced to grow through a terrain in which there are no bands of Büngner, for instance, through tubular chambers grafted in between the proximal and distal nerve stumps.

An undesirable consequence of the lack of specificity in the regeneration pathway of damaged peripheral axons is that fibres regenerating down a long nerve tend all to reconnect to proximal structures, leaving few axons to regenerate distally.

Cut axons frequently branch as they regenerate, particularly at the lesion site, so if the number of regenerating axons distal to the lesion is counted while regrowth is still under way, it will be found to be several times higher than the number of axons proximal to the lesion. This state of affairs continues until axons start to make connections with target structures, when the number of axons starts to decline. There is some evidence that appropriate axonal connections are preferentially preserved over inappropriate ones during this period when some of the many extra regenerated axons withdraw, so this may improve the apparent accuracy of regeneration, since regenerating axons may branch and regrow to several targets, then withdraw the branches that have made mistakes.

The functional results of peripheral nerve repair would be greatly improved if axons could be guided back to their original targets. It is clearly not practicable to match every regenerating axon with its original band of Büngner. However, at a much grosser level, groups of regenerating axons can, under favourable circumstances, be matched with the correct groups of bands of Büngner. Peripheral nerves are divided by connective tissue septa into fascicles, and axons going to a particular muscle or area of skin are concentrated in a particular fascicle near to the target, although they are much more randomly diffused through the nerve further from the target. If the nerve is cut cleanly it is possible for the surgeon to individually reconnect fascicles in the

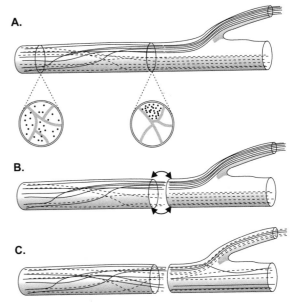

**Fig. 11.5** A. Normal peripheral nerve, showing that axons that will go down a particular branch collect in the same fascicle some way before the branch point. However, further away up the nerve this grouping is lost. B. If individual fascicles can be recognised and reconnected at nerve repair, axons will be guided into the correct branches. C. If fascicles are not reconnected, axons may make contact with the wrong bands of Büngner, and go the wrong target.

proximal stump to their equivalents in the distal stump, and thereby ensure that regenerating axons make contact with a band of Büngner that will take them to the appropriate target (see Fig. 11.5). However, this is only of benefit when the nerve is cut near to the target area, for instance, in the wrist, where most of the axons in a fascicle will normally project to the same target area. It is also important that the injury is a local one, since the fascicular pattern changes over quite short distances, and if a long length of nerve has to be resected it is not possible to match the fascicular pattern in the proximal and distal nerve stumps.

The lack of positional specificity of regenerating axons in the PNS would not matter if the connections in the CNS were sufficiently plastic to allow compensation. However, this does not happen to a significant extent. There is a critical period during development in which the central connections of peripheral nerves are matched up to the correct central connections, but after this period misrouted peripheral nerves do not alter their central connections sufficiently to compensate for major errors of axon pathfinding (Mears and Frank 1996). There is also, as recounted in Chapter 13, considerable central plasticity at the cortical level to allow compensation for incorrect connections in the postnatal period.

## Further reading

Fawcett, J.W. and Keynes, R.J. (1990). Peripheral nerve regeneration. *Annual Reviews of Neuroscience*, **13**, 43–60.

Sunderland, S. (1972). *Nerves and Nerve Injuries*. Churchill Livingstone, Edinburgh.

# 12 | Failure of CNS regeneration

As described in the previous chapter, axons in the mammalian peripheral nervous system (PNS) regenerate well. Axons in the adult mammalian central nervous system (CNS), however, do not spontaneously regenerate, with the result that any injury that cuts axons, such as spinal-cord injury, will not recover. Clearly a central feature of CNS repair will have to be the induction of axon regeneration. In principle, axon growth is a collaborative process that involves a dialogue between the axon and the environment it is trying to penetrate. Whether an axon will regenerate or not, therefore, depends on the regenerative efforts made by the axon, on the inhibitory or permissive molecules in the environment, and on the receptors for these molecules on the axonal surface. In this chapter we will examine these various factors and their effects on CNS axon regeneration.

## Events following lesions of CNS axons

The events that follow CNS damage and axotomy are described in Chapters 1 and 2. To provide a brief recap, the essential features of this process are as follows.

When a CNS axon is cut, it degenerates distal to the cut, as does the myelin surrounding the axons, just as in the PNS. As in the PNS, a proportion of the neurones that have had their axons cut will die, the probability of death being higher the closer to the neuronal cell body is to the damage (see Chapter 2). A proportion of post-synaptic neurones will also die when they lose their synaptic inputs, as discussed in Chapter 1. By contrast, some other neurones do not die, but instead atrophy, losing many of the enzymes associated with neuro-transmitter manufacture and normal cellular function. In addition, when an axon is damaged, many of the synaptic boutons that connect with the cell body are stripped away in a process that involves microglia (Chapter 1). The space that used to be occupied by these boutons is taken over by astrocytic processes, and these probably prevent the connections reforming. In the PNS

the degenerating axonal and myelin debris is rapidly removed by macrophages that infiltrate from the bloodstream, but in the CNS there is little or no recruitment of macrophages from the blood, except in the area of the lesion itself where there has been substantial damage to the blood vessels, with blood cells and plasma entering the CNS. The debris of degeneration is therefore usually removed largely by activated microglia. Although these are cells of the macrophage lineage, divide following injury, and migrate to the injury site, they are not present in nearly such large quantities as macrophages in damaged peripheral nerves, and removal of axonal and myelin debris in the CNS is consequently much slower than in the PNS. There is, therefore, myelin and axonal debris persisting in the CNS for much longer than would be the case in the PNS.

At the site of any CNS lesion there is reactive gliosis, leading to the formation of a glial scar, as described in Chapter 2. The cells that participate in this process are microglia, oligodendrocyte precursors, astrocytes, and meningeal cells. Microglia are the first cells to invade CNS injuries, first being seen in less than 24h, then oligodendrocyte precursors are seen reaching a peak density within 7 days. Both these cell types then decrease in number, and the injury fills up with reactive astrocytes and, where the injury penetrates the meningeal surface, meningeal cells: these two cell types co-operate in the formation of the dense glial scar that is the long-term outcome of a CNS injury. As we will see, all these cell types can produce molecules that are able to inhibit axon regeneration (Eng et al. 1987, Fawcett and Asher 1999). Regenerating axons will, therefore, encounter several cell types, with the type of cell and the nature of the molecules in the CNS environment varying with time.

### Intrinsic regenerative ability versus inhibitory environment

In theory, the failure of CNS axons to regenerate could be due to an intrinsic inability of CNS neurones to regenerate their axons, or to an inhibitory effect of the CNS environment preventing axon growth, or to a combination of these factors. What is the evidence for these two factors?

# The effect of the CNS environment on axon regeneration

There is a large body of experimental evidence, which demonstrates that the environment of the adult CNS is inhibitory to regeneration. There are several different lines of evidence for this conclusion:

## The dorsal root entry zone

Not all axons in the CNS are of CNS origin — sensory axons have their cell bodies in dorsal root ganglia, sending one axonal process into the CNS and one into the peripheral nerves (see Fig. 12.1). The central axonal branch leaves the cell body and travels through the dorsal root, which has the structure and cell types of peripheral nerves, then enters the CNS at the dorsal root entry zone, after which it is surrounded by CNS glial cells. This anatomical arrangement makes it possible to test whether it is the axon or the CNS environment that prevents regeneration. As we have seen in the previous chapter, the peripheral axons of the dorsal root ganglion neurones regenerate well, and this neurone is therefore fully capable of regenerating its axon. Yet the central process of this neurone will not regenerate if it is cut in the spinal cord. Is this because the central process is unable to regenerate at all? This can be determined by injuring the process within the dorsal root itself, where it is surrounded by a permissive environment of Schwann cells. When injured here, the central process regenerates within the dorsal root, but stops growing at the dorsal root entry zone, where the Schwann cell environment of the PNS changes to the astrocytic/oligodendrocytic environment of the CNS, indicating that the CNS environment must be inhibitory to regeneration (Fig 12.1; Carlstedt *et al.* 1989). At this point, the axons first make contacts with the processes of CNS astrocytes (see Fig 12.2). This has been interpreted as showing that astrocytes deliver a stop signal to the regenerating axons, since the nerve terminal undergoes many of the anatomical changes that happen during synaptogenesis (Liuzzi and Lasek 1987). However, this experiment is not quite as simple as it first appears because, as we will see later, there is also evi-

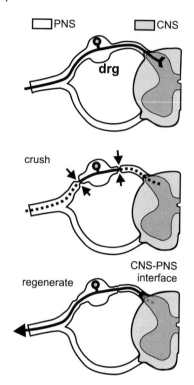

**Fig. 12.1** Crushed peripheral nerves regenerate in the PNS but not in the CNS. In the normal sensory pathway, dorsal root ganglion (drg) neurones send one axonal process to the periphery, one to the spinal cord. If the dorsal root is crushed distal to the spinal cord, sensory axons will regenerate back to the periphery. If the dorsal root is crushed between the drg and the spinal cord, the axons will regenerate towards the spinal cord while they lie in the PNS environment of the dorsal root, but stop when they encounter the CNS environment at the entry zone where the dorsal root meets the spinal cord.

dence that the central process of sensory neurones has a lower regenerative ability than the peripheral process.

## Glial transplant experiments

The experiments above indicate that the CNS/PNS interface is inhibitory to sensory axon regeneration, which suggests that the CNS environment stops regeneration of sensory axons. Thus, PNS neurones will regenerate in the PNS but not in the CNS environment. However, this may not explain why all CNS neurones will not regenerate their axons To find out, it was necessary to do similar experiments with other neuronal types. The environment around damaged CNS axons can be changed from supposedly inhibitory CNS glia to a more permissive environment by transplanting permis-

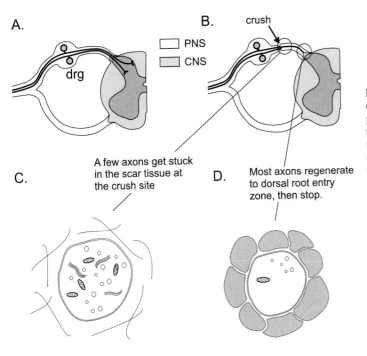

A.

**PNS** □
**CNS** ▨

drg

B. crush

C. A few axons get stuck in the scar tissue at the crush site

D. Most axons regenerate to dorsal root entry zone, then stop.

**Fig. 12.2** Failure of axon regeneration at the dorsal root entry zone. A In the normal sensory pathway, dorsal root ganglion (drg) neurones send one axonal process to the periphery, one to the spinal cord. B If the dorsal root is crushed, sensory axons will regenerate in the Schwann cell environment of the dorsal root; some axons do not grow back beyond the crush site, whereas others regrow until they encounter CNS glia at the dorsal root entry zone. C Axons that get stuck in the fibroblastic scar tissue around the crush site have swollen endings, full of vesicles and cytoskeletal elements. D Axons that stop growing at the entry zone are in contact with astrocytes (*shaded grey*), and the tips undergo anatomical changes similar to those seen in axons that have reached a target. These endings are not to scale, the ending in C is much larger. (Adapted from Liuzzi and Lasek 1987.)

sive materials into the path of cut CNS axons. The obvious tissue to use for this type of experiment is peripheral nerve, which supports the regeneration of peripheral axons, or the Schwann cells over which the regenerating axons grow. An alternative permissive tissue is embryonic CNS tissue, which supports the growth of axons during development. Many experiments have been performed in which either grafts of peripheral nerve, or purified Schwann cells, or embryonic tissue have been grafted in contact with cut CNS axons. For example, Richardson *et al.* (1982) implanted pieces of sciatic nerve to bridge the gap in the transected spinal cord (Fig. 12.3) and used injections of horseradish peroxidase (HRP) to label CNS axons that had grown through the bridge. Whereas the axons of many cells in the distal spinal cord grew into and through the PNS bridge tissue, the axons failed to penetrate back into the CNS on the other side of the transection.

These experiments show that almost all CNS axons can regenerate to some extent in a permissive PNS environment. In the case of peripheral nerve or Schwann cell grafts it is essential that the Schwann cells are alive — grafts of extracellular matrix alone derived from Schwann cells are not effective.

There is a great deal of variation in the vigour with which axons will regenerate, even into the most permissive environments. Almost all the axons that regenerate into Schwann cell grafts come from neurones whose cell bodies are close to the graft interface, and whose axons have therefore been cut close to the cell body. Rat rubrospinal axons, for instance, will regenerate into peripheral nerve grafts inserted into the cervical cord, but they will not regenerate if the graft is inserted further from the cell body in the thoracic cord (Tetzlaff *et al.* 1994). We discuss the mechanisms behind this length dependency later in this chapter. Moreover, some neurones regenerate their axons readily, while others are much less willing to regenerate, even if they are cut near the cell body. An extreme example of this is the Purkinje cells of the cerebellum, which will not regenerate their axons into either Schwann cell or embryonic grafts (Rossi *et al.* 1995). At the other extreme, the neurones of the thalamic reticular nucleus regenerate with particular vigour, and are over-represented in peripheral nerve grafts (Morrow *et al.* 1993).

The reverse form of transplantation has also been done — grafting CNS tissue into a peripheral nerve. The results are as expected from the experiments described earlier, the CNS tissue blocks the regeneration of PNS axons (Giftochristos and David 1988).

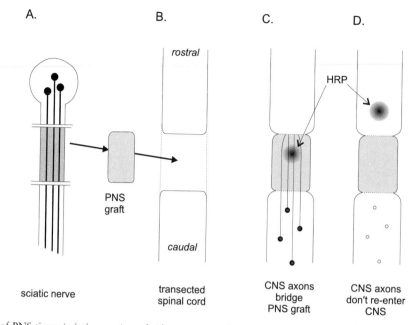

**Fig 12.3** Grafts of PNS tissue (sciatic nerve) can bridge a transected spinal cord. CNS axons in the distal cord will regenerate axons back through the PNS environment of the bridge graft but then fail to grow any appreciable distance further back into the proximal stump of the spinal cord once they encounter a CNS tissue environment. In (C), horseradish peroxidase (HRP) is injected into the PNS graft, labelling host axons that have grown into it. However, the axons are unable to grow out of the graft back into host CNS tissue. Thus, in (D), when HRP is applied in the cord, host neurones on the distal side remain unlabelled.

# Why is the CNS environment inhibitory to axon regeneration?

## Anatomical observations on damaged axons in the CNS

An obvious first step towards working out which CNS glial cells inhibit regeneration, is to look at the damaged CNS and see which types of cell are in contact with cut CNS axons and, therefore, which interactions can occur. As described above and in Chapter 2, the cells available for axons to interact with change with time: thus, immediately after injury there may be blood cells and damaged CNS cells including myelin; a little later blood-derived macrophages and activated microglia will appear to remove dead cells, degenerated myelin, etc.; after approximately 2 days, oligodendrocyte precursors and sometimes meningeal cells invade. The cells present at all times in the damaged brain are astrocytes, oligodendrocyte precursors, and oligodendrocytes. Astrocytes divide in areas of brain injury, and are the main cell type of the mature glial scar (described in

Chapter 2). In this astrocytic matrix there are variable numbers of oligodendrocytes, and of course there is likely to be degenerating myelin, which is removed very slowly in the CNS; oligodendrocyte precursors are recruited in large numbers into lesions over the first few days, then their number declines after about 10 days.

An obvious place in which there is a clearly defined point at which axon regeneration fails is the dorsal root entry zone. As described earlier, when a dorsal root is crushed the central branches of sensory axons are able to regenerate in the Schwann cell environment of the root itself, but regeneration ceases where the axons meet the CNS glial environment at the CNS/PNS interface. Both Thomas Carlstedt and, separately, Frank Liuzzi and Ray Lasek examined the tips of the axons where they stopped growing (Figs 12.1 and 12.2, respectively). They found that the tips of axons that are failing to regenerate are usually found in contact with, and surrounded by, astrocytes. Moreover, they saw that the anatomy of the axon tips is suggestive of an important interaction between axons and astrocytes, which they interpreted as the astrocytes giving the axons a stop signal. This interpretation was based on the different appearance of axon tips that have become trapped in scar tissue in peripheral nerve, and those that have stopped growing in the CNS. Thus when a regenerating axon in a peripheral nerve gets stuck in an area of fibroblastic scar tissue, the axon tip is large and swollen, and full of vesicles and cytoskeletal elements. An axon tip that is failing to regenerate in contact with astrocytes is not swollen, and looks almost like a normal nerve ending, sometimes even containing some synaptic vesicles. One interpretation of this appearance is that the astrocyte has given the axon a signal to stop growing (Carlstedt 1985; Liuzzi and Lasek 1987).

The transition between the PNS and CNS is a rather specialised region — what happens in other parts of the CNS? Observations have not been made in the same detail. However, Steve Davies and Geoff Raisman considered a different model in which they made lesions in the spinal cord so small that there was no anatomically visible disruption of the glial architecture of a white matter tract. Following these lesions, as is often seen in the CNS, there was a small amount of axon regrowth of less than 1 mm, and these axons were seen growing in contact with the longitudinal astrocyte processes that interweave between the axons; but this growth was only seen away from the lesion, the axons would not grow over the astrocyte processes in or very near the lesion. It was not clear whether the axons ever contacted oligodendrocytes. The conclusion was that the normal undamaged CNS environment may not be particularly inhibitory to axon growth, but that injury must cause changes that make the environment inhibitory. The experiment also points to astrocytes as being the main cell type contacted by regenerating axons (Davies *et al.* 1996). Of the other cell types that appear in lesions, it is rare to see axons regenerating in association with the large numbers of meningeal cells that are often seen in spinal-cord injuries, so these may be assumed to be inhibitory. Microglia and macrophages are probably growth promoting, since regenerating axons are seen in lesions that contain largely these cell types. Axonal interactions with oligodendrocyte precursors have not been seen *in vivo*, although there are such large numbers of these cells in lesions between 4 days and 2 weeks after trauma that it would be difficult for sprouting axons to avoid contacting them.

## Interactions of axons with different glial types

If we wish to know which of the cell types is responsible for preventing axon regeneration, the logical step is to look at the interaction of regenerating axons with purified populations of each cell type in turn. This has been done for oligodendrocytes, astrocytes microglia, oligodendrocyte precursors, and meningeal cells. *In vivo* it is much more difficult to do experiments that test whether particular glial types are inhibitory, although there have been experiments in which single cell types have been transplanted, or in which a particular cell type has been removed.

### Oligodendrocytes

Oligodendrocytes in tissue culture repel most types of growing axon. When axons are grown over a surface on which oligodendrocytes have been seeded, they can be seen to avoid growing over the surface of mature oligodendrocytes (Fig. 12.4). Observed under time-lapse video-microscopy, axonal growth cones make contact with the oligodendrocyte, and they are then either paralysed or, more commonly, about 15–45 min after the first contact, the growth cones collapse and retract (Fig. 12.5). The axon may then generate a new growth cone, which will again contact the oligodendrocyte, and the process is repeated (Fawcett *et al.* 1989b).

A different type of assay, which shows a similar result, is to use a section of brain or spinal cord as a tissue culture surface for neurones; in such cultures axons will grow on the grey matter parts of the slice, but neurones adhere poorly and axons grow little on the oligodendrocyte-containing white matter (Schwab 1990). *In vivo*, regions of the CNS can be depleted of oligodendrocytes by injecting an antibody to the oligodendrocyte cell surface together with complement. When this was done in the spinal cord of chick embryos, they retained the ability to regenerate axons in the spinal cord, which normally ceases at the time of myelination, for 2 or 3 days beyond the normal time. Similarly, demyelination of adult rat spinal cord had the effect of allowing a limited amount of axon regeneration (Keirstead *et al.* 1995).

### Astrocytes

The results with astrocytes are more complicated. A monolayer of astrocytes is usually a permissive surface for axon growth. Many different neurones will grow axons rapidly on an astrocyte surface, even if there are oligodendrocytes on it (Fawcett *et al.* 1992). However, astrocyte cultures become less permissive the longer the astrocytes are allowed to mature *in vitro*. Moreover, different types of axon respond to them differently. Axons

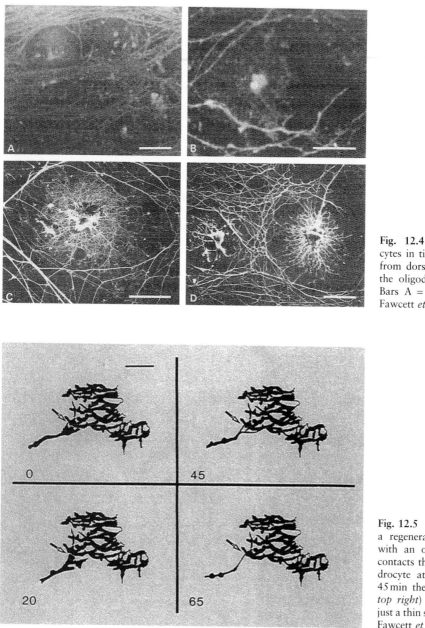

**Fig. 12.4** Axons avoiding oligodendrocytes in tissue culture. Axons regenerating from dorsal root ganglia grow all around the oligodendrocytes, but not over them. Bars A = 100 μm; B,C,D = 50 μm (From Fawcett *et al.* 1989b.)

**Fig. 12.5** Collapse of the growth cone on a regenerating sensory axon on contact with an oligodendrocyte. The axon first contacts the outer margin of the oligodendrocyte at 0 min (*arrow, top left*). After 45 min the growth cone collapses (*arrow, top right*) and withdraws, leaving behind just a thin strand of axon. Bar = 5 μm (From Fawcett *et al.* 1989b.)

regenerating from explants of adult retina, for instance, grow poorly on astrocyte monolayers (Meyer *et al.* 1989). This is particularly the case if the astrocytes have been cultured from the adult optic nerve rather than from their usual source, newborn brain (Bahr *et al.* 1995). However, a monolayer of astrocytes can never be a complete model of an astrocytic scar: in a glial scar, axons have to penetrate a dense tissue of astrocytic processes and the extracellular matrix in between them, which must be a very different process from growth on the surface of a monolayer, particularly, as we will see later, because secreted soluble inhibitory molecules are diluted away in the medium in monolayer culture, but are trapped between the cells in a three-dimensional tissue. If, then, astrocytes are cultured as a three-dimensional tissue rather than as a single layer, regenerating axons penetrate them very poorly (Fawcett *et al.* 1989a) (see Fig. 12.9).

Another astrocytic scar model involves inserting small pieces of filter material into the adult rat brain, then removing it a few days later, together with the astrocytes that attach to it. These astrocytes are also inhibitory to axon growth. Thus, astrocytes can be inhibitory to axon regeneration *in vitro*. Experiments have also been performed on *in vivo* models. The correlation between the position of axons failing to regenerate and astrocytes was described above. Astrocytes have been transplanted into the spinal cord, and also into peripheral nerves, where they either failed to promote or inhibited axon growth. Newborn rat optic nerve is unmyelinated and therefore consists mostly of astrocytes, and this tissue transplanted into a peripheral nerve blocked regeneration. Another test of the regeneration-promoting ability of a predominantly astrocyte environment comes from a mutant rat that has a metabolic defect in oligodendrocytes, and has no oligodendrocytes in parts of its nervous system. Despite there being only astrocytes present, axons still do not regenerate in these rats (Berry *et al.* 1992). Astrocytes can therefore be inhibitory to axon growth *in vivo*.

## Microglia

There has not been a specific study of axon regeneration over microglia in culture. However, astrocyte monolayers, unless specifically purified, have many microglia on their surface, and these do not prevent axon growth (Fawcett *et al.* 1992). Rabchevsky and Streit have performed a direct study on microglia and axon regeneration in the spinal cord *in vivo*, by implanting microglia contained in a tube directly into the cord. This resulted in higher levels of axon regeneration than in control animals (Rabchevsky and Streit 1997). They also observed that a mixture of microglia and astrocytes was more permissive than astrocytes alone. Axon regeneration has also been seen in an environment that is mostly made up of macrophages and microglia, resulting from killing CNS glial cells with an injection of glial toxin (Moon *et al.* 1999). Present evidence therefore suggests that microglia, on the whole, encourage regeneration rather than inhibit it.

## Oligodendrocyte precursors

Although these cells are recruited in large numbers to CNS injuries, there have been no direct estimates of their inhibitory activity. Axons that contact them *in vitro* do not undergo growth cone collapse in the same way as they do when they contact mature oligodendrocytes; yet, as we will see, they produce NG2, a molecule that is extremely inhibitory to axon growth, and other inhibitory chondroitin sulphate proteoglycans.

## Meningeal cells

Meningeal cells *in vitro* are a poor substrate for axon growth, and they also make astrocytes less good at promoting growth (Ness and David 1997). Meningeal cells invade spinal-cord lesions in large quantities and, therefore, cut axons come into contact with them. Even in experiments in which some axon growth has been induced in the spinal cord, the axons generally avoid meningeal cells, suggesting that they are inhibitory to axon growth *in vivo*.

# Inhibitory molecules in the damaged CNS

We have seen that most of the cell types present in the damaged CNS have some inhibitory activity on axon regeneration. What are the molecules that mediate this inhibition? And are these molecules secreted by the cells or dependent on contact with cell surface molecules? There turn out to be many inhibitory molecules produced by the various cell types, and the damaged CNS is probably awash with them.

## Inhibitory molecules on oligodendrocytes

The first inhibitory molecule to be identified on myelin was NI250, recently renamed 'NogoA'. These molecules were characterised by Pico Caroni and Martin Schwab. They first showed that purified myelin was inhibitory to axon growth, and had the effect of causing many types of axonal growth cone to collapse. They then fractionated myelin extracts to find the size ranges that could inhibit axon growth and had growth-cone collapsing activity, then made an antibody, IN-1, which blocked that activity. This antibody makes it possible for axons to grow over oligodendrocytes and (as described in Chapter 22) allows axon regeneration in the damaged CNS *in vivo* (Bandtlow *et al.* 1993; Schwab *et al.* 1993). The receptor for NI250 is not known, but it has been shown that it causes axon growth-cone collapse by acting on axon growth cones via a G protein-mediated release of internal calcium stores. Application of NI250 to an axon causes a rapid and large increase in growth cone calcium, which in turn leads to growth cone collapse.

A major component of myelin is the myelin-associated glycoprotein, MAG. MAG appears to play a major role in myelination, it has the ability to inhibit the growth of many but not all types of axon and, like NI250, is capable of causing growth cone collapse (Mukhopadhay *et al.* 1994; Li *et al.* 1996). The effect of MAG on the growth cone depends on the level of cAMP, the molecule being inhibitory when the cAMP level is low, but promoting growth when it is high. MAG is present on oligodendrocyte cell surfaces, which may suggest a contact-dependent effect on growth cone motility, However, it is also released in a soluble form, and is therefore found widely within the CNS. While MAG is undoubtedly inhibitory to axon growth, it cannot be the only factor preventing regeneration in the CNS, since mice in which MAG has been genetically knocked out have only a minor increase in axon regeneration.

Oligodendrocytes also produce a large extracellular matrix protein called tenascin R, which is present in normal white matter, and is upregulated after damage. This molecule is inhibitory to axon growth (Pesheva *et al.* 1989).

## Inhibitory molecules on oligodendrocyte precursors

While it has not been shown definitively that oligodendrocyte precursors block axonal regeneration, it is very likely that they are inhibitory, since they express the highly inhibitory proteoglycan NG2 on the cell surface. This molecule appears to inhibit growth in two ways: directly via specific interactions of its protein core with neuronal receptors, and through a mechanism that involves the glycosaminoglycan (GAG) chains (Levine 1994; Dou and Levine 1997; Fidler *et al.* 1999). Oligodendrocyte precursors have also recently been shown to produce some of the other inhibitory proteoglycans that appear in CNS injuries, namely neurocan, versican, DSD1/phosphacan. These cells, which are recruited to CNS injuries in large numbers, must therefore be a major source of inhibitory molecules in CNS injuries (Fawcett and Asher 1999).

## How do astrocytes block axon regeneration?

While it is reasonably clear how oligodendrocytes inhibit axon growth, the same cannot be said for astrocytes. The inhibitory molecules produced by astrocytes are chondroitin sulphate proteoglycans, in particular neurocan. Following a CNS injury there is a large upregulation of the amount of chondroitin sulphate around lesions, starting after 4 or 5 days, then remaining high for many weeks. The extent to which this is produced by astrocytes or by oligodendrocyte precursors is not known, but both cell types can certainly produce inhibitory proteoglycans. The chondroitin sulphate is probably carried on several different proteoglycans, since several have been shown to be present in increased amounts around CNS injuries. These include neurocan, phosphacan, versican, brevican, decorin, biglycan, and NG2. Versican and NG2 are produced by oligodendrocyte precursors rather than astrocytes. Most of these proteoglycans have been shown *in vitro* to have some axon growth inhibitory activity.

One of the major astrocyte proteoglycans with inhibitory properties is neurocan. This molecule is strongly upregulated in response to CNS injury. The properties of this molecule probably explain why three-dimensional astrocyte cultures are inhibitory, while monolayers are permissive. Neurocan is secreted in large amounts by cultured astrocytes, but it does not bind to the astrocyte surface and therefore floats away from the upper surface of the cells to be diluted in the medium; it therefore has little inhibitory effect on axon growth. However, in three-dimensional cultures, the inhibitory neurocan is trapped between the cells, and therefore is present in the environment surrounding regenerating axons (Fawcett and Asher 1999).

## Proteoglycans and inhibition

The mode of action of proteoglycans is not well understood. In principle, the proteoglycan molecule can be inhibitory through the actions of its protein core, of the GAG chains, or by a combination of these mechanisms in which the GAG chains are localised to particular sites by the binding of the protein core. Both GAG-chain and protein-core effects have been shown. Thus much of the inhibition of an astrocytic cell line, Neu7, which is used as a glial scar model because of its inhibitory effects on axon growth and its expression of inhibitory proteoglycans (Fig. 12.6), can be removed both by digesting away the GAG chains with chondroitinase, and by removing the strong negative charge of GAG chains by preventing their sulphation. Similarly, reactive astrocytes can be explanted from the damaged adult brain by placing a piece of filter material in the cortex, then removing it some days later with reactive astrocytes

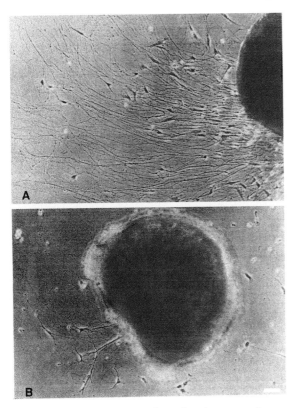

**Fig. 12.6** Axon regeneration from dorsal root ganglia onto extracellular matrix preparations from permissive (A) and inhibitory (B) astrocyte cell lines. A major component of the inhibitory extracellular matrix is proteoglycans, which can block the axon growth promoting properties of laminin. (From Smith-Thomas *et al.* 1994.)

attached. These cells produce inhibitory proteoglycans, and their inhibition can be largely negated by treatment with chondroitinase to remove the GAG chains. In both these models, a major action of the inhibitory proteoglycans is to block the axon growth promoting properties of the extracellular matrix protein laminin, and probably other matrix proteins as well (Smith-Thomas *et al.* 1995; Canning *et al.* 1996). However, chondroitin sulphate proteoglycans can promote growth. DSD1, the mouse form of phosphacan, promotes the growth of axons from embryonic hippocampal neurones, but inhibits growth from sensory neurones, and this property is also GAG-dependent (Garwood *et al.* 1999).

Proteoglycans can also be inhibitory by protein–protein interactions. The most studied, from this perspective, are phosphacan and neurocan. DSD1/phosphacan can bind to L1, N-CAM, tenascin, TAG-1/axonin1, F3/F11, and inhibits axon growth through these interactions. Neurocan binds to Ng-CAM/L1, TAG-1/axonin1, N-CAM and tenascin, and strongly inhibits growth on L1. However, the nature of the interactions between these molecules in the inhibition axon growth are still largely unknown.

# Intrinsic neuronal effects on axon regeneration

The account so far has concentrated on the inhibitory effects of the CNS environment on axon regeneration. However, the axon is not just an innocent bystander that will do whatever the environment dictates. Part of the reason for the failure of regeneration is due to the behaviour of the axons. There are three main properties which affect axon regeneration.

- *Age of the neurone.* Axons regenerating from adult neurones do not grow with anything like the vigour of developing axons, so axons regenerating from adult neurones cannot penetrate tissues that can be penetrated by axons from embryonic neurones.

- *Site of transection.* As mentioned earlier, axons regenerate much more readily if they are cut near the cell body and in many cases will not regenerate, even into a permissive environment, if they are cut more distally.

- *Individual differences between neurones.* Some neurones, even in the adult CNS, are much better at regenerating axons than others.

## The effect of distance on regeneration

There is an important difference between CNS and PNS neurones in the dependence of regeneration on distance. PNS axons will mount a regenerative response of roughly equal vigour wherever they are cut, even at the far end of a long limb. However, CNS axons will only regenerate into grafts of permissive tissue, such as Schwann cell grafts or embryonic CNS grafts, when they are cut near the cell body. This was first seen in the pioneering experiments of Aguayo and his colleagues, when they placed grafts of peripheral nerve into the spinal cord (David and Aguayo 1981; Richardson *et al.* 1982). They saw that many axons originating from spinal cord neurones were able to regenerate their axons into the peripheral nerve grafts, but when they identified those neurones by placing a retrograde nerve tracer into the peripheral nerve graft, they found that all the labelled neurones were very close to the insertion point of the grafts, and few neurones that were distant from the graft had regenerated their axons (see above and Chapter 22).

If only neurones that are axotomised near their cell bodies are able to regenerate into a permissive environment, this presents a major problem for repairing the CNS, since many of the vital axonal pathways that need to be repaired are long. For example, in spinal-cord injuries, many axons are cut long distances away from their cell bodies, such as, *in extremis*, the pyramidal neurones of the motor cortex. There has, therefore, been a major research effort seeking to identify the mechanism(s) behind this phenomenon, and ways to induce regeneration of axons that have been cut far from their cell bodies.

One pathway that has been particularly well-studied is the rat rubrospinal tract, whose axons will regenerate into peripheral nerve grafts placed in the cervical spinal cord, but will not regenerate into the permissive environment of a peripheral nerve graft if it is placed about a centimetre further from the cell body in the thoracic cord (Fig. 12.7). However, if the neurones are stimulated by applying trophic factors to the cell bodies, their regenerative ability can be increased. The trophic factors that are most effective in the rubrospinal tract

are BDNF and CNTF, although other tracts are stimulated to regenerate by NT-3, GDNF, and other factors. Infusions of these trophic factors, whether around the neurones or around the axons, reduce the atrophy of the axons after axotomy, upregulate the expression of the growth-associated protein GAP-43 by the cell body, and restore the ability of the neurones to regenerate their axons when axotomised further from the cell body (Tetzlaff *et al.* 1994).

The experiments in which regeneration of long-tract axons has been achieved in the spinal cord, described in Chapter 22, also mostly rely on the presence of added trophic factors; other effects of trophic factors on stimulating regeneration are described in Chapters 9 and 26. Two examples are experiments in which:

- grafts of fibroblasts to the cord do not induce axon regeneration, but if the fibroblasts are transfected to secrete NT-3 or BDNF, then axons from neurones in the brainstem or motor cortex are able to regenerate into or past them (Xu *et al.* 1995; Grill *et al.* 1997);

- growth of long spinal axons into grafts of Schwann cells has been increased by infusion of trophic factors (Fig. 12.7; Kobayashi *et al.* 1997).

The mechanism behind these behaviours has been partly worked out. There is an exact correlation between the

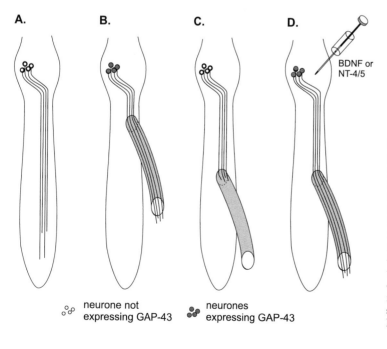

**A.**   **B.**   **C.**   **D.**

BDNF or NT-4/5

neurone not expressing GAP-43

neurones expressing GAP-43

**Fig. 12.7** Regeneration in the rubrospinal pathway. A. Schematic diagram of the intact projection from the brainstem to the spinal cord. B. Axons will regenerate into peripheral nerve grafts placed in the cervical cord, and GAP-43 is upregulated in the neurones. C. If the grafts are placed further from the neurones in the thoracic cord there is no regeneration, and no upregulation of GAP-43. D. Infusion of trophic factors around the neurones, can allow regeneration to occur, even when the peripheral nerve graft is place remote from the cell bodies and site of trophic stimulation. (Adapted from Kobayashi *et al.* 1997.)

ability of neurones to regenerate their axons and expression of the growth-associated molecule GAP-43. Thus, when CNS axons are cut proximally, they rapidly upregulate GAP-43 expression, but when cut distally, they do not. However, PNS neurones upregulate GAP-43 wherever their axons are cut. The neurotrophin treatments that can increase the ability of CNS axons to regenerate when cut distally also upregulate GAP-43 (Kobayashi *et al.* 1997). The properties of GAP-43 are described in Box 12.1. However, GAP-43 expression by itself is not enough to make a CNS axon regenerate if the environment is inhibitory. So when the CNS is damaged, many neurones whose axons have been cut near the cell body will upregulate GAP-43, and its level will remain elevated for some time, but the axons will still not regenerate, presumably because the inhibitory molecules in the CNS environment are sufficiently active to overcome any regenerative response from the axon. For instance, retinal ganglion cells express GAP-43 for weeks after their axons have been cut, but their axons will not regenerate unless they are presented with a peripheral nerve graft into which to do so (Doster *et al.* 1991; Cohen *et al.* 1994). While GAP-43 is an important molecule for axon growth, where it probably plays a part in signalling between the outside environment and the growth machinery in the growth cone, many other molecules are obviously involved, and many of these must have their expression increased by axotomy. There is a complex pathway of growth control that remains to be worked out.

## Mechanisms of action

GAP-43 is a major target of phosphorylation by protein kinase C in the growth cone, and also interacts with calmodulin and with G proteins. The action of GAP-43 on increasing process growth is dependent on its phosphorylation, since when the phosphorylation site is mutated, the molecule does not promote process growth in non-neuronal cells, neither does it cause increased sprouting in transgenic animals. The ability of protein kinase C to phosphorylate GAP-43 is inhibited by calmodulin-binding. The main function of GAP-43 is probably to mediate the effects of cell surface molecules on axon growth, and the ability of N-CAM to promote axon growth is associated with GAP-43 phosphorylation (Meiri *et al.* 1998). The actions of GAP-43 are probably via its interactions with actin and other cytoskeletal molecules, and the phosphorylation state of the molecule can influence cytoskeletal dynamics, including actin polymerisation. With its interactions

with multiple control mechanisms, and its association with the cytoskeleton, GAP-43 is well placed to play a key part in the control of axon growth.

## Effects of neuronal age

Embryonic neurones can be grafted into the adult CNS, and will often then grow axons for some distance through the inhibitory glial environment that blocks regeneration of the animal's own axons. Many types of embryonic neuronal graft have been inserted into various parts of the adult CNS. As described in Chapter 23, many of these are able to grow axons out into the host CNS, and have been able to make synaptic connections, if there are suitable host neurones nearby.

Perhaps the most dramatic examples of long-distance axon growth seen in the adult rat CNS, are when the grafted neurones are not only embryonic but also taken from human embryos (Fig. 12.8). For instance, grafts of rat embryonic substantia nigra implanted into the target site in the adult rat striatum give rise to a halo of axon outgrowth extending up to 2 mm into the host brain (Björklund *et al.* 1993b). However, when implanted homotopically into the adult rat substantia nigra, the axons cannot regenerate connections to distant targets such as in the host striatum (Björklund *et al.* 1993b). By contrast, grafts of human embryonic substantia nigra implanted into the brain of adult rats (which have been immunosuppressed to prevent rejection), are able to grow axons extensively throughout the host brain, restoring projections from the nigra back to the striatum and projecting right down to the upper end of the spinal cord (Wictorin *et al.* 1992). The general result is that when neurones from human embryos are grafted into the smaller rat brain, they will regenerate over longer distances than grafts derived from rat embryos, and the axons grow through both grey and white matter. Since the human embryonic CNS develops over a slower time scale than rodent CNS, the assumption has been that the human embryonic neurones express the genetic programmes associated with axonal growth over a longer time than rodent neurones, and this may mean that the receptors for inhibitory molecules are not expressed, and that the intracellular machinery and signalling mechanisms associated with axon growth are different. However, the observation of growth through both grey and white matter in the xenograft situation suggests that a second factor promoting extensive outgrowth of embryonic grafts from human donors may be that axons derived from human cells are less responsive

# Box 12.1   GAP-43

Several proteins have been identified as Growth Associated Proteins due to the fact their levels are greatly upregulated in neurones and axons during growth and regeneration. Of these proteins GAP-43, a phosphoprotein of 24 kD in its rat form, which runs anomalously at 40–60 kD on SDS polyacrylamide gels due to its low binding of SDS, has received particular attention. GAP-43 (also known as B-50, F1, pp46, 48K4.5) is a major constituent of the growth cone, being found on the inside of the growth cone membrane, is a major target for phosphorylation by protein kinase C, and binds strongly to calmodulin.

## Pattern of expression

GAP-43 is found ubiquitously during development in growth cones, but after development it is down-regulated in most neurones after the completion of synaptogenesis and after critical periods for activity-dependent plasticity are over. However, it continues to be expressed in some neurones in the adult CNS, for instance, the dopaminergic neurones of the substantia naigra. It is also expressed at high levels in neurones iassociated with plasticity, the hippocampus, and limbic system, and in the olfactory system, where axons continue to grow in adulthood (for review see: Benowitz and Routtenberg 1997).

## Expression following axotomy

GAP-43 is upregulated in all axons, peripheral and central, that can regenerate their axons. Following axotomy in peripheral nerves, there is massive upregulation of the protein in both sensory and motor neurones, and levels continue to be high until axons reconnect with their targets, after which expression reduces to baseline levels. The protein is found in the axonal growth cones and, in smaller amounts, in the axons. The pattern of expression after CNS axotomy is more complex: Neurones vary greatly in the extent to which they will upregulate GAP-43 after axotomy. At one extreme, the dopaminergic neurones of the substantia nigra have a high baseline expression, which does not increase after axotomy, while at the other extreme the Purkinje cells of the cerebellum do not upregulate GAP-43 at all after axotomy (Vaudano *et al.* 1995). In between, most neurones show some upregulation, with greater upregulation the closer the axon is cut to the neuronal cell body. For instance, in the descending axons from the red nucleus to the cord, there is upregulation of GAP-43 after axotomy close to the cell body, but not after more distal axotomy (Tetzlaff *et al.* 1994). In the visual system, optic nerve lesions lead to prolonged upregulation of GAP-43 expression. Expression may remain increased for a period of weeks, even in the absence of axon regeneration, but will eventually decrease (Doster *et al.* 1991).

## GAP-43 and axon growth

The presence of GAP-43 in growth cones, and its upregulation in regenerating axons, suggests that the molecule may play a role in axon growth. Direct evidence comes from *in vitro* and *in vivo* experiments. Non-neuronal cells can be transfected with GAP-43, which causes them to produce fine filopodium-like processes all around the cell, the effect being abrogated if the GAP-43 is mutated to prevent membrane-association, or at its phosphorylation site. Axons in which GAP-43 has been knocked out are unable to show an axon-growth response to the adhesion molecule N-CAM. *In vivo*, a GAP-43 knockout has a surprisingly normal CNS, with many axons, but in at least one pathway, the optic tract, axons fail to grow normally, and their growth is arrested at the optic chiasma. Animals that over-express GAP-43 show excess terminal sprouting at the neuromuscular junction and in the hippocampus (Caroni 1997).

## Relationship of GAP-43 expression and axon regeneration

CNS neurones do not normally regenerate their axons, but many can be made to do so if a permissive tissue, such as a peripheral nerve graft, is placed adjacent to the cut axons. All the axons that regenerate come from neurones that have upregulated GAP-43. For instance, in the visual system, regeneration of retinal ganglion cell axons has been induced by attaching peripheral nerve grafts to the cut optic nerve, and the axons that regenerate into these grafts have been labelled with tracers. All the ganglion cells that are labelled with the retrograde axon tracers also show upregulation of GAP-43 (Schaden *et al.* 1994). Even when presented with a permissive environment there is a lot of variation in the regenerative response of CNS neurones. Amongst those that show a particularly vigorous regenerative response are the neurones of the thalamic reticular nucleus, the deep cerebellar nuclei, and the cerebellar climbing fibres. Other neurones, particularly the Purkinje cells of the cerebellum, show no regeneration, even when their axons are given a permissive environment, and these neurones also do not upregulate GAP-43 after axotomy (Zagrebelsky *et al.* 1998). There is thus a good correlation between regenerative response and GAP-43 upregulation after axotomy. This correlation also holds good for the different regenerative responses that occur when most CNS axons are cut close to or far from the cell body. Thus in the case of rubrospinal axons, placing a peripheral nerve graft close to the cell body leads to axon regeneration accompanied with GAP-43 upregulation, while a graft placed further down the cord leads neither to regeneration nor GAP-43 upregulation. However, both regenerative response and GAP-43 upregulation can be enhanced by infusion trophic factors around the neuronal cell bodies (Kobayashi *et al.* 1997).

## GAP-43 *and synaptic plasticity*

The expression of GAP-43 in the adult hippocampus suggests a possible role in long-term potentiation. This is supported by the increased protein kinase C activity, increased phosphorylation of GAP-43 following long-term potentiation, but not after forms of stimulation that do not cause long-term potentiation. The possible role of GAP-43 phosphorylation in long-term potentiation is controversial. Interference with GAP-43 has been shown to affect neurotransmitter release from cells and synaptomes, but no abnormalities in the variations in transmitter release due to protein kinase C activation were seen in GAP-43 knockout animals (Oestreicher *et al.* 1997; Capogna *et al.* 1999).

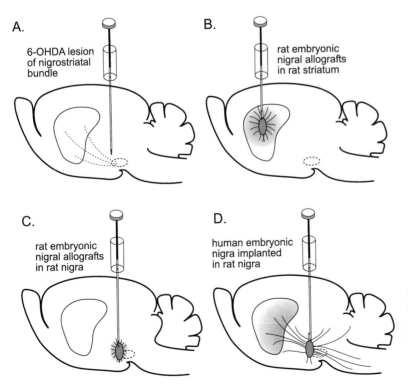

A.
6-OHDA lesion of nigrostriatal bundle

B.
rat embryonic nigral allografts in rat striatum

C.
rat embryonic nigral allografts in rat nigra

D.
human embryonic nigra implanted in rat nigra

Fig. 12.8 The effects of neuronal age on regenerative ability *in vivo*. Grafts of embryonic human substantia nigra grow axons for long distances into adult rat brains D, while equivalent grafts of embryonic rat substantia nigra will only grow axons for small distances C.

to species-specific inhibitory molecules expressed in the rat CNS environment.

Many tissue-culture experiments have shown the same basic phenomenon, that axonal growth from developing embryonic neurones has greater vigour than regenerative growth. Thus, for example, while evaluating an *in vitro* model of axon growth in a glial scar, post-natal sensory axons are unable to regenerate through a three-dimensional tissue made of cultured astrocytes, yet embryonic sensory axons can penetrate this tissue easily (Fig. 12.9; Fawcett *et al.* 1989a). Even when there is no tissue to penetrate or inhibitory cells to grow over, growth of axons from neurones is developmentally regulated. For instance, Purkinje cell axons grow readily from embryonic cells, but as the cells age their ability to grow an axon disappears.

In principle, the differences in the ability of embryonic and adult neurones to grow axons could be due to changes in the internal machinery for axon growth, or due to changes in the molecules that conduct the dialogue between the axon and its environment, particularly the adhesion molecules and receptors for inhibitory molecules. Many molecules recapitulate their embryonic expression pattern in regeneration, and clearly these molecules cannot be responsible for the differences between development and regeneration. However, there are several important molecules whose pattern of expression in regeneration does not recapitulate that seen in development.

Some adhesion molecules, both integrins that mediate interactions with the extracellular matrix, and adhesion molecules that mediate cell–cell interactions, have been shown to be different on regenerating axons from those that were present when the axons grew in embryos, and this may affect the interaction of the axon with its environment. For instance, the adhesion molecule N-CAM has several splice variants and, after development is over, an exon VASE is inserted. The VASE peptide is inhibitory to axon growth, which may partially explain the poor regeneration of axons that express it (Doherty *et al.* 1992). During development some growing axons have been shown to change their adhesion molecules at different times during development, but during regeneration the adult pattern tends to remain.

There are also differences in the molecules inside the axon, which are involved in axon growth. GAP-43 (see Box 12.1) is present in all growth cones during development, and only re-expressed in axons that are able to regenerate their axons. Also of potential importance are the microtubule-associated proteins (MAPs). As an axon grows, a cytoskeleton made up largely of microtubules forms, which is essential to stabilise the structure of the axon. In the absence of a stable cytoskeleton, a long axon cannot grow. Microtubules are made of polymerised tubulin monomers, and in most cells they are constantly forming and depolymerising, with a half-life that can be measured in minutes. Since an axon must remain stable for a long time, the microtubules have to be prevented from depolymerising, and this is achieved by the MAPs. These proteins must play an important part in axon growth, and it has been established that lack of some of them can prevent growth. Some MAPs, expressed in embryos while axons are growing, are different to those found in the adult nervous system. When axons are cut the embryonic MAPs are not re-expressed, and regeneration therefore has to proceed with the adult pattern of MAPs, which may be inappropriate for axon growth (Fawcett *et al.* 1994).

As mentioned earlier, growth factors can greatly increase the vigour of axonal regeneration. However, during initial development an axon cannot be dependent on a target-derived trophic factor, because it is not connected to a target. At around the time when an axon connects to its target, the neurone may start to produce appropriate growth-factor receptors, at which time it becomes critically dependent on the presence of the neurotrophin for survival (Paul and Davies 1995). Axon growth in embryonic neurones is therefore neurotrophin-independent, or dependent on autocrine factors, and this may be a factor in enabling growth through unpromising terrains.

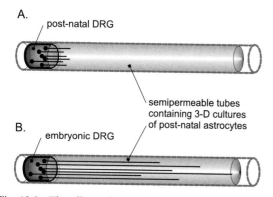

A.  post-natal DRG

semipermeable tubes containing 3-D cultures of post-natal astrocytes

B.  embryonic DRG

**Fig. 12.9** The effects of neuronal age on regenerative ability *in vitro*. A. Axons regenerating from post-natal sensory neurones grow poorly into three-dimensional astrocyte cultures. B. Axons from embryonic sensory neurones are able to regenerate into this tissue.

There must be many other factors, of which we are not at present aware, that change after embryogensis and influence the behaviour of damaged axons. Just how much might be gained by an ability to control these factors is shown by the extraordinary growth of axons from human embryonic grafts into adult rat tissue, shown in Fig. 12.8. If this pattern of gene expression could be re-activated in regenerating neurones, their axons might be able to regenerate through the most inhibitory environments.

## Differences in regenerative ability between neurones

As well as the effects on regenerative response of neuronal age and position of axotomy, different types of CNS neurones vary greatly in their ability to regenerate their axons. This cannot of course be seen in a simple CNS lesion, since none of the axons are able to regenerate. However, if a graft of cells that are permissive to axon growth is placed in a CNS lesion, some axons will grow into it much better than others. Thus a peripheral nerve graft may be placed in the CNS and, after allowing time for axons to regenerate into it, they may be filled with tracer to identify the neuronal types whose axons have grown. When such a graft is placed in the

thalamus, most of the axons were seen to come from the neurones of the thalamic reticular nucleus, and very few from all the other neurones whose axons had been cut (Morrow *et al.* 1993).

Perhaps the most extreme example of a neurone that will not regenerate its axon whatever environment is provided for it, are the Purkinje cells of the cerebellum. When grafts of embryonic cortex or Schwann cells were placed into the cerebellum, into lesions that cut both Purkinje cell and olivocerebellar fibres, the Purkinje cell axons never regenerated into the growth-promoting environment, while the olivocerebellar climbing fibres were seen to grow profusely (Bravin *et al.* 1997).

At the other extreme from Purkinje cells are spinal motor neurones, which are perhaps the best neurones in the CNS at regenerating their axons. When these axons are cut close to their cell body in the spinal cord they can regenerate for a limited distance through CNS tissue to re-enter peripheral nerve tissue. This has been used as the basis of a technique for repairing injuries in which the ventral roots are avulsed from the cord: peripheral nerve tissue is re-implanted into the cord, and the motor axons are able to regenerate into it (Carlstedt 1997).

While the differences in the abilities of axons to regenerate clearly become intrinsic to the neurone, there is

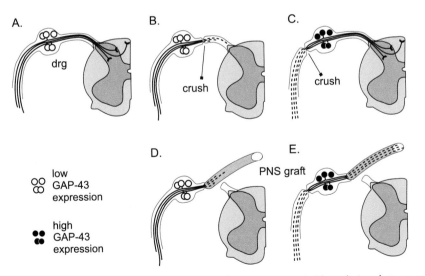

**Fig. 12.10** Regeneration of the central and peripheral branches of sensory axons. A. The unlesioned structures. B. The central branch is crushed within the dorsal root. Some but not all axons regenerate as far as the dorsal root entry zone. C. If a nerve graft is attached to the peripheral root of the sensory ganglion there is rapid and vigorous regeneration. D. However, if a similar graft is attached to the central branch, regeneration is poor and axons do not reach the end of the graft. The regeneration of the central branch can be greatly enhanced if the peripheral branch is lesioned at the same time. (Adapted from Chong *et al.* 1996.)

some suggestion that the CNS environment might instruct this behaviour. This is suggested by the different regenerative abilities of the central and peripheral branches of dorsal root ganglion neurones. The peripheral sensory branch regenerates vigorously when it is damaged (see Fig. 12.10). However, the central branch regenerates with much less vigour, even when it is cut in the peripheral nerve territory of the dorsal root. Crushing the peripheral branch increases the regenerative ability of the central branch, so for some reason damage to the central branch does not activate neuronal axon growth programmes to the same extent as a peripheral branch (Chong *et al.* 1996).

Recently, it has been suggested that the regenerative ability of CNS axons may be down-regulated by a molecule that is inactivated by the IN-1 antibody. The evidence for this comes from the Purkinje cells of the cerebellum, which fail to upregulate axon growth-associated genes, such as GAP-43 and c-jun, when their axons are cut. However, in the presence of the IN-1 antibody, axotomy causes these genes to be upregulated after axotomy, as does blocking axonal transport (Zagrebelsky *et al.* 1998). It is possible, therefore, that the CNS environment produces a retrogradely transported message in CNS axons that causes them to down-regulate their growth programmes.

In general, the differences in regenerative potential between neurones correlates with GAP-43 expression. However, in transgenic animals in which GAP-43 expression has been artificially induced in Purkinje cells, the axons will still not regenerate into Schwann cell grafts, so other mechanisms must be involved as well.

## Summary

The success or failure of axon regeneration is the product of a balance between positive and negative factors. The environment of the damaged CNS contains several inhibitory molecules, produced by astrocytes and oligodendrocytes, and these are sufficient to prevent the regeneration of all the intrinsic CNS neurones. However, experiments in which embryonic human tissue was implanted into the adult rat CNS show that an axon with an extremely high growth potential is able to overcome even these inhibitory effects. At the other extreme, many CNS axons when cut far from their cell body have such little regenerative potential that they will not grow, even in a permissive environment. If axons are to be induced to regenerate in the damaged CNS, the balance must be tilted, by providing a permissive environment and/or increasing the growth potential of the axons. The situations in which this has been successfully accomplished are described in Chapter 22.

## Further reading

Fawcett, J.W. and Asher, R.A. (1999). The glial scar and CNS repair. *Brain Research Bulletin*, **49**, 377–391.

Schwab, M.E. and Bartholdi, D. (1996). Degeneration and regeneration of axons in the lesioned spinal cord. *Physiological Reviews*, **78**, 319–370.

# 13 | Anatomical plasticity

In mammals, after damage to major axon tracts or large areas of neuronal tissue, there is permanent loss of function. Axons will not regenerate, and killed neurones are not replaced. This is in contrast to animals below the evolutionary level of the primitive amphibia, in which there is eventually an almost complete recovery of function, and early mammalian embryos have similar abilities. This is made possible by the regeneration of cut axons, and the replacement of lost neurones. The ability to regenerate central nervous system (CNS) axons over long distances and to replace large numbers of lost neurones is lost in evolutionary terms round the level of the primitive frogs, and in developmental terms around late limb-bud stages in mammalian embryos. However, even the mammalian CNS does have a considerable ability to readjust to functional loss. Thus, immediately after a stroke, patients will often have complete paralysis down one side of the body, but in the ensuing months a large proportion of the lost function may return. Following an incomplete spinal-cord injury, which may initially severely compromise motor function, almost complete functional recovery may occur, even though a large proportion of descending motor axons have been damaged. In neurodegenerative diseases, such as Parkinson's disease, symptoms may not occur until more than 80% of dopaminergic neurones have been lost. Some of the initial recovery from stroke or other traumatic injury is due to the resolution of local oedema and metabolic disturbance, but much of the functional readjustment that occurs after neuronal or axonal loss involves plasticity within the remaining connections.

Two main forms of plasticity have been described, and are discussed in greater detail below. The first is sprouting, in which axon terminals form new branches that grow to, and form connections with, vacant synaptic sites. The second is the functional unmasking of the many silent synapses that exist within the CNS. The local reorganisation and remodelling that these mechanisms subtend is a feature of many parts of the brain throughout life, and the ability to constantly remodel connections is a vital part of the processes of plasticity and learning that are continually going on in the normal brain. In addition, the old dogma that mammalian CNS neurones can never be replaced after they are lost, is looking increasingly shaky. It is now clear that stem cells exist in most parts of the mammalian CNS, which have the ability to differentiate into all forms of neurones and glia, and in two parts of the adult CNS, the dentate gyrus and the olfactory lobes, new neurones are generated throughout adult life.

## Plasticity of connections in the damaged CNS

### Types of regeneration

As described in the previous chapter, long-distance axon regeneration does not occur in the injured adult mammalian CNS. However, the limitations on growth are not absolute, and extensive local axonal sprouting of nerve terminals is a feature of the damaged nervous system. This type of axonal behaviour is an important mechanism behind the functional plasticity that occurs after injury, and there is the possibility that it will be possible to build on this limited mechanism to achieve functionally useful repair. However, the formation of new connections as a result of sprouting can also be maladaptive.

As in the peripheral nervous system (PNS), we need to distinguish axonal regeneration of two distinct types (see Fig. 13.1).

- *Collateral sprouting*. In this type of axonal regeneration, the terminals of intact neurones give rise to sprouts that repopulate synapses vacated by other dying neurones or lost terminals.

- *Regenerative sprouting*. In this type of axonal regeneration, the damaged axon, rather than dying back (retrograde degeneration), gives rise to a growth cone that grows back to re-innervate the denervated target (or possibly another target, which would give rise to aberrant sprouting — see below).

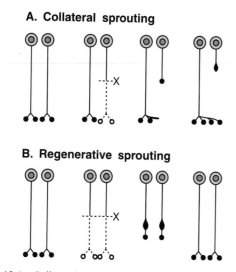

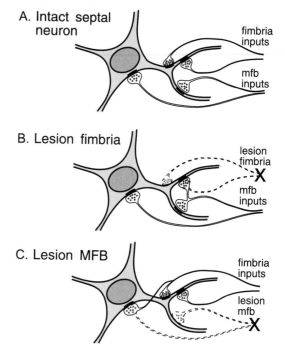

**Fig. 13.1** Collateral and regenerative sprouting in the CNS. A. Collateral sprouting from spared axons after partial lesion. B. Regenerative sprouting of cut axons back to a distant target site. (Adapted from Moore *et al.* 1974.)

## Collateral sprouting in the injured CNS

The first major evidence against the dictum that regeneration cannot occur in the adult mammalian CNS was provided by Geoffrey Raisman, who studied the detailed synaptic rearrangements that took place in response to cutting individual inputs to the septal nuclei in the rat (Raisman and Field 1973). The cells of the lateral septum receive two main inputs: one from the brainstem via the medial forebrain bundle, and the other from the hippocampus via the fimbria (Fig. 13.2). These two inputs can be distinguished in the electron microscope both by the distribution of their contacts on the cell body and dendrites, and by the density of the synaptic vesicles in the two types of nerve terminal. Raisman found that when one input was cut, those terminals degenerated over 1–2 days leading to a temporary reduction (by about 50%) in the total number of synapses on the septal cells. However, over the following 1–2 weeks, the numbers of synapses returned to normal, but now all the synapses were of the type associated with the spared input. Thus, if the medial forebrain bundle is cut, the fimbria projection sprouts new terminals to fill the vacated postsynaptic spaces. Conversely, if the fimbria is cut, the medial forebrain bundle projection sprouts new terminals to fill the vacated spaces. This interpretation was supported not only by the restoration of total synaptic numbers but the appearance of numerous cases of double synapses of a type that was not seen in the normal brain.

**Fig. 13.2** Collateral sprouting of axon terminals on neurones of the lateral septum in response to injury of the axons in the fibre bundles of the fimbria of the medial forebrain bundle (MFB). (Adapted from Raisman and Field 1973.)

The impact of these studies at the time is hard to imagine three decades later. Although a number of other authors had explored issues of regeneration and transplantation during earlier years, those studies were widely ignored. At that time, the *Zeitgeist* was rigid: regeneration simply did not occur in the adult mammalian CNS. Raisman's studies provide the first clear and unequivocal evidence that, under some conditions, plasticity can indeed be observed in the adult CNS. The fact that the PNS and CNS have different regenerative capacities was not in doubt, but the CNS is now seen to be capable of at least some regeneration in some situations, opening the way for the proliferation of research into new possibilities for CNS repair that we have seen in subsequent years.

## *Plasticity and sprouting in the sensory cortex*

The mammalian cortex is divided up into many functional areas, and many of these have some form of topographic map on their surface. These maps are set up during embryonic development, and it might be thought that once established they would be fairly rigid. However, cortical systems retain a remarkable degree of plasticity throughout adult life.

In the early 1980s, Merzenich and Kaas demonstrated that the mapping of the body surface onto the primary somatosensory cortex of the monkey becomes reorganised following peripheral nerve injury. They used electrophysiological recordings to examine the responsiveness of areas of somatosensory cortex following section of the peripheral nerves that projected to that cortical area (see Fig. 13.3; Merzenich *et al.* 1983). The expectation was that when a major sensory nerve is cut, the area of sensory cortex that normally receives an input from the regions of skin supplied by that nerve would be silent, since there is no way that sensory stimuli can now reach that cortical area. However, the finding was quite different. Much of the affected area of cortex was not silent, but rather showed responsive-

ness to stimuli from adjacent areas of skin (which would normally project to adjacent areas of neocortex). For example, when the median nerve is cut, which provides the sensory input from the medial side of the glabrous surface of the hand (i.e. the fleshy palm side, see Fig. 13.3), both adjacent areas on the back of the affected digits, and the more lateral aspects of the palm, come to elicit responses in the area of cortex formerly activated by light touch in the median nerve field. Since these responses are seen immediately after nerve injury, the implication is that there must be, in the normal cortex, existing axonal connections from the thalamus or from neighbouring areas of cortex that are silent, and which are only unmasked when the normal appropriate input is removed. However, if the peripheral nerve lesion removes the input from a large enough area of cortex, there is a silent area in the parts furthest from the boundary with normal unaffected cortex, which is presumably outside the range of the silent connections from neighbouring cortical areas. Over a period of two or

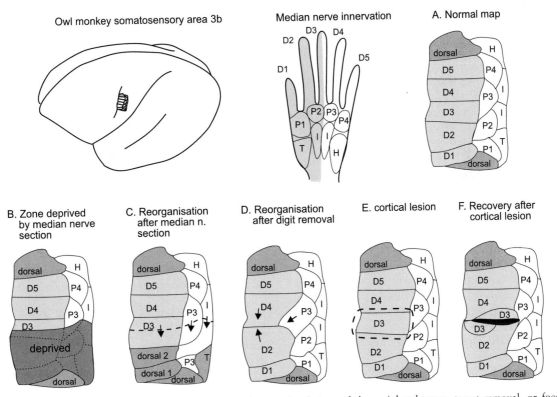

**Fig. 13.3** Reorganisation of the somatosensory cortical map after lesions of the peripheral nerve, target removal, or focal cortical lesion. (Modified from: Merzenich *et al.* 1983; Kaas 1991.) A. Shows a normal map of the digits on the cortex. B. Shows the area deprived of input by median nerve section, and C. the cortical map seen after the reorganisation of the map. A similar remapping occurs in animals that have lost a digit, as in D. E. Shows the area removed in an experimental cortical lesion, and F. the sulsequent cortical reorganisation.

more months, the cortical representation of skin neighbouring the denervated area gradually expands into the silent cortex, until the whole surface of the cortex is responsive to sensory input, and the sensory map has reorganised.

It should be noted that the cut peripheral axons do not regenerate to restore the actual severed connections between the distal receptors and their normal central targets. This is because the Merzenich model involves ligation of the cut nerve ends to prevent such peripheral regeneration. The affected area of the hand, formerly innervated by the median nerve, never restores its sensory input to the CNS and remains anaesthetic. There appears to be very little tendency for the spared sensory terminals of the ulnar and radial nerves (which provide the innervation of the adjacent sectors of the hand) to undergo terminal sprouting, and there is no collateral regeneration to restore the peripheral sensory innervation by a different nerve pathway. Cortical reorganisations similar to those provoked by cutting peripheral nerves can be observed after several different manipulations. One variation is to remove a part of the body rather than denervate it. This has been done by removing whole digits, or the dorsal surface of digits, which leads to the reorganised cortex now coming under the control of the adjacent digits on either side (Fig. 13.3). Another way of provoking reorganisation is to remove an area of cortex. In this case the adjacent areas of spared neocortex reorganise to provide a restricted cortical map for the peripheral fields that have lost their central representation (Fig. 13.3).

These studies indicate a clear capacity for reorganisation of topographical connections in the somatosensory cortex in response to disuse of one set of inputs. If cortical mapping is undertaken immediately after the peripheral nerve lesion, there are seen to be areas of the affected cortex in which the neurones are silent, and which do not appear to have a peripheral target. However, surprisingly, many other neurones throughout the affected area of cortex are seen to respond to stimuli in the adjacent fields that will eventually come to take over the cortical area. This partial reorganisation, whereby some neurones are seen to have receptive fields adjacent to their normal median nerve targets immediately after the lesion, takes place too rapidly for extensive synaptic remodelling, and the effect of the lesion is therefore to 'unmask' a secondary level of organisation. This appears directly analogous to the concept of 'silent synapses' only revealed after a primary input is removed, as described by Deror and Wall (Deror and Wall 1981). In this interpretation, the silent collateral connections are already present at the outset, and the reorganisation over subsequent weeks is considered to be due as changes in the strength of existing synapses.

If this were true, then there would be no requirement to ascribe the cortical reorganisation to any form of anatomical or regenerative sprouting. In fact, Kaas, Merzenich, and colleagues (Wall *et al.* 1986) argue that both types of process are probably operative. There is considerable subsequent reorganisation over a period of weeks, to a point where none of the cortical cells remain unresponsive indefinitely, and the remaining peripheral fields become extensively remapped onto the cortical surface. They argue that it is most plausible to attribute the gradual extension of adjacent target fields to spread into and take over the affected cortical areas as an anatomical rearrangement. Not only is the time course of this pattern of reorganisation more appropriate to a sprouting mechanism; in addition, the occasional observation of a complete translocation of the effective cortical targets of a particular peripheral field is particularly implausible as simply due to a rearrangement of synaptic strengths to activate silent pathways and suppress previously active ones.

## Utility of cortical remapping after injury

Is the remapping that occurs after sensory lesions useful? If it is a response to permanent loss of sensory input, remapping of the cortex will probably make little functional impression. However, there may be real practical benefits after nerve repair and re-innervation of the peripheral targets. Following peripheral nerve repair, many axons make targeting errors and end up projecting to a different muscle or skin area from the one they originally innervated (see Chapter 11). In adults, this leads to considerable functional impairment, because the central nervous system cannot fully compensate for these misconnections. However, children often have much better return of function after nerve injury than adults, yet the accuracy of their nerve regeneration is little better. The mechanism behind this was investigated by the Kaas laboratory (Florence *et al.* 1996), in foetal monkeys. The finding was that after median nerve repair, the axons were as jumbled in the peripheral nerve as would be the case after repair of an older animal, yet the sensory cortical map of body surface was beautifully orderly and topographic. The conclusion is that in young mammals, sufficient plasticity exists within the sensory pathway to allow for remapping of inaccurate sensory connections, but that this capability is lost in adulthood.

## Where does plasticity occur?

An important question is where between the periphery and the cortex is the plasticity occurring? In principle, new connections or unmasked connections could be within the cortex, at the level of thalamo-cortical connections, or even lower. First, it is necessary to distinguish between the changes in cortical representation that occur immediately after deafferentation from the changes involving sprouting and the formation of new connections, which must take longer to establish. Mechanisms for the repression and derepression of synapses within the cortex certainly exist, as we will see, in the motor cortex. These appear to depend on the inhibitory neurotransmitter GABA, and it is likely that the rapid changes that occur after lesioning are based on this mechanism. However, short-term changes in the sensory map also occur within the thalamus. Nicolelis and colleagues showed that numbing of the face in rats caused an immediate change in the responses of the neurones in the ventral posterior medial thalamus (Nicolelis *et al.* 1993). In the longer term, there are a variety of large and permanent changes that must require the formation of new connections.

There are several lines of evidence for formation of new connections within the cortex after lesioning. Florence, Taub, and Kaas have recently made a direct demonstration of massive collateral sprouting in the cortex following forelimb deafferentation, although they could detect no change in the thalmo-cortical connections (Florence *et al.* 1998). In another experiment by Wang and colleagues (1995), in which the cortical representation of three fingers was made to fuse by training animals to use all three simultaneously, no equivalent fusion of the maps of the three fingers could be detected within the thalamus. In experiments in which visual cortex remapping was induced by lesioning the retina, Darian-Smith and Gilbert (1994) showed, by tracing axons from the thalamus to the cortex, that the cortical scotoma was not filled in by sprouting thalamo-cortical axons, but that axons from within the cortex branched into the deprived area. These and other pieces of evidence indicate that extensive sprouting and plasticity can occur within the cortex.

However, there is also evidence that changes to the sensory map after lesions can be due to changes at a lower level. Monkeys with long-standing forearm deafferentation have been mapped at the level of the sensory nuclei in the medulla and at the level of the thalamus, with the finding that major changes also occur at these levels (Florence and Kaas 1995; Jones and Pons 1998). The conclusion must therefore be that sprouting and formation of new connections happen at various levels of the sensory pathway after injury.

## Is cortical plasticity part of normal brain function?

Are these changes in cortical mapping only seen after injury or dysfunction in the nervous system, or is the ability to reorganise following injury the result of a general cortical plasticity mechanism that operates in the normal undamaged CNS? This question has been addressed by looking for cortical plasticity in response to changes in use and function of the fingers and other parts of the body. If disuse of an area of cortex resulting from loss of its peripheral input leads to it being taken over by other inputs, then would unusually intensive use lead to an expansion of the cortical representation? This hypothesis has been tested in a number of experiments, the first being to train a monkey in a task that involves very intensive use of one finger. Following this training, the cortical representation of this area was found to be expanded several-fold (Jenkins *et al.* 1990). Similar changes with use have been reported in other animals and humans. In rats, for instance, the cortical representation of the nipples increases in size during rearing of pups. Reorganisation with use has been seen in humans that use their digits intensively for skilled tasks. Braille readers, for instance, generally use just one finger to read with, and maps of their sensory cortex taken by magneto-encephalography showed that the reading finger had a larger representation than the same finger on the other hand. Players of string instruments use the fingers of one hand to stop the strings, which requires skilled use of individual fingers, while the other fingers are just used to hold the bow. Again, magneto-encephalographic mapping of the cortex shows that the string-stopping fingers have an abnormally large representation, while the fingers of the other hand do not (Elbert *et al.* 1995).

## Patterns of impulse activity control cortical plasticity

What might be the mechanism behind use-dependent cortical mapping? Clearly it involves impulse traffic. The model that is generally accepted is that of the Hebbian synapse, which has been shown to be involved in topographic map refinement during development, in the formation of ocular dominance stripes, and in various forms of synaptic plasticity. The basic rule of the Hebbian synapse is that synaptic strength and stability are determined on the basis of co-incident firing of presynaptic inputs with depolarisation of the post-synaptic cell. Thus if several inputs fire together, they will strongly depolarise the post-synaptic cell, and by doing so will themselves become strengthened. However, inputs that fire out of synchrony with most of the other inputs will be unsuccessful at depolarising the post-synaptic cell, and will as a consequence become weakened. In terms of cortical mapping, the consequence of this type of mechanism would be that cortical neurones would be taken over by active inputs that fire in synchrony with one another. The inputs that fire in synchrony will generally come from neighbouring areas of skin, so this mechanism will ensure that neighbouring areas of skin project to neighbouring areas of cortex, and that the most active inputs win the most cortical cells.

The model makes predictions about mapping of body structures to the cortex, the most important of which is that areas of skin that are stimulated together, and therefore have co-incident patterns of impulse activity, ought to map together on the cortex. Therefore, if two fingers were to be joined together so as to always receive the same sensory input, their maps on the cortex should merge with one another. These predictions have been tested and verified in a number of paradigms. The first was surgically to join two monkey fingers together, and map the cortex some months later. Several experiments of this type were done in the Merzenich laboratory, and they showed that the cortical maps of the joined fingers would fuse together (Clark *et al.* 1988). It has been possible to show a similar phenomenon in humans. Some humans are born with congenital syndactyly, in which one or more fingers are joined. When the sensory cortex of such patients was mapped by magneto-encephalography, the representations of the joined fingers overlapped, but after surgical separation of the fingers they gained their own individual cortical representations (Mogilner *et al.* 1993).

The critical test of the hypothesis that cortical mapping relies on Hebbian rules must be to see whether repeatedly applying simultaneous stimuli to several regions of the normal body surface will induce fusion of the cortical maps of those regions. Wang and colleagues (1995) in the Merzenich laboratory trained monkeys in a task in which they simultaneously touched three finger tips, then the bases of three fingers to a bar.

As predicted by Hebbian synaptic mapping rules, the sensory cortex maps of the three finger tips and three finger bases fused.

## Pharmacological manipulation of cortical plasticity

If, as the above evidence suggests, the mapping rules in the cortex are based on Hebbian synaptic plasticity, it should be possible to prevent plasticity by using pharmacological agents or other manoeuvres that block these forms of plasticity. It has been very difficult to do this type of experiment, because of the long time-scales involved, and because agents that block NMDA channels affect overall cortical excitability and introduce marked non-specific artefacts. However, Garraghty and Muja (1996) have shown that the immediate cortical remapping after peripheral nerve section is prevented by an NMDA blocker. Moreover, in an $\alpha$-CAM-kinase-II knockout mouse, sensory cortical reorganisation in the barrel field (see later) is absent after vibrissa removal. These various pieces of evidence, together with the huge body of evidence showing that Hebbian mapping rules are involved during development and can be paralysed by NMDA blockers, make a convincing case for the involvement of patterns of synchronous impulse activity in plasticity in the adult cortex. However, from a more general point of view, one can ask what mechanisms are responsible for the suppression of silent synapses in the normal brain, and for their derepression in regions of cortex that have lost their normal sensory input. The major inhibitory neurotransmitter in the CNS is GABA, so this is clearly a candidate for the suppression of silent synapses. As we will see below, there is evidence in the motor cortex that GABA is involved in the plastic modulation of synaptic activity.

## *Functional plasticity in the rodent barrel fields*

The rodent somatosensory cortex provides a particularly favourable model for the study of developmental and adult plasticity. A major sensory system for many animals, in particular rodents, is provided by the vibrissae. In keeping with the functional importance of this tactile sensory modality, a large area of the somatosensory neocortex is given over to vibrissa stimulation. In particular, each individual whisker has its own unique representation in the neocortex and can be visualised anatomically. As first described by Woolsey and Van der Loos (1970), a tangential slice through layer IV of the relevant areas of the somatosensory cortex reveals columns or 'barrels' of cells maintaining a similar topographic arrangement to the whiskers on the contralateral snout (see Fig. 13.4).

Accurate one-to-one mapping between individual whiskers and barrel fields in the cortex has been shown both electrophysiologically and using the 2-deoxyglucose technique for metabolic mapping. In this latter case, the rats are injected with radioactive 2-deoxyglucose 45 min prior to sacrifice. The tracer is taken up and concentrated in cells proportional to their utilisation of glucose, which can then be visualised in histological brain sections autoradiographically. Welker and colleagues (1992) studied the effects of whisker stimulation in two ways. First, they glued small pieces of metal onto individual whiskers and then placed the animals in a container within an electromagnetic coil. Busts of 9 Hz current induced an oscillating magnetic field that vibrated the marked whiskers. A substantial increase of 2-deoxyglucose uptake was seen exclusively in the layer IV cells of the associated barrel field in the contralateral neocortex. In the same study, other animals had different subsets of whiskers shaved off unilaterally, and the animals were then allowed to actively explore an enriched novel environment. There was again seen a marked increase in metabolic activity in the contralateral barrel field, but only in the layer IV cells associated with the rows of whiskers that had been left intact, and not in the fields associated with shaved whisker follicles.

The cortical barrel field of mice and rats undergoes marked plastic changes both in development and in adulthood in response to disturbance of sensory afferents. For example, if individual or groups of whiskers are removed at birth, a reorganisation of the affected somatosensory neocortex is seen, involving a shrinking and fusing of affected fields, which can be easily visualised morphologically, as well as physiologically. Some of this plasticity is retained into adulthood. Thus, removal of all but one row of vibrissae results in a 60% increase in the width of the band of associated barrel-field cortex sensitive to activation of the remaining whiskers, as measured by 2-deoxyglucose radiography. The plasticity underlying this increased cortical representation is abolished after noradrenaline depletion (Levin *et al.* 1988) or by the NMDA antagonist APV (Jablonska *et al.* 1995) without changing the basal or stimulus evoked uptake of 2-deoxyglucose *per se*. Although this may in part be due to release of silent synapses, the active induction of GAP-43 mRNA expression suggests that plastic changes in the cortical representation of spared whiskers also involves structural reorganisation, involving synaptic remodelling (Levin and Dunn-Meynell 1993).

## Functional plasticity in the visual system

A major model for the study of developmental plasticity has been the synaptic re-arrangements of connections within the visual system that can occur following disturbance of normal visual experience in young mammals. Indeed, much of the developmental biology of the formation of nerve connections has been worked out in the visual pathways of mammals, chicks, and amphibians. The mammalian visual cortex shows extensive experience-driven plasticity shortly after birth, but (in contrast to the somatosensory cortex, as described

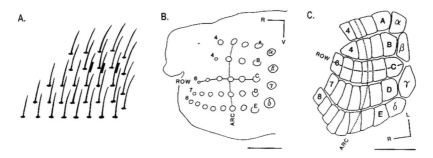

**Fig. 13.4** Barrel fields in somatosensory cortex. A. Distribution of whiskers on the rat snout. B. Position of the whiskers on the rat snout. C. Distribution of the associated whisker barrels in the somatosensory representation in the contralateral cortical layer IV. (From Welker *et al.* 1992.)

above) the plasticity of most visual connections ceases after a critical period. However, the mechanisms responsible for plasticity in the visual cortex are better understood than in any other part of the CNS. Because these mechanisms are probably general to synaptic re-arrangements elsewhere in the CNS, and following injury, it is appropriate to describe them here.

## Ocular dominance columns

A striking feature of the visual pathways in animals (such as cats) with forward-facing eyes — and therefore

extensive binocular overlap — is that the representations of the two eyes are kept separate in the lateral geniculate nucleus and the visual cortex. In the lateral geniculate, the projections from the two eyes occupy alternating layers, whereas in the visual cortex, the inputs from each eye are arranged as alternating ocular dominance columns (Fig. 13.5). However, the relative size of the left and right eye-columns can be altered by depriving one eye of normal visual experience. For example, if visual inputs to one eye are restricted (by suturing the eyelid shut) for several months during a critical post-natal period in a kitten or young monkey,

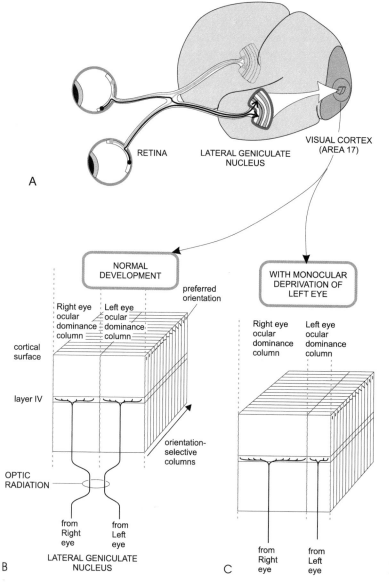

Fig. 13.5 Ocular dominance columns in the visual cortex. A. Distribution of inputs from both eyes via alternating layers in the lateral geniculate nucleus to separate 'ocular dominance' columns in the primary visual cortex (area 17). B. In normal development, the two eyes are represented by ocular dominance columns of approximately equal size. C. Following occlusion of the left eye during a critical period in post-natal development, the cortical representation of that eye is much reduced and the representation of the open eye expands.

the normal development of ocular dominance is altered, enlarging the central representation of the other eye in which vision is retained. When the closed eye was reopened, the monkey had dramatically reduced acuity in the sutured eye. This functional change corresponded to a physiological rearrangement such that the majority of cortical cells were now driven by the non-deprived eye and few neurones could be found that were driven by the closed eye. This electrophysiological shift in ocular dominance to the non-deprived eye (Hubel *et al.* 1977) can be seen anatomically as an expansion in the width of the ocular dominance stripes from the non-deprived eye, and a diminution of those from the deprived eye (LeVay *et al.* 1980).

This cortical plasticity does not occur in adult animals if they are subjected to eyelid suture; the ability of the non-deprived eye to expand its cortical influence is limited to a critical period of post-natal development. Thus, infant macaque monkeys are highly susceptible to monocular deprivation during the first 6 weeks of life. Thereafter, the plasticity of the system declines steadily, and disappears at somewhere between 18 months to 2 years of age. There certainly appear also to be species differences in the duration of the critical period in this system, which Wiesel (1982) has estimated to last in the order of 3–4 months in cats and up to 5–10 years in humans. Does this mean that the visual cortex differs from the somatosensory cortex, in that considerable degrees of plasticity are seen in the sensory cortex into adulthood, while the plasticity of the geniculo-cortical visual projection only shows substantial plasticity around the time or birth? The differences may be less than first appears. The plasticity within the ocular dominance columns involves the geniculo-cortical projection, while, as described earlier, the observed plasticity in the somatosensory cortex is mediated largely by intra-cortical connections. In the visual cortex there is evidence that the plasticity of the intracortical connections also continues after that of the geniculo-cortical connections has ceased.

These experiments clearly demonstrate that experience, especially in the early post-natal period, can influence the structural organisation of a developing part of the CNS. Furthermore, Hubel, Wiesel, and co-workers then went on to analyse the mechanism by which this developmental process may be occurring. Thus, cortical cells could further have their preference changed in the critical period by a process of reverse suturing, in which the sutured eye was opened and the normal eye closed. This reversal in preference was again only possible during the critical period. However, importantly, the

shift in ocular dominance was seen to take place within days of the reversal procedure and before any significant anatomical reorganisation could have taken place. This suggests that the plasticity of the visual cortex during the critical period involves functional as well as anatomical rearrangements. However, it was unclear from these experiments whether plasticity was the result of disuse of an inactive system or competition between the two inputs. Subsequent experiments using binocular deprivation and an experimentally induced squint indicated an answer in favour of competition. In other words, the influence of a given cortical afferent is determined not only by the absolute level of cortical innervation, but also by its influence relative to other competing inputs.

## Ocular dominance column plasticity is controlled by patterns of impulse activity

The changes in ocular dominance were obviously brought about by differences in visual experience between the inputs from the two eyes, and therefore it was a logical step to suppose that blocking action potential activity in the eyes should prevent ocular dominance stripe segregation. Stryker and Harris (1986) showed that stripe formation could be inhibited by blocking impulse activity in the retina with the sodium channel blocker tetrodotoxin. The separation of the projections from the two eyes within the lateral geniculate was also inhibited by blockade of electrical activity.

If two inputs are to be recognised as different to one another there must be some feature that makes this difference recognisable. Experiments in lower vertebrates had already identified a topographic mapping mechanism that relied on co-ordinated patterns of electrical activity in the axons from neighbouring ganglion cells to generate topography. This mechanism could be made inoperative either by blocking impulse activity, or by firing all the retinal ganglion cells in synchrony with stroboscopic illumination, or by blocking NMDA channels on the post-synaptic cells. This same mechanism could also lead to ocular dominance stripes when the terminals from two eyes were made to mix on one optic tectum, since there could be no co-ordinated firing patterns in ganglion cells from two separate eyes. The topographic mapping mechanism in lower vertebrates was therefore identified as obeying Hebbian principles, with correlated patterns of electrical activity and co-incident post-synaptic depolarisation controlling the strengthening and weakening of synaptic contacts (Fig. 13.6). Could the plasticity of ocular dominance stripes

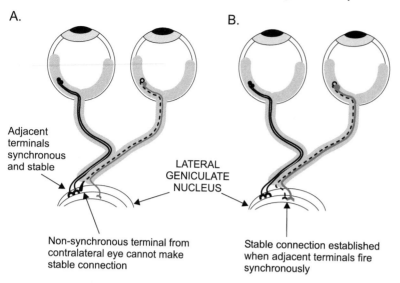

**Fig. 13.6** A Hebbian model for the formation of ocular dominance columns. In the A two neighbouring retinal ganglion cells, which have the same pattern of action potentials map to the same place on the target, and are able to form stable connections. However, the connection from the retinal ganglion cell in the other eye which has formed a connection to the same part of the target does not fire synchronously, and cannot make a stable connection. In the B, this connection has moved to a new site, where there are other terminals that fire synchronously, and it can make a stable connection.

in mammalian cortex be based on the same set of rules?

Various pieces of evidence support the idea for a Hebbian mechanism in ocular dominance stripe formation, although some other competitive interactions probably have added to the basic concept. A clear prediction is that imposition of correlated patterns of activity on all the retinal axons should paralyse stripe formation, since there is now no way of distinguishing one axon from another. This was tested by Stryker and Strickland (1983) by placing stimulating electrodes on the optic nerves of newborn animals, with the finding that stripe formation was inhibited. A second prediction is that ocular dominance column formation should be prevented by blockade of NMDA channels. This is so, but the interpretation of the result is not straightforward, since NMDA-blockade also largely silences all visual responsiveness. A requirement of the hypothesis is that there should be correlated activity in neighbouring ganglion cells. Ocular dominance column formation in many mammals occurs before birth, or before the retina is fully wired up to respond to visual stimuli, so this initially seemed unlikely. However, Carla Shatz and her collaborators showed that the early retina has waves of spontaneous excitation sweeping across it (Meister *et al.* 1991). This is sufficient to underpin the formation of ocular dominance stripes, although their sharpening and maturation requires actual visual experience.

## Synaptic mechanisms in visual cortex plasticity

How might the strengthening and weakening of synapses based on Hebbian principles actually work? Again, the visual system has provided some detailed mechanisms, which may well apply to plasticity in other regions of the nervous system. What is required in order to make the Hebb mechanism work is some form of retrograde signal that is released by post-synaptic neurones when they are strongly depolarised, and which preferentially strengthens the synapses that were active at that precise moment. In hippocampal LTP, nitric oxide is almost certainly one such retrograde message, and because of the similarities between LTP and the forms of plasticity responsible for ocular dominance column formation, nitric oxide is obviously a candidate in the visual cortex. However, Michael Stryker and his colleagues found that blockade of nitric oxide synthesis did not prevent ocular dominance column formation in the kitten (Ruthazer *et al.* 1996). A second family of molecules that plays a part in some forms of LTP is the neurotrophins. Local release of neurotrophins from post-synaptic hippocampal neurones has been shown to be induced by depolarisation, and neurotrophins strengthen presynaptic contacts (Thoenen 1995). Neurotrophins have also been shown to have a major influence on visual cortex plasticity. Brain-derived neurotrophic factor (BDNF) and neurotrophin-4/5 (NT-4/5), which share the same receptor, trkB, can both inhibit the formation of ocular dominance columns, and can change the effects of visual deprivation, while blockade of the trkB receptor inhibits ocular dominance column formation (Cabelli *et al.* 1997). Exactly how the neurotrophins might act is not established. However, one important parameter is that their effect must be specific to active neurones. This has been demonstrated directly for cortical neurones in tissue culture, where BDNF has a dramatic effect on increasing the growth and branching of dendrites, but only in the presence of impulse activity, and the effect is abolished by blocking L-type calcium channels (McAllister *et al.* 1996).

A final important question is why does plasticity cease after the critical period? A possible answer is that the NMDA channels in layer IV of the visual cortex, the layer in which the ocular dominance columns form, decline to a low adult level at the end of the critical period (Catalano *et al.* 1997). As suggested above, NMDA channels are probably central to the mechanism of ocular dominance plasticity, so their disappearance may well be critical. Can plasticity be reactivated? Implantation of embryonic astrocytes into the visual cortex has been reported by Christian Müller to have this effect, the mechanism being at present unknown (Müller 1993).

The mechanisms of synaptic plasticity that we have described above in the visual system must be similar to those active in other parts of the CNS in which it has not been possible to do such detailed experiments. In particular, the unmasking of silent synapses after injury, and the functional plasticity in the sensory cortex described earlier must use similar mechanisms.

## Plasticity in the motor cortex

### Plasticity after injury

So far, we have been looking at plasticity in response to the loss of an input. However, there is also extensive plasticity in the motor cortex in response to loss of a peripheral target after peripheral nerve damage or functional blocking. Donoghue and Sanes showed that forelimb nerve injury in newborn rats resulted in a motor cortex that was extensively reorganised. When they stimulated the area that would normally produce forelimb movement, they got instead movement of the shoulder area, and sometimes the vibrissae (Donoghue and Sanes 1988). This plasticity is not restricted to

newborn animals, however. Jacobs and Donoghue investigated the effects of peripheral nerve transection on the adult rat motor cortex, and they found within hours that stimulation of the area of motor cortex that normally projects to the affected nerve would cause movements of body parts neighbouring the denervated area, which would never normally be stimulated to move by activation of that cortical area (Jacobs and Donoghue 1991). They argued that this plastic change must be due to the unmasking of connections that were already present in the cortex, but which were non-functional. Since the major inhibitory neurotransmitter in the cortex is GABA, they reasoned that it might be possible to unmask these connections in the cortex of normal unlesioned animals by applying a GABA blocker. They therefore applied bicuculline to the cortex, and stimulated. As they predicted, stimulation in the presence of bicuculline caused movement of a larger number of muscles over a more widespread area of the body, suggesting that GABA blockade normally represses inappropriate cortical circuitry. Hess and Donoghue (1994) have since examined slice preparations of motor cortex *in vitro* and shown that the synaptic efficacy of horizontal pathways is increased by GABA blockade. Consequently, a mechanism for the short-term reorganisation of cortical maps based on GABA inhibition certainly exists.

The adult human motor cortex exhibits a remarkable ability to reorganise following peripheral lesions. In recent years it has become possible to obtain fine-grained maps of the topography of the human motor cortex through transcranial magnetic stimulation. Magnetic stimulators can deliver an extremely localised stimulus through the skull to the cortex, and the peripheral motor responses can be monitored. By moving the stimulus point and recording the changing motor effects, a map of the motor area can be constructed. Functional MRI can also be used to image the areas of cortex that are active during motor tasks. These techniques have made it possible to assess the topography of the motor cortex after a variety of peripheral lesions. The results are very similar to those in lower mammals. There is an immediate reorganisation in the motor cortex within minutes of inducing a temporary peripheral nerve block, which is actually enhanced by the widespread cortical activity induced by transcranial magnetic stimulation. This is associated with a decrease in intracortical inhibition, which could be due to a reduction in GABA inhibitory activity (Ziemann *et al.* 1998). Study of patients with long-term peripheral lesions shows that the cortical reorganisation persists, but with changes in the motor threshold that are not seen acutely, which would indicate more permanent changes (Chen *et al.* 1998).

## Plasticity in the motor cortex in response to motor tasks

Plasticity in the motor cortex has obviously not evolved to respond to peripheral nerve lesions. As with the sensory and other cortical areas, the motor cortex has a remarkable ability to reassign cortical area depending on the activities that are required of it. Now that mapping of the motor cortex with transcranial magnetic stimulation is possible, experiments can be done on human subjects to look at cortical remapping as a result of motor tasks. Mark Hallett and his colleagues trained subjects in a piano-playing task, in which they had to learn to play a repeated sequence of notes. While the subjects were learning the task and improving in it, the cortical representation of the muscles involved increased considerably in size, but when the subjects had finally learned the task and could repeat it, the cortical representation shrank again (Pascual-Leone *et al.* 1994). Presumably it is this experience-related plasticity that underlies the reorganisation of the motor cortex after injury.

## *Plasticity in the auditory cortex*

The auditory cortex exhibits very much the same types of plasticity that we have already described in the somatosensory cortex, although there are some features particular to the auditory system. However, a reason for describing these phenomena here is that in the auditory system it has been possible to manipulate and use the plasticity of the adult cortex to repair major and important auditory disabilities.

The auditory cortex exhibits the remapping phenomena that we have described in the somatosensory cortex. However, auditory cortex mapping is according to auditory criteria, and is therefore tonotopic. Just as the somatosensory cortical map fills in areas that have lost their peripheral input after damage to a peripheral nerve, the auditory cortex fills in areas that have lost their tonotopic input when a region of the cochlea is lesioned. Consequently, the cortical area that used to receive an input from the damaged region is now controlled by neighbouring frequencies, which expand into the vacated space (Rajan *et al.* 1993). This has led to the interesting idea that tinnitus may be the equivalent

of the phantom limb sensations that are experienced by patients with limb amputations, and is due to abnormal inputs to a area of cortex that has lost its normal peripheral input. In support of this hypothesis, tinnitus may persist in patients who suffer auditory nerve damage subsequent to developing it, and may therefore be a central rather than peripheral phenomenon. Cortical remapping has been shown in tinnitus patients by magneto-encephalography and PET (Muhlnickel *et al.* 1998). Auditory cortex remapping has also been demonstrated in response to sensory deprivation and training. Thus, for example, monkeys exhibit an expansion in the cortical representations of particular tones following training to respond to those frequencies (Recanzone *et al.* 1993).

## Language-based learning impairment

A group of individuals exists with an inability to learn to understand language, whose auditory system appears to be normal, with normal cochlear performance. It now transpires that these patients with language-based learning impairment suffer from a rather subtle deficit in hearing, in which they are unable to perceive rapid changes in frequency, and cannot therefore hear and interpret the rapidly successive phonetic elements that make up speech (Merzenich *et al.* 1996). It is assumed that this defect is in the cortical areas involved in the processing of sound. Many of these patients may have suffered from a conductive hearing deficit, such as glue ear, at a critical time for the development of auditory skills.

Discovery that the deficit in this group of subjects is in the speed of sound comprehension offers new strategies for treatment. If speech sounds are computationally altered so as to slow down the phonetic elements to an appropriate speed, the subjects can begin to perceive speech. On the basis of this, an attempt was then made to drive cortical plasticity so as to steadily improve the auditory processing ability of these subjects. This was done by constructing a computer game that rewarded the player for correct association of computationally altered spoken words with objects, with rewards being increased for increasing speed of comprehension. The combination of slowing the phonetic elements of speech so that the subjects could perceive them, and demanding attention by rewarding success, led to rapid improvements in auditory performance, to the extent that after 3 months of playing the games daily, children with this particular hearing disability were able to hear normal speech, and having developed the ability to interpret normal speech, the game was no longer necessary since listening to the normal sounds around them was sufficient for further auditory training (Tallal *et al.* 1996). Thus cortical plasticity continuing into childhood was used in a particularly creative way to achieve a form of functional brain repair. A similar form of plasticity and relearning is probably responsible for the ability of patients to learn to interpret the very incomplete and abnormal auditory signals that come from cochlear implants.

# Major CNS functional deficits lead to extremes of plasticity

The greatest challenge to CNS plasticity is probably the death of a large area of the brain that occurs as the result of a stroke. Immediately following a stroke, the patient, if conscious, will frequently have a massive neurological deficit, often involving the whole of one side of the body. Over the ensuing weeks and months there may be a dramatic recovery of function, with the patient often recovering most of the abilities that were lost. This recovery of function must involve several processes. In the first hours after the stroke there is usually substantial local oedema in the CNS, which is responsible for some of the functional loss, and resolution of this oedema must be responsible for part of the recovery. However, recovery continues after the period when oedema has resolved, and this later recovery must be due to the various plasticity mechanisms that we have described earlier in this chapter, namely the unmasking of silent synapses and sprouting.

With the development of functional imaging techniques in the form of PET and fMRI, it is now possible to examine patients who have recovered from a stroke, and ask which parts of the brain have taken over the functions that were lost in the immediate aftermath of the lesion. The results of these studies show an astonishing degree of reorganisation of brain function. For instance, Frackowiak and his colleagues examined patients who had suffered hemiplegic strokes, with well-defined hemispheric lesions. The patients were asked to move their hands, and increases in blood flow in the brain were visualised by PET. When the unaffected hands were moved, the contralateral motor cortex became active, as expected. However, when the affected hand was moved, the normal contralateral motor cortex was damaged, and instead, increased blood flow was seen in the sensorimotor cortex and cerebellum on both

sides, and in various other brain areas that do not normally become active during hand movement. The conclusion was that motor function was taken over by various non-motor areas, and by the other side of the brain (Chollet *et al.* 1991). However, this degree of plasticity is not only seen in those with an actual brain lesion. Mark Hallett and co-workers studied subjects who were blind, and who had learned to read using Braille script. These subjects were seen by PET to be using the visual areas of their brain, the primary and secondary sensory cortex, to process the tactile discrimination tasks involved in Braille reading, but simple touch did not activate these brain areas (Sadato *et al.* 1996). These extreme examples of cortical plasticity cannot simply involve local sprouting in the cortex itself, but must involve a more widespread reorganisation of brain function, including the subcortical regions.

# Sprouting in the hippocampus

The hippocampus has particularly lent itself to studies of the rules of synaptic plasticity and sprouting after CNS lesions. This is because of its regular structure, and because of the layered pattern of inputs to the dendrites of the granule cells in the dentate gyrus and to the pyramidal neurones in the other hippocampal regions. Various histological techniques have made it possible to distinguish the various inputs within these layers, and to see whether their distribution has changed after denervation of a neighbouring region. In the dentate gyrus, in which many of the plasticity experiments have been done, there are two main input layers to the dendrites of the granule cells, called the inner and outer molecular layers (Fig. 13.7). The inner molecular layer contains mostly inputs from the commissural/associational fibres from the contralateral hippocampus and the outer molecular layer contains a major input from the entorhinal cortex on the ipsilateral side, and a much smaller input from the contralateral entorhinal cortex. Both layers contain a cholinergic input from the septohippocampal projection.

## The sprouting response to removal of the entorhinal cortex

Lesions of the ipsilateral entorhinal cortex remove much of the innervation of the outer molecular layer of the dentate gyrus, together with most of the synapses. Starting about 4 days after deafferentation, and complete by

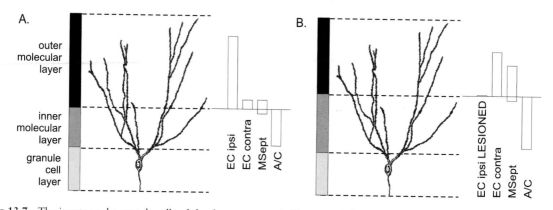

**Fig.13.7** The inputs to the granule cells of the dentate gyrus. A. The normal dentate gyrus. The number of synapses coming from the various inputs is represented as the height of the bars to the right. B. After lesioning of the ipsilateral entorhinal cortex (EC ipsi) the input from the contralateral EC (EC contra) and the cholinergic input from the medial septum (MSept) sprout to increase their number of synapses and the inner molecular layer thickens, but there is no sprouting between layers.

2 weeks, new synapses appear within this denervated area, and by 2 months the density of synapses is almost back to prelesion levels (Fig 13.7B). Lesioning, therefore, initiates a sprouting process, which stimulates the remaining unlesioned innervation of the dentate gyrus to produce new terminals and reoccupy the denervated area. The questions that have occupied many years of research are working out which of the various inputs expand their projections to occupy the vacated space, and what are the rules that govern their sprouting?. The most interesting possibility is that the commissural fibres that are normally restricted to the inner molecular layer sprout outwards into the outer molecular layer, breaking the boundary rules that normally restrict their distribution. The initial evidence suggested that this was the case, because silver impregnations and electron microscopic studies seemed to show commissural terminals in the former terminal zones of the entorhinal connections, and therefore translaminar sprouting (Cotman *et al.* 1973; Zimmer 1973). This suggested that the entorhinal and commissural inputs compete for space at the boundary of their terminal zones, implying that the formation of the boundary itself might be the product of competitive interactions. However, the experiments of Caceres and Steward, and others, have shown that in fact it is the inner layer that expands rather than the commissural fibres expanding beyond it (Caceres and Steward 1983). The granule cell dendrites are remodelled so that their inner zone expands by exactly the same amount as the commissural projection, so that in fact this projection does not expand outside its home territory, rather its home territory expands out-

wards. This fits with *in vitro* experiments with organotypic slice cultures in which granule cell dendrites without an entorhinal input develop longer than normal first-order (commissural/associational recipient) dendrites, and smaller than normal outer (entorhinal recipient) segments, which indicates that the territories of the dendrites are shaped in response to the inputs. The considerable plasticity of the dendrites is shown by taking one of these cultures with atrophied distal dendrites, and co-culturing it with entorhinal cortex, in which case the outer segments now enlarge (Deller and Frotscher 1997). These various detailed studies of the distribution commissural fibres after entorhinal cortex lesions have, therefore, shown that these axons remain restricted to their home layer even when the neighbouring layer is vacated, although there is considerable plasticity in the dendrites that can lead to changes in the thickness of the layers. Where, then do all the terminals that sprout into the denervated outer molecular layer come from? In early studies it was not realised that there is a very small crossed projection from the entorhinal cortex alongside the much larger ipsilateral one. This crossed projection expands greatly when the ipsilateral entorhinal cortex is lesioned, to occupy many of the vacant synaptic sites, and also to return some behavioural functions (Fig. 13.7B).

In addition, there is sprouting of the cholinergic septal input. Both these inputs normally occupy the outer molecular layer, so the laminar boundaries are not breached during these sprouting events. The sprouting that occurs is an expansion of the remaining projections within their normal layer. During development this same rigid laminar organisation of the inputs to the dentate gyrus are also respected. Using organotypic slice cultures of the dentate gyrus, together with slices of the input structures, it is possible to arrange for the inputs to arrive singly or at abnormal times, and they still respect their laminar boundaries, even if the other laminae have no input. The only clear evidence of competition between terminals is therefore within laminae rather than between them. Thus in the inner molecular layer, the commissural and associational fibres compete, and within the outer molecular layer, the ipsilateral and contralateral entorhinal projections, and the septal inputs, compete for synaptic space. At present it is not known what sets the rigid boundary between inner and outer molecular layers. However, there are suggestions that a particular glial cell type, the Cajal-Retzius cells, which are restricted to the outer molecular layer, are involved and, possibly, the protein reelin that they express. When these cells were killed in slice cultures, Del Rio and colleagues (1997) showed that in-growing entorhinal fibres were not restricted to the outer layer. However, inputs to the inner molecular layer did not transgress into the outer layer, so there are clearly other cues as well.

## Sympathetic sprouting in the hippocampus

While the mechanisms behind the forms of hippocampal sprouting describe above are not fully worked out, the mechanism regulating the sprouting of one particular input to the hippocampus, the sympathetic innervation, is better understood. Subcortical cholinergic, noradrenergic, and serotonergic neurones of the regulatory basal forebrain and brainstem, innervate the hippocampus via pathways coursing through the fimbria–fornix. Lesions of the fimbria–fornix denervate the hippocampus of these several input systems. In 1977, Loy and Moore reported the return of a fluorescent noradrenergic innervation of the hippocampus, in particular in the dentate gyrus, several months after a denervating fimbria–fornix lesion of the hippocampus. The new fibres were seen most densely in the areas of the dentate gyrus most extensively deafferented by the transection lesion but, unlike the fine plexus of nerve terminals formed by normal central noradrenergic terminals in the intact hippocampus, they had a distinctive coarse, intensely fluorescent appearance, characteristic of sympathetic fibres. Loy and Moore suggested that this re-innervation was due to spouting of peripheral sympathetic nerve terminals that normally innervate the hippocampal vasculature, rather than being due to sprouting of damaged central noradrenaline neurones (see Fig. 13.8). This they confirmed by showing that the anomalous re-innervation in the dentate gyrus was abolished by making additional lesions of the sympathetic superior cervical ganglion, but was not affected by bilateral lesions of the locus coeruleus, the nucleus of origin of the normal central noradrenergic innervation of the hippocampus.

The anomalous 'sympathetic sprouting' response appears as early as 14 days after the initial lesion, and appears to be stable for many months. However, studies on its specificity have revealed a number of surprising additional aspects to the response. As first described,

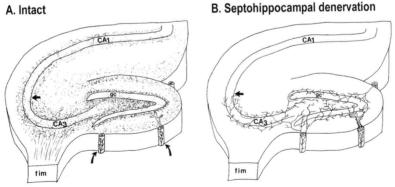

**Fig. 13.8** Sympathetic sprouting in the hippocampus. A. The normal hippocampus receives a rich central noradrenergic innervation originating in the locus coeruleus, and reaching the hippocampus via fibres running through the fimbria. B. Denervation of this central input by cutting the fibres in the fimbria is followed by sprouting of the peripheral innervation of the vasculature and a noradrenergic re-innervation of the hippocampus from this peripheral sympathetic source. (From Crutcher 1987.)

sympathetic sprouting appeared to be a neurotransmitter-specific replacement of lost central noradrenergic fibres by sprouting of peripheral noradrenergic fibres. The septohippocampal lesions first employed to induce sympathetic sprouting, denervate the hippocampus of cholinergic and serotonergic, as well as its adrenergic inputs. It turned out that neither lesions of the locus coeruleus to remove the central noradrenergic neurones specifically, nor lesions of other commissural or entorhinal inputs to the hippocampus, had the capacity to induce sympathetic sprouting, Rather the phenomenon was dependent upon lesions of the septohippocampal pathway, whether in the septum itself or the fimbria fibres, inducing loss of the cholinergic inputs to the hippocampus, and the distribution of sympathetic sprouting matched closely to that of the lost cholinergic inputs (Fig. 13.8; Crutcher *et al.* 1981). Using transplants of sympathetic neurones into the denervated hippocampus of sympathectomised rats, Björklund and Stenevi (1977) proposed that the invasion of the hippocampus by sympathetic or other fibres was under the control of factors released by the denervated targets.

## Sympathetic sprouting is controlled by nerve growth factor

Subsequent studies have shown that this factor is likely to be nerve growth factor (NGF). NGF is the major trophic factor for peripheral sympathetic neurones, which have trkA and p75 on their surface. However, in the CNS, NGF is a major trophic factor for the septohippocampal cholinergic neurones. The hippocampal target areas for the cholinergic innervation produce NGF, and there is a large upregulation of NGF synthesis following cholinergic denervation of the hippocampus (Yu and Crutcher 1995). It is into these regions that the sympathetic fibres sprout. The NGF itself is the major regulator of this sprouting response, since injection of anti-NGF antibodies into the denervated hippocampus completely inhibits the sprouting response of sympathetic terminals (Springer and Loy 1985).

Whether NGF is the sole determinant of sprouting, or whether denervation is also required, is more controversial. When sympathetic ganglia from newborn rats were placed on the hippocampus, together with an NGF infusion, sympathetic axons sprouted throughout the infused region, regardless of whether those areas had been denervated or not. However, in-growth of the endogenous sympathetic fibres only occurs into denervated areas, even in the presence of exogenous NGF (Saffran *et al.* 1989; Scalapino *et al.* 1996).

## Compensatory collateral sprouting in the hippocampus

Lesions of the septohippocampal system have also been employed as a powerful model in which to study collateral sprouting of central neurones in the hippocampus, a response that was first masked by the more obvious sympathetic response. These studies have also allowed an assessment of the functional effects of sprouted fibres. Gage, Björklund, and colleagues were the first to emphasise the fact that the standard fimbria–fornix lesion produces a total denervation of the dorsal and middle parts of the hippocampus of its noradrenergic, serotonergic, and cholinergic innervations, but the ventral pole retains some innervation from all three systems. They used both histochemical stains to visualise, and biochemical assays to quantify, the fact that after such a deafferentation, the nerve terminals in the ventral pole of the hippocampus appear to undergo a substantial sprouting response to expand the density and territory of their innervation into more dorsal parts of the hippocampus (Fig. 13.9).

Since animals with the standard fimbria–fornix lesion involved in these first studies have profound and lasting behavioural deficits, a modification of the model was needed to study the functional role of this type of sprouting in recovery from injury. Gage and colleagues therefore took advantage of the fact that not all of the subcortical innervation to the dorsal hippocampus passes through the fornix and fimbria, a substantial proportion passes in a supracallosal fibre bundle running through the cingulate cortex. Consequently, lesions made through this supracallosal bundle, but sparing the deeper fimbria–fornix fibres, produces a partial denervation of the dorsal hippocampus, which induces marked maze learning deficits but from which the animal eventually recovers. The time course of the functional recovery was protracted over a period of 6 months, similar to the extended time for the collateral sprouting of ventral fibres into the dorsal hippocampus in the full-lesion model. Gage and colleagues therefore considered that the sprouting observed in this model may underlie the functional recovery observed in the partially lesioned rats, and termed this type of long-distance regenerative sprouting through the target 'compensatory collateral sprouting'.

Like the Raisman studies and the sympathetic response, compensatory collateral sprouting involves the sprouting of spared nerve terminals into spaces vacated by a lost innervation. However, in this case it is not only neurotransmitter-specific but it originates from

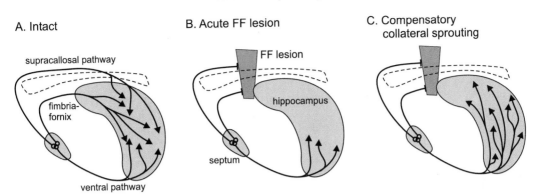

**Fig. 13.9** Compensatory collateral sprouting in the septohippocampal cholinergic system. A. Septohippocampal fibres project to the hippocampus via three main pathways. B. Aspiration septohippocampal lesions remove the dorsal hippocampal innervation arising via the fimbria and supracallosal pathways. C. The ventral pathway sprouts over 3–6 months to provide extensive re-innervation of dorsal hippocampus. A similar pattern of sprouting is seen from ventral noradrenergic innervations arising in the locus coeruleus. (Redrawn from Gage *et al.* 1983.)

the same populations of central cholinergic, noradrenergic, and serotonergic neurones that are lesioned following lesions of the dorsal pathway. An important part of the description by Gage and colleagues is that, whereas regrowth of all three systems is stimulated by the same lesion, each population of cells establishes its own appropriate pattern of terminal of reinnervation.

Although compensatory collateral sprouting is well established in this particular model system, the generality of extensive neurotransmitter-specific fibre regrowth in partially denervated nuclei of the forebrain is not well established, let alone the extent to which it contributes to functional reorganisation and recovery.

## Plasticity of motor and sensory axons in the spinal cord

Spinal-cord injury produces paralysis and anaesthesia that is so permanent, so unchanging, and so rigidly fixed in functional level, that one might be excused for thinking that the cord has little plasticity after injury. However, both sensory and motor axons show considerable plasticity, although less in adulthood than shortly after birth. Even so, in the sensory pathways, some of this plasticity may be maladaptive, not least by contributing to chronic pain syndromes.

### Plasticity in the sensory projections

Plasticity in the sensory projections in the cord has been described as of three main types. The first is the *unmask-*

*ing of silent synapses.* This was first described by Patrick Wall and various collaborators, following cutting of one or more dorsal roots (Deror and Wall 1981). Neurones were found in the denervated regions immediately after denervation that responded to the remaining intact sensory input from dorsal roots higher or lower in the cord, despite the fact that spinal cord sensory neurones at these spinal levels would never normally respond to sensory inputs from dorsal roots so far away. The implication is that sensory fibres in the cord make rather widespread connections, with the inappropriate ones being suppressed. Removal of the appropriate inputs allows the inappropriate sensory inputs to be derepressed.

A similar mechanism may lie behind the increase in the sensitivity to pain that follows inflammation in the skin. Inflamed areas are extremely painful even to light touch, and it has been shown that stimulation of the large A$\beta$ sensory fibres, that normally only carry light touch information, can be interpreted as pain if those fibres come from an area of inflammation. The implication is that there is altered sensory processing in the CNS, such that A$\beta$ fibre information is now interpreted as pain rather than light touch. Baba, Doubell, and Woolf (1999) have shown a physiological correlate to this condition. Pain information is mainly transmitted to neurones in the superficial layers of the dorsal horn, particularly the substantia gelatinosa, via unmyelinated C sensory fibres, and small myelinated A$\delta$ axons, but these neurones do not respond to light touch via A$\beta$ fibres. However, when the skin was inflamed, many substantia gelatinosa neurones started to respond to A$\beta$ input: fine touch could therefore stimulate nociceptive neurones. Baba *et al.* were unable to detect any increased sprouting of Aβ fibres into the substantia gelatinosa, so they ascribe the change to facilitation of normally silent connections of Aβ fibres in the substantia gelatinosa, and to transmitter plasticity in the sensory axons, which gain the ability to secrete substance P after inflammation.

Sensory innervation of the cord shows two additional types of anatomical plasticity. *Regenerative sprouting* can occur along the longitudinal dimension of the sensory input, and between the various layers of the dorsal horn. In the longitudinal axis, sensory axons entering the cord via dorsal roots normally terminate in the same spinal segment, or in the one or two adjoining segments (Fig 13.10). What happens if the neighbouring dorsal roots are cut, so as to create empty synaptic space above or below intact sensory inputs? The result depends on the age of the animal. In adult animals there is little sprouting of the intact projection into the adjacent cord. However, in newborn animals extensive sprouting occurs, resulting in a much enlarged terminal field (Fitzgerald 1985), the period of plasticity ending on about day 5 in rats. However, the lack of sprouting in adult animals can be changed radically by crushing the peripheral nerve, peripheral to the dorsal root ganglion. The peripheral nerve crush completely changes the behaviour of the central processes of the axons, such that they are now able to sprout extensively in a rostrocaudal direction (McMahon and Kett-White 1991). The different effects of axotomy of the central and

peripheral branches of sensory axons has already been described in the previous two chapters on axon regeneration. One important difference is that peripheral axotomy causes upregulation of growth-associated genes, such as GAP-43, while central axotomy does not. It is possible that the upregulation of GAP-43 and other genes by peripheral axotomy may be what enables the central sensory processes to sprout into vacated terminal space (see later).

*Collateral sprouting* of sensory axons can also occur between laminae of the dorsal column. Myelinated Aβ axons, which carry light touch information from low threshold mechanoreceptors, normally only innervate the deeper laminae of the dorsal horn, laminae 3 and 4. Pain fibres carrying information from high threshold mechanoreceptors normally terminate in the superficial layers, particularly the substantia gelatinosa. However the Aβ fibres can be made to sprout into the substantia gelatinosa, and this may be responsible for some chronic pain syndromes, since fine touch fibres will now innervate nociceptive neurones (Fig 13.11). This type of sprouting will occur in response to vacated synaptic space without any extra stimulus. Thus, if the small pain fibres are lesioned with capsaicin, Aβ fibres will sprout into the substantia gelatinosa (Mannion *et al.* 1996). However, Aβ fibres will sprout when the peripheral nerve is crushed even when no synaptic space has been vacated by lesioning. After a peripheral nerve crush, Aβ terminals sprout out into the substantia gelatinosa, and innervate nociceptive neurones (Woolf *et al.* 1992). Pre-

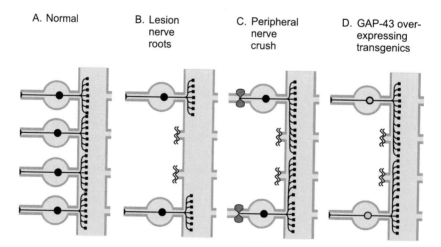

| A. Normal | B. Lesion nerve roots | C. Peripheral nerve crush | D. GAP-43 over-expressing transgenics |

**Fig. 13.10** A. The sensory inputs to the cord via the dorsal roots form a continuous line of terminals in the dorsal columns. B. If some of the dorsal roots are removed, there is little filling in of the vacated synaptic space from the neighbouring roots, except in newborns. C. If peripheral nerves are crushed, the central connections of the dorsal roots can now sprout to occupy vacant synaptic space. D. Overexpression of GAP-43 also increases the sprouting ability of dorsal root axons.

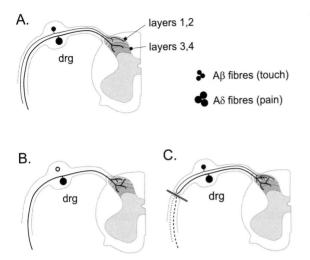

layers 1,2

layers 3,4

drg

Aβ fibres (touch)

Aδ fibres (pain)

B. drg

C. drg

**Fig. 13.11**  Translaminar sprouting in the cord. A. The normal sensory inputs, with the large Aδ fibres projecting to the deeper laminae, and small Aβ pain fibres to the superficial laminae. B. removal of the pain fibres leads to the larger Aδ fibres sprouting into the vacated space. C. Damage to the peripheral nerve leads to the Aδ fibres sprouting into the pain recipient areas even though the pain fibres have not been removed.

sumably the upregulation of growth-associated molecules by the peripheral nerve crush leads to a greatly increased sprouting potential in the central connections, which enables them to take over synaptic space from the pain fibres. This formation of inappropriate connections with nociceptive neurones after peripheral nerve crush may explain the chronic pain syndromes that often follow peripheral nerve damage.

## Sprouting of corticospinal axons in the spinal cord

In adult animals, lesioning of one corticospinal tract does not normally lead to much sprouting of the remaining intact tract across the midline, although there may be sparse sprouting, little of which crosses the midline. However, in newborn animals, Kuang and Kalil (1990) showed that there was extensive sprouting of processes from the intact corticospinal tract across the midline to innervate normal corticospinal recipient regions on the other side of the cord. In the hamster, this plasticity gradually declined to the adult pattern by day 23. Sprouting of descending motor axons in newborn mammals may have a correlate in humans who suffer from cortical damage to one hemisphere in the form of hemiplegic cerebral palsy. Magnetic stimulation obser-

vations on these patients suggest that some of the descending motor fibres on the normal side have sprouted across the midline to control motor neurones on the affected side. This may explain why these patients exhibit 'mirror movements', in which movements of limbs on the normal side sometimes trigger identical movements on the affected side.

## Factors that increase sprouting in the spinal cord

### Age

As described in the previous paragraphs, lesions of the sensory or corticospinal inputs to the cord result in profuse sprouting when lesions are made shortly after birth. However, by 2 weeks after birth, plasticity is much reduced.

### Growth associated proteins

As we have described above, peripheral axotomy stimulates the central terminals of sensory axons to sprout profusely into vacated terminal space, and even causes Aβ sensory axons to sprout into space in the substantia gelatinosa that has not been vacated by removing other inputs. This is associated with an upregulation of the growth associated protein GAP-43 (see Chapter 11) in the sensory neurones. Moreover, expression of GAP-43 is high in newborn sensory neurones and other spinal cord neurones, but declines in the first weeks after birth, at the same time as sprouting diminishes. Is there direct evidence that growth associated proteins can promote sprouting in the spinal cord? This question has been addressed in transgenic mice that overexpress GAP-43 under the control of the Thy 1.2 promoter, which directs expression to mature neurones. In normal mice, as described above, cutting dorsal roots does not lead to a robust sprouting response to occupy the vacated synaptic space from neighbouring sensory roots. However, in the GAP-43 transgenic, the spared sensory inputs sprout strongly, and peripheral nerve section is not needed to promote sprouting (Fig 13.10D). Increased sprouting at the neuromuscular junction and in the hippocampus is also seen in this mouse (Aigner *et al.* 1995).

### Myelin-associated growth inhibitory molecules

As described in Chapter 12, oligodendrocytes produce a range of axon-growth inhibitory molecules. These molecules also have effects on sprouting in the spinal cord. These effects have been examined in two ways. The first is to prevent myelination in part of the cord by irradiation just after birth, which kills the oligodendrocyte precursors that are dividing and myelinating at this time. The second is to use an antibody, IN-1, which neutralises one of the myelin inhibitory molecules, NI-250 (now renamed NogoA). The model in both cases has been to examine sprouting of corticospinal axons across to the other side of the spinal cord or hind-brain above or below the lesion. As described above, after cutting the corticospinal tract in an adult animal, there is little sprouting across the midline from the intact tract. However, in rats that were irradiated at birth there is a robust sprouting response at 3 weeks after birth. (Vanek *et al.* 1998). Sprouting has also been tested in adult rats after treatment with the IN-1 antibody. Section of the corticospinal tract at the level of the pyramids does not, in normal adult rats, lead to sprouting of axons above the lesion to the contralateral red nucleus and basilar pontine nucleus, but in IN-1 treated rats, there was extensive sprouting of corticospinal axons across the midline into these nuclei. There was also an impressive degree of return of corticospinal function (Z'Graggen *et al.* 1998).

## Neurogenesis in the nervous system

Whereas the capacity of amphibians and lower vertebrates to generate new neurones and glial cells after injury has been known for many decades, it was believed until recently that in higher vertebrates the capacity of neurones to divide, either as a part of the normal growth process or in response to injury, has long been thought to be restricted to infancy. However, in recent years it has become clear that mammals possess undifferentiated progenitor cells in most or all parts of their central nervous systems, which have at least the theoretical ability to generate new neurones, and this has raised the possibility that these cells might be manipulated so as to be useful in CNS repair. Moreover, in two regions of the mammalian CNS, neurogenesis continues throughout life.

### Adult neurogenesis in mammals

Even in adult mammals there is a limited level of neurogenesis continuing into adulthood. In a series of

studies undertaken over two decades, Altman and Das used $^3$H thymidine autoradiography to provide a comprehensive analysis of the times of birth of cell populations throughout the nervous system in the rat. From this, comes the clear outcome that virtually all CNS neurones are born during the second half of embryogenesis. However, a few populations of neurones continue to be born into the first weeks of post-natal life, as has been described in a few instances such as subpopulations of neocortical neurones and in the dentate gyrus. What is more surprising is that even in adult mammals there is continuing neurogenesis leading to the birth of two neuronal types, the granule cells of the dentate gyrus, and the neurones of the olfactory bulb. When adult animals are injected with tritiated thymidine, numerous labelled glia and vascular cells (which continue to divide throughout life) are found throughout the forebrain, but very few neurones. However, in 1962 Altman reported that a few labelled cells with the morphology of neurones could be detected in the thalamus and cortex, and that a substantial number of neurones that had divided post-natally could be seen in two areas — in the olfactory bulb, and amongst the granule cells in the dentate gyrus. Subsequent cell-counting studies by Bayer have indicated a 50% increase in the numbers of dentate granule neurones from 1 month to 1 year of age in the rat, suggesting a continuing expansion of cell numbers rather than neurogenesis to replace a turnover of neurones (see Fig. 13.12). Cell division in the subgranular zone of the dentate gyrus goes on into late adulthood, although the number of dividing cells falls to low levels in aged rodents. The differentiation of these dividing cells into dentate granule neurones has been confirmed using a variety of mechanisms including electron microscopy (Kaplan 1981) and immunohistochemical staining for neurotransmitter enzymes, such as glutamic acid decarboxylase (Lubbers *et al.* 1985). Similar populations of dividing cells have now been reported in primate and human dentate gyrus (Eriksson *et al.* 1998; Kornack and Rakic 1999).

The rate of cell division in the dentate gyrus is extremely dynamic. Overall, the rate of division falls with age. However, neurogenesis is affected by a variety of external factors. Gage and his colleagues have shown that the richness of the environment can affect cell division, with mice raised in featureless cages having a lower rate of division, and eventually a smaller number of granule cells than animals raised in a mouse playground, which contained many things to explore (Kempermann *et al.* 1998). Stress also has an effect on rates of cell division (see also Chapter 8). Rodents and marmosets have

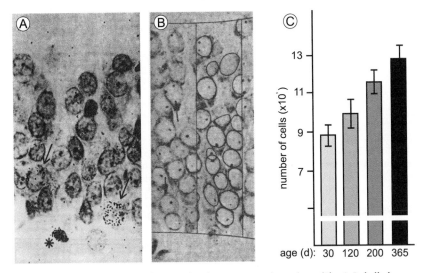

**Fig. 13.12** Neurogenesis and increased cell numbers in the dentate gyrus throughout life. A Labelled neurones in the dentate gyrus after [³H]thymidine injections at 1 month. B Cell depth and density in counting frames in the adult dentate gyrus. C Estimated cell numbers at different ages. (From Bayer *et al.* 1982.)

been exposed to stressful stimuli, injected immediately afterwards with the cell division marker bromodeoxyuridine, then killed after 2 h of labelling time. Even after this short time, dramatic changes in rates of cell division in the dentate gyrus can be detected, with stress decreasing cell division. The major regulatory mechanism appears to be via corticosteroids. Stress causes large increases in corticosteroid levels, and corticosteroids reduce the rate of precursor division in the dentate gyrus, and it may also be that the age-related decrease in the rate of cell division is related to increasing steroid levels with age (Cameron and Gould 1994).

## Ventricular/subventricular precursor cells

Since new neurones can be born in the adult rodent forebrain, the next issue relates to where they come from. Neurones themselves are post-mitotic: they do not undergo subsequent cell division either spontaneously or in response to a stimulus (e.g. injury). Thus, for example, there has been no evidence found for dividing mitotic figures observed in mature neurones. Rather, as described in more detail in Chapter 25, most new neurones appear to divide from defined and localised populations of stem or precursor cells located in the subependymal zone bordering the floor and walls of the lateral ventricles, and in the subgranular layer in the hippocampus. The densest levels of cell labelling are found

the subependymal zone. These progenitor cells are migratory. Cells from the subgranular zone in the dentate gyrus migrate a small distance to produce new neurones in dentate, and having migrated and differentiated these neurones do not divide further. The cells of the subependymal zone migrate for considerable distances to populate the olfactory lobes. Lois and Alvarez-Buyulla (1994) were able to show this both by implanting dividing subventricular precursor cells derived from transgenic mice carrying a neurone-specific transgene into the subventricular zone of non-transgenic host mice, and by injecting cell markers, including ³H thymidine, into the wall of the ventricles (see Fig. 13.13). The transgenic and labelled cells could later be identified as differentiated neurones in the olfactory bulb. When ³H thymidine was injected into the wall of the lateral ventricle, many of the implanted subventricular zone cells were seen to be labelled, indicating continuing cell division, and over the first 6 h after thymidine injection, remained clustered around the implantation site in the subventricular zone of the host. After longer survival times, the cells were seen to migrate in a stream from the wall of the lateral ventricle, rostral and ventral-wards, parallel to the surface of the ventricle, towards the olfactory bulb: the first cells reached the bulb after 2 days, and by 15 days, most labelled cells had reached their olfactory bulb target. The numbers of silver grains marking individual cells decreased at more rostral positions in the stream, suggesting that these precursor cells continued to

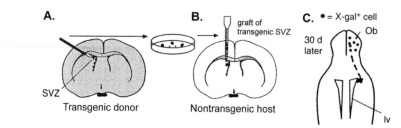

**Fig. 13.13**   Migration of dividing precursor cells of the subventricular zone (SVZ) in a stream from the walls of the lateral ventricle to the olfactory bulb. A. Dissection of SVZ derived from transgenic donor brain in which the cells express the marker gene β galactosidase. B. Implantation of transgenic SVZ graft into SVZ of normal host. C. Subsequent migration of cells from SVZ to olfactory bulb over a 2-week period, visualised by X-gal staining of graft derived cells. (Based on Lois and Alvarez-Buyulla 1994.)

divide *en route*. Only once they had reached the olfactory bulb did the cells stain with an antibody specific for neurones, neurone-specific enolase. At this stage, the cells also acquired a distinctive neuronal morphology.

## Song bird learning

While mammals clearly have some potential to produce new neurones but only do so to a limited extent, there is one well-studied situation in which higher vertebrate species regularly generate large numbers of neurones. The males of many species of song birds develop rich and varied song patterns during the spring breeding season. Each male will develop its own complex and distinctive pattern, which in many species (such as zebra finches or canaries) will change from year to year.

Fernando Nottebohm (Nottebohm 1991) and colleagues have undertaken a series of studies identifying the structural organisation in the brain necessary to represent such complex motor patterns and associated with these changes in species-specific behavioural skills.

- The motor nuclei necessary for song, the hyperstriatum ventrale pars caudalis (HSVc) and the nucleus robustus archistiatalis (RA), are three- to four-fold larger in volume in singing males than in female.

- The volumes of these nuclei were found to increase in the spring and decrease in the autumn, associated with the cycle of song activity during the breeding season.

- Their volumes correlated with the richness and complexity of the individual male's song patterns. Furthermore, these two variables also correlated with testis weight suggesting that the cortical complexity may be hormonally regulated. This was tested by treating female canaries with testosterone, which

resulted in an increase in the size of HSV and RA, and the development of a male-like song.

In order to identify the source of expansion in HSV nuclear volume, the testosterone-treated canaries were injected with thymidine to label dividing neurones (Fig. 13.14; Goldman and Nottebohm 1983). When the birds were sacrificed 3–4 weeks later, a large number of thymidine labelled neurones were seen in the HSV, suggesting that the expansion of nucleus size was due to the division of new neurones (i.e. neurogenesis) in the adult brain. Interestingly, when the birds were killed 1 or 2 days after thymidine injection, labelled neurones were not seen in the HSV, but rather heavy labelling was seen in the overlying ventricular zone with many labelled endothelial and glial cells. This suggests that the new neurones divide from a population of precursor cells located in the ventricular margins of the hyperstriatum, which then migrate into and populate the expanding HSV.

## Progenitor differentiation *in vitro* and *in vitvo*

One of the key events in the development of the field of CNS precursor biology over the last decade, has been the identification of progenitor cells with the capacity to divide even in adulthood, and the development by Reynolds and Weiss (1992) of techniques to make the cells proliferate in culture. As elaborated in greater detail in Chapter 25, it has been possible to culture progenitors from almost all parts of the CNS, that have the ability to differentiate into the three main neuronal cell types: astrocytes, neurones, and oligodendrocytes.

This has led to several important new concepts. Initially it was found that cells from embryos with the

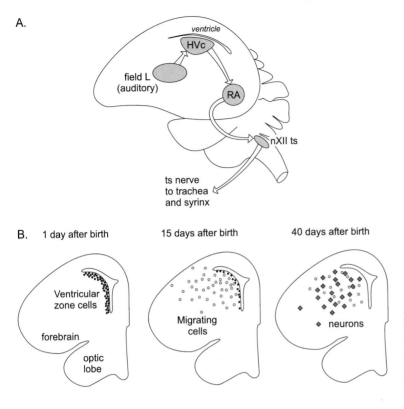

A.

B. 1 day after birth     15 days after birth     40 days after birth

**Fig. 13.14**  A. Location of the main vocal learning centres in the canary brain (see text). B. Migration of thymidine-labelled newly differentiated neurones into the dorsal forebrain. (Based on Goldman and Nottebohm 1983.)

properties of undifferentiated and multipotential progenitors could be cultured from embryonic CNS, and stimulated to divide more or less indefinitely by EGF or FGF-2. It was then found that similar cells could be cultured from the adult brain, mainly from subependymal zone or hippocampus. These cells appear to be genuinely multipotential, in that if they are labelled they can subsequently be shown to have generated oligodendrocytes, astrocytes, and neurones in the brain (see Chapter 25). Not only can these progenitors generate several cell types, but it appears that when progenitor cells are transplanted into host animals, the type of cell into which they will differentiate is determined not by where the progenitor came from but also by its surroundings. This is well established for progenitors derived from the embryonic CNS, which have been transplanted into several sites in the embryonic, newborn, and adult CNS. The cells possess a substantial degree of developmental plasticity, those implanted into the hippocampus turn into hippocampal neurones, and so on. However, while progenitors transplanted into the embryonic CNS will migrate widely, and produce many different types of neuronal and glial cell, the ability of the CNS to instruct progenitor cell differ-

entiation into neurones declines with age. In the adult CNS, the regions that can instruct progenitors towards a neuronal fate are those areas in which neurogenesis is still continuing, namely the hippocampus and olfactory bulb. If grafted to other regions, progenitors tend either to differentiate into astrocytes or die (Gage *et al.* 1995; Brustle *et al.* 1997). The general rule is that the fate of grafted progenitors is determined not by the position of origin of the cells, but by the place into which they are grafted. Thus progenitors grafted into the pathway of cells migrating from the subependymal zone to the olfactory bulb, will migrate and differentiate into olfactory neurones (Suhonen *et al.* 1996), progenitors from whatever source grafted into the hippocampus will become hippocampal neurones.

## Progenitors in the damaged CNS

If there are progenitors in most parts of the adult mammalian CNS, then the question arises as to why they do not replace the cells that are lost when the CNS is damaged. Certainly, similar cells in lower vertebrates are able to replace damaged neurones. Although traumatic injury in the mammalian brain does induce a massive increase in cell division, double-labelling studies indicate that this is entirely attributable to dividing precursor cells and glial cells that differentiate into different classes of reactive glia. However, under natural circumstances, the mammalian CNS injury response apparently does not include the formation of new neurones as part of a natural repair process. Is this because the progenitors that are present in the mammalian CNS fail to be recruited into CNS injuries, or is because they are recruited but then fail to generate replacements for the cells that are lost?

The evidence is mixed. In spinal-cord injuries there is direct evidence for the recruitment of progenitor cells into injuries. Johannson and co-workers (1999) have made an extensive study of precursor behaviour in the spinal cord. By a combination of labelling techniques, and by culturing clones of cells derived from single precursors, they showed that the ependymal cells lining the central canal are true CNS stem cells, in that they can generate the three major forms of CNS cell type (Fig. 13.15). The ependymal cells divide slowly and generate a population of progenitors, which lie next to the ependymal layer. When the spinal cord was damaged, the rate of division of the ependymal and subependymal cells increased, and some of the cells migrated away from the central canal into the lesion. However, instead of replacing lost cells, the progenitors differentiated into astrocytes, which formed part of the glial scar.

It is not clear whether subependymal cells in the brain are recruited into CNS lesions some distance away; at the time of writing, the evidence is conflicting. Various other studies in which progenitor cells have been grafted into CNS injuries have shown them differentiating into scar astrocytes. However, there are several circumstances in which implants of progenitor cells have replaced lost CNS cells. The first is in demyelination. Progenitors grafted into demyelinated regions have generated new oligodendrocytes (see Chapter 24). The second instance applies when the progenitor cells are not endogenous cells that have migrated into the lesion, and not cells that have been expanded *in vitro*. Instead, progenitor cell lines have been derived by immortalisation of stem cells with oncogenes, either *myc* or SV40T. These cells can be grafted into the undamaged CNS, and will survive in an undifferentiated state. However, when the CNS is damaged, the cells migrate to the injury site. In several experiments, Evan Snyder, who made one of these cell lines, has shown that they have a remarkable ability to replace neuronal cells that have been lost. For instance, if the cells of the progenitor line are placed in

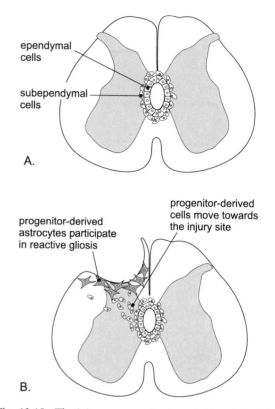

**Fig. 13.15** The injury response in the spinal cord. A. The uninjured cord. The ependymal cells cycle slowly, and represent a stem-cell population, while a population of subependymal progenitors derived from them are also dividing. B. After injury, both the subependymal cells and the ependymal cells increase their rate of division, and their progeny migrate towards the injury site. However, they do not replace the lost neurones, all the migrating cells turn into astrocytes. (After Johansson *et al.* 1999.)

the spinal cord, and a lesion is made that kills motor neurones, then the progenitors can differentiate into neuronal cells with many of the properties of adult motor neurones, while in the cortex the cells were able to replace neurones in the adult cortex that were killed be photolysis (Snyder *et al.* 1997). This research raises several important questions about the response of progenitors to CNS injury, which need to be resolved.

- Are CNS progenitors recruited to all CNS injuries?

- If the CNS retains the ability to instruct progenitors to replace cells that have been lost, as suggested by Snyder's results, why do endogenous progenitor cells, or progenitors expanded *in vitro* fail to respond?

- What are the signals that make stem cells in injuries turn into astrocytes?

If the damaged brain can still direct stem-cell differentiation towards those elements that have been lost through damage, then the task of repairing the CNS will be much easier than it will be if those signals no longer exist.

If precursors are present, and if they will not generate new neurones, it is possible that the environment of the mammalian CNS in some way represses those precursors that are present.

## Summary

In summary, neurones of the adult mammalian nervous system do have a greater plasticity than was once believed. Following axonal injury, adult axons can undergo both collateral and regenerative sprouting under the correct signals, and the adult glial environment can support quite extensive regrowth of some classes of central axons, for example, those derived from embryonic neurones. Similarly, the former belief of a complete absence of neurogenesis in the adult CNS is now known not to be absolute, and there do appear to be resting populations of progenitor cells with the capacity to divide, proliferate, and differentiate into neurones in response to the right signals. Nevertheless, in normal circumstances, none of these features appears to provide the basis for a regenerative response for repair of the CNS in response to injury. Nevertheless, they open the way for developing new strategies for promoting repair and reconstruction of damage in the central nervous system, which are now providing a major impetus for novel approaches to treatment, as explored in the remaining chapters of this volume. First, however, we must explore a second form of plasticity that might underlie recovery of function, the biochemical adaptation of spared neurones in response to injury in ways that can compensate for the neurones that are lost.

## Further reading

Craig, C.G., Tropepe, V., Morshead, C.M., Reynolds, B.A., Weiss, S., and Van der Kooy, D. (1996). *In-vivo* growth-factor expansion of endogenous subependymal neural precursor cell-populations in the adult-mouse brain. *Journal of Neuroscience,* **16**, 2649–2658.

Crutcher, K. (1987). Sympathetic sprouting. *Brain Research Reviews,* **12**, 203–233.

Jenkins, W.M. and Merzenich, M.M. (1987). Cortical remodelling. *Progress in Brain Research,* **71**, 249–267.

Kempermann, G. and Gage, F.H. (1999). New nerve cells for the adult brain. *Scentific American,* **280**, 48–53.

# 14 | Biochemical plasticity

Another mechanism whereby neurones can adapt to damage is by changes in the electrophysiological, biochemical, and neurotransmitter activities of the cells. Many events can alter the neurotransmitter phenotype of central nervous system (CNS) neurones. For instance, most neurones down-regulate their neurotransmitters and the enzymes that make them after axotomy or other forms of damage. Neurotrophins tend to cause neurones to upregulate their neurotransmitter phenotype or even change it, and neurotrophins often prevent the down-regulation of neurotransmitter phenotype after damage. There are so many examples of these types of behaviour that it would not be sensible in this book to try and detail them all. However, there are two particular experimental models in which neuroplasticity of this type has been analysed in detail, and we will describe them. These model systems are the nigro-striatal dopamine system of rats, and the expression of neuropeptides, cholinergic, and adrenergic phenotype in sympathetic neurones. However, the dynamic changes seen in these models are likely to apply much more widely in the CNS.

## The nigro-striatal lesion model

The dopaminergic nigro-striatal pathway projects from the substantia nigra to the neostriatum. The neostriatum is involved in the highest levels of motor control. It has been known for several decades that stimulant drugs, such as amphetamine, increase dopamine release in the striatum and produce an overactivity syndrome in both animals and humans, involving excessive activation of all aspects of behaviour. Conversely, drugs that reduce dopamine levels in the striatum (such as reserpine) or that block dopamine receptors (such as haloperidol), produce a profound suppression of voluntary behaviours. Indeed, the dopamine antagonists constitute a leading class of major tranquilliser drugs for psychiatric use, and dopamine-uptake inhibitors are a major class of antidepressant.

The dopamine system can be lesioned in experimen-

tal animals with a variety of selective toxins, such as 6-OHDA or MPTP. If the lesions are made bilaterally, such lesions are debilitating. Small lesions reduce general activity levels (hypokinesia), whereas after larger lesions the animals cease to make any voluntary movements at all (akinesia). When placed into its cage, the lesioned rat adjusts itself into a stable hunched posture and simply maintains that position indefinitely. This syndrome is not due to an inability to move *per se*, since if the animal is dropped or flipped onto its back it shows an efficient vestibular righting reflex. Rather, it appears to suffer a general inability to initiate any voluntary action. This includes such life-sustaining functions as eating and drinking, and if left to itself the animal will neither eat (aphagia) nor drink (adipsia), and will die within a few days of inanition (Zigmond and Stricker 1972; Marshall *et al.* 1974).

## Recovery from 6-hydroxydopamine lesions

In 1973, Zigmond and Stricker made total forebrain dopamine lesions in rats by injecting 6-OHDA into the lateral ventricles, but then kept the rats alive by tube-feeding several times a day with a palatable and highly nutritious liquid diet. They made the remarkable observation that the rats would eventually recover the ability to eat and drink, although it could take several months of intensive nursing care before the animals could sustain themselves without help. Moreover, the recovery appeared to progress through a systematic series of stages whereby the animals first nibbled at highly sweet, moist foods, and only later would they sample dry foods, or drink water as an adjunct to eating (see Fig. 14.1). Eventually, most, if not all, of the rats reached the stage where they could maintain themselves on normal lab chow and water. Body weight typically remained low and the animals never recovered the ability to regulate their food and water intake in response to internal challenges (such as a disturbance of cellular fluid balance following injection of hypertonic saline) (Stricker and Zigmond 1976).

The ability of the animals to respond in the recovery phase appears to depend on external factors (like the palatable taste of the food, or drinking in response to a dry mouth when eating dry food), rather than to an internal need (hunger or thirst or level of weight loss).

A very similar syndrome had previously been well described following lesions in the lateral hypothalamus

(Teitelbaum and Epstein 1972). However, the demonstration that this general motivational syndrome could be essentially reproduced by lesions in just one pathway of the forebrain, at the same time as the anatomical, pharmacological, and physiological tools were becoming available to dissect the functions of identified neurones of the brain, opened the way to understand not only the syndrome but the mechanisms of recovery.

## Biochemical plasticity in dopamine pathways

Following a series of studies detailing the 6-OHDA syndrome and its recovery, in 1976 Stricker and Zigmond proposed an integrated theory to account for behavioural recovery after extensive damage of central catecholamine neurones, which involved the dynamic regulation of surviving presynaptic nerve terminals to compensate for the loss of other terminals. As illustrated in Fig. 14.2, Stricker and Zigmond proposed a variety of mechanisms that could be responsible for the partial recovery from the 6-OHDA syndrome, spanning mechanisms that could increase transmitter release to increased transmitter sensitivity. The possible mechanisms were: that surviving terminals may increase their synthesis of dopamine, dopamine release may increase for a given level of depolarisation of the nerve terminal, the presynaptic firing rate of the neurones may increase, further increasing synaptic release of dopamine; reduced re-uptake may increase the duration of dopamine availability in the synaptic cleft and allow diffusion to adjacent receptors from which presynaptic input is lost; and,

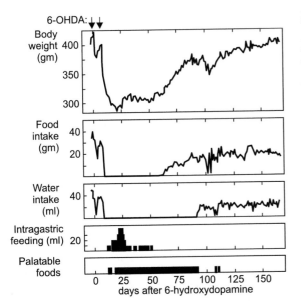

**Fig. 14.1** Recovery of eating and drinking after general forebrain dopamine depletion. (Redrawn from Zigmond and Stricker 1973, with permission.)

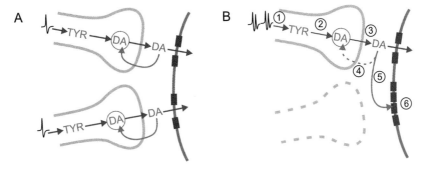

**Fig. 14.2** Biochemical plasticity following nigro-striatal lesions. A Two intact dopamine terminals on a nigro-striatal neurone. B Following partial loss of terminals, others upregulate to restore normal levels of striatal dopaminergic activation, by (1) increased cell firing, (2) increased dopamine synthesis, (3) increased dopamine release, (4) reduced dopamine uptake, (5) diffusion to deafferented synapses, (6) development of receptor supersensitivity. (Redrawn from Zigmond and Stricker 1984.)

finally, the cell receptors themselves may increase in sensitivity to the receptor ligands. Although at the time this theory was largely speculative, substantial evidence has subsequently been accumulated for most of these compensatory processes.

## Increased dopamine synthesis

Dopaminergic nerve terminals have a limited dopamine storage capacity, and post-mortem assay of striatal dopamine concentration is routinely taken as a measure of the numbers of surviving terminals. The enzyme tyrosine hydroxylase (TH) is the rate-limiting enzyme in presynaptic dopamine synthesis, catalysing the conversion of tyrosine to DOPA to dopamine. Although TH levels in the striatum also decrease after a 6-OHDA lesion, they do not do so to the same extent as the loss of dopamine itself (Fig. 14.3). As a consequence, the TH:dopamine ratio increases after 6-OHDA lesions, which suggests an increase in the rate of dopamine synthesis in the remaining nerve terminals spared by the lesion.

## Increased dopamine turnover

The major metabolite of dopamine is dihydroxyphenylacetic acid (DOPAC). In exactly the same way as we have just seen with TH, the DOPAC levels in the striatum also decrease after a 6-OHDA lesion, but again they do not do so to the same extent as the loss of dopamine itself, and the DOPAC:dopamine ratio increases after the lesion (see Fig. 14.3). This indicates an increased number of extracellular metabolite molecules per rate of release from the nerve terminal, indicating an increase in the levels of turnover and release.

## Reduced dopamine re-uptake

The dynamics of dopamine re-uptake are disturbed after nigro-striatal lesions. Kinetic analysis suggested a reduction in the maximum velocity of uptake, which correlated well with loss of dopamine levels (i.e. it was proportional to the loss of dopamine terminals). By contrast the affinity of the re-uptake channel was not seen to change.

## Changes in cell firing rates

Grace and Bunney (1984a, b) have found that some nigro-striatal dopamine neurones remain in a relatively quiescent, inactive state, while others exhibit spontaneous activity and fire in essentially two different modes: single-spike firing and burst firing. They proposed that during single-spike firing, autoreceptor activity would be minimised and tyrosine hydroxylase activity maximised — conditions that favour accumulating stores of dopamine in the presynaptic terminal. By contrast, burst firing of neurones is likely to lead to a massive depolarisation release of dopamine from the nerve terminals, followed by feedback inhibition of the neurone. They suggested that burst firing would enable the neurones more effectively to generate spikes in response to an excitatory influence.

In a subsequent investigation, Hollerman and Grace (1990) showed that 6-OHDA partial lesions of the nigro-striatal pathway resulted in a reduction in the numbers of inactive nigro-striatal neurones and an increased percentage of burst firing in the spared neurones. This suggested that the remaining neurones adapt their electrophysiological firing patterns to maximise the amount of dopamine released. However, perhaps surprisingly, these compensatory changes only occurred when the loss of the nigral dopamine cells exceeded 95%, whereas smaller lesions resulted in few changes in the patterns of cell firing. This suggests that changes in firing patterns are only likely to be involved in compensatory plasticity and relatively advanced stages of denervation.

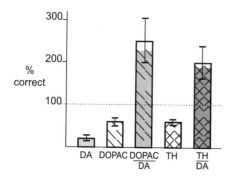

**Fig. 14.3** Biochemical changes after intraventricular injections of 6-OHDA in rats. Abbreviations: DA, dopamine; TH, the synthetic enzyme tyrosine hydroxylase; DOPAC, the primary dopamine metabolite, dihydroxyphenylacetic acid. (Redrawn from Zigmond *et al.* 1984.)

## Receptor supersensitivity

Changes in the sensitivity of dopamine receptors after denervation was first proposed by Ungerstedt to account for the effects of dopamine-stimulant drugs on the motor asymmetry produced by unilateral lesions of the nigro-striatal pathway. Ungerstedt and Arbuthnott (1970) injected 6-OHDA into the nigro-striatal pathway on just one side of the brain. The animals initially show a marked postural bias and spontaneous turning, but this acute effect of the toxin rapidly recovers. However, if the animal is activated, either by a stress (such as placing it in a shallow tray of cold water) or by a stimulant drug (such as amphetamine), the animals exhibit a motor asymmetry, one aspect of which is a characteristic turning response (rotation) towards the side of the lesion. The animals turn head-to-tail in tight circles for the duration of the drug action or of the applied stressor. This is typically interpreted as reflecting a stimulation of dopamine release, producing a functional activation of the striatum and its motor outputs on the intact side of the brain but not on the side of the lesion (Fig. 14.4). The rate at which animals turn under amphetamine correlates well with the extent of the lesion. As a consequence, rotation has become a popular non-invasive test to characterise the completeness of unilateral lesions and the effectiveness of alternative treatments to alleviate damage, such as neural transplantation (see Chapter 23).

Not surprisingly, the precise mechanism of drug action and why it is translated into a particular behavioural phenomenon, turns out to be more complicated than proposed in the original Ungerstedt model. Nevertheless, the basic interpretation that rotation primarily reflects a differential level of dopamine activation of the intact and lesioned sides still stands. The unexpected result in these studies came about when considering the effects of dopamine receptor agonists, such as apomorphine, on rotation. Ungerstedt found that when given a peripheral injection of apomorphine, animals with unilateral lesions turned not towards the side of the lesion, but in the opposite direction (Ungerstedt 1971b). He proposed that since contralateral rotation must reflect a differential activation of the striatum on the lesioned side, there must be an increase in the responsiveness of dopamine receptors on spared striatal neurones following loss of their dopaminergic inputs. This suggests a dynamic plasticity of dopamine receptors in response to a loss of their normal dopamine input: the receptors become *supersensitive* to any residual dopamine molecules or other ligands. The plausibility of this interpretation is enhanced by the fact that the phenomenon of supersensitivity takes several weeks to develop fully, and the animals then become sensitive to very low doses of agonist drugs, well below the levels to produce any detectable effects in intact animals.

Although this hypothesis of receptor supersensitivity was first proposed to account for behavioural data, the phenomenon has subsequently been confirmed using neurochemical binding assays and receptor autoradiography. These have confirmed that supersensitivity develops in D2 dopamine receptors in response to deafferentation, and reflects changes in both the affinity and numbers of receptors (Creese *et al.* 1977). Moreover, we can see similar dynamic changes in the sensitivity of dopamine receptors after pharmacological treatments:

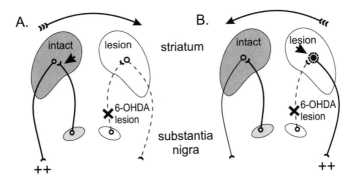

**Fig. 14.4** The Ungerstedt rotation model. The unilateral 6-OHDA lesion removes the dopamine inputs to the striatum but leaves intact the intrinsic striatal neurones bearing the post-synaptic dopamine receptors. A. Stimulant drugs (e.g. amphetamine) or other stressors stimulate dopamine release in the intact striatum (arrow head), and induce rotation in the direction ipsilateral to the side of the lesion (*curved arrow*). B. Dopamine agonist drugs (e.g. apomorphine) have a greater activation of the lesioned striatum due to their direct action on supersensitive receptors on post-synaptic neurones (*arrow head*) and induce turning in the contralateral direction (*curved arrow*). (Based on Ungerstedt and Arbuthnott 1970.)

for example, when animals are treated chronically with neuroleptic drugs (e.g. haloperidol), they show increased responsiveness to low levels of agonist treatments.

## Mechanisms and limits of recovery

In the Stricker and Zigmond model, recovery depends on *sparing* of at least a few of the nigro-striatal dopamine neurones to take over the functions of those lost. Indeed, the *extracellular* levels of dopamine in the 6-OHDA lesioned striatum, as measured with a micro-dialysis probe, can approach 100% of normal levels, even when the number of dopamine cells lost from the substantia nigra and the depletion of the total (pre-dominantly intracellular) level of striatal dopamine is as high as 90%.

Recovery may also appear to imply a degree of *redundancy*. The fact that an animal may compensate well for a partial loss by the remaining neurones sustaining normal levels of food and water intake may seem to suggest that the dopamine system is so important for regulating fundamental life-supporting processes that animals have evolved an excess of dopamine neurones over and above the number necessary for efficient performance. However, the fact that the recovered animals still exhibit residual deficits when challenged, suggests that the full system may be utilised in the intact animal for the most precise aspects of regulation of motivated behaviours. Similar degrees of redundancy are seen in many other parts of the nervous system. For instance, some patients who have received spinal-cord injuries may have almost normal motor and sensory behaviour, even though many long spinal-cord axons have been disrupted.

It is noteworthy that some plastic processes (such as changes in dopamine synthesis, release, metabolism, and re-uptake) appear to operate with relatively incomplete lesions, whereas others have little effect until the lesions are quite advanced. Thus rats only show good agonist-induced rotation (and inferred development of receptor supersensitivity) when depletions approach 90% and the changes in electrophysiological firing patterns may not appear until the denervation reaches the 95% level (Hefti *et al.* 1980). Not only does this suggest that only a subset of the proposed mechanisms actually contribute to the recovery process in most partial lesions, but other studies (in particular ones related to the side-effects of anti-parkinsonian drugs) have suggested that the later developing changes may actually impair, rather than enhance, recovery.

## Dopaminergic plasticity in Parkinson's disease

The timing of onset and progress of Parkinson's disease almost certainly owes as much to a failure of biochemical plasticity as it does to the progress of the underlying lesion. No sooner had the basis of Parkinson's disease as a profound loss of dopamine neurones been identified than it was noticed that the underlying anatomical loss of dopamine cells, and the associated biochemical dysfunction, had usually already progressed to a relatively advanced stage (typically around 70–80%) before the very first symptoms become apparent (Bernheimer *et al.* 1973). An acute lesion of similar size in an animal, for example, by giving MPTP to a monkey (see Chapter 6), will result in a profound debilitation, even though the animal will largely recover in subsequent weeks. This suggests that with a slowly progressing disease like Parkinson's disease, the intrinsic plasticity can fully compensate for partial cell loss. It is only when those compensatory processes themselves approach their limits that symptoms become apparent.

At the earlier stage, when an animal appears to be recovered from an acute lesion, or in a pre-symptomatic patient with Parkinson's disease, deficits can still be exhibited if the compensatory processes are themselves challenged. For example, a rat that has recovered normal eating, drinking, and locomotion after a partial 6-OHDA lesion, remains hypersensitive to the dopamine synthesis inhibitor α-methyl tyrosine. A low dose of α-methyl tyrosine, which has no detectable effect in a normal rat, will induce profound akinesia, aphagia, and adipsia in a rat that had apparently recovered fully from an earlier dopamine-depleting lesion (Zigmond and Stricker 1973). Similarly, it is a familiar observation of clinicians that newly diagnosed patients first develop or notice symptoms when tired, stressed, or otherwise run-down.

## Efficacy and side-effects of l-DOPA

The treatment of Parkinson's disease was revolutionised in the mid-1960s by the introduction of the dopamine precursor drug, L-DOPA, which to this day remains the mainstay of pharmaceutical therapy for this disease. The advantage of L-DOPA over dopamine itself as a direct replacement therapy, is that the latter does not cross the blood–brain barrier (see Chapter 6). In its usual formulation, L-DOPA is given in combination with carbidopa, an antagonist of L-DOPA, which also does not cross the blood–brain barrier, but blocks the rather marked peripheral side-effects of L-DOPA on the cardiovascular system.

At its simplest, L-DOPA is metabolised in the brain to dopamine, and hence provides a direct replacement therapy for the striatal dopamine lost in the disease process (Fig. 14.5A). However, the therapeutic action of L-DOPA is believed in large part to be dependent upon an interaction with the residual populations of spared nigro-striatal dopamine terminals. The drug is accumulated in spared terminals, increasing the availability of stored dopamine for regulated release and re-uptake. As such, the drug promotes the compensatory plasticity of the spared intrinsic system, and extends its function when those plastic processes reach their limit, rather than acting as an independent source of receptor ligand. Indeed, dopamine synthesis and metabolism takes place within a few minutes, so that as the disease progresses and there are fewer and fewer intrinsic terminals to regulate L-DOPA metabolism, the balance between efficacy and side-effects of the drug breaks down: there is an initial surge of excess dopamine formed extracellularly, over-stimulating the receptors to pronounced dyskinetic side-effects, followed by a rapid waning of the effects as all the available drug is metabolised away (see Fig. 14.5B; Marsden and Parkes 1977). The attempt to identify and regulate an effective therapeutic dose between swings from dyskinetic 'On' states to ineffective 'Off' states represents one of the major clinical challenges for managing advanced Parkinson's disease.

It is likely that the late development of receptor supersensitivity may also contribute as much to the problems as to therapeutic compensation in Parkinson's disease. The dyskinesias characteristic of the peak dose–response to L-DOPA are akin to the stereotypies associated with amphetamine overdose. Moreover, in animals the development of similar side-effects can block the therapeutic effects of dopaminergic drugs after acute lesions. Thus, for example, Marshall and Ungerstedt found that the profound aphagia induced by bilateral 6-OHDA lesions could be alleviated by giving L-DOPA during the first week after lesion (Ljungberg and Ungerstedt 1976). However, thereafter, with the development of receptor supersensitivity, no dose of the drug could be found that was sufficient to activate the animals from akinesia without at the same time producing such debilitating stereotypies that the animals were unable to drink.

The recognition, that receptor supersensitivity may be a fundamental contributor to the side-effects of existing drug therapies has led to an intensified search for strategies to inhibit its development. One major strategy relates to the pharmacological data that the side-effects are due to an acute over-stimulation on a background of receptor changes due to chronic under-stimulation. Consequently, a number of alternative drug delivery systems are being investigated that would provide slow release for longer term stable delivery of L-DOPA, in the belief that this would inhibit development of supersensitivity (see Fig. 14.5C; Poewe and Granata 1997). A slow-release system may also have other advantages, such as allowing delivery of compounds that are metabolised too rapidly in the body to allow an effective duration of action, such as the receptor agonist apomorphine, which has been widely used in animal

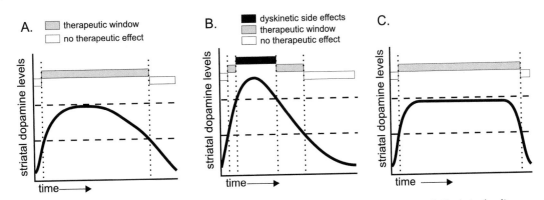

Fig. 14.5 Schematic illustration of the changes of efficacy of a single dose of L-DOPA over time. A. Early in the disease, extra-cellular levels of L-DOPA are regulated by residual terminals, providing therapeutic benefit over a prolonged period. B. As the disease progresses, the therapeutic window between no effect and dyskinetic side-effects of excessive levels of drug becomes increasingly difficult to titrate. C. A slow-release preparation may provide L-DOPA within a stable therapeutic window over prolonged periods of time, even in advanced patients.

experimentation, but the 20–30 min of drug action has been considered too brief for single-dose formulations. However, recent evidence using 'apomorphine patches' to allow delivery of the drug by cutaneous absorption has renewed therapeutic interest in this classic research compound.

## Functional compensation by other systems?

Another challenge has come through the suggestion that other systems may contribute to recovery by a process of adaptation. It has been known for a long time that 6-OHDA lesions have remarkably little effect when made in neonatal animals, in contrast to the marked debilitation caused by this toxin in adult animals. Bruno and colleagues (1987) observed that neonatal lesions producing up to 98% loss of striatal dopamine were accompanied by a marked increase in the concentration of serotonin in the striatum, and proposed that compensatory sprouting of serotonergic systems may take over the functions normally sustained by dopamine pathways as a developmental adaptation, if the disturbance was sustained during in early life.

This observation provides one aspect of a more general phenomenon that, in many situations, comparable damage appears to produce less functional disturbance if sustained in infancy. This is the so called *Kennard principle*, named after the findings of Margaret Kennard in the 1930s, that damage in the motor cortex of infant monkeys produced less lasting impairments than when damage of similar extent was made in the motor cortex of adults (Kennard 1936, 1942). Finger and Stein interpret this phenomenon in terms of involving two distinct aspects of plasticity. First, that the immature brain by virtue of being in a state of flux and less specifically organised, has greater capacity for physiological plasticity than is true later in life once the systems are more fixed and established. At a second level, the younger organism may have a greater capacity for behavioural adaptation and the flexibility for adopting new behavioural strategies to overcome the limitations imposed by damage.

The second aspect of the data on the effects of neonatal 6-OHDA lesions relates to whether the correlation with an increase in serotonin systems represents a true explanation of the milder functional deficits and the more complete apparent recovery, even with rather complete lesions that have been reported in many of these animals. If so, then we would predict that lesions of the raphé-striatal system (e.g. by using the selective serotonergic toxin 5,7-dihydroxytryptamine) or pharmacological blockade with a serotonergic antagonist

(e.g. flufenazine) should re-instate the full syndrome of aphagia, adipsia, and akinesia in neonatally lesioned adult rats. This has not been shown. Rather, the neonatally lesioned rats, which apparently develop normally, still have marked deficits in adulthood on a range of sensitive cognitive and motor tests, and they are exquisitely sensitive to very low doses of the dopamine synthesis inhibitor $\alpha$-methyl tyrosine, which will induce the full aphagia, adipsia, and akinesia syndrome, lasting several days until dopamine stores can be repleted (Rogers and Dunnett 1989). These findings indicate that the failure to ever develop marked motivational or regulatory impairments in animals given neonatal 6-OHDA lesions is due to the remarkable plasticity of the residual dopamine system (which may comprise no more than 1% of the normal complement of nigral dopamine neurones) to upregulate to a level where it can sustain normal tonic levels of dopaminergic activation of the striatum. Nevertheless, the upregulated system remains at the limits of its capacity throughout the animals' life and the animals remain highly sensitive to any stress or disturbance.

# *Neurotransmitter plasticity in sympathetic neurones*

The autonomic nervous system is mostly clearly divided into cholinergic neurones for the parasympathetic nerves, and noradrenaline for the sympathetic. However, there are a few inconsistencies, one of which is the cholinergic sympathetic nerve supply to some sweat glands. The neurones supplying these sweat glands are in normal sympathetic ganglia, the majority of the cells in which are adrenergic. Moreover, these neurones are adrenergic during early development until their axons make contact with the sweat glands. Only after contact with sweat glands do the neurones change to a cholinergic phenotype.

From these developmental considerations, we may ask: do the sweat glands instruct the axons to become cholinergic? The answer is, yes (see Fig. 14.6). A variety of transplant, tissue culture, and other experiments have shown that the plantar sweat glands must secrete a factor that causes embryonic sympathetic neurones to assume a cholinergic phenotype (Landis and Keefe 1983). Along with the change from an adrenergic to a cholinergic phenotype, the neurones also increase their production of several neuropeptides, particularly vasoactive intestinal polypeptide (VIP), substance P, and galanin. This is such a clear example of developmental regulation of transmitter phenotype that this system has become a standard model system in which to do experiments on the mechanisms of developmental plasticity, which are consequently better understood here than elsewhere.

The model took a further step towards being relevant to the subject of this book when it was found that sympathetic adrenergic neurones undergo major changes in their transmitter phenotype, not only during development but also in response to peripheral nerve injury (Fig. 14.6B). Axotomy causes an increase in VIP, substance P, galanin, and neurokinin A levels in the neurones, and a decrease in tyrosine hydroxylase (Hyatt-Sachs *et al.* 1993). These appear to reflect exactly the same changes that the neurones undergo when changing from an adrenergic to a cholinergic phenotype in development, so the possibility arises that the same signals might be released in development and after nerve injury to cause a similar change in axotomised neurones.

The search for the active factors in the control of sympathetic phenotype was greatly aided by the fact that it was possible to construct an *in vitro* assay, in which co-culture with sweat glands or with sweat-gland extracts would cause sympathetic neurones to express cholinergic markers. By looking for the presence and activity of a large number of possible trophic molecules, leukaemia inhibitory factor (LIF) was identified as a candidate, in that it was produced in foot skin at the right time, and could induce cholinergic changes in neurones. However,

when a LIF knockout mouse was examined, it was found that the innervation of the foot sweat glands was entirely normal, and cholinergic (Rao *et al.* 1993). This put paid to the theory that LIF is the relevant factor during development, and at the time of writing it appears that sweat glands produce another factor, sweat gland factor (SGF), released by sweat glands in response to noradrenaline and at present unidentified, which largely controls cholinergic differentiation *in vivo*. However, the LIF knockout mouse had one very important abnormality, which was that the normal 40 times upregulation of VIP after axotomy was almost absent, as was upregulation of the other neuropeptides. It appeared, therefore, as if LIF was the key molecule that causes the changes in neurotransmitter phenotype after axotomy. LIF is released at the site of nerve injury, and it is also upregulated in the glial cells of autonomic ganglia after axotomy, the controlling factor possibly being interleukin 1, which is released at most injury sites (Sun and Zigmond 1996). However, upregulation of VIP and other peptides in sympathetic neurones does not happen if LIF is simply applied to unlesioned sympathetic ganglia. Axotomy is also required, and the reason for this is that nerve growth factor (NGF), which sympathetic axons will acquire from their target areas, antagonises these changes. A combination of LIF- and NGF-blocking antiserum is therefore sufficient to induce VIP upregulation, even in the absence of axotomy. LIF acts on the neurones via a cell surface receptor, which

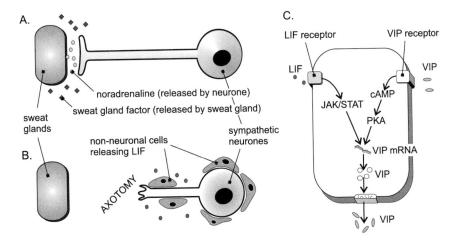

**Fig. 14.6** Neurotransmitter plasticity in sympathetic neurones. A. When sympathetic axons first contact sweat glands, their secretion of noradrenaline causes the sweat gland to secrete sweat gland factor. This in turn will convert the adrenergic neurone to a cholinergic phenotype. B. After axotomy of sympathetic axons, the glial cells start to secrete leukaemia inhibitory factor (LIF), which acts on the neurones to increase their production of vasoactive intestinal polypeptide (VIP) and other peptides. C. Signalling mechanisms for the control of VIP synthesis in sympathetic neurones. LIF upregulates VIP production, and VIP itself has an autocrine feedback.

signals via the JAK/STAT signalling pathway, but levels of VIP are also affected by cAMP levels. Even an apparently very simple example of biochemical plasticity, therefore, involves a complicated set of signalling events.

## Biochemical plasticity and pain

A system in which the various concepts discussed above have practical significance is the pain pathways of the spinal cord. As outlined in Chapter 5, skin inflammation causes an increase in pain sensitivity, such that light touch to inflamed skin causes a sensation of pain. A major contribution to this increased sensitivity comes from a change in the function of the A$\beta$ light touch sensitive axons, which in response to peripheral inflammation start to secrete the pain-associated neurotransmitter substance P, and which also gain a greatly increased ability to depolarise nociceptive neurones in the substantia gelatinosa of the cord through an increase in synaptic efficacy. The mechanisms behind these changes are unknown. Another major issue in chronic pain management is the phenomenon known as deafferentation pain. It seems logical that removing sensory inputs to the cord should lead to complete anaesthesia of the affected region. However, this is not always so, and sometimes the patient will report unpleasant and painful feelings from the supposedly deafferented area. The source of this pain must be central, and it is therefore extremely difficult to treat. The probable cause is an increase in the sensitivity of nociceptive neurones that have lost their normal input, and have become hypersensitive to other abnormal inputs as a result.

## General applicability of biochemical plasticity

The dopaminergic pathway, in which much of the evidence for biochemical plasticity and consequent functional recovery has been worked out, is one of several pathways in the CNS that take the form of widely distributed connections. In this and other similar pathways, such as those containing adrenergic, serotonergic, and cholinergic fibres, the individual axons have large terminals that connect to many neurones. Individual point-to-point synaptic connections may be less important than the general levels of transmitter in the extracellular space. It is in these widely distributed pathways that one would expect biochemical plasticity to be most effective at mediating recovery from injury. However, there are other pathways, such as the cortico-spinal tract or the visual pathway, in which precise connections between individual pre- and post-synaptic cells are essential for normal function. In these latter types of pathways, biochemical plasticity is unlikely to be a major factor in recovery from injury, and synaptic plasticity will be the major mechanism.

## Further reading

Patterson, P.H. and Nawa, H. (1993). Neuronal differentiation factors/cytokines and synaptic plasticity. *Cell*, **72** (suppl.), 123–137.

Zigmond, M.J., Abercrombie, E.D., Berger, T.W., Grace, A.A., and Striker, E.M. (1990). Compensations after lesions of central dopaminergic neurones: some clinical and basic implications. *Trends in Neuroscience*, **13**, 290–296.

# 15 | Remyelination

## By Robin Franklin

Demyelination is unusual in the spectrum of pathological processes that affect the central nervous system (CNS) in that it may be followed by a spontaneous regenerative process. This process, termed remyelination, involves re-investing demyelinated axons with new myelin sheaths (or internodes), and has been described in a number of experimental models, as well as in naturally-occurring demyelinating disease — most notably the acute lesions of multiple sclerosis (Prineas *et al.* 1993a). Remyelination allows the axon to transmit action potentials by saltatory conduction, a property that is lost in demyelination (Fig. 15.1; Smith *et al.* 1979).

Although lengths of demyelinated axon may acquire the ability to conduct by continuous or non-saltatory conduction, this form of conduction is less rapid and less 'secure' (i.e. more vulnerable to small changes in the environment, such as temperature) than the saltatory conduction permitted by remyelination. Moreover, some demyelinated axons do not conduct action potentials due to an imbalance between densities of sodium and potassium channels. There is emerging evidence from clinical observations and experimental data that remyelination is an important reason for recovery of functional deficits that arise due to demyelination (Fig. 15.2; Jeffery and Blakemore 1997). Its unusual status as a spontaneous regenerative process in the CNS and its role in recovery of function make remyelination a particularly fascinating area of brain repair from both a biological and clinical perspective.

If remyelination is a spontaneous consequence of demyelination, why is it that some demyelinating diseases (such as the chronic, progressive form of multiple sclerosis) have such an unfavourable outlook? The reason for this is in part due to the inconsistent nature of remyelination, and there are many occasions where remyelination fails or occurs to an inadequate extent (e.g. Prineas *et al.* 1993b). This phenomenon has given remyelination research an added impetus, since there are clinical situations where enhancement of remyelination, either by the reactivation of the inherent process or by transplantation of myelinogenic cells, may have significant therapeutic benefits.

## What does remyelination look like and how can it be identified?

Remyelination was first described in the 1960s by Richard and Mary Bunge. Using the technique of cerebrospinal fluid (csf) barbotage, in which csf was removed from and then re-injected into the rat cisterna magna, they observed a process in the underlying white matter of initial myelin loss followed by the appearance of new myelin, albeit with a slightly different staining quality (Bunge *et al.* 1961).

The emergence of other experimental models of CNS demyelination and remyelination, and in particular the so-called gliotoxic models developed by William Blakemore in Cambridge in the 1970s and 1980s, enabled this process of myelin restoration to be studied in greater detail (Table 15.1). An important technical development was the improvement of methodologies for tissue fixation, which accompanied the increasing use of the electron microscope by experimental biologists, for it was at the ultrastructural level that a key feature of remyelination was first described. In normal myelination there is a stable relationship between myelin sheath thickness (i.e. number of wraps of myelin or myelin lamellae) and internodal length, both of which are determined by the axonal diameter. A characteristic feature of remyelination is that, although the relationship between thickness and length is preserved, the relationship to the axonal diameter is altered, with the result that the new myelin sheath is thinner and shorter than the original myelin sheath (Fig. 15.3; Blakemore 1974). Thus, remyelinated axons have thinner and shorter internodes than one would expect for their diameter. The characteristic thin myelin sheaths of remyelination can be readily identified by light microscopy and electron microscopy in well-fixed, resin-embedded tissue (Fig. 15.4), and this feature explains the paler quality of

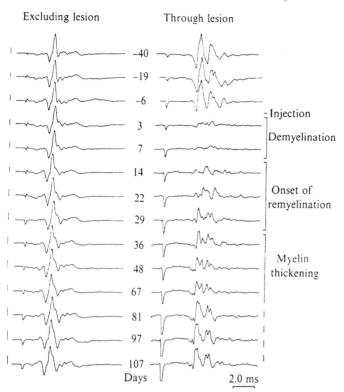

Excluding lesion          Through lesion

-40
-19
-6
- Injection
3
- Demyelination
7
14
22          Onset of
remyelination
29
36
48          Myelin
thickening
67
81
97
107
Days          2.0 ms

**Fig. 15.1** Restoration of secure conduction following CNS remyelination. This figure shows saphenous nerve compound action potentials at different times during a lysolecithin-induced demyelinating/remyelinating lesion in the dorsal funiculus of a cat. (From K.J. Smith *et al.* 1979.)

**Table 15.1**   Commonly used toxin-induced models for studying CNS remyelination

| Agent | Mode of delivery | Species | Mechanism of action | Comments |
|---|---|---|---|---|
| Cuprizone | Orally | Mouse | Not known | Creates demyelination in cerebellar peduncles, corpus callosum and internal capsule which undergoes oligodendrocyte remyelination |
| Lysolecithin | Direct injection | Any | Membrane pore formation (myelin forming cells particularly susceptible) | Creates demyelinating lesion, which in the spinal cord, is mainly remyelinated by oligodendrocytes |
| Ethidium bromide | Direct injection | Any | DNA intercalating agent; non-specific cell toxin, which kills oligodendrocytes and astrocytes in white matter | Creates demyelinating lesion, which in the spinal cord, is mainly remyelinated by Schwann cells |

areas of remyelination with conventional myelin stains. The new sheaths continue to undergo a degree of remodelling for many months, but never regain the dimensions of the original sheaths. It is worth noting that thin myelin sheaths in transverse sections of white matter tracts do not always indicate remyelination, since there are situations, such as chronic compression, where the myelin sheath can become thinner (usually in the paranodal region) without the axon ever becoming

completely demyelinated. This phenomenon is called partial demyelination and may reflect compromised oligodendrocyte function. Although appearing similar in transverse section, the two situations can be distinguished by longitudinal sectioning, where myelin sheaths of normal internodal length but of variable thickness indicate partial demyelination, while shorter internodes of uniform thinness indicate remyelination (see Fig. 15.5).

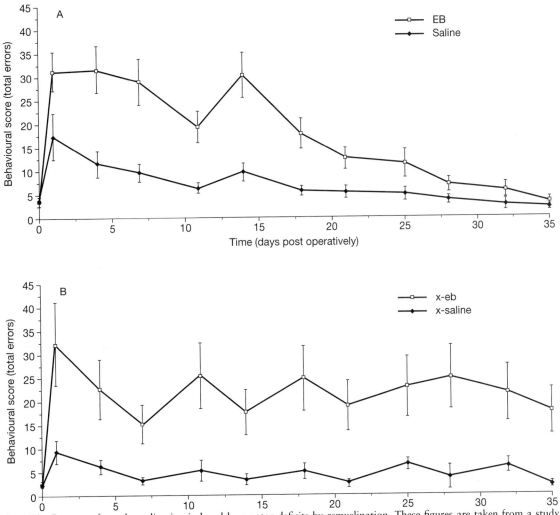

**Fig. 15.2** Recovery from demyelination-induced locomotor deficits by remyelination. These figures are taken from a study in which ethidium bromide (EB) lesions are induced in the dorsal funiculus of rats trained to walk across a beam. A Following demyelination the rats exhibit locomotor deficits which are scored (the higher the score the greater the degree of deficit). Following demyelination animals recover their locomotor function with a time course commensurate with remyelination of the lesion. B The belief that this recovery is due to remyelination is lent support by the failure of recovery if remyelination is blocked by X-irradiation. (From Jeffery and Blakemore 1997.)

## The cellular and molecular mechanisms of remyelination

Despite numerous morphology-based studies over the last several decades, our knowledge of the molecular and cellular mechanisms of CNS remyelination remains rather scant. Nevertheless remyelination is widely-accepted to involve three stages (Fig. 15.6):

- *generation* of progenitor oligodendrocytes by division;

- *migration* of these cells into and within areas of demyelination;

- *engagement* of demyelinated axons and differentiation into a myelinating phenotype.

Although evidence in support of this model continues to emerge, remarkably little is known about the molecules involved in its orchestration. The process of remyelination is in many ways a recapitulation of the initial process of myelination that occurs during development, in that both involve the generation, migration,

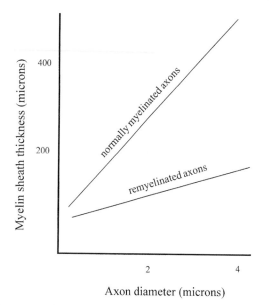

**Fig. 15.3** The relationship between myelin sheath thickness and axon diameter in normally myelinated fibres in the superior cerebellar peduncle of normal adult mice and in remyelinated fibres following demyelination with cuprizone. (Redrawn from Blakemore 1974.)

and differentiation of myelinating cells. Consequently, we can look to developmental studies to provide clues to understanding remyelination (Fig. 15.7). There is now a wealth of information on the developmental biology of the oligodendrocyte lineage, and on the molecules (e.g. growth factors and extracellular matrix molecules), which govern their behaviour and bring about myelination (see Box 15.1). An important point to emerge from these studies is that as one progresses along the lineage from oligodendrocyte progenitor to mature myelinating oligodendrocyte, the cells become less responsive to mitogens and less motile. Thus, the highly proliferative and motile oligodendrocyte progenitor differentiates into the non-motile and non-dividing mature oligodendrocyte. Since proliferation is a key feature of remyelination, there is *a priori* good reason to believe that immature stages of the lineage will be primarily responsible for repopulating an area of demyelination. This view is supported by available evidence from experimental and clinical studies in which oligodendrocyte lineage cells have been identified ultrastructurally or immunocytochemically.

Whilst it is clear that a proliferating population of oligodendrocyte progenitors is required for remyelina-

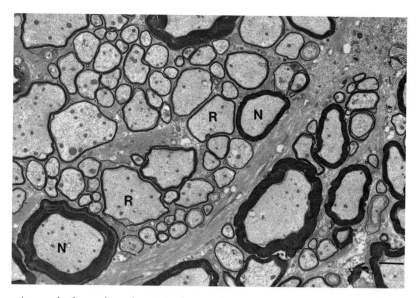

**Fig. 15.4** Electron micrograph of remyelinated axons in the rostral cerebellar peduncle of a mouse following cuprizone-induced demyelination. Compare the relative thickness of the myelin sheath in a normally myelinated axon (N) with a remyelinated axon (R). Scale bar = 1.2 μm.(Kindly provided by Professor Bill Blakemore.)

tion, an issue of continuing controversy is the identity of the parent cell from which the remyelinating cell is derived. One possibility is that these cells are generated from oligodendrocytes within the intact tissue that surrounds an area of demyelination. However, the evidence

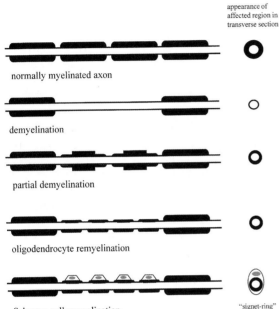

appearance of affected region in transverse section

normally myelinated axon

demyelination

partial demyelination

oligodendrocyte remyelination

Schwann cell remyelination

"signet-ring"

**Fig. 15.5** Diagrammatic summary of the histological appearance of demyelination, partial demyelination, and remyelination.

that myelinating oligodendrocytes can undergo division is very slight. In a number of elegantly executed studies, Samuel Ludwin and his colleagues showed that these cells were able to incorporate tritiated thymidine but it was not unequivocally established that these cells underwent cell division (Ludwin and Bakker 1988). Even if they were to do so, it would appear to be an event of sufficient rarity to make the myelinating oligodendrocyte an unlikely major source of remyelinating cells.

A separate piece of evidence in support of the mature oligodendrocyte as the parent cell of the remyelinating cells has come from tissue-culture studies. Oligodendrocytes, identified with the marker O1, appear able to 'back-differentiate' and assume the phenotype of a less mature stage of the lineage akin to that of the remyelinating cell (Wood and Bunge 1991). However, clear evidence for this position is hard to obtain because of the difficulty in identifying myelinating cells *in vitro* as mature oligodendrocytes, i.e. cells that had synthesised and maintained myelin sheaths prior to their extraction from the animal, since the process of extraction itself causes them to lose their processes. Although cells expressing proteins associated with myelin sheaths (such as myelin basic protein, MBP, and proteolipid protein, PLP) can be recognised in culture, it is difficult to know whether these cells reached this late stage of maturity before or after culturing. If it were the latter (in other words, cells that have differentiated *in vitro* from less mature stages of the lineage), then their behaviour may not be representative of the *bona fide*

## *Remyelination recapitulates myelination ?*

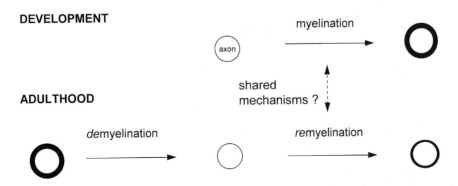

**Fig. 15.6** Remyelination and myelination are similar in that they both have the shared objective of investing a naked axon with a new myelin sheath. It is reasonable to suppose, therefore, that they may also share many common mechanisms. The extent to which this is true still remains to be established, and differences do exist. The concept has nevertheless proved a useful 'working hypothesis'.

## Box 15.1  **The rodent oligodendrocyte lineage**

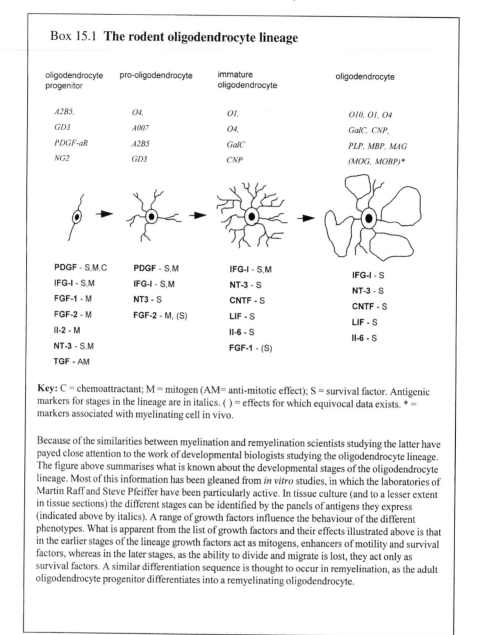

| oligodendrocyte progenitor | pro-oligodendrocyte | immature oligodendrocyte | oligodendrocyte |
|---|---|---|---|
| *A2B5,* | *O4,* | *O1,* | *O10, O1, O4* |
| *GD3* | *A007* | *O4,* | *GalC, CNP,* |
| *PDGF-aR* | *A2B5* | *GalC* | *PLP, MBP, MAG* |
| *NG2* | *GD3* | *CNP* | *(MOG, MOBP)\** |

| | | | |
|---|---|---|---|
| **PDGF** - S,M,C | **PDGF** - S,M | **IFG-I** - S,M | |
| **IFG-I** - S,M | **IFG-I** - S,M | **NT-3** - S | **IFG-I** - S |
| **FGF-1** - M | **NT3** - S | **CNTF** - S | **NT-3** - S |
| **FGF-2** - M | **FGF-2** - M, (S) | **LIF** - S | **CNTF** - S |
| **II-2** - M | | **II-6** - S | **LIF** - S |
| **NT-3** - S,M | | **FGF-1** - (S) | **II-6** - S |
| **TGF** - AM | | | |

**Key:** C = chemoattractant; M = mitogen (AM= anti-mitotic effect); S = survival factor. Antigenic markers for stages in the lineage are in italics. ( ) = effects for which equivocal data exists. * = markers associated with myelinating cell in vivo.

Because of the similarities between myelination and remyelination scientists studying the latter have payed close attention to the work of developmental biologists studying the oligodendrocyte lineage. The figure above summarises what is known about the developmental stages of the oligodendrocyte lineage. Most of this information has been gleaned from *in vitro* studies, in which the laboratories of Martin Raff and Steve Pfeiffer have been particularly active. In tissue culture (and to a lesser extent in tissue sections) the different stages can be identified by the panels of antigens they express (indicated above by italics). A range of growth factors influence the behaviour of the different phenotypes. What is apparent from the list of growth factors and their effects illustrated above is that in the earlier stages of the lineage growth factors act as mitogens, enhancers of motility and survival factors, whereas in the later stages, as the ability to divide and migrate is lost, they act only as survival factors. A similar differentiation sequence is thought to occur in remyelination, as the adult oligodendrocyte progenitor differentiates into a remyelinating oligodendrocyte.

myelinating oligodendrocyte. An intriguing possibility is that cells, which *in vitro* have some of the features of a mature oligodendrocyte, may exist as non-myelinating cells within the CNS, and that these cells may give rise to the remyelinating cell. For example, it has recently been shown that some oligodendrocyte progenitors obtained from adult CNS can express O1, a marker previously thought to be exclusive to mature oligodendrocytes.

A more likely candidate for the remyelinating cell is the adult oligodendrocyte progenitor that persists in the adult CNS (Gensert and Goldman 1997; Carroll *et al.* 1998). This cell is similar to (and indeed is derived from) the developmental oligodendrocyte progenitor. The

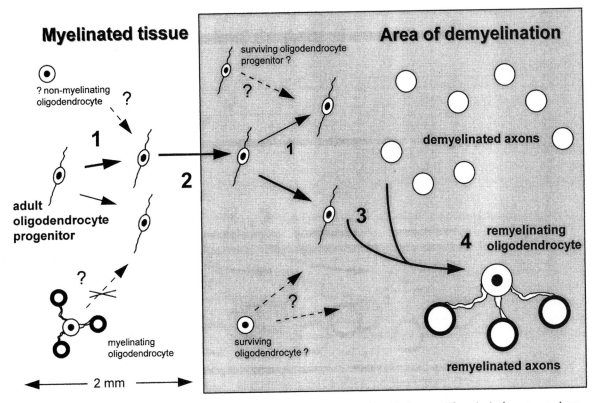

**Fig. 15.7** Possible mechanisms of oligodendrocyte remyelination are illustrated in this diagram. The principal events are: 1 proliferation; 2 migration; 3 engaging of a demyelinated axons by an oligodendrocyte lineage cell; and 4 the differentiation of the remyelinating cell into a myelinating oligodendrocyte. The sequence of events for which most evidence exists is indicated with the *thicker arrows*. Other less likely mechanisms are indicated in *dotted-line arrows*. The extent of the non-demyelinated tissue around a lesion from which remyelinating cells can be recruited is approximately 2 mm for gliotoxin-induced demyelination in the rat.

adult oligodendrocyte progenitor was first identified in tissue-culture preparations of adult rat optic nerve by Charles ffrench-Constant and Martin Raff (1986). It differs from its neonatal forebear in being less motile and in having a slower cell turnover. This somewhat sluggish cell is itself an inappropriate cell for remyelination. However, if these cells are exposed to combinations of growth factors (such as they might encounter in the inflammatory milieu of a demyelinating lesion), they can be goaded into faster turnover and greater motility (Wolswijk and Noble 1992). Their ability to change properties in this manner is precisely what one would expect from cells that lie dormant in a stable environment for most of their existence but which must respond vigorously in the event of a demyelinating episode.

Although adult oligodendrocyte progenitors have been extensively studied *in vitro*, less is known about their abundance and distribution *in vivo*, not least because of the lack of any suitable histological markers. The recent identification of the platelet derived growth factor (PDGF $\alpha$) receptor and NG2 (and to a lesser extent GD3) as markers of oligodendrocyte progenitor in tissue sections means that the dynamics of the adult oligodendrocyte progenitor's response to demyelination can now be studied.

It has recently been demonstrated that remyelinating cells are generated from a very narrow rim of tissue surrounding an area of demyelination (Fig. 15.5; Franklin *et al.* 1997; Keirstead *et al.* 1998a). From this we can draw two conclusions.

- Extensive migration of remyelinating cells into areas of demyelination does not occur. This conclusion is consistent with the observation that upregulation of the pro-migratory substrate PSA-NCAM is limited around areas of demyelination (Oumesmar 1995).

- The restricted area from which remyelinating cells are derived means that these cells may be prone to exhaustion if called upon to provide cells for extensive or repeated episodes of remyelination.

An alternative form of remyelination has been suggested for situations in which demyelination occurs due to damage to the myelin sheath, but where the associated oligodendrocyte survives. Thus, there are cells in acute multiple sclerosis plaques that are positive for the myelin/oligodendrocyte glycoprotein (MOG) marker, and consequently are thought to be surviving oligodendrocytes (Brück *et al.* 1994). In this situation, it is argued that the surviving oligodendrocyte may recover to the extent that it is able to re-form new myelin sheaths. However, there is emerging evidence from experimental models that surviving oligodendrocytes are unable to contribute to remyelination and it may indeed be the case that an oligodendrocyte that has already myelinated can not do so for a second time (Keirstead and Blakemore 1997).

The process of identifying the molecules involved in orchestrating remyelination has only recently begun. The concept that '*remyelination is a recapitulation of myelination*' has already been introduced and has been a guiding principle in remyelination research (Fig. 15.6). A great deal is now known about the molecules mediating myelination and this information has provided useful clues to understanding remyelination. For example, there are many growth factors that function as mitogens, chemoattractants, survival factors, and modulators of differentiation in myelination (see Box 15.1). Given the importance of all of these functions to the repair process, different growth factors almost certainly play important but as yet ill defined roles in remyelination. This view is supported by the ability of a growth factor antagonist to inhibit spontaneous remyelination following lysolecithin-induced demyelination (Fig. 15.8; McKay *et al.* 1997). On the other hand, it is clear that the two events are not identical. For example, thyroid hormone, which is crucial to normal myelination, does not appear to be so for remyelination. Nevertheless, of the plethora of growth factors involved in myelination, at least three, insulin-like growth factors (IGF-I), fibroblast growth factor (FGF-1), and platelet derived growth factor (PDGF), have increased levels of expression during remyelination (e.g. Komoly *et al.* 1992). There are still a great many

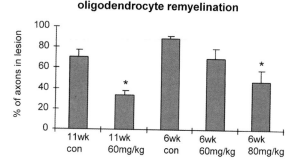

**oligodendrocyte remyelination**

**Fig. 15.8** Systemic administration of the growth factor antagonist trapidil causes a significant decrease in the extent of oligodendrocyte remyelination following lysolecithin-induced demyelination of the rat dorsal funiculus. Note that a dose of 60 mg/kg is sufficient to cause this decrease in 11-week-old rats, but that a higher dose of 80 mg/kg is required for 6-week-old rats, perhaps reflecting a more robust growth factor response in the younger animals. There is no significant difference in the extent of Schwann cell remyelination between any of the groups. con = saline treated controls. (From J.S. MacKay *et al.* 1997, with permission.)

other oligodendrocyte development-associated growth factors, such as FGF-2, ciliary neurotrophic factor (CNTF), NT-3, and GGF-2, whose role in remyelination has yet to assessed.

## Demyelinated CNS axons can be remyelinated by Schwann cells

As one would expect, demyelinated CNS axons are usually remyelinated by oligodendrocytes. However, there are situations where demyelinated CNS axons are remyelinated by Schwann cells, the myelinating cell of the peripheral nervous system (PNS). Schwann cell remyelination, like oligodendrocyte remyelination, restores saltatory conduction to demyelinated axons, and can be distinguished from oligodendrocyte remyelination by a number of criteria. Antibodies against the peripheral myelin protein P0 (Fig. 15.9) can be used to identify Schwann cell myelin, while in well-fixed, resin-embedded tissue the proximity of the Schwann cell body to its single myelin internodes give the Schwann cell–axon unit a distinctive 'signet-ring' appearance in transverse sections (Figs 15.5 and 15.10). Ultrastructurally, the Schwann cell is surrounded by a basal lamina and produces myelin with a slighter greater interlamellar periodicity than central myelin.

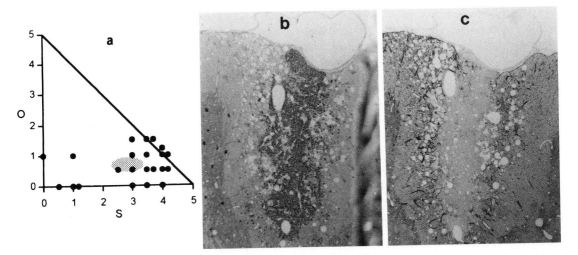

**Fig. 15.9** Following injection of ethidium bromide into the dorsal funiculus of the adult rat spinal cord, a focal area of demyelination is created where the local oligodendrocytes and astrocytes are destroyed but the *en passage* axons remain intact. a These axons are remyelinated partly by oligodendrocytes (*y*-axis), but to a much greater extent by Schwann cells (*x*-axis) on account of the absence of Schwann cells. b P0 immunocytochemistry indicating extensive Schwann cell remyelination of axons following ethidium bromide-induced demyelination. c An adjacent section to that in b, immunostained with the astrocyte marker glial fibrillary acidic protein (GFAP), indicates that the Schwann cell remyelination is confined to areas from which astrocytes are absent.

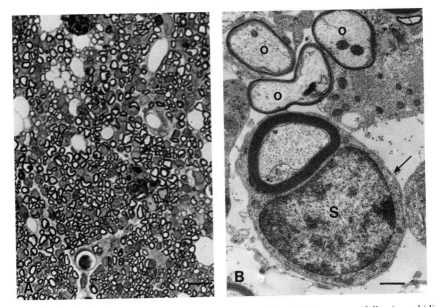

**Fig. 15.10** A Schwann cell remyelination of axons in the rat spinal cord white matter following ethidium bromide-induced demyelination. Note the characteristic 'signet ring' appearance that is apparent at the light microscopic level in resin-embedded osmicated tissue stained with toluidine blue (*arrows*) Scale bar = 25 μm. B Electron micrograph of a CNS axon remyelinated by a Schwann cell (S). Note the presence of a basal lamina surrounding the cell (*arrow*). Three oligodendrocyte-remyelinated axons can also be seen (o) Scale bar = 0.7 μm.

What are the circumstances that allow Schwann cell remyelination to occur? The key issue in determining whether a demyelinated axon is remyelinated by an oligodendrocyte or a Schwann cell is the presence or absence of astrocytes. The boundary between CNS and PNS is defined by astrocytes forming the glia limitans. In pathological situations,where this boundary is disrupted (such as following the injection of gliotoxins, or in the more aggressive forms of multiple sclerosis), then demyelinated axons become available for remyelination by Schwann cells as well as by oligodendrocytes (Blakemore 1976; Itoyama *et al.* 1985). When demyelinating lesions lack astrocytes, remyelination is predominantly achieved by Schwann cells. This occurs for two reasons: first, because oligodendrocytes require a minimal astrocyte presence to provide both a cellular substrate for migration and appropriate growth factors for their differentiation; and second, because Schwann cells have a much greater proliferative capacity than the more fragile oligodendrocyte progenitor.

Although they are presumed to originate from the PNS, the actual source of remyelinating Schwann cells in the CNS has never been fully identified. In spinal-cord lesions, it is often assumed that they are derived from the nearby spinal roots. However, since Schwann cell remyelination can occur in lesions buried within the depths of brain white matter, an alternative view is that the non-myelinating Schwann cells that ensheath the autonomic fibres associated with the CNS vasculature constitute the major source, not only in the brain but also the spinal cord. Indeed, Schwann cell remyelination is often found spreading out from blood vessels, although this could be because they use the vessels as a route of migration rather than as their source.

## Remyelination in multiple sclerosis

The presence of thin myelin in multiple sclerosis lesions was observed many years ago when it was thought to indicate incomplete or on-going demyelination. However, it was not long after the description of remyelination in experimental models that it became apparent that remyelination also occurred in multiple sclerosis lesions (Prineas *et al.* 1993a). Evidence of remyelination can be found in a substantial minority of acute foci of demyelination, either seen as a rim of repair around the edges of a lesion or involving the entire area, giving rise to lesions classically described as 'shadow plaques' or *Markschattenherde*. Shadow plaques con-

stitute an attractive anatomical substrate for the clinical recovery that characterises the remitting/relapsing form of multiple sclerosis. Schwann cell remyelination can occur in the more aggressive forms of multiple sclerosis lesion characterised by concurrent damage to astrocytes (Itoyama *et al.* 1985).

The new myelin of remyelination is susceptible to the same pathological process that caused the loss of the original myelin sheath, and so the same area of white matter can be the target of more than one successive episodes of demyelination. Careful examination of pathological material, together with experimental data, suggest that remyelination of the same area of tissue becomes less efficient with each wave of demyelination (Stidworthy-Johnson and Ludwin 1981; Prineas *et al.* 1993b). Eventually the ability to remyelinate is exhausted, especially if a single area is exposed to a sustained rather than a repeated demyelinating stimulus, and the lesion persists as a demyelinated focus. Such a sequence of events may underlie the characteristic plaques of chronic multiple sclerosis in which demyelinated axons reside in a dense matrix of astrocytic processes. There is some evidence to suggest that there is axonal loss within chronic plaques, which together with the absence of myelin lead to persistent clinical impairment.

Strategies for enhancing remyelination in multiple sclerosis by promoting remyelination and glial cell transplantation are developed further in Chapter 24.

# *Further reading*

Ludwin, S.K. (1988). Remyelination in the central nervous system and the peripheral nervous system. In *Advances in Neurology*, Volume 47, (ed. S.G. Waxman), pp. 215–254. Raven Press, New York.

Ludwin, S.K. (1997). The pathobiology of the oligodendrocyte. *Journal of Neuropathology & Experimental Neurology*, **56**, 111–124.

Pfeiffer, S.E., Warrington, A.E., and Bansal, R. (1993). The oligodendrocyte and its many cellular processes. *Trends Cell Biology*, **3**, 191–197.

Raine, C.S. and Traugott, U. (1985). Remyelination in chronic relapsing experimental allergic encephalomyelitis and multiple sclerosis. In: *The pathology of the myelinated axon*. (ed. M. Adachi, A. Hirano, and S.M. Aronson), pp. 229–275. Igaku-Shoin, New York.

Woodruff, R.H. and Franklin, R.J.M. (1997). Growth factors and remyelination in the CNS. *Histology & Histopathology*, **12**, 459–466.

# Section IV
## Clinical assessment of brain damage

# 16 | *Coma*

## *With Barbara Wilson*

## Introduction

Coma accounts for approximately 3% of emergency hospital admissions, with causes ranging from the potentially treatable, such as epilepsy and certain drug overdoses, to severe trauma and vascular insults, which will be fatal or leave the patient with irreversible brain damage. However, coma can be regarded as a potentially dangerous condition with a fatal outcome in a high proportion of patients. Accurate assessment is important for institution of the most appropriate therapy.

## What is coma?

The definition of coma is one that has caused a certain amount of confusion over the years. Coma can be defined as an absence of consciousness, and consciousness is itself difficult to define, although a narrow definition of consciousness can be given as 'a state of awareness of one's self and one's environment'. The *Encyclopaedia Britannica* defines coma as 'unconsciousness from which one cannot be aroused'. However, for medical purposes this is inadequate, as it ignores the variation of coma depth, which is an important part of coma assessment. A widely accepted definition by Teasdale and Jennett (1976) states that coma is where the patient gives 'no verbal response, does not obey commands and does not open the eyes spontaneously to stimulation'. Despite variations of precise definition, there is general agreement that patients in coma show no evidence of independent cognitive functioning.

In addition, a number of other important disturbances of consciousness are sometimes used ambiguously with reference to coma. These include confusion, clouding of consciousness, and stupor. The ambiguity arises because these terms are also used in everyday language, and as such possess a variety of meanings. In addition, these terms may be used rather differently in general medical and psychiatric practice. In medical terms, confusion (or 'acute confusional state') and clouding of consciousness refer to patients who are unable to think with usual clarity, speed and precision, and who are unable adequately to use cues from their environment. Stupor is a state whereby patients are minimally active in terms of mental and physical activity and can only be roused for short periods of time by repeated vigorous stimuli.

The terms of wakefulness, confusion, stupor, and coma present a continuum, so some health workers would argue that these definitions are not meaningful. However, others would argue that the degree of consciousness at presentation lends important clues to diagnosis and so in practice these terms do continue to be widely used.

There are a number of important related conditions of disturbed consciousness, which deserve separate mention. 'Persistent vegetative state' (PVS) is a condition that follows a period of deep coma. Patients appear initially to be recovering from coma, in that they open their eyes (initially to a stimulus and eventually spontaneously with cycles of apparent wakefulness and non-wakefulness) and start to exhibit eye movements. However, there is no progression beyond this state. The eye movements are not directed, and the patient is mute, inattentive, and unaware. Other movements of the limbs or trunk are reflex and postural only.

Coma and PVS must be distinguished from other conditions in which a patient is motionless and unresponsive but able to perform cognitive processes. Such a condition is the 'locked-in syndrome'. This is most commonly due to a lesion in the basis pontis, which leaves the somatosensory and ascending neuronal systems responsible for wakefulness intact, but destroys the corticospinal and corticobulbar pathways so that the patient is left able to see and hear and with normal cognition, but is unable to respond. The importance of recognising this condition is obvious, in that these patients are often fully aware and normal cognitively. Careful examination may reveal that the patient is able to respond by eye movements alone. A number of ancillary investigations may be used in an attempt to distinguish these conditions from coma. Such investigations include EEG recording and PET scanning, both of which may provide evidence of likely ongoing cognitive function.

## Causes of coma

A summary of the causes of coma are shown in Table 16.1. Of patients presenting to hospital in coma, the majority (around 80% in most series) are due to alcohol or drug overdose, trauma, or stroke. A further 10% are due to epilepsy, secondary to diabetes (hypo- or hyperglycaemic coma) and infections such as meningitis, and a couple of per cent are due to medical conditions such as pneumonia or cardiac disturbances. Obviously, the cause of the coma is important, both in terms of treatment (patients in hyperglycaemic coma may recover following infusions of insulin and fluids) and outcome (the outcome would usually be better in patients with coma due to epilepsy or secondary to drug or alcohol overdose, compared to coma due to stroke or trauma). Predictors of outcome are outlined below. Assessing the cause of coma requires a battery of tests including brain imaging, a metabolic blood screen to uncover such conditions as diabetes, and assessing the patient's metabolic state, which may become deranged in coma.

**Table 16.1**   Causes of coma

| Type of coma | Disorders |
| --- | --- |
| Coma with neurological signs indicating focal brain disease | Brain tumour |
|    Intracerebral haemorrhage, thrombosis, or embolism | |
|    Subdural heamatoma or abscess | |
|    Brain abscess | |
|    Hypertensive encephalopathy | |
| Coma without focal signsbut with meningism | Meningitis |
|    Subarachnoid haemorrhage | |
| Coma with no focal signs and no meningism | Alcohol intoxication |
|    Drug intoxication (in particular barbiturates and opioids) | |
|    Carbon monoxide poisoning | |
|    Anoxia, e.g. following a cardiovascular event | |
|    Hypoglycaemia, such as may occur following administration of insulin | |
|    Diabetic coma, secondary to *hyper*glycaemia | |
|    Other metabolic causes such as uraemia, | |
|    Idiopathic epilepsy | |

## Assessment of coma

Given the lack of response to stimulation, coma is likely to be perceived as a passive state, although Tsubokawa (1991) cautions against this view and suggests that coma should be considered as an active inhibitory process rather than a passive one. The main factor in determining whether a patient responds or not may depend on the type of stimulation given. Bricolo *et al.* (1980) also remind us that in prolonged coma, when staff may believe that no change is occurring, careful observation shows that many behavioural responses are present. Wilson *et al.* (1999) corroborated this finding through detailed observation of 88 severely head-injured patients during, and shortly after, the period of coma. They recorded 147 different items of behaviour, at least seven of which could be seen prior to the return of consciousness. This led Wilson *et al.* to argue for more detailed and objective assessment of comatose patients, particularly those who are slower to recover consciousness.

Over the years a number of scales have been devised to assess coma. These range from scales primarily devised as research tools, such as the Munich Coma Scale (Brinkmann *et al.* 1976), to those designed to assess responses to coma-stimulation programmes, such as the Western Sensory Stimulation Profile (Ansell and Keenan 1989). The scales also vary in their utility at different stages of recovery. Some scales are exclusively confined to the comatose period (e.g. the Grady Classification of Stupor and Coma by Fleischer *et al.* 1976), while others not only cover the comatose period but extend the assessment beyond the coma to the recovery of orientation in space and time (e.g. Rancho los Amigos Scales by Malkmus *et al.* 1980). Horn *et al.* (1993) discuss the strengths and weaknesses of ten of the most widely used coma scales.

Despite the variety of assessment procedures, the one in most widespread clinical use is the Glasgow Coma Scale (GCS) (Table 16.2; Teasdale and Jennett 1974, 1976). It is simple, objective, and precise, requiring the assessor to observe and record three categories of behaviour, namely eye opening, verbal responses, and motor responses. Within each section, the worst possible response is scored as 1 and the best 4, 5, or 6, depending on which category is being measured. The operational definition usually adopted is that a combined

## Box 16.1 The principles of diagnosing brain death

The diagnosis of brainstem death requires a number of criteria to be fulfilled by two independent medical doctors, one of whom is a neurologist. Two assessments are made by a consultant neurologist, and another consultant or senior registrar is usually present to act as a witness. Respiratory disconnection is usually supervised by an anaesthetist and witnessed by the assessors.

The diagnosis of brain death is not normally considered until at least 6 h has elapsed from the onset of coma, although in the case of anoxia or cardiac arrest this should be 24 h.

The cause of the irreversible brain damage needs to be established and the reasons why it is irremediable. The time of onset of the coma needs to be known.

Preconditions have to be met. These include: exclusion of hypothermia, drugs, metabolic-endocrine abnormalities to be contributing causes, neuromuscular-blocking drugs (such as those given during an anaesthetic) must not have been given within the preceding 12 h. If the rectal temperature is 35 °C, the patient must be warmed and reassessed.

Once all of these conditions have been met, brainstem function can be assessed as follows.

1. There should be the absence of cerebral functions (the patient is unreceptive and unresponsive).

2. Absence of brainstem functions. This is judged by:

   — the lack of spontaneous eye movements;
   — the mid-position of the eyes;
   — the lack of response to oculocephalic and caloric testing;
   — dilated or mid-position fixed pupils;
   — the paralysis of bulbar muscles;
   — the lack of decerebrate response to noxious stimulation;
   — the lack of spontaneous respiratory effort.

3. The irreversibility of 1 and 2. This is judged to be present by repeating the tests 6 h later, although if a clear history of an intracerebral event is absent, or there are no facilities to exclude the presence of drugs that could affect consciousness, then a period of 72 h is required.

Many centres also require the recording of a flat EEG trace to confirm the absence of cerebral activity.

**Table 16.2** The Glasgow Coma Scale (GCS): circle he most appropriate number for each of the three categories

| Eyes open | Best verbal response | Best motor response |
|---|---|---|
| 1. Never | 1. No response | 1. No response |
| 2. To pain | 2. Incomprehensible sounds | 2. Extension (decerebrate rigidity) |
| 3. To verbal stimuli | 3. Inappropriate words | 3. Flexion abnormal (decorticate rigidity) |
| 4. Spontaneously | 4. Disorientated and converses | 4. Flexion withdrawal |
| | 5. Orientated and converses | 5. Localises pain |
| | | 6. Obeys |

score of 8 or less means that the patient is in coma. However, the value of a combined score in this way is not universally felt to be useful. For example, some patients may score 4 for opening eyes spontaneously, 3 for flexing to pain, and 2 for making incomprehensible sounds, giving a total of 9, but are still unable to obey a command and thus would not necessarily be considered to be out of coma. In addition, a patient could be out of coma, but fail to score 9 because a tracheostomy tube prevents speech, swollen eye lids prevent eye opening, or fractured limbs in plaster prevent limb movements. Watson *et al.* (1992) also describe abuses of the GCS by medical staff. For example, they report instances where the GCS was completed on the basis of previous recordings, and instances where the sheet was not filled in at the specific time or was completed incorrectly when the recording was stopped too soon. This is not a criticism of the scale itself, but of its misuse.

Obviously, no test is perfect, and to simply record a total score may be considered a misuse of the scale.

Indeed, even the authors of the scale warn against this (Jennett and Teasdale 1977). A more useful approach is to record the three categories of response separately; this enables a rapid and accurate picture of the patient's conscious level. Despite these reservations, the GCS is easy to understand and enables comparisons in individual patients to be make across time using different raters, and also allows comparison of data between centres.

In practice, once a patient can obey a command it is clear that a message has been received, understood, and acted upon, and that coma is not present. However, care must be taken to use appropriate commands for those in, or emerging from, coma. For example, 'open your eyes' is not a good command as the subject may open his eyes to the sound of a human voice rather than to the command itself. Equally, 'squeeze my hand' should be avoided as the tester may simply be eliciting a grasp reflex. An unequivocal response may be elicited by such commands as 'blink three times' or 'touch your nose'. Following a simple command is the highest scoring item on the GCS motor section and is probably the most specific for a patient emerging from coma, as eye opening is frequently observed in comatose patients, even those who later die without emerging from the coma (Wilson *et al.* 1999). Equally, meaningful speech may not be achieved until well after the end of coma for a number of reasons, including the presence or after-effects of tracheostomy tubes, or the presence of dysphasia, dyspraxia, and dysarthria. However, obeying a simple command can be adjusted so that even these patients can perform successfully.

## Prediction of coma outcome

Early prediction of the outcome of coma in individual patients is desirable for both humane and economic reasons. The patient's family need an assessment of likely outcome so that they can prepare themselves both in psychological and social terms, and the health-care team need the prediction so that the patient's management can be planned. In addition, decisions regarding institution of some very expensive or life-saving therapies have to be made on the basis of which patients are most likely to benefit, as such therapies are only available in a setting of finite health resources.

For the reasons given above, there has recently been considerable interest in the development of predictive indicators (for review see: Diringer 1992). However, especially when informing patients' relatives, advice based on such indicators must always be qualified, in that all cases require a prolonged period of observation

before a more precise prediction can be given in individual cases.

In assessing the likely outcome of coma, it can conveniently be divided into medical (hypoxic/ischaemic injury, metabolic disturbances, drug overdose, infections, tumour) and traumatic coma. For both, the absence of brainstem reflexes early on is a reasonably reliable predictor of poor outcome. In fact, for medical coma, it has been shown that just two brainstem reflexes — pupillary reflexes and vestibulo-ocular reflexes — can predict the outcome of coma, in that 92% of patients with absent vestibulo-ocular reflexes, and 100% of patients with absence of both, died (Mueller-Jensen *et al.* 1987). A comparison of clinical scales, EEG recordings, and metabolic screens has shown that clinical scales are the strongest predictors of outcome (Edgren *et al.* 1987). Despite some wide variations, the findings of Evans (1987) is useful, and has shown that unconsciousness for 3 weeks or more will rarely allow a person to achieve independent existence.

---

> ## Box 16.2   Initial assessment of the patient in coma
>
> 1. History from relatives or witnesses may give important information as to the nature of the coma, e.g. a history of trauma, epilepsy, or depression suggesting a drug overdose, may be vital pieces of information.
>
> 2. Immediate assessment of the patient is principally that of cardiovascular status to determine whether life-saving measures, such as assisted ventilation, are required.
>
> 3. General medical examination, including temperature (to look for fever as an indicator of infection or hypothermia as a cause of coma), and detailed cardiovascular examination to look for clues as to the cause of coma.
>
> 4. Detailed neurological examination, including assessment of Glasgow Coma Scale (see below).
>
> 5. Ancillary tests to establish the cause of coma. These include blood tests to establish underlying metabolic defects and drug overdose, scanning to explore the possibility of intracerebral lesions, and may include other tests such as lumbar puncture.

# Management of patients in coma

## Physical management

Immediate/early management of coma requires supportive measures and possible specific therapies to reverse coma, if appropriate. Early physiotherapy is also important to avoid pressure sores, reduce the risk of chest infections and thrombosis, and lessen potential complications such as limb contractures through disuse.

If coma becomes prolonged, the management of patients requires that health workers and relatives are responsible for all the physical and mental needs of the patients, as they are unable to be responsible for any of these functions themselves. This includes attempting to assess and treat the presence of pain and discomfort, which patients cannot communicate. Thus day-to-day care of such patients must take account of all details, such as monitoring fluid input and output, bowel movements, monitoring the patients' metabolic state, and care of the skin and pressure areas. With more prolonged periods of coma, feeding may be instituted via a percutaneous gastrostomy. Patients in prolonged coma or PVS may need this degree of care for months or even years.

## Sensory stimulation programmes

In addition to caring for the patient's physical needs, there has been increasing interest recently in caring for the patient's cognitive recovery, even before consciousness has returned. Should patients in coma be stimulated in an attempt to reduce the depth and duration of coma or should they be allowed to recover in their own good time? The answers to these questions are not clear and findings are controversial. Programmes differ in intensity, duration, and in the nature of the stimulation provided, and many of the research studies are methodologically flawed. On the one hand, we know that environmental deprivation can have deleterious effects on animals (Le Winn and Dimanescu 1978) and that both animals and humans benefit from a stimulating environment (Mitchell 1990). On the other hand, Wilson *et al.* (1999) suggest that some of the behaviour problems seen in patients recovering from coma are the result of over-arousal. When too many people or too much noise is present, patients may become agitated and difficult to manage. Reducing the stimulation by dimming the lights, decreasing the noise level, and only allowing one person in the room at a time may lead to a reduction in agitation. Wood *et al.* (1993) express similar views

when they argue for sensory regulation rather than sensory stimulation.

Wilson and McMillan (1993) have reviewed 14 studies of coma-stimulation programmes, classifying them according to whether evaluation was by means of outcome statistics, behaviour change, or physiological measures. The authors note that the studies raise a number of methodological issues, including the lack of a clear definition of coma, the need for control subjects and reasonable sample sizes, control for spontaneous recovery, and the need to investigate functional changes systematically. The review concludes that, on balance, there is evidence for the efficacy of sensory stimulation programmes in reducing the duration of coma and in altering the behaviour of comatose patients, although the relevance of these effects for everyday function is unclear.

## Can learning still occur in coma?

Learning without awareness has been demonstrated in certain patient groups. For example, amnesic subjects can demonstrate normal or nearly normal learning on implicit memory tests when performance does not depend on the active recollection of the learning experience (e.g. Schacter 1987; Baddeley 1990; Tulving and Schacter 1990). Such learning can also occur in subjects with no neurological abnormality (e.g. Davey 1987). Neither of these groups of subjects, however, are unconscious, so cannot be directly compared to patients in coma. Perhaps a closer comparison is with anaesthesia, where there is some evidence of learning while under the effects of anaesthetic drugs (e.g. Millar and Watkinson 1983; Andrade 1995; Bennett *et al.* 1985).

Although a number of reports exist of coma stimulation or coma-arousal programmes (for review see: Wilson and McMillan 1993), studies looking at learning during coma are rare and we know of only two published studies. The first, by Boyle and Greer (1983), looked at three patients, all of whom were in protracted coma. One had sustained a cerebrovascular accident, one anoxic damage, and one severe head injury. Operant conditioning procedures were used in an attempt to teach compliance to verbal requests. Music was used as a positive re-inforcer. Only the head-injured patient showed a definite increase in response to verbal requests.

The second study, by Shiel *et al.* (1993), reported three experiments to demonstrate that patients in coma following traumatic head injury can learn simple tasks. Initial observations showed that comatose head-injured patients made a variety of responses when a cloth was placed on their faces. A cloth on the face was one item used as part of a battery to assess recovery from coma. The item was taken from the cognitive section of the Portage Developmental Checklists (Bluma *et al.* 1976) for the assessment of pre-school children with severe learning difficulties. Some of the head-injured patients removed the cloth while still in coma. A typical sequence might be for the patient to first become quiescent when a cloth was placed over the face, then to become agitated, and finally to remove the cloth.

Following these preliminary observations, Shiel *et al.* (1993) employed a more systematic procedure to investigate the ability of comatose patients to learn. Backward chaining (Yule and Carr 1987) was the teaching strategy employed. In the first experiment, five patients learned to remove the cloth while still in coma. The second experiment was in part a replication of the first but with three patients who were more deeply comatose at the start of the study. In addition, an increased number of prompts was provided. In the third experiment, two patients were taught to carry out other tasks using the same backward-chaining technique. One learned to switch off a buzzer and one learned to reach out to take a note from the tester.

These three experiments demonstrate that some patients can learn to make reliable responses to specific stimuli without concomitant change in the level of coma. Such learning has both theoretical and practical relevance. Theoretical implications include the role of conscious awareness in learning and the process by which comatose patients learn. Practically, it might be possible to harness such learning to prevent some commonly observed complications of severe head injury, such as contractures, which develop because of the adoption of certain postures.

Further research should not only address the theoretical issues of learning in coma but seek to provide guidelines about the nature, timing, and frequency of rehabilitation procedures in the early stages following head injury.

## Rehabilitation of the post-coma patient

Following a period of coma, the victim may return to normal living or, more commonly, will be left with a degree of disability ranging from the trivial to a serious level of disability requiring constant care throughout day and night. However, it is well to remember that even very mild degrees of cognitive under-functioning may render a patient incapable of performing his or her usual standard at work, and thus may result in stress, depression, and self-harm, or result in loss of the job. Rehabilitation aims to minimise residual handicap in physical, cognitive, social, and economic terms (for review see Chamberlain *et al.* 1995). For example, problems such as limb contractures can turn a potentially mobile patient into an immobile one, and prove extremely expensive in both social and economic terms. Unfortunately, as rehabilitation of this large group of patients (head injury is 35 times more common than spinal injury) is expensive and rehabilitation services are generally Cinderella services, the economics of treatment is a prominent issue.

## *Further reading*

O'Brien, M.D. (1990). Management of major status epilepticus in adults. *British Medical Journal*, **301**, 918.

Pallis, C. (1999). ABC of brain stem death. The arguments about the EEG. *British Medical Journal*, **286**, 284–287.

Plum, F. and Posner, J.B. (1980) *Stupor and Coma*. Davis, Philadelphia.

Wilson, B.A. (1997). Cognitive rehabilitation: how it is and how it might be. *Journal of the International Psychological Society*, 3, 487–496.

Wilson, B.A. (1998). Recovery of cognitive functions following non-progressive brain injury. *Current Opinion in Neurobiology* 8, 281–287.

# 17 | Motor, sensory, and autonomic function

## With Charlotte Behan and Roger Barker

## Principles

In this chapter we discuss the clinical approach to assessing damage to the motor, sensory, and autonomic systems based on the functional anatomy of these pathways. For clarity we describe them separately, although it is important to emphasise that damage is rarely restricted to a single system, and that in health full function depends on the proper integration of all of these systems. Clinical assessment is focused on localising, as far as possible, the nature of the neurological lesion, which can be best understood in relation to the functional anatomy. In addition, the extent and cause of the deficit coupled to additional information, such as the age, race, sex, and even occupation of the patient, all need to be taken into account in assessing the disorder. Indeed, the pattern of deficits may be suggestive, although rarely pathognomic, of a particular type of pathology. For example, in multiple sclerosis (MS) the demyelinating plaques have a predilection for certain sites, such as the cervical spinal cord, brainstem, and optic nerves. Thus, damage to these regions in a young Caucasian adult would prompt investigations to look for evidence of MS, although a number of less common diseases, such as sarcoidosis, may present similarly.

The importance of identifying the nature of the underlying lesion is to understand the pathology, which in turn determines prognosis as well as influencing management and long-term follow-up. However, with the growing emphasis on clinical trials of emerging therapies, detailed clinical assessment is essential for recording the safety and efficacy of new interventions, and related to this is the use of careful longitudinal assessment to document the natural history of progressive disease. The latter is an essential prerequisite to a proper understanding of such conditions.

In this chapter, the initial discussion concentrates on the anatomical substrate underlying elements of the motor, sensory, and autonomic systems, both within the central and peripheral nervous systems, and explains how this relates to clinical assessment. There then follows a discussion on how this clinical assessment is applied as a research tool, in conjunction with supplementary investigations, to quantify the degree and rate of progression of neurological deficits for a number of specific conditions — MS, Parkinson's disease (PD), and Huntington's disease (HD) — and how this can be used to evaluate new therapies.

A detailed discussion of the neurological examination and underlying neurobiology lies beyond the scope of this chapter; the interested reader is referred to the further reading list at the end of this chapter.

## Motor function

The control of all movements — postural, reflex, and volitional — is accomplished through the integrated action of a large number of cortical and subcortical structures. These structures form a motor hierarchy with sensory feedback at each level, with the final common pathway being the motor neurone and the muscle it innervates (see Fig. 17.1). It is therefore clear that the division of the CNS into motor and sensory systems is largely arbitrary, and in this respect it is often unclear when a highly processed sensory stimulus becomes a cue for a movement. That having been said, it is clear that damage to different parts of the nervous system may yield characteristic motor deficits as described below.

As can be seen from Fig. 17.1, the motor system is complex and most likely operates in a hierarchical fashion. Lesions to different parts of this system result in different, often overlapping, types of motor deficit. For example, damage to the cerebellum affects co-ordination, and lesions to the basal ganglia produce slowness of movement and abnormalities of posture, but neither type of lesion produces actual weakness or major reflex changes in the limbs. In contrast, damage to the motor cortex and its descending pathways does not affect the repertoire of movements except in so much as it causes weakness and changes in muscle tone. This latter disruption often produces a pattern of weakness that is described as 'pyramidal' in nature, which is something of

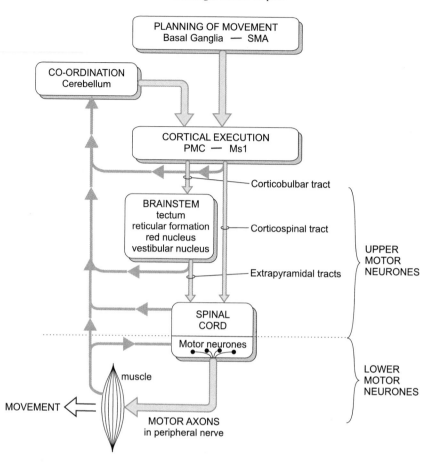

**Fig. 17.1**   Overview of motor function. This figure illustrates the major structures and pathways involved in the planning, execution, and modulation of a motor action. The final common pathway is from the spinal cord (or brainstem) motor neurone to the muscle it innervates, and this is termed the 'motor unit'. A complete lesion at the peripheral nerve level will cause complete paralysis of the part of the muscle it innervates (lower motor neurone lesion), whereas lesions at a higher level tend to produce a more complex motor disorder with spasticity and a lesser degree of weakness (upper motor neurone lesion). Abbreviations: SMA, supplementary motor area; PMC, premotor cortex; Ms1, primary motor cortex.

a misnomer as both pyramidal and extrapyramidal tracts are typically involved. Furthermore, the term extrapyramidal disorders is erroneously attributed to abnormalities within the basal ganglia, despite the fact that these structures have no direct input into the extrapyramidal tracts. These terms are therefore misleading, but nevertheless are widely used in clinical practice.

## Descending motor pathways: upper and lower motor neurone lesions

Weakness can be produced by lesions to the large motor neurones in the primary motor cortex and their descending pathways, or by lesions of the motor neurones of the ventral horns of the spinal cord and brainstem. The characteristic deficits are quite different for these two types of lesion, which are referred to as 'upper' and 'lower' motor lesions, respectively (see Figs 17.2 and 17.3). An 'upper motor neurone' lesion results in weakness of a spastic type (see Fig. 17.3) and is typically seen with strokes and in MS. In contrast, loss of 'lower motor neurones' and their projections onto muscle cells occurs in a number of diseases (see Fig. 17.2) and produces quite a different picture. The lower motor neurone lesion is characterised by weakness and wasting of the section of muscle deprived of its input, and the loss of tendon reflexes. In addition, a muscle deprived of its input also has a tendency to fasciculate, which can be

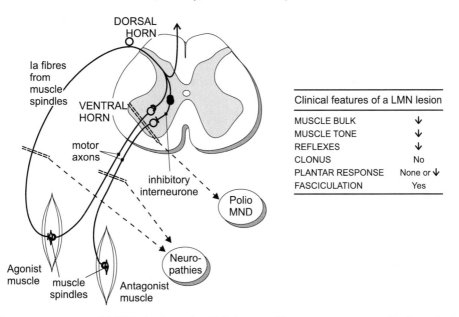

| Clinical features of a LMN lesion | |
| --- | --- |
| MUSCLE BULK | ↓ |
| MUSCLE TONE | ↓ |
| REFLEXES | ↓ |
| CLONUS | No |
| PLANTAR RESPONSE | None or ↓ |
| FASCICULATION | Yes |

**Fig. 17.2** A lower motor neurone (LMN) lesion is one in which the ventral horn motor neurone and/or its projection to muscle is damaged. Tendon reflexes depend on the sensory input from the muscle spindle (Ia fibres) via the dorsal horn to the ventral horn motor neurone, which in turn innervates the same agonist muscle, as well as providing an inhibitory input (via an inter-neurone) to antagonistic muscles. Thus, a lesion in either the sensory or motor arm of the reflex may lead to loss of the tendon reflex. The clinical features of lower motor neurone damage are listed. MND, motor neurone disease

seen with the naked eye as multiple, minute, rippling contractions. The combination of both upper and lower motor neurone lesions is unusual in clinical practice, and when it does occur, it is typically in the context of motor neurone disease (MND).

There are a number of descending influences on the ventral horn motor neurone, which are illustrated in Fig. 17.3, of which the largest is the corticospinal or pyramidal tract. Approximately one-third of the fibres in this tract originate in the primary motor cortex (Ms1) in the precentral gyrus of the frontal lobe, with another third from the premotor area, immediately anterior to Ms1, and the final third from areas 1, 2, and 3 in the primary somatosensory cortex (Sm1). However, these latter corticospinal neurones probably have more of a role in regulating the transmission of afferent sensory information throughout the dorsal column nuclei (see below). The corticospinal fibres descend through the posterior limb of the internal capsule to reach the ventral portion of the mid-brain and then the pons, where they separate into small bundles coursing between the pontine nuclei. The fibres regroup in the medulla to form the pyramids, two bundles on the ventral surface of the medulla, and hence pyramidal system. At this stage the fibres are uncrossed, but at the

junction of the medulla and spinal cord the majority decussate and descend in the dorsal parts of the lateral columns to form the lateral corticospinal tracts, with a smaller uncrossed tract descending in the ventral columns (ventral corticospinal tracts). The lateral corti-cospinal tracts synapse ipsilaterally on the motor neu-rones supplying the distal muscles, whilst the much smaller ventral uncrossed fibres synapse bilaterally on neurones supplying the axial muscles.

In addition to the corticospinal tract, a number of brainstem nuclei (in particular the reticular formation, tectum, and vestibular and red nuclei) also project down the spinal cord as the extrapyramidal tracts, and are important for proximal and postural muscle control. However, the rubrospinal tract is more involved with the distal musculature, a role it fulfils in conjunction with the lateral corticospinal tract. Furthermore, a number of other brainstem structures are important in movement, especially locomotion, one example being the pedunculopontine nuclei, which have a complex relationship with these tracts and the motor neurones they innervate.

Damage to neurones or fibres in these descending pathways produces the so-called 'upper motor neurone' lesion. This term refers to damage in the motor cortex

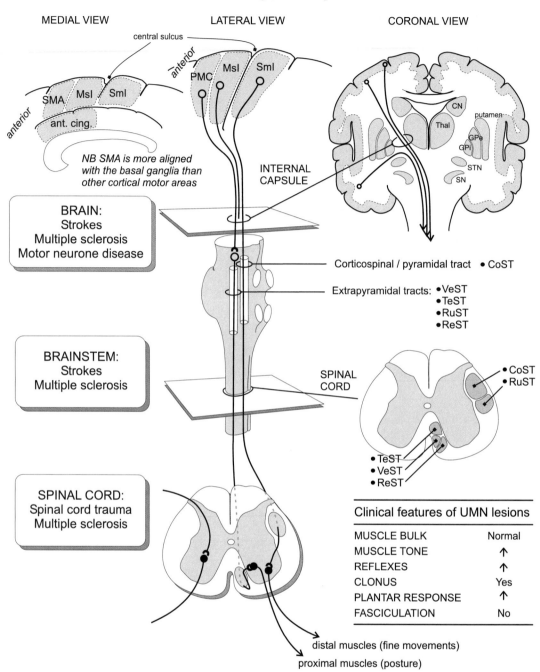

**Fig. 17.3** Schematic representation of cortical motor areas and descending motor pathways, illustrating the crude anatomy of this system and some typical lesions affecting it at various levels. The corticospinal tract and rubrospinal tract form the lateral descending motor pathways, which preferentially innervate those motor neurones controlling distal muscles and are thus important in the control of fine movements. In contrast, the tecto-, vestibulo-, and reticulospinal tracts form the ventromedial descending motor pathways responsible for controlling proximal muscles and thus, posture. Abbreviations: SMA, supplementary motor area; PMC, premotor cortex; Ms1, primary motor cortex; Sm1, primary somatosensory cortex; ant cing, anterior cingulate motor areas; CN, caudate nucleus; Thal, thalamus; STN, subthalamic nucleus; GPe, globus pallidus, external segment; GPi, globus pallidus, internal segment; SN, substantia nigra; VeST, vestibulospinal tract; RuST, rubrospinal tract; TeST, tectospinal tract; CoST, corticospinal tract; ReST, reticulospinal tract; UMN, upper motor neurone.

and its projections at any level down to their synapse onto, but not including, ventral horn neurones. These extensive projections clinically tend to be treated as a unit because any damage affecting this system removes the inhibitory input on the lower motor neurones. This results in weakness of a spastic type, with increased basal muscle tone and exaggerated reflexes with clonus, although muscle wasting is not a prominent feature, and so a spastic limb is stiff and clumsy. This is typically seen in advanced MS, where there are demyelinating plaques throughout the descending pathways.

## Cerebellum and co-ordination

Inco-ordination may be produced by lesions at a number of sites, including damage to the sensory path-ways, motor pathways, vestibular system, and cerebellum. The cerebellum, in addition to being important in the co-ordination of movements, is also concerned with the regulation and control of muscle tone, eye movements, and posture (see Fig. 17.4). In broad terms, lesions of the cerebellum in humans give rise to loss of muscle tone, ataxia of volitional movement, and disorders of equilibrium and gait, as well as dysarthria and eye movement abnormalities (characteristically nystagmus). Lesions of the cerebellar cortex give rise to inco-ordination of the ipsilateral arm and leg, whilst lesions of the vermis produce truncal and gait ataxia with relatively well-preserved limb function. The most severe and enduring deficits are caused by lesions to the superior cerebellar peduncle or dentate nucleus, and are often characterised by tremor.

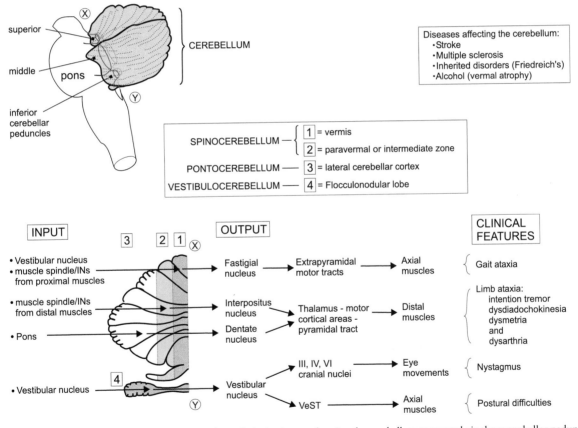

**Fig. 17.4** (*Top*) A schematic sagittal section through the brainstem showing the cerebellum connected via three cerebellar peduncles. (*Bottom*) Schematic representation of the cerebellum in which this structure has been pressed into the page such that the cerebellar tonsil (Y) lies at the bottom of the figure and the anterior medullary velum (X) at the top. The cerebellum is best considered in terms of a series of functional systems, each of which has a unique input and output. Thus, the spinocerebellum has intimate connections with the spinal cord, whilst the pontocerebellum is more associated with the cerebral cortex via the pons and the vestibulocerebellum with the vestibular nucleus. VeST, vestibulospinal tract; INs, interneurones.

In cerebellar damage, motor programmes are degraded and the predictive control of movement patterns are also lost, which can result in ataxia, or incoordination. This manifestations of cerebellar damage are:

- intention tremor: this describes rhythmical movements, typically of the hand, as a target is approached;

- dysdiadochokinesia: this is a defect of rhythmical movements, which is best seen when attempting rapid alternating hand movements;

- asynergia: this describes the inappropriate and fractionated recruitment of muscles;

- dysmetria: abnormal excursion of movements;

- nystagmus: involuntary rhythmic movements of the eyes;

- dysarthria: abnormality of speech production — in cerebellar disease this is usually either slurred or broken, giving the so-called staccato speech

- gait ataxia: the characteristic gait being wide based, swaying and lurching with patients having great difficulty maintaining balance.

Many diseases and disorders may affect the cerebellum, including alcohol, drugs, MS, and inherited cerebellar degeneration, such as Freidreich's ataxia.

## The basal ganglia and extrapyramidal disorders

The basal ganglia have no precise anatomical definition, so that although the term is most often used to include the caudate and putamen (neostriatum), the globus pallidus (which consists of internal and external segments: GPi and GPe, respectively), the substantia nigra (pars reticulata, SNr, and pars compacta, SNc), and the subthalamic nucleus (STN) (see Fig. 17.5), some authors may extend this to include other structures such as the red nucleus, amygdala, or insular cortex. In addition, there is a ventral extension of the basal ganglia that includes the nucleus accumbens and is thought to have more of a role in cognitive and emotional processes.

The connections of the basal ganglia can be thought of as a series of 'loops', which run in parallel to each other (Alexander and Crutcher 1990), although still allowing for communication between the loops. The main receiving region of the basal ganglia is the neostriatum, with the dominant input being from the cerebral cortex, whilst the main outflow is from the GPi and SNr to the premotor cortical areas. In addition, the basal ganglia project to the pedunculopontine nucleus, which is thought to be involved in locomotion, and the superior colliculus, which is involved in eye movements.

At the simplest level, the major basal ganglia connections divide into cognitive, motor, and limbic loops (see Fig. 17.5, *bottom*). The cognitive loop is through the caudate to the prefrontal cortex, the motor loop is through the putamen to the premotor cortex and supplementary motor area, and the limbic loop involves the ventral striatum and prefrontal cortical areas. In addition, there are two notable internal loops within the basal ganglia (see Fig. 17.6): the striato-nigral-striatal loop, with the latter being the dopaminergic projection that degenerates in Parkinson's disease; and a second loop from the GPe to the STN, which in turn projects to the GPi and SNr. The dopaminergic loop modulates the flow of cortical information through the striatum, whilst the STN loop controls the activity of the inhibitory outflow nuclei of the basal ganglia.

Superimposed on these loops is an additional organisational feature, which relates to the internal structure of the neostriatum, and consists of 'patches' or 'striosomes' that are deficient in acetylcholinesterase (AChE), and the 'matrix', which is rich in AChE (Graybiel 1984, 1995). In general, the striosomes are associated with the dopaminergic nigro-striatal pathway and prefrontal cortex and amygdala, whereas the matrix is more involved with sensorimotor areas. However, how this relates to the loops is unclear.

PD and HD are the best characterised of the basal ganglia diseases in terms of symptomatology and the relationship of structure to function. In PD, the primary pathological event is the loss of the dopaminergic nigro-striatal pathway. This pathway has overall an inhibitory influence on striatal projection neurones, such that its loss will ultimately lead to activation of the STN. In PD it is now known from *in vivo* electrical recordings and functional imaging in patients, that the STN and the projection from GPi to the thalamus are overactive, which increases the inhibition of the thalamus and thus the neocortex, leading to the hypokinesia of PD (Hutchison 1994, 1998; Jenkins 1992). In HD, the striatal projection neurones to the GP themselves degenerate, thus reducing activity in the same circuit and resulting in a reduction of the inhibitory output of the basal ganglia to the thalamus, and the overactivation of

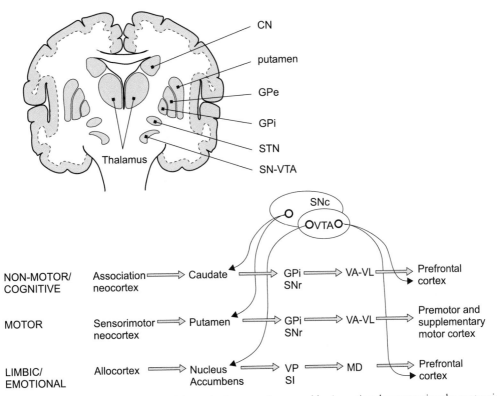

**Fig. 17.5** Anatomy of the basal ganglia. (*Top*) Schematic diagram of a coronal brain section demonstrating the anatomical location, and composition of the basal ganglia. (*Bottom*) The major motor and non-motor basal ganglia circuits and their dopaminergic innervation from the substantia nigra and ventral tegmental area. Abbreviations: CN, caudate nucleus; STN, subthalamic nucleus; GPe, globus pallidus, external segment; GPi, globus pallidus, internal segment; STN, subthalamic nucleus; SN(c/r), substantia nigra (pars compacta/ pars reticulata); VTA, ventral tegmental area; VA–VL, ventroanterior and ventrolateral nuclei of the thalamus; MD, mediodorsal nucleus of the thalamus; VP, ventral pallidum; SI, substantia innominata.

motor cortical areas leading to hyperkinesia (Penney 1996). However, it is important to note that, whilst this argument is internally consistent in terms of simplified wiring diagrams such as that in Fig. 17.6, these explanations ignore other connections, which may turn out to be as important.

## Clinical assessment of motor function

The overall assessment of patients with abnormalities of the motor system is given in Fig. 17.7. In essence, the patient is examined for abnormal movements, gait, and muscle bulk, before a more detailed examination is undertaken. This latter part involves an assessment of eye movements, speech, muscle tone, power, co-ordination, as well as the status of the reflexes and the plantar responses.

## Sensory function

The somatosensory pathways are responsible for conveying different modalities such as touch, proprioception, temperature, and pain from the periphery to the CNS. Somatic sensation is mediated via a number of specialised receptors, which are distributed throughout the body, and which relay their information to the CNS (afferent nerves) via axons that travel in the peripheral nerves, which also contain motor axons (efferent nerves). The afferent sensory nerves have their cell bodies in the dorsal root ganglia and pass information to the spinal cord via the dorsal root, whilst the efferent motor fibres have their cell bodies in the ventral horn. These two sets of fibres unite just outside the spinal cord to form the peripheral nerves.

After entering the spinal cord, the afferent nerves

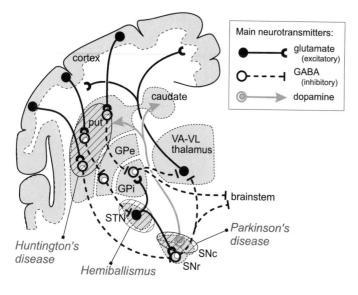

**Fig. 17.6** Functional connections of the basal ganglia. This is a simplified illustration of some of the major connections of the basal ganglia demonstrating the inhibitory outflow via the thalamus, and the GPe–STN–SNr/GPi excitatory control of this outflow. The nigro-striatal dopaminergic and striato-nigral projections are also illustrated. The primary site of pathology in PD is the loss of the nigro-striatal dopaminergic pathway, and in HD is the loss of the striatal projection neurones. Abbreviations: put, putamen; GPe, globus pallidus, external segment; GPi, globus pallidus, internal segment; STN, subthalamic nucleus; SN(c/r), substantia nigra (pars compacta/ pars reticulata); VA–VL, ventroanterior and ventrolateral nuclei of the thalamus.

carrying information relating to the different sensory modalities separate, and the information is conveyed to the brain by anatomically distinct pathways. Fibres carrying information for touch, proprioception, and vibration ascend ipsilaterally in the dorsal white matter of the spinal cord, as the dorsal columns (see Fig. 17.8). Their first synapse is in the caudal medulla in the cuneate (for upper thoracic and cervical sections) and gracile (for lower thoracic, lumbar, and sacral sections) nuclei. The axons then cross the midline as the internal medial arcuate fibres and ascend through the brainstem as the medial lemniscus. In the thalamus they synapse again in the ventroposterior nucleus, which in turn projects primarily to the primary somatosensory cortex (Sm1), which is located in the post-central gyrus and depths of the central sulcus. Projections to the cortex are somatotopically organised with the representation of the face, ventral and lateral to that of the arms, legs, and trunk. Representation at the cortical level is not proportionate to the corresponding body surface area, but to the skin sensory receptor density, such that the perioral region and fingertips have the largest cortical representation.

Nerve fibres carrying pain and temperature sensation, after entering the spinal cord, travel a few segments only before synapsing in the dorsal horn grey matter in laminae I and V–VII. Most fibres then cross anterior to the central spinal canal and ascend in the anterolateral pathway to synapse in a number of supraspinal sites, including the reticular formation, midbrain, and thalamus (both ventroposterior, and intralaminar nuclei).

The thalamic projection is then to a number of cortical sites, including the primary and secondary somatosensory areas, as well as the prefrontal, anterior cingulate, and insular cortex. In addition, there are projections to other structures, such as the basal ganglia and hypothalamus.

The consequences of losing somatosensory sensation can be seen in a relatively pure form in the sensory polyneuropathies, in which the sensory nerve fibres in multiple peripheral nerves are damaged. In most polyneuropathies, all modalities are involved, although one modality is usually affected out of proportion to the others. For example, some pathological processes principally affect the large myelinated fibres, so that touch, vibration, and proprioception are the main modalities affected, whereas others damage small unmyelinated fibres, thus affecting pain and temperature. Such neuropathies can result in negative or positive symptoms, where negative symptoms refer to the loss of sensation and positive symptoms are often described as 'tingling' or 'burning' and are termed 'paraesthesias'. These latter symptoms may result from deranged transmission of sensory information, perhaps due to hyperexcitability of abnormal nerves or from 'cross-talk' between abnormal axons. They may be trivial and barely noticeable, but they may be extremely uncomfortable and even painful, sometimes causing the patient even more distress than the negative symptoms.

Polyneuropathies usually result in a characteristic distribution of abnormal sensation with the extremities (especially lower limb) being involved first, although

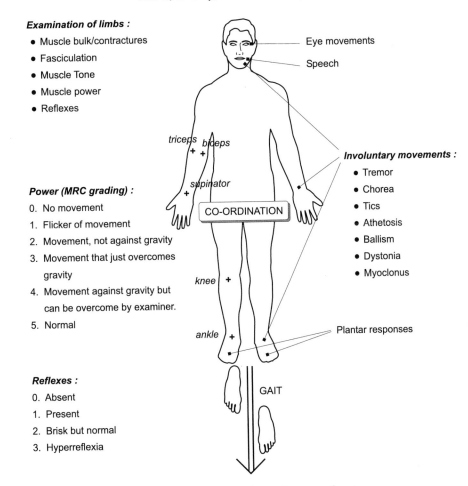

**Fig. 17.7** The principles of assessing motor function.

with progression of disease, the symptoms spread centrally. This is called a 'glove and stocking' distribution, for obvious reasons, and it probably develops because the distal portions of nerves, which are furthest from the cell body, are the most susceptible to damage from disorders of cell metabolism and transport.

The result of losing touch, vibration, and proprioception are well illustrated by demyelinating neuropathies, where the large myelinated nerves, carrying these modalities, are affected. Typically, touch sensation is lost in the toes and fingertips, producing a sensation of numbness and difficulty with fine motor tasks such as doing up buttons and handling a pen. Braille readers may find that they are no longer able to use this mode of communication if loss of touch sensation is profound. With loss of sensation in the soles of the feet, a patient's gait is affected such that they tend to lift their feet high

with each step and stamp the foot on the ground. The reason for this is that the fine adjustments made by feeling contact with the floor are lost. Gait is also disturbed by impairment of proprioception, because feedback of information from the muscle spindle and joint receptors is disturbed. This is termed a 'sensory ataxia' (see also cerebellum) and is particularly noticeable in the dark when visual cues are also removed, such that the patient is left relying solely on vestibular information.

If the small unmyelinated pain fibres bear the brunt of the damage, a somewhat different pattern emerges with the predominant sensory, disturbance, being that of pain and temperature. Prolonged analgesia in the extremities may lead to trophic ulcers, which occur because the body's main safeguard against prolonged contact with noxious agents, i.e. pain, is impaired.

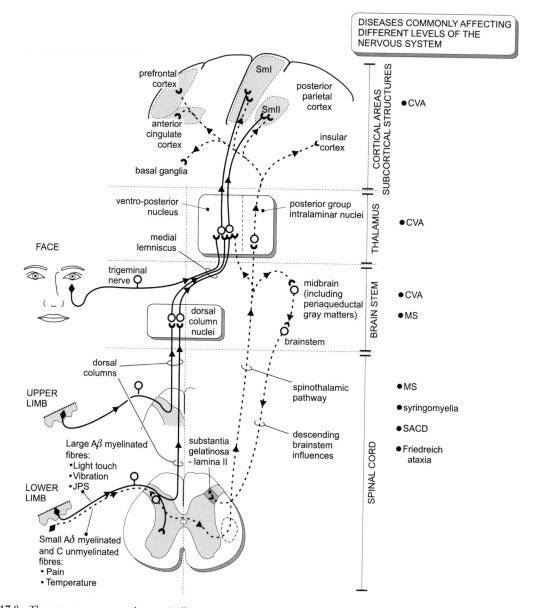

**Fig. 17.8** The somatosensory pathways. Different sensory modalities are registered by different peripheral receptors and are carried by different types of axons. Nearly all mechanoreceptor information travels via large myelinated axons, and most nociceptive information via small myelinated or unmyelinated axons. Once nerve fibres have entered the spinal cord, the pathways for touch and proprioception are anatomically distinct from those for pain and temperature. Touch and proprioception travel via the dorsal column–medial lemniscal pathway and pain and temperature via the anterolateral, mainly spinothalamic, pathway. The separate nature of the two pathways is important in determining the pattern of sensory loss with spinal-cord damage. The pathways for touch and proprioception are ipsilateral up to the level of the medulla, whereas the pathways for pain and temperature cross the midline soon after entering the spinal cord. The projections are somatotopically organised throughout, although this is less true for pain, where the projections are more diffuse—especially at supraspinal levels. Both systems synapse in the ventroposterior thalamus, although onto separate populations of projection neurones. However, there is almost certainly processing between the modalities at this and other levels, which may alter the character of the deficit depending on the anatomical site. Abbreviations: Sm1, primary somatosensory cortex; SmII, secondary somatosensory cortex; JPS, joint position sense; CVA, cerebrovascular accident (stroke); MS, multiple sclerosis; SACD, subacute combined degeneration of the cord with vitamin B12 deficiency.

Probably for similar reasons, joints in the region may also be damaged and these are known as 'Charcot' joints.

The extent to which the two main sensory pathways in the spinal cord are affected by disease depends on the type of lesion. This is summarised in Fig. 17.9, which clearly illustrates that these pathways are separate entities at this level.

Damage to the primary somatosensory cortex (Sm1), or its thalamocortical projections, impairs a patient's ability to make sensory discriminations. The primary modalities of touch, vibration, and pain remain relatively intact, but joint-position sense is almost always disturbed and a variety of other sensory discriminatory functions are impaired. For example, patients are able to perceive the sensation of a small blunt pointer on the skin, but have difficulty distinguishing between two points placed a small distance apart. Normally it is possible to distinguish between two points 3–5 mm apart on the fingertips, but in a patient with a cortical lesion affecting the region representing the hand, this can be considerably impaired. Other sensory discriminations

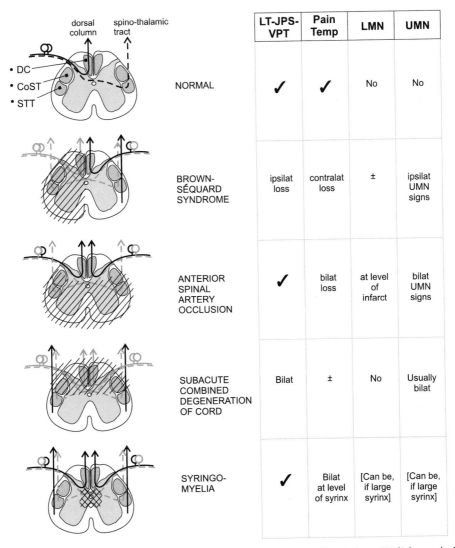

| | LT-JPS-VPT | Pain Temp | LMN | UMN |
|---|---|---|---|---|
| NORMAL | ✓ | ✓ | No | No |
| BROWN-SÉQUARD SYNDROME | ipsilat loss | contralat loss | ± | ipsilat UMN signs |
| ANTERIOR SPINAL ARTERY OCCLUSION | ✓ | bilat loss | at level of infarct | bilat UMN signs |
| SUBACUTE COMBINED DEGENERATION OF CORD | Bilat | ± | No | Usually bilat |
| SYRINGO-MYELIA | ✓ | Bilat at level of syrinx | [Can be, if large syrinx] | [Can be, if large syrinx] |

**Fig. 17.9** Summary of spinal-cord lesions and their sensory and motor deficits. Abbreviations: LT, light touch; JPS, joint position sense; VPT, vibration perception threshold; LMN, lower motor neurone lesion; UMN, upper motor neurone lesion; DC, dorsal column; CoST, corticospinal tract; STT, spinothalamic tract. Shaded area shows extent of damage.

include the ability to interpret touch without the aid of other sensory systems. Objects can normally be identified by touch and texture with the eyes closed, but with a lesion in the contralateral somatosensory areas, again especially in the region of the hand, this may be impossible despite the presence of near normal primary modalities. This inability to distinguish objects by touch is called astereognosis. Indeed, lesions placed in the posterior parietal cortex can lead to a neglect of sensory stimuli in the contralateral limbs (sensory inattention).

In the anterolateral system, conveying pain and temperature, the diffuse nature of the supraspinal projections makes it hard to attribute perception of these modalities to any specific CNS site. It is almost certainly the case that the conscious awareness of pain occurs only when pain impulses reach the thalamocortical level. The precise roles of the thalamus and cortex in this function are not yet fully understood. Pain can occur due to lesions of the thalamus as first described by Déjerine and Roussy in 1906 when they documented a series of patients with intractable pain resulting from vascular lesions to the CNS, all of whom had lesions in the thalamus at autopsy. Central pain can result from damage to a number of ascending pain structures, but damage to the thalamus is probably the most common site. There has been a trend in the literature towards the concept of separation of the awareness and localisation of pain (said to be a function of the parietal cortex) from the awareness of the nature and quality of the pain linking it to its emotional context (said to be a function of the thalamus and its connections with the limbic system). However, this is almost certainly an oversimplification.

Damage in the periphery, as well as the CNS, can lead to the generation of chronic pain conditions. For example, in reflex sympathetic dystrophies, relatively trivial peripheral damage can result, in susceptible individuals, in chronic pain as a result of abnormal alpha receptors being expressed on the nociceptors. This therefore leads to the abnormal activation of nociceptors by noradrenaline released from sympathetic nerve endings, which has meant that such conditions have traditionally responded to local sympathectomies. Furthermore, there is mounting evidence that damage to the peripheral nervous system resulting in chronic pain syndromes is mediated by a host of structural and functional changes within the central pathways, both at the level of the spinal cord/dorsal horn, and supraspinal sites. Such changes almost certainly underlie phantom limb pain, which refers to the pain experienced by amputees in the missing limb.

---

**Box 17.1   Routine investigations used to aid the motor and sensory clinical assessment**

*Imaging*

- CT scanning.

- MRI scanning of brain and spinal cord.

*Neurophysiology*

- Nerve conduction — measures speed and size of the electrical signal down both sensory and motor nerves.

- Electromyography — records the activity within muscles and is particularly helpful in distinguishing lower motor neurone lesions from primary muscle diseases.

- Visual evoked responses — measures the speed and size of the electrical signal along the visual pathway.

- Electroencephalogram — measures electrical activity within the brain through series of scalp electrodes.

- Somatosensory evoked potentials — measures the speed and size of the electrical signal along a sensory pathway from the arm or leg to the sensory cortex.

- Thermal thresholds — subjective measure of small fibre response to changes in skin temperature.

---

## Autonomic nervous system

The autonomic nervous system consists of nerve cells and processes that innervate internal organs, blood vessels, and skin, and can be divided into sympathetic, parasympathetic, and enteric systems. The former two have opposing actions on the various organs, as described below, and are involved in processes that are not usually under voluntary control (see Fig. 17.10). CNS control of the sympathetic system is by a number of brainstem structures, which in turn receive a controlling input from the ventromedial hypothalamic area. In contrast, the parasympathetic system receives its controlling input from the lateral hypothalamic area. These descending pathways influence the cell bodies of the pre-ganglionic sympathetic neurones in the intermediate part (lateral horn) of the spinal cord from T1 to L3, and the cell bodies of the preganglionic parasympathetic neurones in the brainstem and sacral cord. Post-ganglionic cell bodies of the sympathetic system are found in a 'chain' adjacent to the spinal cord, whereas the post-ganglionic cell bodies of the parasympathetic system are found adjacent to, or within, the wall of the organ they supply. In addition, the sympathetic nervous system uses noradrenaline as its post-ganglionic transmitter, whereas the parasympathetic system uses acetylcholine, with both systems using acetylcholine as the preganglionic transmitter.

Damage to the autonomic nervous system may result from a number of causes and can be a generalised or localised deficit. Generalised autonomic failure may occur as a consequence of damage to central CNS structures, such as in primary autonomic failure or multisystem atrophy (MSA), as well as part of a peripheral neuropathic process as seen in Guillan Barré syndrome or diabetic neuropathy. The full constellation of symptoms includes orthostatic and post-prandial hypotension (faintness on standing, exercising, or after eating a larger meal), loss of the usual variation of heart rate (e.g. loss of the usual tachycardia on exercise), urinary urgency and incontinence, and bowel disturbances, impotence, loss of sweating and pupillary responses.

In some circumstances, localised damage to the autonomic nervous system occurs and the deficits can be predicted according to the site of damage. Whilst a generalised process is likely to lead to a full set of symptoms, a more localised lesion, such as may occur in the spinal cord in multiple sclerosis, will produce predominantly bladder and bowel disturbance. Although it is important to remember that bladder function is con-

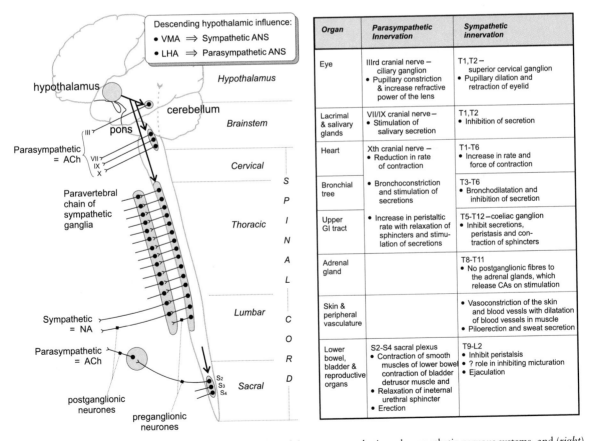

| Organ | Parasympathetic Innervation | Sympathetic innervation |
|---|---|---|
| Eye | IIIrd cranial nerve – ciliary ganglion • Pupillary constriction & increase refractive power of the lens | T1,T2 – superior cervical ganglion • Pupillary dilation and retraction of eyelid |
| Lacrimal & salivary glands | VII/IX cranial nerve – • Stimulation of salivary secretion | T1,T2 • Inhibition of secretion |
| Heart | Xth cranial nerve – • Reduction in rate of contraction | T1-T6 • Increase in rate and force of contraction |
| Bronchial tree | • Bronchoconstriction and stimulation of secretions | T3-T6 • Bronchodilatation and inhibition of secretion |
| Upper GI tract | • Increase in peristaltic rate with relaxation of sphincters and stimulation of secretions | T5-T12 – coeliac ganglion • Inhibit secretions, peristasis and contraction of sphincters |
| Adrenal gland | | T8-T11 • No postganglionic fibres to the adrenal glands, which release CAs on stimulation |
| Skin & peripheral vasculature | | • Vasoconstriction of the skin and blood vessls with dilatation of blood vessels in muscle • Piloerection and sweat secretion |
| Lower bowel, bladder & reproductive organs | S2-S4 sacral plexus • Contraction of smooth muscles of lower bowel contraction of bladder detrusor muscle and • Relaxation of ineternal urethral sphincter • Erection | T9-L2 • Inhibit peristalsis • ? role in inhibiting micturation • Ejaculation |

**Fig. 17.10** This schematic illustrates (*left*) the organisation of the parasympathetic and sympathetic nervous systems, and (*right*) a table of the major innervation of organs and their function. VMH (vendiomedical hypothalamic area; LHA lateral hypothalamic area; CA catecholamine.

---

## Box 17.2    Tests of autonomic function

### Bedside testing

- Pupillary response to light.

- Postural blood pressure readings (should not normally drop more than 30 mmHg for systolic and 15 mmHg for diastolic).

- Heart-rate response to standing (normally increases 10–30 beats per minute).

- Sweat test using quinizarin powder.

- Valsava manoeuvre with ECG monitoring — there should be a rise of heart rate with respiration and a further rise with the Valsava manoeuvre.

### More complex testing

- Baroreflex sensitivity with changes in posture using a tilt table.

- The cardiovascular response to meals is assessed by giving the patient a liquid meal and monitoring blood pressure and heart rate.

- Bladder function can be assessed using cystometrography.

- GI motility can be measured by barium meal.

- Pupillary testing using agents that act on the sympathetic or parasympathetic synapses.

---

trolled by a number of other pathways, which are summarised in Fig. 17.11.

# Research tools

In order for the clinical examination to be useful in research, features of it must be standardised so that comparisons can be made across time and between examiners. This is not only helpful in describing the natural history of the condition, but critical to investigating experimental therapies. However, such an approach has an inherent problem in that there is often variability between different examiners, creating interrater differences. These differences need to be minimised in order for meaningful data to be collected and col-

lated, and a number of protocols have now been developed that try to minimise this — often with training videotapes to help standardise the assessment procedure. The adoption of such protocols has the advantage of allowing studies to be conducted under 'standardised' conditions in a number of different centres. Thus such protocols have been developed, for example, for neural transplants and other neurosurgical interventions in both HD and PD (see below).

The research tools described below have been developed for a series of specific conditions, but the principles employed can be extrapolated to a number of other neurological disorders. However, the elements that make up the research protocol must be relatively easy to apply and quantify, and sensitive to the core pathogenic events, as well as the therapeutic intervention. The tests that form the core assessment programme need to be applied longitudinally in patients, whilst minimising any practice effect. The initial assessment requires a relatively long run-in period in order for a stable baseline to be obtained, given that most patients with neurological disorders show day-to-day variability. Furthermore, the tests should ideally be given under identical conditions, e.g. 'off' therapy first thing in the morning for patients with PD. Ideally the complete assessment protocol should be done using a series of different approaches including historical information, clinical examination with neuropsychological, and neuropsychiatric assessments, where appropriate, along with imaging and neurophysiological measures.

The adoption of assessment protocols for interventional therapy requires that clear end-points are defined, which are encompassed by this assessment protocol. These are in the form of primary end-points, and a series of secondary, less important, end-points. In such circumstances the need for control patients is helpful, given the placebo effect of such therapies and the variable natural history of the untreated condition. Finally, the assessments need to include measures of activities of daily living, as well as quality of life, as there is only limited use in assessing the effect of treatments on clinical measures if this does not translate into a functionally meaningful impact on the patient's life.

The discussion will now concentrate on a number of specific CNS disorders and their assessment.

## Multiple sclerosis (MS)

MS is an inflammatory disorder of the CNS of unknown aetiology that characteristically affects the myelinated axons within the brain and spinal cord of young adults

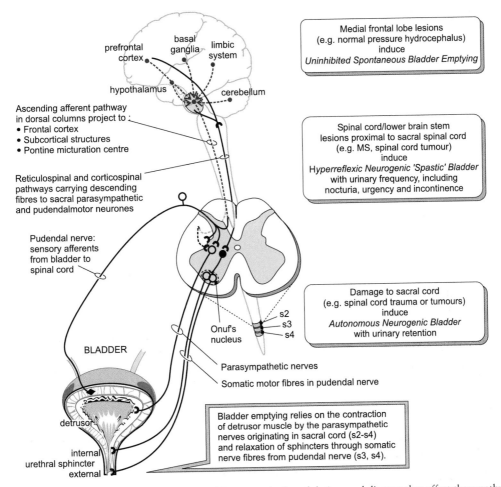

**Fig. 17.11** The normal innervation of the bladder and its supraspinal modulation, and diseases that affect these pathways and their effects on micturition.

(see Chapter 4 and Appendix 6). The disease varies from individual to individual but, in general, several patterns of disease progression are seen (Lublin and Reingold 1996).

1.  Relapsing–remitting disease is the commonest form of MS and is characterised by episodes of inflammation at different sites and times within the CNS, with spontaneous recovery, with or without deficits, thus producing the following subgroups:

    (a)  some of these patients have a benign form of the condition with only sensory and visual relapses and little in the way of deficits;

    (b)  others experience neurological relapses but, in this instance, recovery is less complete and in

time patients accrue deficits and enter a secondary progressive phase;

    (c)  a further subgroup accrue deficits from their first relapse.

2.  Primary progressive disease is a non-relapsing, progressive disorder that typically affects the spinal cord of late middle-aged patients.

The recognition of these different forms of MS is crucial in any assessment programme, as the natural history will vary according to the type of disease and by so doing will influence the effect of any therapeutic interventions. For example, the treatment may be designed to primarily reduce relapse rate without an effect on disability, and thus patients with primary progressive MS would be inappropriate for such a study (e.g. interferon-β; Thompson *et al.* 1997).

This issue of monitoring disease progress and the effects on intervention has gained prominence over the years as newer therapies have appeared for MS. One approach of late has been the possibility of repairing the demyelinated plaques by transplanting cells capable of remyelination (Duncan 1999). One cannot hope to repair all the lesions, but some are symptomatically very disabling and found at strategic CNS sites, such as the spinal cord, optic nerves, and cerebellar peduncles. These lesions therefore represent the most likely target for transplantation and are currently the focus of active investigation (see Chapter 24). The assessment of lesions at each of these sites is detailed below and combines clinical examination, neurophysiology, and MRI imaging protocols.

## Optic nerve

The optic nerve is prone to inflammation in MS (optic neuritis), which can lead to permanent damage and loss of function. This can be measured clinically by the loss of visual acuity, although a more sensitive test in early disease is the loss of colour vision. In addition, the clinical assessment can be supplemented by the visual evoked responses (VER), which is the cortical response to a patterned visual stimulus. Demyelination within the optic nerve leads to a slowed, small-amplitude response, which varies according to the extent of demyelination and axonal loss. The clinical and neurophysiological abnormalities can then be correlated with the anatomy of the optic nerve as assessed using fat-suppressed MRI (Miller *et al.* 1988). This technique allows for the assessment of plaques within the optic nerve, as well as the possibility of calculating their cross-sectional area, which offers a measure of axonal loss within this nerve (Youl *et al.* 1996).

## Spinal cord

The spinal cord is susceptible to inflammation in MS, which can affect ascending sensory and descending motor pathways, thereby producing a constellation of signs and symptoms (see above). These can be recorded in terms of clinical signs and quantified using a variety of instruments, including the Ashworth Tone Scale (Haas 1996), Medical Research Council MRC grading of muscle power (John 1984), and timed 10-m walking tests (Schwid *et al.* 1997), as well as by detailed mapping of sensory skin disturbances. Such clinical assessment can be supplemented with neurophysiological measures

of sensory pathway integrity using somatosensory evoked potentials from the arm or leg, and motor pathway function using central motor conduction time following magnetic stimulation of the motor cortex (Hess *et al.* 1987). This in turn can be correlated with the number of lesions in the spinal cord using a variety of MRI protocols, as well as the cross-sectional spinal cord area (a surrogate marker of axonal loss; Losseff 1996).

## Cerebellar peduncles

Plaques within the superior cerebellar peduncle are typically associated with tremor which can be especially disabling. However, the quantification of tremor is difficult, as it can vary according to fatigue, temperature, and anxiety, which can be exacerbated by invasive monitoring processes and therefore simple functional tests often give the most consistent results. Such tests include the Nine Hole Peg test (Goodkin *et al.* 1988); spiral drawing (Bain *et al.* 1993); and the amount of water remaining in a jug held for 30 s (Nakamura *et al.* 1993). The use of accelerometers to study the frequency of the tremor are often not of value, and thus the only other test of value in assessing cerebellar peduncle lesions is MRI imaging (Nakamura *et al.* 1993).

Overall, the MS patient has deficits at multiple CNS sites and so, whilst the above assessments are helpful for specific lesions, an overall assessment of the patient is required and a number of different clinical rating scales have been developed for MS. Perhaps the best known of these is that developed by John Kurtzke in the 1950s (Kurtzke 1961), in which he described eight functional systems with scores for each, leading to a composite expanded disability status score (EDSS) (see below):

However, other systems have been devised, of which a recent one is the Guy's Neurological Disability Scale (Sharrack and Hughes 1999), which uses disability scores in separate categories including mental, visual, speech, swallowing, upper and lower limb function, bowels, bladder, sexual function, fatigue, and a separate category to cover 'other' disabilities (e.g. pain and vertigo). In addition, less quantifiable aspects of the patients health can be addressed using handicap scores, one example of which is the Cambridge Multiple Sclerosis Basic Score (CAMBS) (Mumford and Compston 1993), which incorporates a patient's own perception of his/her degree of handicap using a simple visual analogue scale.

Overall, the judicious use of specific assessments,

## Box 17.3   Expanded Disability Status Scale (EDSS)

Developed by J.F. Kurtzke (1955), the EDSS assesses eight functional systems (pyramidal; cerebellar; brainstem; sensory; bowel/bladder; visual; cerebral; and others)

The EDSS measures disability on a scale from 0 to 10 in 0.5-step increments excluding 0–1:

0     indicates normal neurological examination;

1–1.5   indicates a diagnosis of MS but no obvious disability;

2–3.5   indicates minimal to moderate disability in one or more functional systems;

4–5.5   indicates relatively severe disability in one or more functional systems. with decreased mobility;

6.0    and above, indicates progression of disease initially requiring constant assistance through to total dependence and confinement to bed;

10.0   death due to MS.

## Box 17.4   Summary of the UPDRS

Each question scores from 0 (normal) to 4 (maximally severe symptoms), except for complications of therapy where many of the questions require a 'yes' or 'no' answer. The rating scale divides into six main sections:

(1) mentation, behaviour and mood;

(2) activities of daily living (on and off treatment);

(3) motor examination (on and off treatment);

(4) complication of therapy in the past week:
   (a) dyskinesias;
   (b) clinical fluctuations;
   (c) other complications;

(5) modified Hoehn and Yahr staging:

Stage 0:   no sign of disease;
Stage 1:   unilateral disease;
Stage 1.5: unilateral and axial involvement;
Stage 2.0: bilateral involvement with no impairment of balance;
Stage 2.5: mild bilateral involvement with recovery on pull test;
Stage 3.0: mild–moderate disease, some postural instability, physically independent;
Stage 4.0: severe disability, still able to walk or stand unassisted;
Stage 5.0: wheelchair-bound or bed-bound unless aided;

(6) Schwab and England activities of daily living scale (0–100%; 100%: normal and 0%: vegetative).

coupled to an overall disability and quality of life score, is helpful in the study of patients with MS, with the caveat that the appropriate phenotype of MS must be selected for inclusion in the study.

## Basal ganglia disorders

Research tools have been designed both to study the features and progression of two basal ganglia diseases, namely PD and HD, and have been used as documentation for the purposes of establishing the effect of interventions. One extensively used tool is the Unified Parkinson's Disease Rating Scale (UPDRS) (Fahn *et al.* 1987). This tool comprises a series of scales that cover important aspects of the history and examination of patients with PD (Lang 1996). The battery consists of scales to assess pertinent aspects of the history, including drugs and their side-effects, and an examination (see Box 17.4 for a summary). It has been well-validated over a number of years (van Hilten *et al.* 1994; Marder *et al.* 1994; Martinez-Martin *et al.* 1994; Louis *et al.* 1996; Stebbins *et al.* 1998), and has been used in the evalua-

tion of both surgical interventions (Ghika *et al.* 1998; Krack *et al.* 1998; Hauser *et al.* 1999; Kondziolka *et al.* 1999; Samii *et al.* 1999) and drug therapies (Wermuth 1998; Linazasoro *et al.* 1999; Pinter *et al.* 1999).

An equivalent tool has been developed for the study of a second basal ganglia disorder, Huntington's disease. The Unified Huntington's Disease Rating Scale (UHDRS) (Kieburtz *et al.* 1996b) is newer, but has also been shown to be valid as an assessment tool for the relevant features of HD, and appears to be appropriate for repeated administration during clinical studies. It has been used for assessment in studies of drug intervention in HD (Kieburtz *et al.* 1996a; van Vugt *et al.* 1997; Kieburtz 1999), as well as the natural history of the condition (Siesling *et al.* 1998). The UHDRS comprises four domains of clinical performance in HD:

motor, functional capacity, cognitive functions, and psychiatric abnormalities (see Box 17.5 for summary).

Both the UPDRS and the UHDRS are parts of larger batteries developed for assessment of patients undergoing neural transplantation. The way in which answers are recorded (yes/no or a number on a scale) make trans-

---

## Box 17.5   UHDRS

Every section of the UHDRS requires identification of the rater, as in large multidisciplinary clinics more than one person may complete the assessment, e.g. the cognitive assessment may be performed by a psychologist and the motor assessment by a neurologist. Rater identification is important in the estimation of tool reliability in each centre. The UHDRS comprises the following.

1.  A structured history, which includes demographic data, past and current general health status, brief psychiatric history, family history, onset of symptoms (the date of onset and class of initial symptom is assessed according to the patient, relative, and rater to obtain as accurate an estimate as possible). Responses are entered as yes/no answers except where dates etc are required.

2.  Medication, including doses, at each visit.

3.  Details of genetic analysis and whether the patient and family are aware of results.

4.  Cognitive assessment including verbal fluency, symbol digit modalities test, and Stroop interference test. Results are entered as raw scores.

5.  Behavioural assessment: mood symptoms, especially those relating to HD such as depression and obsessive/compulsive behaviour, are assessed by the rater according to clinical impression from the patients and informants' reports. Symptoms are rated on a scale of 1 to 4 as follows: 0, absent; 1, slight; questionable; 2, mild; 3, moderate; 4, severe. The rater is also asked to comment as to whether the patient is confused, demented, depressed, and requires pharmacotherapy for depression.

6.  The motor section comprises examination of ocular pursuit, saccade initiation, saccade velocity, dysarthria, tongue protrusion, finger taps, pronation/supination hand taps, the Luria tri step test, arm rigidity, overall bradykinesia, maximal dystonia, maximal chorea, gait, tandem walking, and the retropulsion pull test. The rater is required to estimate severity on a precisely defined five-point scale of 0 to 4 for each of the above (e.g. tongue protrusion: 0, can hold tongue fully protruded for 10 s; 1, cannot keep tongue fully protruded for 10 s; 2, cannot keep tongue fully protruded for 5 s; 3, cannot fully protrude tongue; 4, cannot fully protrude tongue beyond lips). Weight at each visit is also recorded.

7.  Functional scales. Three scales are completed.

    (a) Functional assessment. Twenty-five questions to which the answer is yes/no. These assess the subjects ability to perform or partake in a range of activities of daily living from the ability to continue in employment and drive, to getting out of bed without help.

    (b) Shoulson and Fahn independence scale. This rates the current level of the subjects independence from 100, indicating no special care, to 10, indicating tube feeding and total bed care.

    (c) Functional capacity. This assesses the degree to which a subject is able to function normally at work, handle personal financial matters, domestic chores, activities of daily living, and the overall care level.

It is also recorded whether the above assessments were obtained from the patient alone or also from an informant, and an overall impression of change (compared to the last assessment) is recorded separately from the patient and the rater.

fer of information to a computerised data base straightforward. The first battery to be put together in this way was the 'The core assessment program for intracerebral transplantation' for evaluation of PD (now known as CAPIT-PD) (Langston *et al.* 1992), and this has been followed by 'The core assessment program for intracerebral transplantation in Huntington's disease' (CAPIT-HD) (Quinn *et al.* 1996). Although these batteries were originally designed to provide minimum standards for the longitudinal assessment of patients receiving intrastriatal neural transplants of human foetal tissue, they are eminently suitable for other surgical interventions (Duff and Sime 1997; Kazumata *et al.* 1997; Shannon *et al.* 1998).

The need for these assessments arose for several reasons.

- Many conditions, but PD in particular, are variable on a day-to-day basis. This necessitates longitudinal patient assessment to understand the nature of baseline measurements on an individual basis. A major part of CAPIT is to define timing parameters, e.g. in CAPIT-HD a pre-operative assessment of 1 year is mandatory.

- Following a neural transplant, there is a prolonged period, which may be up to a year in PD, during which the transplanted tissue grows, develops, and makes connections. Thus it is necessary to define minimum follow-up periods, 2 years in the case of CAPIT-HD.

- The practical constraints of transplanting primary human foetal tissue dictate that it is only possible to transplant a handful of patients in any one centre per year. Thus, the study of this intervention has to be via a multicentre effort, and this makes the design of a standard protocol essential to allow meaningful comparison of results between centres.

We will concentrate on the CAPIT-HD battery, which is also discussed in the following two chapters. It consists of the UHDRS, described above, which is largely a motor and functional assessment with minimal cognitive and behavioural testing; an extensive battery of neuropsychological tests (discussed in Chapter 18); comprehensive neuropsychiatric tests (discussed in Chapter 19); and imaging (see Fig. 17.12). The imaging comprises mandatory PET and MRI images immediately pre-operatively and at 2 years, and ideally also 12 months pre-operatively. This imaging looks at the anatomical integrity of the graft (MRI), as well as functional measures such as the extent of dopamine receptor binding (e.g. raclopride binding on PET scanning). This latter measure is especially helpful as it gives an *in situ* measure of the functional capacity of the graft to restore and repair neuropharmacological systems, which in the case of PD has been shown to correlate well with functional recovery as assessed clinically.

The major aspects of the CAPIT-HD are shown in Fig. 17.12; an essential aspect of the battery is specification

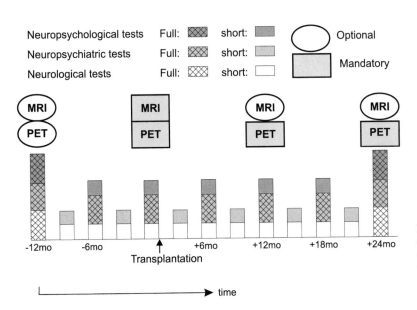

Fig. 17.12 The timing of neurological, neuropsychological, and neuropsychiatric test batteries and imaging in the CAPIT-HD protocol. This is the updated form of this battery. Quinn et al. 1996.

of the timing for the reasons given above. It is also important to recognise that these batteries comprise an agreed international minimum and that many centres also employ additional tests.

## Conclusions

The accurate assessment of the motor, sensory, and autonomic nervous systems relies on a knowledge of their functional anatomy and the nature of the disorders that can affect these systems. This understanding of the conditions affecting the CNS and PNS is essential in planning interventional therapies, although the heterogeneity of many neurological conditions needs recognising for such therapies to be accurately assessed. Indeed, the need to develop standardised assessment protocols is now gaining prominence, especially as newer, more experimental therapies become available. This is especially true in the emerging field of neural transplantation, where the benefit of any therapy develops slowly, such that long-term reproducible assessment is required to gauge the success, or otherwise, of the therapy.

## Further reading

Barker, R.A. and Barasi, S. (1999). *Neuroscience at a Glance*. Blackwell Scientific, Oxford.

Kandel, E.R., Schwarz J.H., and Jessell, T.M. (2000). *Principles of Neural Science*, 4th *edn*. McGraw-Hill Companies Inc.

Adams, R.D. and Victor, M. (1993). *Principles of Neurology*. McGraw-Hill, New York.

# 18 | *Cognition*

## *By Andrew D. Lawrence and Barbara J. Sahakian*

## *Introduction*

The aim of this chapter is to outline the role of cognitive testing as an outcome measure in evaluating treatments for dementia, with a particular emphasis on neural transplantation strategies. We begin with a brief overview of issues in the diagnosis of dementia. We then review the desirable characteristics of instruments for evaluating dementia treatments, followed by a discussion of one particular battery: that used in the CAPIT-HD neural transplantation programme, in order to demonstrate the application of the principles of cognitive assessment to a clinical research setting.

## *Dementia: nosological issues*

Dementia is 'an acquired syndrome of decline in memory and other cognitive functions sufficient to affect daily life in an alert patient' (Small *et al.* 1997). There are many ways of classifying dementia and one means of classification is given in Table 18.1. There have been significant advances in dementia diagnosis since the term first came into use in the seventeenth and eighteenth centuries (Berrios 1987). However, inconsistent operational definitions have resulted in confusion in the nosological system. Four major criteria have been used to define various types of dementia (e.g. Alzheimer disease versus Huntington's disease) and subtypes (e.g.

**Table 18.1** Classification of dementia. This table illustrates a classification of dementia according to whether the patient has other signs of a general medical or neurological condition

| Type of dementia | Examples of classes and specific causes |
| --- | --- |
| Dementia associated with other medical condition. | Alcohol-related dementia<br>Nutritional deficiency (such as Wernicke-Korsakoff's syndrome, and Pellagra)<br>Endocrine disorders (such as hypothyroidism, and Cushing's syndrome)<br>Inflammatory and infective disorders (such as syphilis, AIDS, and sarcoidosis)<br>Toxins<br>Drugs |
| Dementia in which the disease appears to be primarily neurological, but in which there are neurological signs other than the dementia itself. | Neurodegenerative conditions (such as Huntington's disease, cerebrocerebellar degeneration, and progressive supranuclear palsy)<br>Metabolic diseases (such as the lipid storage diseases)<br>Infections (such as Creutzfeldt-Jakob disease)<br>Stroke<br>Brain trauma (such as chronic subdural haematoma and cerebral contusion)<br>Space occupying lesions (such as brain tumour)<br>Normal pressure hydrocephalus<br>Disorders leading to anoxia |
| Conditions in which dementia appears to be the only evidence of neurological or medical disease. | Alzheimer's disease<br>Pick's disease<br>Some cases of AIDS |

different variants of Alzheimer disease and frontal lobe dementia) of dementia. According to Stuss and Levine (1996), these are:

(1)  site of the maximum structural changes in the brain;

(2)  histopathology;

(3)  clinical symptomatology;

(4)  aetiology.

Of these, location of major pathology in the brain has been the most frequently used scheme to classify the dementias. Dementias such as Alzheimer's disease (AD), which are considered to affect the cortical mantle most significantly have been labelled 'cortical dementias', which have been further subdivided into frontal, central, and posterior dementias(Cummings and Benson 1992). Disorders such as Huntington's disease (HD) and Parkinson's disease (PD), on the other hand, are classified as subcortical dementias, since the major pathology is in subcortical regions (Cummings and Benson 1992). However, this system of classification has come in for heavy criticism, not least because of the lack of specificity in such a distinction. For example, the major neurotransmitter lesion in Alzheimer's disease is subcortical, whilst Huntington's disease patients have been shown to have considerable cortical pathology, even in relatively earlier stages of the disease. Classification via histopathology, clinical symptomatology, and aetiology has also been subjected to much criticism (Brown and Marsden 1988; Lawrence and Sahakian 1996; Stuss and Levine 1996). At present then, there is no integrated nosological system for the classification of dementia. This lack of a comprehensive dementia nosology does not alter the fact that diagnoses of the dementias are required for both clinical treatment and research protocols. Stuss and Levine (1996) suggest that a convergence of classification criteria are necessary for improved dementia diagnosis. This suggestion is echoed by the proposals of the International Working Group on Harmonization of Dementia Drug Guidelines (Antuono *et al.* 1997). They propose that diagnosis of dementia should go through several phases, which would act as a series of progressively finer filters. The initial phase, conducted on the basis of evaluation of clinical symptoms and medical history, would include almost everyone who meets the criteria for dementia. The next phase would add a number of clinical tests to improve specificity and reduce false positives. Subsequent levels of evaluation would include structural and/or functional

imaging, and genetic markers, which would further categorise patients for particular purposes. No single criterion at present can provide diagnostic certainty. However, evidence converging from multiple sources greatly increases the specificity and stability of prediction (Stuss and Levine 1996; Antuono *et al.* 1997).

# Theoretical and empirical issues in the development and use of assessment tools

As cognitive decline is the defining symptom of dementia, objective assessment of the cognitive functions impaired in dementia is central to diagnosis, patient selection, and assessment of treatment efficacy (Sahakian 1990). Clinical cognitive neuroscience has emerged within recent times as an important clinical discipline (Margolin 1992), and one of the major contributions of the discipline has been the development of standardised cognitive test batteries. However, the properties by which to judge the utility of a particular cognitive test battery, as an outcome measure in clinical trials, are still much contested. Traditionally, the psychometric constructs of reliability and validity have been the criteria by which any such instrument was to be judged. There are no single indices of 'validity' or 'reliability'. It is not true that a test has inherent 'validity', a test that is valid under one set of conditions may not be valid under another set of conditions. 'Validity' can be broken down into three main types: content validity, criterion validity, and construct validity (see Box 18.1; Lemke and Wiersma 1976; Nunally 1978; Morley and Snaith 1992).

## Reliability

The reliability of an instrument is concerned with the replicability of measurement. Test–retest reliability is established by administering the test to two groups of subjects at different time points, and correlating the scores obtained. A low test–retest reliability does not necessarily imply that a measure is poor, but that it is sensitive to a number of factors. For example, measures of executive function often have poor test–retest reliability, but this follows by definition: 'The function of the executive system is to facilitate adaptation by making itself redundant' (Burgess 1998). If tests do have low test–retest reliability, then it is important to have alternate, equivalent forms of the test available.

## Box 18.1   Determining test validity

The validity of psychometric tests is determined according to four main criteria (Morley and Snaith 1992; Lemke and Wiersma 1976; Nunally 1978).

### Content validity

Content validity is concerned with whether the instrument in question adequately probes the specific domain(s) one requires. Arguments about the content validity of instruments are thus inextricably linked with theories about what one is trying to measure, and hence there are no empirical measures of content validity.

### Criterion validity

Criterion validity determines whether a measure discriminates between individuals who are known to differ on a marker external to the measure itself. Criterion validity is often presented in terms of the sensitivity and specificity of the measure in question. The sensitivity of a measure is defined as the proportion of positive cases correctly identified, the specificity is the proportion of negative cases identified. Sensitivity and specificity are not fixed values, but will depend on the cut-off score of a particular measure. Receiver operating characteristic (ROC) curves are plots of the sensitivity (true positive rate) of a particular measure versus the false positive rate (100% specificity). ROC curves can be used to determine the impact of selecting a particular cut-off score on the sensitivity and specificity of a measure, and can aid in determining the efficiency of different tests to discriminate between cases.

### Construct validity

Construct validity relates to the theoretical underpinnings of a test, and is evaluated by demonstrating that certain explanatory constructs account for performance on a test. The most important factor in construct validity is thus the explicitness of the theory behind the test in question. To have good construct validity, there must be a strong, well articulated theoretical rationale underpinning the measure, and there must be evidence of a consistent pattern of findings over a whole range of studies.

### Reliability

The reliability of an instrument is concerned with the replicability of measurement. Test–retest reliability is established by administering the test to two groups of subjects at different time points, and correlating the scores obtained. A low test–retest reliability does not necessarily imply that a measure is poor, but that it is sensitive to a number of factors. For example, measures of 'executive' function often have poor test–retest reliability, but this follows by definition: the function of the executive system is to facilitate adaptation by making itself redundant (Burgess 1998). If tests do have low test–retest reliability, then it is important to have alternate, equivalent forms of the test available.

Another form of reliability is the internal consistency of a measure, which relates to the reproducibility of measurement across different items within a test. There are a number of internal consistency measures available, all of which are obtained by inter-correlating subjects' scores on individual items within a test.

---

Another form of reliability is the internal consistency of a measure, which relates to the reproducibility of measurement across different items within a test. There are a number of internal consistency measures available, all of which are obtained by inter-correlating subjects' scores on individual items within a test.

A number of assessment tools, most especially clinician-rated interview-based methods, cannot be assessed using the above measures. In this case, reliability can be assessed by comparing the ratings of two independent observers (usually by computing some form of correlation coefficient) to determine the extent to which they agree in their observations (Lemke and Wiersma 1976; Nunally 1978; Morley and Snaith 1992), termed inter-rater reliability.

## Extensions to the standard psychometric approach

In several important recent articles, it has been strongly argued that the psychometric constructs of 'validity' and 'reliability' are insufficient criteria by which to judge the utility of cognitive test instruments in special populations, such as the elderly (Mohs 1995; Milberg 1996). For example, Mohs (1995) and Demonet *et al.* (1997) have argued that, in addition to meeting criteria for validity and reliability, cognitive instruments must also meet certain 'practicality' or 'pragmatic' criteria, such as being brief enough to be well tolerated by patients.

The most thorough review of criteria that any cognitive test battery designed for use in clinical trials has been provided by Milberg (1996). In this paper, Milberg strongly makes the case that the relative merits of any cognitive test instrument represent a compromise between the various demands of psychometry and practicality. Milberg argues that the properties of assessment techniques will be increasingly shaped, not simply by advances in cognitive neuroscience theory, but by the forces of demographics and economics. With advances in medical technology and public health policy increasing the expected life-span of people in industrialised nations, the incidence and prevalence of late-life disorders of cognition have increased dramatically in the later half of this century, and are expected to continue rising well into the twenty-first century (Milberg 1996). Thus, more individuals will require the assessment of cognitive functions, while resources available for health care are becoming increasingly limited. Milberg (1996) makes the argument that these circumstances demand that cognitive assessment techniques are designed to be as efficient as possible, where efficiency is defined as the ratio of 'useful' information obtained to time/cost. Thus, in addition to the traditional concepts of validity and reliability, efficiency is an important criterion by which cognitive assessment instruments should be judged.

Milberg also laments the lack of a theoretical context behind the use of most cognitive assessment batteries. He claims that the developers/users of clinical assessment tools have been mainly concerned with criterion validity rather than interpretative/theoretical (i.e. content/construct validity) issues. For example, a great many neuropsychological assessment tools, such as the Wechsler Adult Intelligence Scale, were not designed to be tests of neural function *per se*, but have been appropriated by neuropsychologists for such a purpose. Further, other measures, such as the Halstead-Reitan Battery, have their origins in outdated anti-localisationist theories of neural function, but have persisted in use because of their validity as measures sensitive to 'organic brain dysfunction'. Such tests do not reflect clinically relevant theoretical advances in our understanding of psychological processes, such as memory

systems (Parry and Hodges 1996) and executive or control processes (Owen *et al.* 1998). Thus, the sensitivity and specificity of an assessment tool to the presence of brain damage are not enough to ensure that an instrument is constructed in an optimally interpretable fashion, or that the levels of sensitivity and specificity obtained have been obtained in a maximally efficient manner. Similar arguments have been made by Cipolotti and Warrington (1995) who state that, 'Before approaching a neuropsychological assessment it is necessary to have a theoretical structure on which to base and interpret the different levels of disturbance that can arise as a result of cerebral damage'.

The dominant paradigm (Kuhn 1970) in neuropsychology and cognitive neuroscience today is the localisationist paradigm. Although not without its critics (Farah 1994; Kosslyn 1996), it is broadly accepted that there is a high degree of functional specialisation in the brain, and that brain damage can selectively disrupt some components of the cognitive system. Furthermore, it is accepted that broad functions, such as memory, language, and attention, can be broken down into more basic processing elements (what has been termed the 'modularity approach to the analysis of complex skills'; Cipolotti and Warrington 1995) and that these more basic elements are candidate descriptions for neural function. Although the precise natures of these basic cognitive functions are not resolved, there is sufficient consensus within the literature to inform clinical assessment practice. Even a division into such seemingly procrustean categories as language, memory, visual and space perception, attention, and executive function, would be a useful starting point. Within each broad domain, tasks should be constructed that reflect the current understanding of underlying psychological processes. For example, memory measures should allow separation of encoding/retrieval/monitoring functions and assess separate information-domains (e.g. spatial/visual); measures of attention should assess selective, divided, and sustained attention, etc.. This type of specificity in assessment tools is particularly important because of the increasing recognition that dementia is not a unitary syndrome within or across aetiologies: even though broad patterns can be distinguished, patients with similar underlying pathologies may vary widely in the neural distribution of the causative lesion and hence in the behavioural manifestations of those lesions (Stuss and Levine1996; Lawrence 1997). It is vital that cognitive assessment tools are sensitive to such biological and cognitive variability.

Although some clinicians might argue that such cognitive specificity is of little clinical relevance, this is not the case. There is emerging evidence to suggest that domain-specific measures are better predictors of activities of daily living than are global measures of cognitive severity, and determining with specificity which areas of cognitive dysfunction strongly predict impaired day-to-day functioning will be of importance in informing patient management and rehabilitation strategies, including neural transplantation strategies (Weintraub *et al.* 1982; Lawrence 1997; Plaisted and Sahakian 1997).

In addition to these efficiency and content/construct validity criteria, several authors have argued that certain 'practicality' criteria are important when assessing measures that are applied to patients with dementia (Mohs 1995; Milberg 1996; Demonet *et al.* 1997). Perhaps the most important of these is that the tests are brief enough to avoid fatigue effects and enjoyable so that patients do not become frustrated or distressed during testing.

In classic psychometric theory, a measure's reliability is assessed in three ways: internal consistency (e.g. split-half reliability), temporal stability (test–retest), or inter-rater reliability (Morley and Snaith 1992; Lemke and Wiersma 1976; Nunally 1978). However, internal consistency measures may be affected by patient fatigue, distractibility, mood, and measurements of temporal stability may be limited due to diurnal variations in symptoms and because symptom severity changes over time. It has therefore been argued that the reliability of cognitive assessment tools to be used in clinical trials of dementia be determined within the clinical context in which the measure is being used. The goal should be to 'optimise reliability as it empirically affects test validity and efficiency' (Milberg 1996).

A final feature of tests judged to be important by Milberg (1996) is that tasks should cover a wide range of ability, while avoiding ceiling effects in young, healthy individuals and floor effects in the dementing elderly.

The above considerations led Milberg (1996) to propose seven criteria by which any cognitive assessment tool for use in dementing individuals be judged (see Box 18.2).

These requirements for cognitive assessment batteries had been presaged somewhat by the work of Stephen Ferris (1992) on psychological testing in dementia patients. Although less specified than Milberg's arguments, he reached somewhat similar conclusions regarding the requirements for psychological testing in dementia. His requirements are:

---

## Box 18.2   Milberg's (1996) criteria for cognitive assessment batteries

1. *Neuropathological sensitivity/specificity.* The ability to distinguish patients who show evidence from independent biological markers (e.g. neuro-imaging/genetic data) of a particular neuropathological entity.

2. *Cognitive domain specificity.* Measures should be relatively homogeneous and designed to assess different cognitive domains. The choice of these domains should be justified on both biological and psychological grounds.

3. *Construct or process specificity.* Tasks included in the battery should assess empirically and theoretically justified variables that reflect the information processing demands specific to each domain. The tasks should reflect the most recent understanding of cognitive processes.

4. *Functional specificity.* Tasks included in the battery should be relevant to a patient's daily functional abilities.

5. *Contextually appropriate reliability.* Reliability for a given measure should be estimated for the clinical population and within the assessment context the task is likely to appear. Task length may be titrated to optimise the reliability of a measure as it will actually be used.

6. *Age appropriate item difficulty.* The tasks included in the battery should be appropriate in form and difficulty level for healthy adults in the age range of the patients being assessed.

7. *Efficiency.* The battery should be as brief as possible given the constraints outlined above.

---

- sample the full range of relevant cognitive functions;

- sensitivity to deficits of ageing and dementia;

- sensitivity to longitudinal change;

- difficulty range appropriate to severity of patient sample;

- equivalent forms for repeated administration;

- reasonable duration;

- sensitivity to treatment effects;

- good reliability;

- good validity (in relation to brain pathology or symptoms relating to activities of daily living (ADL).

These lists raise important issues for clinicians to consider, and any test battery that satisfied all of these constraints would certainly be admirable. However, it would be wrong to dismiss a battery simply on the grounds that it fails to satisfy all of Milberg's or Ferris's criteria. Test batteries should be evaluated with respect to the question the clinician wants to answer.

In addition to the criteria set out by Milberg and Ferris, which are applicable to all clinical trials that involve cognitive assessment as an outcome variable, The International Working Group on Harmonisation of Dementia Drug Guidelines (Ferris *et al.* 1997) have produced a position paper on the use of objective psychometric tests as outcome measures in clinical trials of AD, to which the interested reader is referred.

## Putting principles into practice

The cognitive assessment battery of the CAPIT-HD programme provides a model for principled cognitive assessment as part of a multicentre brain-repair study (Quinn *et al.* 1996). As cognitive dysfunction is core to the symptomatology of Huntington's disease, and is a stronger predictor of activities of daily living than is the involuntary movement disorder (Brandt and Butters 1996), it was imperative that a detailed, theoretically motivated assessment protocol was implemented when clinical trials of brain-repair strategies, especially the use of intracerebral transplantation techniques, were begun. The component elements of this battery were chosen with regard to the above principles, that is, they were chosen to have contextually appropriate reliability; to have neuropathological sensitivity and specificity; to have cognitive-domain specificity and construct specificity; to be sensitive to longitudinal change; to be of the appropriate difficulty range to avoid floor and ceiling effects; and to be efficient. As Huntington's disease is characterised by a dysexecutive syndrome, memory deficits, impaired attention, and reduced psychomotor speed (Brandt and Butters 1996; Lawrence *et al.*

1998b), the tests in particular examine these domains of cognition. In addition, a comprehensive neuropsychological assessment of premorbid ability; general intellectual level; language; and perception is provided, so that a detailed cognitive profile can be constructed for individual patients.

### The full CAPIT-HD battery

This battery is administered at entry to the programme and then annually. Testing is arranged over several sessions, in order to avoid fatigue and interference effects (i.e. to satisfy Millberg's 1996 efficiency criteria).

The instruments for assessing cognitive function in the CAPIT-HD protocol fall into two broad categories (Ferris 1992; Mohs 1995; Ferris *et al.* 1997).

1. Global cognitive assessment tools, which use performance subtests to assess a variety of relevant cognitive symptoms and provide a total score that represent a composite index of the magnitude of cognitive impairment. These instruments are generally used to confirm the presence of dementia, to select cases for research protocols, and to monitor change in clinical trials.

2. Objective neuropsychological/psychometric tests. These tests are useful in documenting significant decline in cognitive function, determining patterns of cognitive function, evaluating the rate and manner of cognitive decline, and assessing treatment effects. The greater breadth and sensitivity of these tests in comparison with more global scales makes objective psychometric tests especially useful in early clinical trials when the nature and effect size of a new treatment are not fully known. Such sophisticated instruments are particularly important in the context of novel treatment strategies, such as neural transplantation techniques.

The CAPIT includes both types of instrument.

## Global cognitive assessment tools

### The Mini Mental State Exam (MMSE)

The classic and most widely used clinical rating scale in dementia trials is the Mini-Mental State Examination (MMSE) (Cockrell and Folstein 1988). This instrument assesses orientation, recall, praxis, calculation, and language with a score range of 0 (maximal impairment) to 30 (no impairment), and usually takes 10–15 min to administer. Although the MMSE is designed to produce a rating of global cognitive status, it contains some tasks that could be classified as 'domain specific'. The major strengths of the MMSE are that it is quick and easy to administer, it is within the capabilities of older adults, and it yields a single summary score that can be used as the primary cognitive outcome measure for a clinical trial. Its major weaknesses are that it is too brief, so that separate cognitive domains are not assessed thoroughly or systematically, nor do they reflect conceptual details of the particular domains in question. For example, the tasks assessing memory cannot be separated in encoding/retrieval components. Thus the subcomponents of the MMSE do not easily lend themselves to being assessed as independent cognitive functions, although this has been attempted (Brandt *et al.* 1988). In addition, the MMSE is subject to ceiling effects and is not particularly sensitive to the early stages of dementia and to changes in mental status in individuals with high premorbid IQ levels (Milberg 1996). Scores on the MMSE have been shown to be strongly influenced by, for example, linguistic capabilities (Reisberg *et al.* 1997). Furthermore, the MMSE has no alternative forms, resulting in enhanced susceptibility to practice effects. Nevertheless, the MMSE remains a useful tool for rating the severity of global cognitive dysfunction, allowing comparison across a large number of studies which have used this instrument.

## Mattis Dementia Rating Scale (DRS)

An optional clinical rating scale of global cognitive function is the Mattis Dementia rating Scale (DRS) (Mattis 1976). The DRS consists of five subscales measuring attention, initiation and perseveration, conceptualisation, construction, and memory. The items are administered in hierarchical fashion, such that if a patient is unable to complete simple items, they do not receive more complex ones. The total score ranges from 0 (maximal impairment) to 144 (no impairment), and the test takes up to 45 min to administer. The major strengths of the DRS are its broad coverage of the relevant cognitive domains, the inclusion of items designed to assess attention and executive function, and its ability to distinguishing different patterns of dementia, i.e. it meets Millberg's (1996) criteria for neuropathological and cognitive domain specificity. Its major weakness is the lack of alternate forms.

# Assessment of current and premorbid IQ

## National Adult Reading Test (NART)

The National Adult Reading Test (NART) is a measure of premorbid optimal level of functioning based on the overlearned skill of reading. The NART, developed by Nelson (1991), which consists of 50 irregular words, has become one of the most commonly used measures of premorbid intelligence. One of the major limitations of this test is that it cannot be used with those who have poor literacy skills or in patients with obvious problems of speech production or with dyslexia. In addition, it has been claimed that patients with dementing disorders may not present with preserved irregular word reading (Cipolotti and Warrington 1995). Consequently, these patients present with difficulties in reading the NART words, resulting in erroneous low estimates of their premorbid IQ. In the cases of early dementia, when language skills are relatively unimpaired, however, it has been shown that the NART remains stable over time and can be used as a predictor of the premorbid optimal level, i.e. it has good process specificity (Cipolotti and Warrington 1995).

## Wechsler Adult Intelligence Scale-Revised (WAIS-R)

The Wechsler Adult Intelligence Scale-Revised (WAIS-R) (Wechsler 1981) is considered to be one of the core measures for evaluating general intellectual ability. It involves six verbal and five non-verbal subtests that sample various skills. These subtests are thought to measure various mental abilities, including both a generic knowledge base and the ability to solve new cognitive problems. Verbal and performance IQs are determined from the use of the Wechsler Scales. It has been suggested that such scales have little value as regards the localisation of a lesion or the identification of specific cognitive deficits (Warrington *et al.* 1986). Nevertheless, the WAIS-R is the most often used psychological test of intellectual functioning and is a cornerstone for most neuropsychological batteries. The full WAIS-R is excessively long, and so does not meet Millberg's (1996) efficiency criteria. Therefore, a variety of short forms of the WAIS-R have been developed to minimise frustration and fatigue on the part of the patient, several of which show good validity (Randolph *et al.* 1993). In the CAPIT-HD protocol, a shortened form consisting of vocabulary, comprehension, similarities, digit span, block design, object assembly, and picture arrangement is recommended.

# Memory

Memory is not a unitary construct, but rather is better described as a collection of distinct and independent components, each of which is associated with different neural structures. At a course level of analysis, a distinction can be made between short- and long-term memory. Short-term memory consists of the immediate retention of a limited amount of information, which will rapidly decay if not refreshed. Long-term memory retains larger amounts of information for longer periods. Short- and long-term memory can be further divided into particular informational domains (e.g. verbal, visual). Long-term memory can also be divided broadly into declarative and non-declarative systems. Non-declarative memory retains information that affects behaviour but is not available for conscious recollection (e.g. motor skill learning). Declarative memory retains information that can be consciously accessed. Declarative memory can be further subdivided into episodic and semantic memory. Episodic memory contains information relating to temporally dated episodes and the relationship among them (e.g. remembering a list of words). Semantic memory relates to the organised knowledge of concepts and facts about the world (e.g. knowing that Paris is the capital of France). These different domains of memory are assessed to a certain degree in the CAPIT-HD battery, thus meeting Millberg's (1996) construct specificity criterion.

## Digit span

Verbal short-term memory span is assessed using the digit span subtest from the WAIS-R (Wechsler 1981), which requires the repetition of a progressively lengthening string of digits. Both forward and reverse span are measured. Visual memory span is assessed using the Corsi Blocks (Milner 1970), which requires the subject to tap a progressively lengthening sequence of blocks.

## Hopkins Verbal Learning Test (HVLT)

Episodic memory is assessed using the HVLT. This word-learning task (Rasmussen *et al.* 1995) comprises a list of 12 high-imagery concrete nouns randomly organised into three semantic categories. After presen-

tation, the subject is tested for immediate free recall. The same list is presented for two more trials to assess list learning. Delayed free recall is assessed after 30 min, followed immediately by a recognition test. Six alternative forms are available.

## Rivermead Behavioural Memory Tests (RBMT)

The Rivermead Behavioural Memory Tests (RMBT) (Wilson *et al.* 1985) consists of a series of tests held to have ecological validity or, as Milberg (1996) would put it, good functional specificity. In addition to assessing immediate and delayed recall, and recognition, it assesses prospective memory. It comprises remembering an appointment, remembering a belonging, picture recognition, immediate and delayed story recall, face recognition, immediate and delayed tracing of a short route, remembering to deliver a message, orientation, and remembering a name. The test takes 20–30 min to administer. It has four parallel forms and is translated into all major European languages.

## Conditional Associative Learning Test (CALT)

The CALT requires the learning of a series of arbitrary associations between a set of stimuli and a set of responses. Training is by a trial-and-error procedure, during which the subject performs the various responses when a given stimulus is presented and the experimenter provides feedback until the correct response is performed. This task has been shown to be sensitive to the cognitive deficit of Huntington's disease.

# Language

Again, language is not a unitary function. The most useful dichotomy is to consider spoken and written language separately (McCarthy and Warrington 1990). Due to the nature of the movement disorder in Huntington's disease, assessment of written language is problematic, and so the CAPIT battery focuses on assessing two areas of spoken language: comprehension and retrieval.

## Token Test (short form)

One of the most commonly used tests of sentence comprehension is the Token Test (De Renzi and Vignolo

1962). This test uses tokens of different shapes, sizes, and colours, and the patient is given an oral instruction with progressively more complex non-redundant sentences. The 36-item short form of the token test is used in the CAPIT-HD battery. Educationally standardised normative data are available.

## Boston Naming Test (short form)

To evaluate word retrieval, picture-naming tests can be used. The 60 picture item standard Boston Naming Test, which comprises line drawings of objects, is divided into two alternate forms comprising odd- and even-numbered items, respectively. Research has shown these forms to be equivalent (Mack *et al.* 1992).

# Visuo-perceptual function

## The Visual Object and Space Perception battery (VOSP)

Two major, dissociable systems of complex visuospatial perception have been identified — that subserving space perception and that subserving form perception. Furthermore, each of these may fractionate into sub-components. A basic screening and comprehensive assessment of space and form perception is provided by the Visual Object and Space Perception battery (Warrington and James 1991). This test assesses various aspects of object or space perception, with the involvement of other cognitive skills being minimised, e.g. praxis skills, and thus has good domain specificity.

# Attention and psychomotor speed

## Symbol Digit Modalities Test (SDMT)

This is a version (Spreen and Strauss 1998) of the Digit Symbol subtest from the WAIS, and is considered to require rapid shifts of attention and also taps psychomotor processes. It differs from Digit Symbol in that the subject writes the digits rather than the symbols. As with the Digit Symbol test, the subject has 90 s to write as many correct responses as possible. Norms and test–retest data are available (Mitrushina *et al.* 1998). Scores on the SDMT have been shown to correlate significantly with functional neuro-imaging indices of striatal neuronal loss in HD (Brandt and Butters 1996), and so this test has some validity in relation to neuropathology in HD.

## Reitan Trail Making Test (TMT)

This is a test of speed for visual search, attention, mental flexibility, and motor function. It requires the connection, by making pencil lines, between 25 encircled numbers randomly arranged on a page in proper order (part A) and of 25 encircled numbers and letters in alternating order (part B). In the CAPIT-HD protocol, only 90 s are allowed for each, and the score taken as the number of correct responses achieved in this time period. Four alternate forms are available for repeat testing, although practice effects of significant magnitude have not been reported (Mitrushina *et al.* 1998). This test has also been shown to correlate with functional imaging indices of striatal metabolism in HD (Brandt and Butters 1996; Lawrence 1997), and so has some validity in relation to neural pathology in HD.

# Executive function

The term 'executive function' refers to those processes by which an individual optimises his/her performance in multicomponent tasks. As with memory, executive function is not a unitary construct, and a variety of attempts have been made to fractionate the subcomponents of the 'executive' (Robbins 1996; Burgess 1998). These different processes include the ability to respond flexibly and appropriately in altered circumstances, efficient scheduling of behaviour and attentional resources, as well as the suppression of inappropriate responding, the use of strategies to enhance mnemonic function, and the formulation of new plans of action (Robbins *et al.* 1998). Although not cast in any particular theoretical framework, the CAPIT-HD battery recommends that use of a variety of tests that have been considered to tap these different components of executive function. These tests have been shown to be sensitive to the pronounced dysexecutive syndrome of HD, even in early disease; are related to neuro-imaging indices of the primary striatal neuropathology in HD; and are related to everyday functioning of HD patients, as measured by Activities of Daily Living scales (Brandt and Butters 1996; Lawrence *et al.* 1998b).

## Verbal fluency

The Controlled Oral Word Association test (Benton 1968) is a useful test of executive function, which places demands upon the patient's ability to generate an appropriate strategy without any external stimulus. This test involves the production of words beginning with a given letter within a limited amount of time (60 s). In English, the letters F, A, and S are used, corresponding to low, medium, and high frequencies of occurrence within the English language. French, German, Italian, and Spanish equivalents are available. Scores on letter fluency in HD have also been shown to correlate with functional neuro-imaging indices of striatal neuronal loss (Lawrence *et al.* 1998b). In addition, semantic category fluency is assessed. This involves naming as many exemplars from a given semantic category (e.g. animals) as possible in 60 s. Norms for these tests are available (Mitrushina *et al.* 1998).

## Stroop test

The Stroop colour-word test (Macleod 1991) is used clinically to assess a specific aspect of executive function, i.e. selective inhibition. It requires a subject to inhibit an automatic reading response in favour of a less-well rehearsed, competing colour-naming response. In the CAPIT-HD protocol, a modification of the Stroop test is employed. It comprises three sections: naming colour rectangles (red, green, or blue), reading colour words written in black, and naming the colour of the ink of incongruent colour words. Each test comprises 100 stimuli presented on a card. The test is scored as the number of correct responses and number of errors made in 45 s. Studies have shown low, but significant test–retest reliability for the Stroop (Mitrushina *et al.* 1998). It also has some validity in HD, as performance on the Stroop has been shown to correlate with structural neuro-imaging indices of striatal atrophy (Brandt and Butters 1996; Lawrence 1997). However, there is some controversy about how best to control for possible contributions of differences in basic reading ability to Stroop interference scores. The interested reader can find a discussion of these issues in (Mitrushina *et al.* 1998).

## Wisconsin Card Sorting Test (WCST)

The Wisconsin Card Sort Test is the classic test of cognitive flexibility (Milner 1963). Three dimensions are used for classification of a series of cards (number, colour, and shape). The patient is required to sort the cards according to one dimension and, having maintained the classification for a criterion number of trials, is subsequently required to shift to each of the other dimensions in turn (six shifts in total). The Nelson short form of the WCST is used in the CAPIT-HD battery, in

which patients are explicitly informed of a change in sorting criterion, rather than the examiner simply saying 'wrong' to a previously correct choice. Performance on the WCST in HD has been shown to correlate with functional neuro-imaging indices of striatal metabolism (Lawrence *et al.* 1998b), so again, the WCST has some validity in relation to neural pathology in HD.

## Cambridge Neuropsychological Test Automated Battery (CANTAB) — visual discrimination learning/attentional set-shifting

In addition to the above tests, the CAPIT-HD protocol includes, as an option, the visual discrimination/attentional set shifting test from the CANTAB battery (Fray and Robbins 1996; Fray *et al.* 1996).

The CANTAB battery is a computerised system with detailed automatic recording of response accuracy and speed made via a touch-screen apparatus. The results are instantly available, and standardised scores can be produced from a large pool of normative data. These tests have a number of theoretical and practical advantages, and indeed meet the majority of criteria set in the introductory section for cognitive assessment tools. The tests have strong theoretical underpinnings, being designed to reflect recent theoretical developments in the cognitive neuroscience of memory, attention, and executive functions and are specifically designed to facilitate cross-species comparisons between rats, primates, and humans (Roberts and Sahakian 1993). The tests are graded in nature, allowing for a wide range of ability; have satisfactory levels of test–retest reliability, with some reaching correlations of better than 0.9; and longitudinal data are available for both healthy volunteers and several patient groups. There are five equivalent versions available and the tests have been used successfully in a number of cross-cultural studies, as tests of language are deliberately not included to make the tests genuinely cross-cultural in nature (Maruff *et al.* 1996). Importantly, with respect to the present discussion, the tests have been shown to be sensitive to neural pathology in Huntington's disease (Lawrence *et al.* 1998), as well as to activities of daily living (Lawrence *et al.* 1999), and are sensitive enough to discriminate preclinical cognitive decline in different dementia types (Lawrence *et al.* 1998; Sahakian *et al.* 1995).

For the CAPIT-HD protocol, the use of the visual discrimination learning/attentional set-shifting task has been recommended. This is a test of executive function modelled on the Wisconsin Card Sorting Test (WCST) (Roberts and Sahakian 1993). Although an excellent clinical test of cognitive flexibility, the WCST is a pragmatically validated test, rather than being theoretically derived, and hence it suffers from a number of confounds, such as tapping a variety of potentially dissociable cognitive processes, in addition to executive processes. Thus, by Milberg's criteria, it is lacking somewhat in terms of cognitive domain specificity and process specificity (as indeed are the other tests of executive function in the CAPIT-HD battery). The CANTAB version of this test addresses such problems by initially using a much simpler task. In this way, the cognitive requirements of the task can be assessed independently and then their relative contribution to any deficit can be assessed as the test builds to a higher level of complexity that requires more sophisticated skills. The stimuli are constructed with only two perceptual dimensions, those of shape and line. Starting with simple shape discrimination and reversal, the subject proceeds to tests of distraction where irrelevant lines are introduced, first adjacent to the shapes and then superimposed upon them. Once training to the shape through several reversals is complete, and the irrelevance of the lines has been established, one of two different types of shift occurs. Initially, there is an intra-dimensional shift, whereby novel exemplars of the stimuli are used, but with shape still the relevant dimension. In this way, there can be no carry over of a tendency to respond to the stimuli from the first stage of the test. When discrimination has been established to these new stimuli, an extra-dimensional shift occurs in which, again with new stimuli, the line finally becomes relevant, and the previously changed shape is irrelevant. It is this stage that is formally equivalent to the category shift of the WCST but, by comparison of the two types of shift, the CANTAB test yields a pure measure of attentional set-shifting uncontaminated by confounds of perseveration to particular stimuli and distraction. The stages of the test are illustrated in Fig. 18.1; Fig. 18.2 shows representative results of the test. The test appears extremely sensitive to the cognitive deficit of HD. Early in the course, HD patients have difficulty with attentional set-shifting, and later-stage patients have problems even at the simple reversal stage of discrimination (Lawrence *et al.* 1998). Of particular interest is that genetically identified asymptomatic individuals exhibit deficits on the test at a stage prior to the development of overt clinical movement disorder (Lawrence *et al.* 1998).

Of note in a neural-transplantation context, similar discrimination learning impairments are seen in trans-

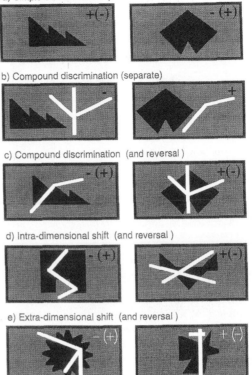

**Fig. 18.1** Schematic representation of the CANTAB visual discrimination learning/attentional set-shifting task. Reversal refers to a reversal of the contingencies, such that the correct and incorrect stimuli are unpredictably swapped. The stimuli are presented randomly with respect to spatial location. (a) Simple discrimination between shapes. (b) and (c) Compound discrimination, in which the white lines are introduced as distractors. (d) and (e) Dimensional shifts are implemented with unexpected changes to novel exemplars of both shape and line; with intra-dimensional shift, shape remains relevant (one of the new shapes is correct, regardless of its pairing with line); with extra-dimensional shift, line becomes relevant (one of the lines is correct, regardless of its pairing with shape).

genic mouse models of HD, suggesting that discrimination learning paradigms may have a particularly important role to play in monitoring the effectiveness of treatments for HD at both the experimental and clinical stages of evaluation. A major advantage of the CANTAB visual discrimination learning/attentional set-shifting task is that analogous versions are available for use with primates, and can be used to monitor the effects of, and help refine procedures for, substitutive therapy using foetal striatal grafts on cognitive function in primate models of HD. These findings highlight the

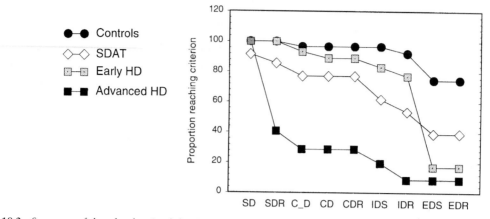

**Fig. 18.2** Summary of data for the visual discrimination learning/attentional set-shifting task in groups of patients with early HD (*shaded squares*), advanced HD (*black squares*), probable DAT (matched for dementia severity with advanced HD patients) (*open diamond*), and age and IQ-matched controls (*black circles*). Abbreviations: SD, simple discrimination (i.e. shapes or lines only); SDR, simple reversal; CxD, compound discrimination (both shapes and lines present); CD, compound discrimination (shapes with lines superimposed); CDR, compound reversal; IDS, intra-dimensional shift; IDR, intra-dimensional reversal; EDS, extra-dimensional shift; EDR, extra-dimensional reversal.

advantages of a theoretically motivated, comparative approach to cognitive assessment.

An important future development in cognitive assessment will be to combine functional neuro-imaging with theoretically driven cognitive testing; an approach that, in due course, could be used to map the restoration of functional neural circuitry following neural transplantation. Again, the CANTAB visual discrimination learning/attentional set shifting task may prove useful in this case, as the neural structures underlying performance on this task in healthy volunteers have been recently mapped out (Rogers *et al.* in press).

### CAPIT-HD short battery

The short battery comprises a subset of the full battery. It is administered at one-yearly intervals in between administration of the full battery. It is comprised of the following tests, which are considered to be most sensitive to longitudinal change in HD: MMSE, span, RBMT, HVLT, CALT, verbal fluency, Stroop, WCST, and SDMT.

At six-monthly intervals, the cognitive tests of the UHDRS (The Huntington's Study Group 1996), verbal fluency (letters), Stroop, and SDMT are administered.

## Conclusions

In this chapter, we have outlined the arguments relating to the design of cognitive assessment batteries. Following a discussion of the constructs of classic psychometric theory and detailing some of its deficiencies, we focused on the criteria laid down by Milberg and Ferris as the standards by which any cognitive assessment battery should be judged. We then described the CAPIT-HD battery, as an example of a cognitive test battery in which a principled design stance was taken at its inception, and described the utility of such an approach in the setting of a clinical trial. We believe that such a principled approach can inform the design of other cognitive assessment batteries for use in a wide variety of brain repair programmes.

# 19 | *Psychiatric assessment*

## *With G.E. Berrios, E.S. Paykel and A. Wagle*

## Introduction

Brain disease of whatever nature can give rise to mental symptoms and disorders that, on occasions, may interfere with the assessment, treatment, rehabilitation, and recovery of the underlying disease. Good practice enjoins clinicians to evaluate and manage these complications. This is easier said than done. Evaluation often requires suitable psychometric tools and questionnaires, and on occasions this cannot be separate from research; management should include neurobiological and psychosocial information, and be skilful enough to dovetail with the ongoing medical management.

During the acute disease, alterations of consciousness and cognition (e.g. stupor, confusion, and delirium) (see Chapter 16) are commonest and may cloak all other mental changes. As consciousness clears up, changes in mood and thinking, anxiety, irritability and other neurotic symptoms, personality changes, hallucination, and dementia-like states may be revealed (see Chapter 18). The severity and duration of these symptoms varies according to age, gender, education, genetics, laterality and nature of lesions, premorbid personality and the nature of the underlying disease. The fact that during acute disease the brain responds with a surprisingly limited set of dysfunctional behaviours (Bonhoeffer 1910; Hoche 1912; Redlich 1912) makes mapping of psychiatric disorders onto brain sites a difficult task. As the subject comes to terms with the changes in his life and fortune, and chronicity sets in, maladaptive behaviours often appear, which magnify and perpetuate any earlier mental symptoms and cause havoc with management. The nature and neurobiological status of these behaviours remains beyond understanding.

This notwithstanding, the time-honoured way of classifying psychiatric complications of brain disease is still followed:

(1) 'distortions' of known function;

(2) new behaviours released by the disease; and

(3) reactive psychological states, based on meanings and symbols, putatively the result of negotiations between impaired subjects and the environment.

The devil, however, is in the detail and most clinical accounts combine all three explanations. Even harder, is to transfer neuropsychological insights into management routines or to agree on the standards of *evidence* required to accept such insights in the first place. As things stand, evidence comes from correlations obtained in cross-sectional studies carried out on 'clinical samples'. The relevant variables are all proxies. Some represent putative brain functions (e.g. changes in blood flow as captured by neuro-imaging); others abnormal behaviour (score variances representing severity of mental symptoms or disease). This model is at the basis of prototypical papers of the type 'Mental state M in disease X'. The yawning logical gaps and methodological and statistical flaws bedevilling this model are such that the kind of evidence it generates would not be accepted in any other science. This state of affairs should not make us self-complacent, for even if the correlations obtained could be shown to be legitimate, their interpretation remains equivocal (Berrios and Quemada 1990).

For reasons of space, this chapter will discuss only some of the principles guiding clinical practice and research in this field, and then deal with the psychiatry of brain trauma, vascular insult, and Huntington's disease (the latter in more detail), in order to illustrate how the type and expression of the psychiatric complications is modulated by different patterns of disease. By psychiatric 'complications' is meant here mental symptoms (e.g. hallucinations, delusions, sadness, confusion, obsessions, irritability, aggression, etc.), syndromes (e.g. delirium, dementia, affective disorder) and less often 'diseases' (schizophrenia, mania, etc.) (Table 19.1). According to the rules governing psychiatric diagnosis, isolated mental symptoms and syndromes are likely to be far more common than full mental diseases.

**Table 19.1**  Main psychiatric disorders

| Psychiatric disorder | Definition and description |
|---|---|
| Affective disorders | In affective disorders changes in mood, general vitality and activity are the central feature<br>'Depression' may include low mood, pessimist thoughts, feelings of worthlessness and guilt, slowness or agitation, anxiety, anhedonia, suicidal ideas, apathy, an attentional and other subtle cognitive deficits. Somatic features may be prominent: loss of appetite, libido, weight, and poor sleep.<br>**Mania** is characterised by heightened mood, increased activity, self-important ideas, and occasionally delusions and hallucinations. |
| Schizophrenias and paranoid states | The schizophrenias comprise a group of disorders sharing clusters of positive and negative symptoms. The former include delusions, hallucinations, made feelings, thought insertion, withdrawal, thought disorder. The latter a reduction and or impairment of survival functions such as cognition, activity, interest in the environment, attention, capacity to enjoy things, judgement, executive functions, etc. Typically, the schizophrenias affect young people although it can occasionally be seen after the fourth decade of life. A prominence of negative symptoms predicts bad outcome to treatment. |
| Neuroses | The classification of these disorders is still controversial, and classically includes anxiety, phobias, obsessive-compulsive diseases, hysteria, 'reactive' affective states, and hypochondriasis. |
| Personality disorders | This group of disorders refer to rather fixed personality types that lie outside the accepted range for normal behaviour patterns and comprise: paranoid, cyclothymic, schizoid, explosive, obsessive-compulsive, and hysterical disorders, etc. |

# *The psychiatric assessment of brain disease*

The psychiatric examination of subjects with brain disease includes a *longitudinal* assessment of emotions, volitions, cognitions, personality, coping mechanisms, and their psychosocial and neuropsychological context. It requires that the skills of the psychiatrist be modified and adapted to the singularities of each neurological disease. Psychiatric and neuropsychological assessment, although complementary, are different activities.

## How?

The psychiatric evaluation of the subject with brain disease concerns a person and his social context which, whilst in hospital, must include the medical and para-medical team looking after him. Both the physical and mental state of the patient must be recorded in detail, rather that in short-hand categories, as these are wasteful of information. To say that the patient believes that he is 'seeing shadows by his bed, which talk to him and are trying to kill him' is very different from saying that he has got composite paranoid hallucinations. Neurological patients often complain of experiences that

cannot be recognized in terms of conventional psychiatric categories. These must be acknowledged and recorded rather than dismissed or fitted into some Procrustean category. For example, if the patient is complaining of strange changes in the perception of time, which make him somehow disconnected from his environment, it is no good saying that he is 'depersonalising'.

Baselining behaviour on the first contact is essential. This can be done descriptively or by means of psychiatric instruments. Composite behaviours and psychomotor routines (writing letters, shopping, cooking, taking a taxi, etc.) must also be evaluated, as there is evidence that 'molecular' behaviours alone are not good predictors of ecological competence. There is, however, little guidance in the literature as to which composite behaviours are more predictive. The areas on which some knowledge exists include self-care, independent living, academic achievement, and vocational functioning (Miller 1984).

Examination of family context and social network provides information on premorbid personality, family resources, and the expectations of key carers. The premorbid behaviour of the patient is often idealized by relatives, and finding out what the person 'was really like' can take a great deal of detective work. This information, however, is essential to understanding the magnitude of mental change and to organize social re-entry.

## When?

Assessments carried out too early, particularly when the patient is non-responsive, confused, disorientated or with marked attentional impairment, yield little psychiatric information. At this stage, interloping mental events, e.g. hallucinations, tend to be fleeting, difficult to ascertain on direct questioning, have to be surmised from expressions and behaviours, and as a rule are forgotten by the patient. Paranoid delusions and misidentification syndromes are equally fleeting. Irritability, agitation, and aggression (common causes of referral to the psychiatrist), do not necessarily suggest specific lesions (the proverbial temporal love irritation!) but result from states of 'sensory hyperæsthesia' (causing intolerance to noise, light, and touch, and the feeling that one is overloaded with sensations), reduced capacity to concentrate, and drowsiness. Patients thus affected may develop veritable subclinical confusions sufficient to cause irritability, impair social orientation, and damage the ability to recognize that any ongoing malaise may be the result of an odd bodily position or full bladder.

Very early assessments will often find the patient suffering from reveries or '*mentisme*', i.e. a form of dreaming in wakefulness characterized by unbridled images and thoughts (sometimes frightening in nature), which combine with real perceptions and undermine hold on reality (Heuyer and Lamache 1929). In the subject with acute brain disease, disorientation tends to be persistent and even when correct answers are obtained, the psychiatrist must continue looking for *behavioural disorientation*, which disables the reading of social cues and environmental landmarks (e.g. not responding to the status of others, not finding the toilet, being unable to return to bed, etc.) (Berrios 1982).

Assessments carried out too late have to deal with new confounders. Grief at the realization of the seriousness of the disease, side-effects of medication, dysphasia and other language disorders, etc., will distort the information. Erratic oscillations of mood (Schoenhuber and Gentilini 1988; Middelboe *et al.* 1992). Maladaptive behaviours may also complicate the picture, such as acting-out leading to self-harm, sulking and withdrawing from social interaction, abnormal interactions with members of the staff, misinformation by those who want the patient moved onto another ward, and so on. Once again, the psychiatrist should

resist interpreting these behaviours as resulting from 'temporal lobe or limbic system lesion' or 'emotional incontinence of frontal lobe origin' and look at the broader picture.

Understanding psychological turbulence is not easy, particularly when communication problems preclude a full mental state examination. Differentiating grief from major depression in the diseased brain can be difficult. Mourning subjects may also show feelings of worthlessness and guilt (which in the neurological patient have been considered as indicators of real depression) (Berrios and Samuel 1987). This is why short assessment visits at different times of the day, rather than one long session, will provide more information on circadian variations and behavioural phenocopies (i.e. temporal coincidence of complaints each caused by different aetiology).

The best time to carry out the baseline assessment is usually when the periods of lucidity are long enough (in the case of the brain-damaged patient this is when he is out of post-traumatic amnesia). The problem is that both these periods of lucidity and post-traumatic amnesia (PTA) are difficult to evaluate in themselves.

## Where?

Assessment venues vary according to whether the psychiatrist is part of the neurological team (i.e. has an office in the ward) or whether he is a visiting consultant. A visiting psychiatrist has often little idea of the ward set-up and of the past history of the patient, or there may be little information in the casenotes. The patient may not be able to give a history, or the key worker or relatives may not be present. The psychiatrist may gain a misleading impression of a greater disturbance, particularly if the patient is hostile (has not been told that he will 'be seeing a psychiatrist' or cannot remember) or is embarrassed (e.g. if the interview is conducted in an open ward).

The psychiatric evaluation fulfils diagnostic, management, prognostic, and (sometimes) research purposes. Informing relatives of the current state and outcome, demands psychiatric skills. *Faute de mieux*, the psychiatrist is often cast in the role of senior medical informant. Telling relatives about outcome entails more than uttering probability statements ('there is a 20% chance that the patient will return to his job'). Relatives must be given clear and sympathetic descriptions of how the patient will behave at home, of any changes in mood, level of dependence, sexual behaviour, and ability to deal with his own children.

To improve matters the psychiatrist should make sure that:

(1) a room is available (sister's office is not good enough, for it is often is the busiest place in the ward and the telephone rings all the time!);

(2) the patient is ready at the appointed time (and not having a lengthy investigation done so that there are 5 min left for the psychiatric assessment);

(3) a key informant is available; and

(4) someone from the neuro-team is at hand to discuss the case.

Subjects with brain disease, whether brain-damage, multiple sclerosis (MS), epilepsy, Parkinson's disease (PD), or Huntington's disease (HD), become fatigued easily and tend to be distrustful — particularly because they fear that calling the psychiatrist is the first step towards a mental hospital admission. They may say little during the first interview and not before they have been re-assured. It is always useful to have a word with the ward social worker (who will provide a reliable, social, and family assessment), and the physiotherapist and speech therapists (who have assessed the patient's attitudes, stamina, and motivation).

The reason for the referral gives the psychiatrist important clues as to what might be going on. In order of importance, the commonest reason for such referrals are:

- *behavioural acting out* (which may include angry outbursts or disinhibited behaviour, e.g. sexual advances to nurses);

- *uncooperative behaviour* (refusal to take medication or to participate in physiotherapy);

- '*depression*' (the subject is reported as crying, threatening suicide, looking withdrawn or not thriving);

- help with a surgical or medical *decision* (is the patient consenting enough to have intervention X?);

- and, less often, *research*.

## What for?

The distinction between assessment for *management* and *research* is a useful one, although in conceptual terms there may be little difference. Assessments, regardless of their purpose, occur within constraints determined by:

(1) the validity and reliability of the mapping systems for mental symptoms and categorisation systems for mental diseases;

(2) a body of correlations expressing putative contacts between these mappings and the brain on the one hand and society on the other; and

(3) social warrants supporting the validity of psychiatry as a profession.

These three levels set the boundaries to all forms of assessment, regardless of their objective. There is no deeper science in assessing for research than there is for management. The difference is determined by the way in which the clinician makes use of the belief and knowledge database at his disposal. For example, when assessing for management, he or she may rely more on hearsay, soft social data, and categories such as 'understanding', which may not be used in the sort of 'objective' description demanded by scientific correlations. The crucial question in a way is whether the use of special structured instruments actually adds to the validity of the information obtained. This debate has not yet been settled.

The Neuro-liaison team at Addenbrooke's hospital (Cambridge, UK) follows the same neuropsychiatric assessment protocol regardless of whether it is for management or research (Table 19.2).

# The psychiatry of traumatic brain damage

Although psychiatric morbidity plays a crucial role in the personal and social impact caused by head injury (Mifka 1976), it is often neglected, for epidemiological studies tend to report neuropsychological and psychiatric data together. Likewise, little is known about the long-term prognosis of psychiatric morbidity, namely the proportion of patients that remain intermittently psychotic, depressed, or obsessional years after their injury. Because diagnostic criteria and evaluating instruments change over time, long-term studies of this nature are difficult to implement. In addition, the age and severity ranges of the head-injured population has changed over time. Until 30 years ago, most patients were stable adults with occupational head injuries; currently, the highest proportion is constituted by young people (many with personality or drug problems) (Parmelee *et al.* 1989) with severe injury. There is little

**Table 19.2** Cambridge Computerised Assessment for Neuropsychiatry Clinics and Neuro-Liaison Services

(IMPORTANT: ALL *CORE* TESTS MUST BE APPLIED)
Name:............................ Date:.............. Short ID:........

| | Computer code | Tick if applied |
|---|---|---|
| **General:** | | |
| General Health Questionnaire: | GHQ | ○ |
| Insight | INS | ○ |
| Personality Deviance Scale | PER | ○ |
| **Affective Disorders:** | | |
| Hamilton Depression Scale (observer rated) | HDS | ○ |
| Profile of Mood States | POMS | ○ |
| Irritability Scale | IRR | ○ |
| Hospital-Anxiety Depression Scale | HAD | ○ |
| Mania Scale | MAN | ○ |
| Beck Depression Inventory | BECK | ○ |
| Geriatric Depression Scale (*for older than 65*) | GDS | ○ |
| **Cognitive:** | | |
| Attention Test | ATT | ○ |
| Signal Detection Memory Test | SIGNAL | ○ |
| Metamemory Test | MET | ○ |
| Cognitive Failures Questionnaire | CFQ | ○ |
| **Neuroses:** | | |
| Obsessions interference / resistance | OCD | ○ |
| Obsessive–Compulsive Disorder | MOC | ○ |
| Hypochondria Scale | HYP | ○ |
| Zung Anxiety Scale | ZG | ○ |
| Phobias Scale | PHO | ○ |
| Dissociative Behaviours Questionnaire | DIS | ○ |
| Self-evaluation Questionnaire (Form Y-1) | STAI | ○ |
| Self-evaluation Questionnaire (Form Y-2) | STAI2 | ○ |

(NB: please apply other relevant instruments according to findings in interview)

doubt that advances in resuscitation techniques (Lee *et al.* 1990; Cohadon *et al.* 1991; Miller 1991) have contributed to the survival of the seriously injured. Each year, in a region with a population of around 3.5 million people (e.g. the size of East Anglia or Greater Manchester), around 140 people will survive moderate to severe brain trauma. They then will join a population of up to 70 000 disabled survivors, most of whom have a normal life expectancy (Medical Disability Society 1988).

Helmets and car belts have contributed to creating a different type of 'brain-injured' subject. In the immediate wake of the accident, many may show no detectable neurosurgical signs and only complain in the middle term of chronic headache, fatigue, dizziness, reduced libido, and irritability. Some of these subjects will in due course engross the ranks of the so-called 'post-concussional syndrome' or 'mild head injury' patients

(Bruyn and Lanser 1990; Bohnen and Jolles 1992; Fenton *et al.* 1993).

Little is known about what increases the risk of developing psychiatric complications. There is some evidence that the latter correlates with duration of PTA, i.e. the period following a brain injury for which the patient has no memory (Steadman and Graham 1970; Lishman 1973). Psychiatric morbidity seems also to be associated with marked attentional, language, and memory impairment, although these very deficits may cloak the presence of mental symptoms. More practical predictors are history of alcohol abuse and premorbid psychiatric illness.

## Course

The coma caused by the injury is followed by disorientation, fluctuating confusion, irritability, restlessness, and agitation, over-reactivity to stimuli, and inversion of sleep rhythms. This veritable delirium occupies the early part of the post-traumatic amnesia. Fleeting hallucinations and delusions, often paranoid in nature, may also be present during this stage of the disease but tend to be underdiagnosed, for patients often enough conceal their presence (fearing that they are 'going mad'). Rarer neuropsychiatric complaints include beliefs that parts of the body or surroundings have been duplicated, delusions of memory, confabulations, and misidentification phenomena (e.g. the patient may believe that his wife is an impostor looking exactly like her).

As the confusional state and capacity for communication improve, the subject becomes accessible to assessment. In addition to psychiatric symptoms, he might have impairments of higher cortical functions ranging from mild memory problems to a severe state of cognitive disorganisation. In the brain-injured, there tends to be a rapid improvement during the first few months and then a gradual one over the next 5 years. In few cases, no improvement is seen and dense states of so-called 'traumatic dementia' can set in (Feher *et al.* 1988). It has now been repeatedly suggested that mild trauma might accelerate pre-existing cognitive decline (Mazzuchi *et al.* 1992) or precipitate Alzheimer's (Rudelli *et al.* 1982; Clinton *et al.* 1991) and Pick's disease (Kosaka *et al.* 1980).

## Affective symptoms

Whether overt or covert, agitation and anxiety are pervading in subjects with brain injury. Starting early, the symptoms may get worse as the patient gains insight into his condition. It has been suggested that agitation is related to dysattention (Corrigan *et al.* 1992) and anxiety correlates with the severity of neuropsychological impairment (Bornstein *et al.* 1989). This means that, in practice, a modicum of anxiety is omnipresent and must be dealt with.

Risk of depression is increased by about ten-fold in traumatic head injury (Gualtieri and Cox 1991; Silver *et al.* 1991; Fedoroff *et al.* 1992); and hence about 42% of subjects will suffer from this condition during the first year after injury (Fedoroff *et al.* 1993). Jorge *et al.* (1993b) have suggested that earlier forms of depression are a direct manifestation of the lesion, whilst latter forms result from psychosocial factors. Family history of affective disorder seems to play a lesser role in the development of depression than of mania (Robinson

1988). When matched for site of lesion, however, brain injury sufferers seem to have *less* depression than stroke patients (Robinson 1981).

In the context of brain damage, depression may be difficult to distinguish from chronic hopelessness and grief (Tadir and Stern 1985). Behavioural phenocopies, i.e. coincidences of features each generated by a different aetiology, also lead to over-diagnosis (Berrios and Samuel 1987; Berrios and Dening 1990). It has been claimed, however, that DSM III-R criteria for depressive episode are an adequate tool for diagnosed (Jorge *et al.* 1993a) (see Box 19.1). Others have used the DSM III-R category 'organic mood syndrome' for the same purpose. In this regard, it has been claimed that cases falling under this category are more difficult to treat! (Barnhill and Gualtieri 1989). Depression is also considered as a late complication in both 'post-concussion syndrome' (Szymanski and Linn 1992) and whiplash

---

### Box 19.1   Definitions and mechanisms of head injury

Head injury results from the sudden application of a physical force to the head resulting in injury to the brain. Other terms used to describe head injuries are listed below.

- *Blunt or non-penetrating injuries.* Even though the skull is not penetrated, such injuries may induce loss of consciousness, and result in gross and widespread brain damage.

- *Penetrating injuries.* High-velocity missiles penetrate the skull and brain, or less frequently the skull is subject to a crush injury. In these injuries the patient may suffer serious or even fatal injury without preceding loss of consciousness.

- *Concussion.* Violent shaking or jarring of the brain with transient functional impairment with no definition of underlying nerve cells. The existence of this condition has not been confirmed by animal experiments nor clinical studies.

- *Contusion.* This literally means bruising of the brain and is a rather loose term in clinical use.

injury (Ettlin *et al.* 1992). 'Severe depression' can appear *de novo* 3 years after the injury (Burke *et al.* 1990).

Patients who do not improve after antidepressant treatment have been found to have received their injury in an assault, and to have abused alcohol before the event (Dunlop *et al.* 1991). Depression predicts a bad response to rehabilitation (Ryan *et al.* 1992); indeed, it has been reported to correlate with fatigue, which is a known obstacle to rehabilitation (Walker *et al.* 1991).

## Schizophrenias-like states

Regardless of severity, brain-injured subjects may experience delusions or hallucinations and, less frequently, functional psychoses. The significance of these complaints depends upon premorbid personality, extent and type of lesion, and stage of recovery. During the post-injury confusional state, hallucinations are fleeting and probably non-specific (Muller 1974; Ferrey and Gagey 1987). During recovery, when cognitive grasp and orientation have been regained, hallucinations have to be taken seriously as they may be the only manifestation of seizural activity. Thus, Varney *et al.* (1992) found that in 25 head-injured patients the presence of olfactory hallucinations correlated with theta bursts on the EEG. More rarely, hallucinations may be the result of conversive and dissociative mechanisms released by the injury. It is said that in such cases the hallucinations are rich, detailed, and ever-changing.

The prevalence of delusions in head injury remains unknown. Achte *et al.* (1991) reported that 28% of a sample of 3000 war veterans with moderate or severe brain injury were suffering from paranoid delusions, the commonest types being jealousy and fear of being sexually betrayed. Delusions occurring in the wake of head injury are often bizarre. For example, Young *et al.* (1992) reported the case of a 24-year-old man with a right temporo-parietal injury who developed a belief that he was dead (Cotard's delusion); and Kellner and Strian (1991) described the case of a 65-year-old man who, after a traumatic haemorrhage in his left basal ganglia, developed the bizarre delusion of having 'artificial tubes implanted into his body'. There is some evidence that a schizophrenia-like state (Box 19.2) may occasionally develop in head injury. It has also been suggested that brain injury may contribute to schizophrenia in later life (Box 19.3). Fenwick *et al.* (1985) studied 17 subjects from the College of Psychic studies and found that they had experienced more 'mystical experiences' and 'psychic sensitivity' than controls, and that

they also had a significantly more frequent history of head injury.

## Behavioural and personality changes

Since the nineteenth century it has been known that changes in character and personality may result from brain injury, particularly when the frontal and temporal lobes are involved (Welt 1888, quoted in Bumke 1947; De Mol 1981; Stuss and Gow 1992). Premorbid personality traits and history of drug abuse increase the risk of personality change. Objective assessment of such

---

### Box 19.2   Evidence for schizophrenia-like state in head injury

In 14 389 head-injured patients, Davison and Bagley (1969) reported that 'traumatic insanity' (a concept wider than schizophrenia) occurred with a prevalence of 2.24%. This figure significantly exceeds chance expectation. Furthermore, there was an association with temporal lobe lesions. The commonest mechanism was severe closed head injury.

Recent research has confirmed the above finding.

(1) A follow-up study of 291 head-injured subjects found nine cases of 'schizophreniform psychosis' (Roberts 1979).

(2) Thomsen (1984) found eight cases of schizophrenia and one of schizophreniform psychosis in a sample of 40 severe close head-injuries.

(3) Nasrallah *et al.* (1981) have reported a case with good premorbid history and no family history who developed schizophrenia-like state after head injury.

(4) Based on the description of six cases, De Mol *et al.* (1982) have suggested that young men are more prone to developing a form of traumatic psychosis whose clinical presentation is no different from that of conventional schizophrenia. Interestingly, severity of injury does not seem to be a relevant factor.

---

### Box 19.3 Head injury as a causal factor in schizophrenia

- The presence of early head injury seems to be a factor in the development of schizophrenia-like states in adolescents (O'Callaghan *et al.* 1988).

- Patients with schizophrenia are claimed to have a significantly higher rate of childhood head trauma than controls with mania, depression or no mental disorder (Wilcox and Nasrallah 1987).

Against this, other authors have claimed that early brain damage may *protect* against schizophrenia (Lewis *et al.* 1990). Nasrallah and Wilcox (1989) have attempted to tease out the respective contribution of genetic and head-injury factors, and concluded that the latter seems more important in males. This contradicts older findings that the presence of 'alien tissue' (small focal tumours, hamartomas, and focal dysplasia) in the temporal lobe is more likely to cause schizophrenia-like states in the female (Taylor 1975).

---

### Box 19.4 Biological markers in neuropsychiatry

Need for, and general problems of, biological markers in psychiatry:

| | |
|---|---|
| Depression | Dexamethasone suppression test (doubtful validity) |
| | Receptor status (classical) |
| | Platelet serotonin uptake (classical) |
| Scanning | PET studies (classical) |
| | Functional MRI (growing) |
| | EEG and Brain cartography (classical) |
| | Response to Transcranial Magnetic Stimulation (growing) |

---

## The psychiatry of cerebrovascular disorder

This section deals with the psychiatric sequelae of both large vessel disease (stroke), aneurysmal haemorrhage, and small vessel pathology, (e.g. Binswanger's disease and systemic lupus erithematosus (SLE) vasculitis).

### Affective symptoms

Depression is reported in stroke with a frequency ranging between 25% to 70% (Starkstein and Robinson 1993). Important issues, however, remain unresolved, not least that of the validity of the diagnosis of 'depression' itself (Ross and Rush 1981; Primeau 1988). Over-diagnosis seems a problem here and is accounted for by the use of the wrong diagnostic criteria and instruments. Time of assessment, type of sample, and training of assessor all seem to contribute to inflating the data. Indeed, when these variables are controlled rates of reported depression fall sharply (Agrell and Dehlin 1989; Egelko *et al.* 1989; House *et al.* 1989, 1991; Parikh *et al.* 1988; Sharpe *et al.* 1990).

Stroke patients diagnosed as depressed cannot often be separated from controls on the basis of the dexamethasone suppression test (Box 19.4) although non-suppression seems to correlate with stroke severity regardless of whether depression is present or not (Reding *et al.* 1985; Olsson *et al.* 1989; Dam *et al.* 1991; Grober *et al.* 1991). Growth hormone response to

---

changes is not easy, for no reliable tools are available. 'Design fluency' and performance on the Wisconsin card-sorting test are often used as proxy variables but such usage makes the assumption that 'personality' is related to the frontal lobes. Personality change has a particular negative impact on rehabilitation.

### Other mental changes

Head-injured subjects show a variety of mental changes whose nature is, on occasions, elusive and challenging of conventional psychopathological categories. For example, the frequency of obsessional behaviour seems increased in head injury, as is that of untriggered laughing and crying, maudlinism, apathy, anhedonia, and alexithymia. Sleep changes, ranging from secondary narcolepsy to major disturbances of sleep architecture with fitful sleep or insomnia are not uncommon. Lastly, reductions in sexual drive and libido, changes in sexual object, and disinhibition can be seen.

desipramine has been reported as blunted in stroke subjects, suggesting diminished alpha-2 adrenoreceptor function (Barry and Dinan 1990); and platelet serotonin uptake seems also significantly reduced in post-stroke depressives (Barry *et al.* 1990). In at least one unmedicated subject, PET-measured cortical serotonin-2 receptors were reported to increase by 25% pari passu with clinical improvement (Mayberg *et al.* 1991). In an earlier study, the same research group found that, in non-depressed stroke subjects, non-damaged areas had greater cortical binding of serotonin-2 receptor than damaged areas, and that this differential was more marked for right-hemisphere strokes. Mayberg *et al.* (1988) concluded that depression may be due to a failure to up-regulate serotonin receptors after stroke, and that the biochemical response of the brain may be different depending upon what hemisphere was involved.

Some studies have reported more depression in left/anterior strokes (Morris *et al.* 1992); others in right-sided strokes (Williams *et al.* 1986; Danel *et al.* 1989; Finset *et al.* 1989); yet others have found no association at all (Rosse and Ciolino 1985; House *et al.* 1990) or only differences in severity (Sinyor *et al.* 1986). These contradictory results may be partly explained by the biases causes by the fact that the studies have been carried out in stroke survivors and in subjects with preserved communicational abilities (Zerfass *et al.* 1992).

## Other mental changes

As the acute confusional states that accompany the early stages of stroke subside, isolated delusions and hallucinations may be uncovered. Emotionalism, unmotivated crying, pathological display of affect, and distorted expression of emotions are also common. For example, Borod *et al.* (1985) have reported that subjects with unilateral right-sided damage use facial expression and intonation less frequently than subjects with left-sided lesions.

Anderson (1990) reported a typical case of Koro in a white British subject with a non-dominant temporo-parietal stroke. Peroutka *et al.* (1982) reported the case of a man with right temporo-parietal stroke who presented delusions and hallucinations; and Levine and Finklestein (1982) described delayed psychosis in eight subjects with similar right-sided lesions. Price and Mesulam (1985) described agitation, paranoid delusions, hallucinations, and lack of appropriate concern in five subjects with infarcts in the right hemisphere. Danel *et al.* (1992) have reported delusions in a left-

lenticular infarction with right frontal involvement, and Assal and Bindschaedler (1990) delusional disorientation in a patient with left hemisphere stroke. Based on five subjects, Rabins *et al.* (1991) suggested that subjects are more prone to developing schizophrenia-like psychosis when they have pre-existing subcortical atrophy and right-sided strokes.

In general, therefore, it would seem that delusions of various types may appear in the wake of a variety of brain insults affecting either hemisphere or the mid-line (Cummings 1985). Cutting (1990), in turn, has suggested that lesions affecting the right temporal hemisphere generate delusional beliefs at a rate higher than chance. Meyendorf (1976) found in a sample of 150 subjects undergoing heart surgery that those who developed psychosis after cerebral embolism had a significantly higher family history of psychiatric illness.

Arteriosclerotic pathology of basal small vessels causes lacunar destruction of white matter and this, on occasions, may be accompanied by subcortical slowness and mild memory impairment, a syndrome that has been called 'Binswanger's disease' (Janota 1981). Hallucinosis, mania, disinhibition, and change in personality complete the condition (Englund *et al.* 1989; Coffey and Figiel 1991). Cerebral small vessels may also be involved in SLE. Thus about 40% of SLE patients are known to have a degree of central nervous system involvement, and up to 50% exhibit cognitive impairment (Van Dam 1991); a smaller number will also show delusions, hallucinations, and affective changes (Giang 1991).

# The psychiatry of Huntington's disease

The relationship between psychiatric morbidity and HD is complicated by conceptual problems relating to, amongst other things, the definition of the psychiatric morbidity itself and the method of its capture. There is little space in this chapter to explore such issues in depth (Berrios and Samuel 1987; Berrios and Dening 1990; Berrios and Quemada 1990) but some essential points need to be highlighted.

First, there is the question as to whether the relationship between psychiatric morbidity and all neurological diseases can be subsumed under a single model. Empirical evidence thus far would suggest that the relationship between mental symptoms and neurological diseases, which are non-progressive, and those which are progressive seems to be different. Hence, it might make sense to construct different interactional models in relation to each neurological disease. Second, the actual nature of the relationship between mental symptoms and neurological disease is unclear and several possibilities need to be considered. For example, the mental symptoms may be 'caused' directly by the neurological lesion or they may be 'triggered' in some other way by the presence of the neurological disease. Alternatively, they may arise or be present coincidentally. In addition, it may not be clear whether such mental symptoms are in fact isolated symptoms, or syndromes or diseases. Third, there is the issue concerning the sorts of mental symptoms seen in the context of neurological diseases and whether these constitute the 'same' phenomena as those seen in psychiatric practice. Lastly, one may ask if the symptoms 'caused' by the neurological lesion should be considered as concomitants of the disease or as a defining part of it: in other words, when do psychiatric symptoms become essential to the definition of a given neurological disease? We believe that views in this area are mostly controlled by history and tradition (i.e. the fact that some diseases have been considered as 'neurological' since they were constructed during the inenteenth century) and more empirical research, including the search for real phenotypes, is required. One way of investigating the latter is by seeking correlations between CAG repeats and mental symptoms (see below) (Berrios *et al.*, in press).

## Prevalence

The prevalence of conventional psychiatric disorder in HD ranges from 25% to 80% (Harper 1991). This wide range is likely to result from variations in diagnostic routines. Thus, because single symptoms such as irritability, anger/hostility (Baxter *et al.* 1992), apathy, and delusions of persecution (Pflanz *et al.* 1991), or excessive worrying and somatic complaints (Ball *et al.* 1974; Webb and Trzepacz 1987) tend to be more common in HD than full-fledged mental diseases, the severe application of DSM-IV or ICD-10 criteria will yield lower rates of psychiatric morbidity than if a symptom-orientated data capture is implemented. Partly to deal with this problem, the suggestion has been made that a dimensional symptom-based approach should be used (Caine and Shoulson 1983). Under-diagnosis may also result from the fact that HD patients (like sufferers of other neurological disorders) issue mental complaints that are not recordable, for they do not match conven-

tional clinical categories: for example, HD patients may experience strange disturbances in their perception of time, emotions, and insight, or show rigidities of thinking and behaviour for which no name has yet been coined. The fact that absolute onset of HD remains difficult to determine may also contribute to the loss of psychiatric information. This is because there is some evidence that 'psychiatric' morbidity in the form of emotional disturbance and change of personality may appear very early in the development of HD (Lyon 1962; Dewhurst *et al.* 1969; Wallace and Hall 1972).

Lastly, it cannot be ruled out that, on occasions, over-diagnosis also contributes to the wide-ranging prevalence figures. In this sense, a proportion of the 'morbidity' captured by psychiatric instruments, particularly when applied cross-sectionally, is likely to be constituted by behavioural phenocopies (Berrios and Samuel 1987).

## Affective disorders

Since very early it has been known that affective (mainly depressive) symptoms are common in HD (Hamilton 1908). Oliver (1970) found depressed mood, lack of interest, subjective feelings of inability to cope, and tiredness in 18% of his patients. In the West of Scotland survey, Bolt (1970) identified depressive symptoms in 29% of female and 20% of male patients, but no gender effect on suicidal behaviour. Mattson (1974) reported depressive symptoms in 16% of his sample. Wallace and Hall (1972) and Brothers and Meadows (1955) have also commented on the high frequency of depressive symptoms in HD patients. Dewhurst *et al.* (1970) found depression with anxiety and obsessional traits, and anxiety states (including secondary neurasthenia, depressive and hysterical symptoms) in 36% of their patients.

Interestingly, early studies rarely report full-blown depressive psychoses or bipolar states. For example, Saugstad and Odegard (1986) in Norway identified only one case of 'depressive psychosis' and six cases of depression of 'moderate severity' in their case review of 199 inpatients admitted between 1916 and 1975. Mattson (1974) remarked that 'depressive-anxious states' was less common (15%) than 'schizophrenic-paranoid state' (17%) or personality disorders (24%). Bolt (1970) reported that 'affective psychoses' were less common (17%) than 'schizophrenia and paranoid psychoses', the latter forming the largest psychiatric diagnostic group in her sample.

On the other hand, earlier studies had reached different conclusions: Davenport (1916) noted that manic-depressive psychosis was commonly associated with HD but suggested that this association might affect only certain pedigrees. In 102 patients, Dewhurst *et al.* (1969) found affective states and psychoneuroses (*n* = 20) to be the commonest psychiatric diagnoses. A similar conclusion was reached by Bickford and Ellison (1953). With the exception of Bolt (1970), who reported two cases of mania, no other study mentions either mania or hypomania.

In the last 20 years, studies based on modern diagnostic criteria and prospective follow-up have concluded that the 'affective syndrome' seems commonest. McHugh and Folstein (1975) followed up eight psychiatric inpatients and found 'an affective disorder that affects a considerable proportion and can mimic in every way manic-depressive illness'. Caine and Shoulson (1983) followed up 30 patients for 2–6 years and classified 'behavioural disorders' using DSM III criteria and a structured diagnostic interview. They found dysthymic disorder (*n* = 6) and major depressive disorder (*n* = 5) to be the commonest psychiatric disorders (37%). No diagnosis of bipolar disorder was made. Perhaps the most persuasive evidence for the high prevalence of affective syndromes in HD comes from a remarkable study by Folstein *et al.* (1983) involving 88 HD patients, who were assessed using a structured interview (the NIMH Diagnostic Interview Schedule — DIS), including the spouse as an informant, together with a clinical psychiatric evaluation, a review of all obtainable case notes; and, in 46 cases, personal longitudinal follow up of 1–7 years. They found a high prevalence (41%) of affective disorders, of which 32% were depressive and 9% bipolar disorders In the Maryland study, Folstein *et al.* (1987) found that the prevalence of affective disorder was 33%. Recent retrospective studies (Pflanz *et al.* 1991; Shiwach 1994) report a prevalence of depression of 53% and 39%, respectively. CATEGO analysis of their data by Pflanz *et al.* (1991) classified two-thirds of cases into the available affective diagnosis categories.

Authors have also reported that depressive symptoms can precede the onset of chorea (Bolt 1970; Dewhurst *et al.* 1970; Mattson 1974). For example, Folstein *et al.* (1983b) reported that in 70% of cases, depression preceded the onset of chorea by an average of 5 years; that high figure dropped to 41% and 32%, respectively, when depressive reactions, grief, etc., were excluded. In an interesting study, Mindham *et al.* (1985) compared matched samples of HD and Alzheimer's disease patients on psychiatric morbidity prior to the onset of dementia. Although numbers were small and Alzheimer's patients were significantly older, the HD group showed twice as many cases with major affective disorders; the authors concluded that there was a specific relationship between HD and major affective disorders. This disorder seems to respond to ECT (Ranen *et al.* 1994; Lewis *et al.* 1996). Folstein *et al.* (1983a) studied prevalence of affective disorders among 112 offspring of 34 HD patients. They concluded that affective disorder in the offspring was associated with the presence of similar symptoms in the HD parent, and was unrelated to earlier family disorganization. There were no cases of mania.

Thus 'depression' seems far more common than mania. Its aetiology, however, is likely to be multiple. In addition, the high prevalence figures quoted may be partially spurious.

- Over-diagnosis can be caused by the use of instruments not designed to yield categorical discrimination (e.g. the Hamilton Depression Scale and the Beck Depression Inventory, which are not diagnostic instruments and should not be used in patients suffering an organic disorder).

- A host of affective symptoms can be caused by grief and reactional syndromes resulting from faulty learning, living in a HD home, and so on.

- Behavioural phenocopies are not infrequent in HD. They are caused by combinations of the early mood changes seen in HD dementia together with motor, cognitive, and anxiety symptoms due to a variety of aetiologies (Mindham *et al.* 1985).

Once these obvious causes of over-diagnosis are excluded, the researcher is left with a core of cases to which the brain changes of HD are relevant. Thus, a relationship seems to exist between affective symptoms and the atrophy and neo-striatal neuronal loss seen in HD (Marsden 1982; Weinberger *et al.* 1988). The basal ganglia-thalamo-cortical circuits are known to play an important role in the generation and monitoring of motor and cognitive plans and emotional sets. In regard to the latter, rich connections have been described between the caudate with the limbic system (Saint-Cyr *et al.* 1995). It has been suggested that in HD the affective disorder relates to the part of the neostriatum damaged earliest, viz. dorsal-medial caudate (Peyser and Folstein 1990).

## Suicide

In his description of the disease, George Huntington commented on the 'tendency to suicide', which he considered to be one of the major features of the illness (Huntington 1872). Since then many studies (Reed and Chandler 1958; Dewhurst *et al.* 1970) have confirmed this to be the case. Suicide occurs more frequently in the early stages of the illness, but its rate increases again in the 50–69-year-group, where it is eight times higher than in general population (Schoenfeld *et al.* 1984). In addition to age, other risk factors include absence of offspring, family history of suicide, unmarried state, contact with other HD sufferers, living alone, and depression (Lipe *et al.* 1993).

## Schizophrenia-like states

Before the 1970s, there was a tendency to report a high incidence of schizophrenia and paranoid psychoses. For example, the rates reported by Bolt (1970) and Saugstad and Odegard (1986) were 15% and 20%, respectively; and the corresponding figure for the diagnosis 'schizophrenic-paranoid state' reported by Mattson (1974) was 17%. These studies were mainly retrospective and used looser diagnostic criteria.

On the other hand, Oliver (1970) reported only a 6% of schizophreniform 'symptoms' (e.g. paranoid delusions, ideas of reference, bizarre behaviour — described as 'queerness and irrational behaviour'); and in the study by Dewhurst *et al.* (1970), only 7% of patients had an initial diagnosis of schizophrenia. More recent studies have tended to confirm that schizophrenia is uncommon in HD. For example, Webb and Trzepacz (1987), using DSM-III diagnostic criteria, did not find a single patient with such diagnosis in their sample of 10 patients. Folstein *et al.* (1983b, 1987) using similar diagnostic criteria and the DIS, found that only 3% and 6%, respectively, of their patients had schizophrenia, compared with 41% and 33%, respectively, with affective disorders. Caine and Shoulson (1983), using DSM-III criteria found only three out of 30 patients with schizophrenia; two other patients showed acute onset psychoses following discontinuation of neuroleptics, presumably prescribed for the motor disorder. In the study by Jensen *et al.* (1993), none of 37 HD patients showed the disease at the moment of discharge, although 11% of patients (*n* = 4) were thought to be 'psychotic' at the time of admission. Using the PSE-CATEGO classification, Pflanz *et al.* (1991) found that the commonest psychotic features were delusions of persecution (23%) but the symptoms were seen in association with dementia or 'non-specific psychoses'; nuclear, catatonic, residual syndromes, and incoherent speech occurred only in 2–6% of patients. A study of 110 HD patients from 30 families by Shiwach (1994) found that only three patients (2.7%) had schizophrenia; although retrospective, this study applied a strict methodology.

Discrepancies between early and later studies are likely to relate less to changes in the psychiatric morbidity of HD than to vicissitudes of the diagnosis of schizophrenia. This variability was compounded by the retrospective nature of reports (Bolt 1970; Mattson 1974; Saugstad and Odegard 1986; Pflanz *et al.* 1991; Shiwach 1994); by biases inherent in the sample studied, for example, of inpatients whose admission may have been motivated by the presence of psychoses in the first place (Mattson 1974; Saugstad and Odegard 1986); and by a past tendency to over-diagnose schizophrenia (Cooper *et al.* 1972) on the basis of oddities of behaviour, difficult interpersonal relationships, and persecutory ideas. Indeed, writing 'odd letters' was sufficient for such a diagnosis in at least one case (Oliver 1970). Lastly, in regards to HD patients there is the additional issue of co-morbidity (psychosis and a brain disease) and the assumption made that the former has been caused by the latter. Under the DSM system, psychotic symptoms in HD come under the rubric of 'organic mental syndrome' or 'organic mental disorder' (Webb and Trzepacz 1987). Not all authors, however, have operated under these constraints (Caine and Shoulson 1983; Folstein *et al.* 1983, 1987) and made used of other diagnostic categories. This inconsistency of usage may lead to much variability in reported rates for a disease.

Schizophrenic and paraphrenic symptoms can predate the motor disorder (Mattson 1974; Saugstad and Odegard 1986; Bolt 1970; Oliver 1970). It is now believed, however, that most of these clinical states do not constitute schizophrenia and according to the predominant symptom are called 'delusion-hallucinatory states' (McHugh and Folstein 1975), 'hallucinatory states which do not meet all research criteria and did not respond to phenothiazines' (Folstein *et al.* 1979), 'hallucinosis — sometimes called schizophrenia, specially in mental hospital records, in the absence of clear delusions' (Folstein and Folstein 1983b); and 'delusionary and hallucinatory states, particularly in young women, where schizophrenia may have appeared before dementia' (Folstein and McHugh 1983). First-degree relatives of HD have a variable incidence of schizophrenia. While Mattson (1974) did not find a single case among 31 first-degree relatives of three HD probands, Saugstad and Odegard (1986) reported four families from a series of 135 families in which 'several' relatives were diagnosed as suffering from schizophrenia. Using two families in a small case-control study, Tsuang *et al.* (1998) concluded that family history of schizophrenia-like symptoms may segregate with the HD gene. Watt and Seller (1993) found a 10% prevalence of schizophrenia in affected patients, but not a single case among subjects at 50% risk of HD.

It seems likely therefore that some of the schizophrenia-like syndromes seen in HD are related to the underlying brain pathology. In this regard, it has been suggested that the general motor disorder model could be used to explain the generation of schizophrenia: an intact nigro-striatal pathway would continue releasing approximately 'normal' quantities of dopamine, which would over-stimulate a reduced number of target striatal neurones and cause the motor disorder of HD (Spokes 1980; Marsden 1982); a similar mechanism in the meso-limbic system could generate schizophrenia-like symptoms.

## Obsessive–compulsive disorder

Obsessive–compulsive disorder (OCD) is rarely reported in HD. Dewhurst *et al.* (1970) observed 'obsessional features' in 7% of their patients. In their 6-year follow-up, Caine and Shoulson (1983) and Folstein *et al.* (1983) made no mention of it. Since then, only six patients have been reported exhibiting this comorbidity: three cases by Cummings and Cunningham (1992) and Tonkongy (1989), and three by Marchi *et al.* (1998). The latter are interesting for they belonged to a pedigree where OCD occurred before the onset of HD. All six cases are phenomenologically convincing and not merely repetitive or stereotypical behaviour. Marchi *et al.* (1998) also speculated that the HD gene might contribute to the overall clinical picture of OCD or OC-related disorders; and that the gene (or one of the genes) for OCD and OC-related disorders may be physically close to HD gene. Cummings and Cunningham (1992) observed that OCD is more commonly associated with frontal and striatal disease. Because similar lesions can be observed in HD, it has been suggested that the latter could become a experimental model for OCD; in practice, however, patients with idiopathic OCD and HD differ in terms of their profile of cognitive dysfunction (Martin *et al.* 1993).

## Personality disorder

Behavioural and personality disorders are often mentioned in HD but much variability seems to exist in the description and criteria adopted for diagnosis (Shepherd and Sartorius 1974). This makes trans-historical comparison difficult. Early studies (Rosenbaum 1941; Chandler *et al.* 1960; Brothers 1964) reported an increased incidence of disturbance of 'temperament' in HD patients — especially in the prodromal phase of the illness. According to later studies (Oliver 1970; Bolt 1970; Dewhurst 1970; Mattson 1974; Saugstad and Odegard 1986), 'personality deviation' ranges from 10% (Bolt 1970) to 35% (Saugstad and Odegard 1986). Striking in all these clinical descriptions is the preponderance of affective symptoms. Patients are described as 'emotionally unstable', 'moody', 'excitable', 'quarrelsome', 'childish' (Oliver 1970), 'difficult', 'unpleasant', 'excessively strict' (Bolt 1970), 'anxious', 'depressed', 'inadequate' (Dewhurst *et al.* 1970), 'apathetic', 'suspicious', 'irritable' (Shiwach 1994), 'hysterical' and 'neurotic' (Mattson 1974). Authors have also commented on personality changes, which 'sometimes resulted in alcoholism and criminal behaviour' (Mattson 1974) and antisocial behaviour including 'violence, lying, thieving, cruelty to young children and acting as a con-man' (Oliver 1970). Other authors (Saugstad and Odegard 1986) seem to have included in their description states redolent of paranoid psychosis and schizophrenia. Prevalence figures obtained by means of modern diagnostic criteria yield lower rates: for example, using DSM-III criteria, Folstein *et al.* (1983, 1987) found only 2% and 5.9% prevalence of 'antisocial personality disorder', respectively; and none of the cases in the sample by Caine and Shoulson (1983) meet criteria DSM for personality disorder, although two showed 'antisocial personality changes' and two 'paranoid behaviour'.

As it is the case with other forms of psychiatric morbidity, these lower rates probably result from the more stringent diagnostic criteria in use but the type of samples (severe hospital cases versus outpatients) studied and the wider availability of tranquillizing medication may also be important factors. Thus, symptoms such as irritability, moroseness, querulousness, anxiety, and depression were interpreted in early studies as pertaining to personality changes. The concept of 'choreopathy' (Kehrer 1928; Panse 1942), first put forth by German psychiatrists, is worth mentioning in this respect. It encompassed the gamut of personality changes occurring in HD, as well as any premorbid abnormal personality that might have been present long before the onset of motor symptoms. The 'choreopathic' patients were either 'callous, instinctual or irritable' or 'hyperthymic, depressives, anxious, fantastic or hysterical'; and had a prevalence of between 20% and 80% (Panse 1942; Huber 1981). In regard to the role of management in the prevalence decline mentioned above, it is interesting to remark that in the sample reported by Caine and Shoulson (1983), five out six patients improved on antidepressants.

One problem with using the DSM system is that the first manifestations of personality disorder should occur by adolescence and a proportion of HD patients might not meet this criterion. For example, two of the patients in the series of Caine and Shoulson (1983) developed their antisocial personality changes after age of 30 and 2–3 years after the onset of movement disorder. Folstein et al., in their Maryland survey (Folstein et al. 1987), did not make explicit age of onset in their cases with antisocial PD. The category 'organic personality disorder' (Wallace and Hall 1972; Shiwach and Norbury 1994) might help in this regard, as it would be reasonable to assume that the personality changes seen in either the prodromal phase or after the establishment of HD are 'organic' in nature (Weinberger et al. 1988; Aylward et al. 1998) and would include cognitive inflexibility, poor planning and reduced initiative reflecting impaired performance on neuropsychological tests of executive and frontal lobe functions (Hodges et al. 1990; Hanes et al. 1995; Lange et al. 1995).

Behavioural and personality disorders seen several years prior to the onset of HD are difficult to link to HD, for environmental explanations may loom larger in these cases. Indeed, in their study of offspring of HD patients, Folstein et al. (1983) showed that disorders of conduct beginning in adolescence and sometimes continuing into adult life as antisocial personality disorder, were closely related to the social disorganization which occurred most often in large families, where the affected parent's symptoms began early and the unaffected parent could not maintain the family structure. Equally telling in this regard is the finding by Dewhurst (1970) of behavioural disorders in spouses and unrelated family members who had no risk of inheriting HD.

## Alcohol abuse

Alcohol abuse can be studied as a separate category of dysfunction or as part of the affective or personality disorders. We shall use the latter strategy here. Early studies reported high rates of alcoholism in HD (Hans

and Gilmore 1968; Oliver 1970); for example, Dewhurst (1970) quoted a 20% incidence. However, in her survey in the West of Scotland (an area 'where alcoholism and heavy weekend drinking are common'), Bolt (1970) reported excessive drinking in only 13 out of 334 cases. Mattson (1974) suggested in passim that alcohol problems may be responsible for some of the 'personality changes' shown by his Swedish sample. Saugstad and Odegard (1986) reported that in 8% of subjects alcoholism was a problem and that in most cases it might be related to 'personality deviation prior to admission to hospital'. Similarly Hughes (1925) and Spillane and Phillips (1937) found 'little evidence' of alcoholism in their probands.

The prevalence figures in more recent studies (Folstein et al. 1983, 1987) range from 10% to 15%. A study specifically dedicated to the question in hand has found that the prevalence of current or past alcohol abuse is about 16%; in this sample there was a preponderance of males, and cases had a family history of alcohol abuse; alcohol abuse was accompanied by depression and had usually started before the onset of motor symptoms; however, the overall rate of alcohol abuse among HD patients was not higher than that of the local community (King 1985).

## Irritability, aggression, and intermittent explosive disorder

Despite its frequent occurrence in HD (Baxter et al. 1992), irritability (anger, hostility, etc.) have not yet been systematically explored despite the fact that instruments are available (Snaith et al. 1978). Brothers and Meadows (1955) found 'quick temper and irritability' in 70% of their HD patients, particularly when psychiatric symptoms preceded chorea. In her Scottish survey, Bolt (1970) noted that up to 50% of patients showed 'some degree of ill humour ranging from irritability to actual violence'. Of the patients seen by Dewhurst et al. (1970), 7% also showed 'irritability, restlessness and neurotic symptoms'. They also reported that violence and social deterioration accounted for half of the HD admissions. Oliver (1970) observed that emotional instability manifested as 'irritability, quarrelsomeness, tantrums, violent outbursts or abusiveness' was the most frequent personality change. Pflanz et al. (1991), in their retrospective study of 86 HD cases, using the PSE-syndrome check-list, found irritability to be present in 20% of men and 30% of women. Shiwach (1994) noted irritability together with suspiciousness and apathy as part of the personality change seen in

HD, but did not give its prevalence. Of the 30 cases followed up by Caine and Shoulson (1983), two patients fulfilled criteria for intermittent explosive disorder. Four out of 10 patients seen by Webb and Trzepacz (1987) had a past history of explosive disorder, though none had the current diagnosis in the cross-sectional examination. During their Maryland survey, Folstein *et al.* (1987) concluded that up to 31% had shown intermittent explosive disorder during the course of their illness and that white subjects had a greater prevalence (34%) than black subjects (20%).

Aggression can be seen in later stages of HD. Shiwach and Patel (1993) reported that, among patients in a nursing home, 26% showed mild aggression, while 11% showed moderate aggression. Aggression was equally common in men and women and rarely resulted in injuries to patients or others. Burns *et al.* (1990) measured irritability and apathy in 26 HD and 31 Alzheimer's disease patients and their relatives; both groups showed the same level of irritability (58%) but there was significantly more aggression in the HD group (59% versus 32%); in HD, irritability was reported as related to premorbid 'bad temper'.

In summary, the rates at which aggression and irritability are seen in HD at rates suggest that the relationship is not a random one. These behaviours appear early (Oliver 1970; Dewhurst *et al.* 1970; Shiwach and Patel 1993) in the course of the disease and are more often present in carriers than in non carriers (Berrios *et al.*, in press) and in males than in females (Tamir *et al.* 1969).

## Apathy

After dementia, apathy is the most common symptom of HD (Mattson 1974; Folstein *et al.* 1987). Caine *et al.* (1978) noted that, 'when left alone most seemed content to sit and do nothing; many watched television for hours. Those who were more cognitively impaired rarely initiated any activity'; when stimulated, however, some of their patients were able to get going. In a later study, Caine and Shoulson (1983) divided apathy into two types — 'pervasive' and 'situational', the latter, disappearing when stimulating inputs were present. As the disease progressed, apathy became more pervasive and insight was lost. Burns *et al.* (1990) found that the prevalence of apathy was the same in HD and Alzheimer's disease (48%) and that apathy did not correlate with cognitive impairment; however, when the samples were matched for dementia, the HD group was more apathetic. Depression may be an explanation for

apathy (Schulterbrandt *et al.* 1974) but none of the patients in the Burns *et al.* sample was thus affected.

Apathy has been often described in the context of subcortical dementia (Huber and Paulson 1985). Whether viewed as a part of personality change or as a specific syndrome ('situational apathy'), in HD, apathy seems to increase pari passu with dementia and is correlated with neuropsychological (Caine and Shoulson 1983) (arousal, attention, concentration) and neuropathological changes involving the frontal lobes (Bamford *et al.* 1995; Aylward *et al.* 1998).

## Sexual dysfunction

Sexual behaviour is altered in HD. For example, Dewhurst *et al.* (1970) reported hyper-sexuality in 12% of men and 7% of women; and Oliver (1970) found three cases of 'uncontrolled sexual advances' and three more who indulged in 'sodomy, incest and masturbation in front of their own children'; cautioning that this may be an underestimate! A recent study (Fedoroff *et al.* 1994), specifically assessed frequency and type of sexual disorder in 39 HD patients and 32 partners. They found that 82% of patients and 66% of their partners had one or more sexual disorder, the commonest in fact being hypoactivity. In addition, patients also exhibited paraphilic disorders. Impotence is commonly reported among male HD patients (Folstein 1989).

Reduced libido seems a common dysfunction and this may be neurobiological in origin or relate to medication, affective disorder, and perhaps marital discord and rejection. In general, inferior frontal cortex and medial striatal region and amygdaloid nuclei are known to be involved in other disorders showing hypersexuality (Gorman and Cummings 1992); these very structures (striatum and frontal cortex) are damaged in HD and it is tempting to associate them to the sexual disorders reported in this condition.

## Sleep disorder

HD patients often complain of sleep disturbance. In mild cases of HD, sleep may be normal (Hansotia *et al.* 1985). Sleep disturbance begins to appear in moderately advanced disease. Abnormal movements may decrease, but never completely disappear in sleep. Sleep efficiency is nearly always poor with a high prevalence of wakefulness after sleep onset and increased number of arousals (Silvestri *et al.* 1995). REM sleep is often reduced, as is slow wave sleep (Shiwach and Patel 1993). A recent study that used the carer's questionnaire, found that 88% of patients were reported as suffering from restless legs, excessive daytime somnolence, and early waking (Taylor and Bramble 1997).

## Iatrogenic mental symptoms

Antipsychotics, antidepressants, anxiolytics, and anti-epileptics are often prescribed in HD and all are capable of causing subtle (or less subtle) cognitive, motor, and affective changes of their own. For example, Carbamazepine is associated with generalized impairment in cognitive functions, and when $Na^+$ levels are less than 120 mEq/l, even encephalopathy (Pendlebury *et al.* 1989; Steinhoff *et al.* 1992). Stupor has been reported with sodium valproate with isolated increased levels of blood ammonia; and even a reversible dementia-like syndrome (Betts *et al.* 1982). Neuroleptic medication, prescribed to suppress movements and 'control' aggression, can also cause behavioural and cognitive side-effects. The former can mimic psychiatric disorders. Delirium has been reported with sedating anticholinergic drugs such as chlorpromazine or thioridazine (Brown and Larson 1993).

Akathisia, a subjective sensation of restlessness associated with difficulty in remaining still, is a common side-effect of neuroleptics, with prevalence ranging from 20% to 75% (Van Putten *et al.* 1984). Patients suffering from akathisia are often misdiagnosed as experiencing agitation and aggression, and are treated with even higher doses of neuroleptics, which can make akathisia worse, particularly in the HD patient. A persistent form, tardive akathisia, has also been reported and can make its debut after many months or years of treatment with dopamine receptor blockers. There is a pharmacological distinction between acute and tardive akathisia: neuroleptic discontinuation or dose reduction improves the former but exacerbates the latter.

All traditional neuroleptics, especially those with higher potency, are capable of causing parkinsonian side-effects, which can present as amotivation, apathy, slowing and sometimes depression. Rarely, the neuroleptic-induced super-sensitivity psychosis may develop following long-term treatment with antipsychotic medication, where increasing doses of medication are needed to maintain the antipsychotic effect (Jain *et al.* 1988).

Cognitive changes, including memory deficits and delirium, have been reported with all antidepressant medication. Of the agents currently in use, tricyclic antidepressants have the highest incidence of cognitive side-effects, which are probably dose related (Bye *et al.*

1978). Hypnagogic and hypnopompic hallucinations in the absence of delirium have also been observed in association with tricyclic antidepressants (Hemmingsen and Rafaelsen 1980). Amongst newer antidepressants, a potentially life-threatening side-effect associated with serotonergic antidepressants is the 'serotonergic syndrome', consisting of mental changes, restlessness, myoclonus, hyper-reflexia, fever, chills, diarrhoea, and hypertension. It occurs most often when serotonin reuptake inhibitors and monoamine oxidase inhibitors are administered together or in close succession (Feighner *et al.* 1990). Benzodiazepines produce somnolence, confusion and anterograde amnesia — all of which are more likely to occur in the elderly, with intravenous administration, or in patients with hepatic dysfunction (Lader 1995). Acute withdrawal of benzodiazepines may produce anxiety, tremor, or delirium (Foy *et al.* 1995). Outbursts of aggressive, hostile behaviour during treatment with various benzodiazepines have been reported, which may be more common with alprazolam (Strahan *et al.* 1985). Anticholinergic medication, frequently prescribed in conjunction with neuroleptics, can cause temporary deficits in memory, particularly in elderly patients, as well as delirium (also called the central anticholinergic syndrome) characterised by restlessness, euphoria, irritability, confusion, delusions, and hallucinations (Goetz and Cohen 1994).

## Symptoms and trinucleotide (CAG) repeats

The relationship between mental symptoms in general and trinucleotide repeats has become the focus of interest following the availability of the predictive genetic test for HD. So far, no firm correlation has been found between CAG repeats and psychiatric symptomatology (Campodonico 1996; Weigell-Weber *et al.* 1996; Zappacosta *et al.* 1996). CAG length correlates with some aspects of the disease: e.g. age of onset and severity of motor disorder (Andrew *et al.* 1993; MacMillan *et al.* 1993); 'clinical progression' (Illarioshkin *et al.* 1994; Brandt *et al.* 1996); neuropathological changes (Penney *et al.* 1997); and 'severity' of cognitive deficits (Snell 1993; Jason *et al.* 1997), although not all studies have found a link between cognitive deficits and CAG repeats (Lawrence *et al.* 1998).

In regard to psychiatric symptomatology and CAG repeats, a few studies have explored this specifically. Zappacosta *et al.* (1996) found no correlation between CAG repeats and patients' scores on the Brief Psychiatric Rating Scale (BPRS), Hamilton Depression Rating Scale (HDRS), and Hamilton Anxiety Rating Scale

(HARS). Based on case records and applying DSM criteria, Weigell-Weber *et al.* (1996) divided symptomatic HD patients into four categories ('personality change', 'depression', 'psychosis' and 'non-specific alteration') but again found no significant correlation between the categories and the size of the CAG expansion. In retrospective studies based on information from case notes, Andrew *et al.* (1993) and MacMillan *et al.* (1993) likewise found no correlation between their patient groups and CAG repeats. In the former study, patients were divided into groups according to the presentation at the age of onset, the 'psychiatric' group consisting of patients presenting with psychosis or depression. In the latter study, patients were divided into 'motoric' and 'psychiatric' ('behavioural/cognitive') groups but no further information was provided about 'psychiatric' groups. On the other hand, Illarioshkin *et al.* (1994) reported a significant positive correlation between CAG repeat length and the rate of progression of psychiatric features. However, the 'psychiatric' features in this study were assessed on the basis of the Mini Mental State Examination, and hence, might be more usefully considered as 'cognitive'.

Given the known association between motor symptoms of HD and CAG repeats, the reported *lack* of association between the latter and psychiatric morbidity requires exploration. One explanation is that in the studies reported so far, correlations have been weakened by the poor quality of psychiatric information obtained either from casenotes or interviewing patients who are neurologically and cognitively impaired (Campodonico *et al.* 1996; Weigell-Weber *et al.* 1996). This does not seem to be the case, for our group has recently reported a study where no significant correlation was found between CAG repeats and psychiatry — even when the psychiatric profiles were painstakingly mapped by means of a computerized battery (Berrios *et al.*, in press).

Another explanation is that the wrong type of sample is being studied. In this regard, there is evidence that the correlation between CAG repeat length and motor symptoms is driven by the larger expansion sizes (MacMillan *et al.* 1993). Subjects thus affected, however, tend to present with juvenile onset HD. In consequence, samples including patients older than 30 may not contain enough variance to yield significant correlations between CAG repeats and motor symptoms (Reed 1993). This may also explain the absence of correlations between CAG repeats and cognitive impairment reported by Lawrence *et al.* (1998b) and Andrew *et al.* (1993). Jason *et al.* (1997), on the other hand,

have found a correlation between 'lower cognitive performance' and CAG repeats, but unfortunately do not quote CAG length ranges; the same lack of information affects studies that have reported no association between psychiatry and CAG repeats (Campodonico 1996; Weigell-Weber *et al.* 1996; Zappacosta *et al.* 1996).

Yet another explanation pertains to a putative signal/noise ratio in regards to the aetiology of the psychiatric morbidity itself. This is assumed to be constituted by mental symptoms directly related to either gene or brain lesion (signal) and by 'reactive' mental symptoms (noise) (Paykel 1978). A predominance of noise would attenuate the signal, reduce variance, and diminished the chances of identifying a significant correlation between CAGs and mental symptoms.

## Summary and conclusions

Psychiatric morbidity of varying severity may accompany the acute and chronic stages of most neurological disorders. Because psychiatric complaints rarely achieve critical mass they can be missed out if morbidity is reported in terms of rigid systems, such as the DSM-IV classification. In this regard, it is advisable to analyse the psychiatric aspects of neurological disease in terms of individual 'mental symptoms'. Neurological diseases offer a varied context for the development of psychiatric symptoms and hence need to be treated individually. Models for some are available in the literature (Berrios and Samuel, 1987; Berrios and Dening 1990; Berrios and Quemada 1990; Berrios *et al.* 1995).

The capture of mental symptoms in the general context of neurological disease is bedevilled by problems. At the individual level, the question of whether a patient is sad, suicidal, apathetic, or hallucinated, etc., can be usually resolved. Inferences obtained from comparisons of samples, however, are rarely useful in clinical practice. Part of the problem is that the information included in current 'evidence-based' exercises has been obtained by instruments not designed for use in neurological subjects.

Neurological patients do suffer from a number of mental symptoms, which can be recognized and named and from others which cannot and which are either set aside or forced into some Procrustean category. Salient amongst the known mental complaints are those involving affect. On occasions, the complaints may achieve sufficient critical mass to be called a 'depressive episode'. Anxiety is usually pervading and states of temporal alexithymia, apathy, fatigue, and disordered control of emotions quite common. The identification of these symptoms can be particularly difficult if the patient is also depressed or cognitively impaired. Less frequent are psychotic disorders and again all depends upon definitions. Hallucinations and delusion-like ideas and odd behaviours are not uncommon, and it matters little whether or not these complaints meet DSM-IV criteria. In the clinical context, the presence of such symptoms and their effect on personality and behaviours is important for it may determine whether the patient can be discharged early or whether the family is able to look after him or her. Other complaints, such as sexual dysfunction and sleep disorder, may also get in the way of adaptation to the disease and often remain hidden. Thus they are not an uncommon cause of rejection by spouses. Apathy can be confused with stubbornness or depression and severely affect everyday functioning.

Lastly, there is the issue of iatrogenesis. As the number of medical practitioners participating in the care of neurological patients increases, more medication is prescribed. Their accumulation increases the likelihood of side-effects. Unfortunately, no specific studies exist as to whether neurological patients are specially susceptible to the various chemical groups. This seems to be the case, for example, with tricyclic antidepressants and neuroleptic medication, which at lower doses may cause or worsen apathy, motor and mental slowing, confusion, hallucinations, irritability, and eating disorders.

It is only through a detailed knowledge of the neuropsychiatry of individual neurological disorders and of their pharmacotherapy, together with a full understanding of individual, family and social circumstances, that effective overall management plans can be tailored for each case. All concerned with neuropsychiatry should work towards this desideratum.

# Section V
## Pharmacology and rehabilitation

## Introduction

Many neurological disorders lead in the long term to disability through dysfunction of various parts of the nervous system. Discussion of newer drug therapies that have been developed to slow disability in neurodegenerative disorders by theoretically retarding the primary pathophysiological disease process is to be found in Chapter 7. Discussions on neural transplantation therapies and rehabilitation of the disabled patient are to be found in Chapters 21 and 23.

In this chapter we shall discuss these aspects of neurological disorders using an anatomical approach which broadly defines the following areas:

(1) the association areas of the cerebral cortex, their subcortical connections, and limbic system structures causing cognitive deficits as well as epilepsy;

(2) the basal ganglia and their associated nuclei causing disorders of movement;

(3) the cerebellum and its connections causing incoordination or ataxia;

(4) the bulbar musculature causing problems with swallowing and speech;

(5) the spinal cord reflexes, and their descending modulatory inputs from the brain, mediating bladder and bowel emptying;

(6) the limbs with either:

    (a) the development of spasticity due to interruption of the inhibitory descending supraspinal motor pathways; or

    (b) the development of a flaccid paralysis due to damage to the lower motor neurone and/or is axon;

(7) the sensory pathways, including the peripheral nerves causing either:

    (a) positive sensory symptoms such as parathesiae or pain; or

    (b) negative symptoms such as numbness with loss of light touch, proprioception and pain and temperature sensibility;

(8) the subcortical brainstem nuclei mediating affective disorders and disorders of sleep;

(9) the brainstem respiratory centres and respiratory musculature causing hypoventilation;

(10) the brainstem cardiovascular centres and autonomic nervous system causing orthostatic hypotension and cardiac arrhythmias.

Although these symptom groupings are dealt with separately, in reality they are often combined, which is perhaps best illustrated by patients with the chronic CNS inflammatory disorder, multiple sclerosis (MS). In this condition (see Chapter 4) there are relapsing and remitting episodes of inflammation and demyelination, which over time can lead onto progressive disability secondary to axonal loss (Waxman 1998). It is, therefore, not uncommon for patients 10–15 years into the disorder to have a combination of an 'unstable bladder', spasticity with reduced mobility, parathesiae, slurred speech, and occasional swallowing difficulties. In this chapter we shall explore each of these disabilities, primarily in terms of their physical and pharmacological management.

## Cognitive deficits and epilepsy

Many of the neurodegenerative conditions of the central nervous system involve those structures that are involved in cognitive processes, most notably the cerebral cortex, limbic system, and their associated nuclei along with the basal ganglia. The nature of the cognitive deficit is dependent on the site that is primarily affected, for example, memory with medial temporal lobe structures (Squire and Zola-Morgan 1991). Many of these deficits are not amenable to drug therapy, given that the disease process actually destroys that part of the brain normally subserving that function. However, in some instances cognitive behavioural strategies can be developed, especially in the context of acute fixed deficits (e.g. head injuries) and involves the use of various aids, for example, the Neuropager in patients with amnesic syndromes (Wilson *et al.* 1997). However, many patients with more widespread chronic progressive cognitive deficits do not benefit from such an approach and are best managed by reducing the amount of conflicting information to which they may be exposed. This approach entails maintaining a familiar environment, where confusing and changing sensory inputs are avoided and well-established behavioural patterns can be followed (Taylor and Lewis 1993). It is also important to exclude any underlying depression or affective disorder, which may be primary or secondary to the ongoing degenerative process, as this can be a significant adverse factor in patients with cognitive abnormalities. Indeed, on occasions severe depression can present as an apparent dementing process (pseudodementia).

Drug therapies for cognitive deficits are largely disappointing, although some agents may produce limited benefit for the patient. These include the use of the dopamine agonist bromocriptine in deficits of attention (Fleet *et al.* 1987), acetylcholinesterase inhibitors for Alzheimer's disease (Rogers *et al.* 1998; Rogers and Friedhoff 1998); and drugs that activate the dopaminergic network in Parkinson's disease (see Table 20.3; Lang and Lozano 1998). In all instances these drugs are designed to restore failing neurotransmitter pathways, irrespective of the underlying disease process. Thus they are normally of benefit only in the earlier or milder stages of the disease.

In some patients, cortical damage may cause epileptic seizures, which may be focal or generalised depending on the site and extent of the insult. In general, epileptic seizures are more a feature of acute CNS insults (head injury, cerebrovascular accident (CVA)) than neurodegenerative diseases, and when secondary to focal cortical injury they can be extremely difficult to manage. Drug therapy for epileptic seizures is complex and lies outside the scope of this book, but the main anticonvulsants are listed at the end of this chapter.

# Movement disorders

Many chronic disorders of the CNS generate movement disorders, of which there are many different types (see Table 20.1). The management of these conditions is complex and a list of the various drugs that are commonly used in these conditions are listed in the Table 20.3.

## Parkinsonism

Selective degeneration of neurones within the nigrostriatal tract and the concomitant striatal dopamine deficiency is believed to be the basis of idiopathic Parkinson's disease (PD) (reviewed in: Schapira 1999). Although other neurotransmitter systems are affected in PD, these changes are thought on the whole to be secondary to the dopaminergic deficiency. This specific biochemical defect in PD has therefore meant that L-DOPA is generally accepted to be the most effective available treatment for this condition (Lang and Lozano 1998a). Endogenous L-DOPA is synthesised from tyrosine by the

**Table 20.1** Different types of movement disorders and common diseases causing them

| Disorder | Description | Diseases |
|---|---|---|
| Parkinsonism | Bradykinesia; tremor; rigidity | Idiopathic Parkinson's disease (PD); Drug-induced PD; Parkinsonian plus syndromes |
| Tremor | Rhythmical oscillatory movement, typically of upper limb | PD, essential tremor; anxiety/thyrotoxicosis |
| Chorea | Involuntary, rapid, dance-like movements | Huntington's disease (HD); drug induced with L-DOPA in PD |
| Ballism | Sudden, large flailing movements of a limb | Vascular lesions of the subthalamic nucleus |
| Dystonia | Sustained abnormal posture of a part of the body, typically limb or head | When focal, usually idiopathic; when generalised, more often inherited, e.g. HD |
| Myoclonus | Brief, electric-shock like movement, typically of hands | Myoclonic epilepsy; metabolic abnormalities; Creutzfeldt–Jakob disease |
| Tics | Abnormal complex habitual movement of body, including voice | Gilles de la Tourette syndrome |

enzyme tyrosine hydroxylase (TH), and L-DOPA is then converted into dopamine (DA) by DOPA decarboxylase in the dopaminergic neurones. DA is then stored in vesicles and released at the nerve terminal in the striatum following depolarisation, with an additional site of release being the substantia nigra itself. The released DA then diffuses across the synaptic cleft and binds to a range of DA receptors, especially the D2 receptor in the striatum, and a post-synaptic response (which can be either inhibitory or excitatory in nature) induced.

The maximum benefit from L-DOPA is seen in the early stages of treatment. It is widely accepted that exogenous L-DOPA, taken up by the remaining nigro-striatal neurones, is converted intraneuronally to DA in order to exert its therapeutic action. Although this may be a simplification, it does help explain the common clinical observation that the benefit of L-DOPA is rarely well sustained, since the slow and continued loss of nigro-striatal neurones means this uptake and conversion becomes increasingly erratic with disease progression (Stocchi *et al.* 1997).

Comparable benefit to that achieved by L-DOPA can sometimes be obtained with dopaminergic agonists, such as bromocriptine, lisuride, pergolide, apomorphine, and ropinirole (Swanson 1994; Lang and Lozano 1998). These drugs stimulate dopamine receptors directly and so have theoretical advantages over L-DOPA, since they are not necessarily dependent on the presence of residual intact dopaminergic striatal neurones (Hely and Morris 1996). In addition, the avoidance of L-DOPA early on in the disease by the use of dopamine agonists appears to delay the onset of the dyskinetic 'on–off' problems, which characterises prolonged L-DOPA use (Swanson 1994; Stocchi *et al.* 1997; The Parkinson's Disease Consensus Working Party 1998).

Other non-dopaminergic drugs may be useful in the treatment of parkinsonism. Anti-cholinergic agents, such as ophenadrine, benzhexol, and benztropine, were developed in the light of the beneficial effects of belladonna extracts discovered in the nineteenth century. Their role has become a rather secondary one since the introduction of L-DOPA, but they are still useful in selected patients, particularly those in whom tremor is the predominant symptom. Rigidity is also reduced but there is rarely a useful influence on bradykinesia. Efficacy of these anti-cholinergic agents is explicable in terms of reducing enhanced activity within the striatal cholinergic interneurones that occurs secondary to loss of the dopaminergic input in PD. In advanced cases, the normally undesirable reduction of salivation with anti-cholinergic agents may be useful when sialorrhea is troublesome. Unfortunately, the elderly parkinsonian population is particularly susceptible to the toxic effects of anti-cholinergic drugs, and confusional states not uncommonly necessitate their withdrawal.

It should be emphasised that there are a number of other causes of parkinsonism, which by virtue of their pathological involvement of the basal ganglia include clinical features similar to those seen in idiopathic PD. However, most of these conditions have more extensive pathological changes involving other CNS structures with appropriate signs and symptoms. Of particular significance are a group of conditions known as the parkinsonian plus syndromes (Quinn 1997). In general, these patients respond poorly to therapy, in part because the pathological process is more extensive and not simply confined to the nigro-striatal pathway, and this therefore means that these diseases are not amenable to surgical therapies, including transplantation.

## Tremor

The most useful classification of tremors is clinical and based on the circumstances in which they are seen, and so are generally of three types: static, postural, and action tremors. Static tremor occurs when a relaxed limb is fully supported at rest. Postural tremor appears when a part of the body is maintained in a fixed position and may also persist during movement. Kinetic or action tremor occurs specifically during active voluntary movement of a body part. If the amplitude of such an action tremor increases as goal-directed movement approaches its target, this is often termed an intention tremor.

Physiologic tremor has a frequency in the 7–11 Hz band and is typically symptomatic in states of increased sympathetic nervous activity through stimulation of peripheral $\beta_2$-adrenergic receptors in muscle. The fine postural tremors associated with stress and anxiety states, thyrotoxicosis, and delirium tremens fall into this category and usually respond to beta blockers (Bain 1993).

Symptomatic postural tremors occur in association with a wide range of neurologic disorders and can be shown to differ from physiologic tremor by frequency analysis. Most have a dominant peak at about 6 Hz, including that of PD, although the postural tremors seen in association with multiple sclerosis and certain cerebellar lesions are somewhat slower.

Essential heredofamilial tremor is the commonest example of a symptomatic postural tremor (Bain *et al.*

1994). It may begin at any age and usually increases with time, often starting in one upper limb before becoming bilaterally symmetric over the course of many years, and often involving the head, jaw, tongue, and larynx and, less commonly, the legs and eyes. Its inheritance is usually autosomal dominant with variable penetrance, but sporadic cases also occur. The dominant frequency ranges from 6 to 12 Hz; there is no known histopathology, although recent functional imaging studies have pointed towards the cerebellum as the probable site of origin. It often shows a striking sensitivity to alcohol, and is best treated with propranolol, although primidone and benzhexol have also been used with rather less effect.

PD provides the most common, and most classical, example of symptomatic resting tremor, which attenuates during active movement and characteristically commences in one upper limb. Drug therapy for PD may help the tremor, although anti-cholinergic drugs are anecdotally thought to have a preferential effect on this feature of the disease (see above; Comella and Tanner 1995).

Kinetic or action tremor becomes evident only on voluntary movement of a body part. In fact most patients with postural tremors also show some element of an action tremor. This also occurs in cases of parkinsonism, when the action tremor shows the same frequency characteristics as the cogwheel phenomenon. The best known form of action tremor, however, is that known as intention tremor, which is seen in cerebellar disorders and has a dominant frequency of 4–5 Hz. This is perhaps most commonly seen with multiple sclerosis, where the tremor may be so severe as to prevent any useful activity with the affected limb. In such circumstances, the tremor is often present with any movement and is termed a rubral tremor, although this name is misleading as the pathology is not within this structure but in the cerebellar outflow to the thalamus. It is therefore more accurately termed a midbrain tremor and is often refractory to treatment, although some patients benefit from weighted wrist bands and/or clonazepam, propranolol, isoniazid, or thalamotomy (see below).

The surgical treatment of tremor has been undertaken in a number of conditions with variable success, and of late, thalamic ablative lesions have been superseded by the use of deep brain stimulators (Blond *et al.* 1992; Goldman and Kelly 1992). Indeed the tremor, along with other features of PD, is now managed effectively in the advanced stages of the disease by either pallidal or subthalamic stimulation (reviewed in: Speelman and Bosch 1998). In general, the best patients for these types

of intervention are young, with severe incapacitating and preferably unilateral tremor, unresponsive to medical treatment. Bilateral procedures carry a risk of severe dysarthria and mental change, and are seldom justified in the case of ablative lesions.

## Chorea

As a generalisation, ballism and chorea share a number of common features. There is usually demonstrable pathologic abnormality affecting the subthalamic nucleus in ballism or corpus striatum in certain cases of chorea e.g. Huntington's disease (HD) (Mark 1997; Marshall and Shoulson 1997). The treatment of both of these conditions is often unsatisfactory, as the mainstay of therapy are DA-depleting drugs, such as reserpine or tetrabenazine, or DA-receptor antagonists, such as the phenothiazines or butyrophenones. However, these drugs often produce a number of side-effects (see Table 20.3), whilst often only having marginal effects on the underlying movement disorder. Furthermore, surgical intervention is never warranted, although the possibility of neural transplantation for HD may lead to a re-evaluation of this statement.

## Dystonia

Our knowledge of the mechanisms underlying athetosis and dystonia is inadequate and indeed the pathophysiology may even be identical in the two disturbances. Athetosis occurs almost exclusively in children, when it is assumed to result from brain damage during difficult delivery and is often accompanied by other neurologic abnormalities, including spasticity and mental retardation. The striatum sometimes has a distinctive marbled appearance (status marmoratus) caused by hypertrophied myelinated nerve fibres and gliosis. No consistent structural abnormality has been detected in either focal or generalised dystonia, although caudate, thalamic, and pallidal lesions (especially the globus pallidus, internal segment, GPi) have all been associated on occasions with the development of dystonia (Berardelli *et al.* 1998). Because of the spectacular acute dystonias that may occur following administration of neuroleptic drugs, and by analogy with other movement disorders, an alteration in central DA transmission has been postulated, but firm evidence for this is lacking. Unlike the choreas, only a few patients with dystonia derive worthwhile benefit from dopaminergic antagonists, whilst agonists have been reported as helpful in other individuals.

At present the pharmacology of dystonia and athetosis is unknown and their drug treatment correspondingly unsatisfactory, although a combination of anti-cholinergic drugs, benzodiazepines, and dopamine-depleting drugs or dopamine-receptor antagonists, is often tried with moderate success (Marsden and Quinn 1990). One notable exception is the dopa-responsive dystonia (or Segawa's syndrome), which is an autosomal dominant condition that begins in the first decade of life with a marked diurnal variation of a lower limb dystonia. It can be associated with other movement abnormalities, such as a tremor, postural retrocollis, and bradykinesis, but because of its predominant leg involvement it can be mistaken for cerebral palsy. The genetic abnormality underlying this disorder has now been elucidated and results in a defect in GTP cyclohydrolase I, an enzyme important in the activation of the dopamine synthetic enzyme, TH (Ichinose *et al.* 1994). These patients therefore have a normal number of dopaminergic neurones but a reduced turnover of dopamine that can be corrected by the administration of low doses of L-DOPA. This treatment is dramatically effective and not associated with the development of long-term side-effects, such as dyskinesias. It is therefore recommended that any child or young adult with either a dystonia or 'cerebral palsy' be given a therapeutic trial of L-DOPA.

Surgery for dystonia, especially when it is focal, is now rarely indicated — although this is being re-evaluated given the resurgence of neurosurgery in general for movement disorders (Jankovic 1998). However, the increasing use of botulinum toxin in the treatment of focal dystonias has radically altered the approach to treatment of these conditions. Indeed botulinum toxin injections are now also being used with some success in cases of chronic spasticity (see below), as well as in some task specific tremors (Jankovic 1994). However, whilst botulinum toxin can be useful in focal dystonias, the more generalised dystonias are not amenable to this form of treatment and a combination of agents is often required to gain some form of control, but even then the results are disappointing.

### Myoclonus

Sudden brief-like muscular contractions, myoclonus, can derive from a number of CNS sites including cortex, subcortical brainstem sites, as well as within spinal cord itself (reviewed in: Brown 1996). It can occur as part of an inherited epileptic syndrome (e.g. Unverricht–Lundborg disease); following a fixed CNS insult such as

after cardiopulmonary arrests (post-anoxic myoclonus), and in certain neurodegenerative processes (e.g. Creutzfeldt–Jakob disease). In addition, myoclonic jerks are commonly seen in metabolic disorders and thus any patient with this type of movement disorder should be investigated in this respect.

In all cases, the myoclonic jerks are often precipitated by sensory stimuli and normally represent the synchronous discharge of many motor units. The treatment for myoclonic jerks is pharmacological and includes sodium valproate in epileptic myoclonic syndromes, whilst benzodiazepines and piracetam and more commonly used in the non-epileptiform myoclonic conditions.

## Cerebellar problems

There is no effective treatment for cerebellar problems, except that tremors generated by disordered output of the cerebellum may be amenable to drug and surgical interventions (see above). Therefore, the management of patients with cerebellar dysfunction is designed towards issues of safety — walking aids, swallowing advice, and so on (see below). Anecdotally, amantadine and 3,4 diaminopyridine have been reported to offer some patients benefit but this is normally only in terms of a transient, marginal improvement (Bever 1994; Botez *et al.* 1996). Furthermore, acquired nystagmus has been reported to respond to gabapentin, and to a lesser extent, baclofen (Averbuch-Heller *et al.* 1997).

Finally it is important to remember that the worsening state of a patient with cerebellar disease may have an aetiology outside that of the underlying pathological process. For example, many patients with chronic neurological disorders will be on anti-convulsant drugs that can disrupt the cerebellum, especially at high doses. Furthermore, in MS it may represent an acute inflammatory episode and as such high-dose intravenous methylprednisolone may be of value.

## Bulbar dysfunction

The normal functioning of the bulbar musculature in swallowing and speech relies on its normal innervation from the lower cranial nerves, which in turn receive a descending pathway from both cerebral hemispheres. A unilateral hemispheric lesion is therefore without effect, but bihemispheric damage (e.g. in CVAs, motor neurone disease (MND)) leads to a pseudobulbar palsy with difficulty in speech and to a lesser extent swallowing.

**Table 20.2** Bulbar and pseudobulbar palsy: clinical features and common causes

|  | Bulbar palsy | Pseudobulbar palsy |
|---|---|---|
| Tongue | Weak, wasted, fasciculating | Spastic |
| Jaw jerk | Absent | Exaggerated |
| Common causes | • MND<br>• Polio<br>• Structural lesions of lower brainstem<br>• Myasthenia gravis<br>• Some forms of muscle disease | • MND<br>• Bihemispheric strokes<br>• MS |

Damage to the cranial nerve nuclei and/or their motor axons creates a bulbar palsy (see Table 20.2), with, again, difficulties in speech and, more significantly, swallowing. Bulbar palsies are seen commonly with MND, polio and structural lesions of the lower brainstem. In addition some extrapyramidal disorders such as PD (see above) can cause profound slowing of the oropharyngeal musculature contraction, which leads to drooling and difficulty swallowing with the production of a quiet monotonous voice.

Problems with swallowing can vary but typically take the form of either nasal regurgitation of liquid and/or food, or choking on attempted swallowing, which, if severe, can lead to aspiration pneumonia. The initial assessment of the patient with bulbar problems requires a detailed history and examination, with special attention to the competence of the facial and orolingual/pharngeal musculature, as well as pharyngeal sensation. Radiographic assessment of swallowing is best done using videofluoroscopy of a barium swallow in the presence of a speech therapist (Hughes and Wiles 1998).

The problem once identified is normally best managed by modification of the diet and advice on swallowing technique, as there is often little in the way of pharmacological intervention that is of benefit. Although in the case of PD, l-DOPA is of value and acetylcholinesterase inhibitors (e.g. mestinon) have been recommended in MND, although the evidence that this helps is minimal (Langton-Hewer 1995).

In some cases, swallowing is compromised to the point that either the patient is receiving insufficient calorific intake or is at too great a risk of aspiration pneumonia. In these situations a percutaneous endoscopic gastrostomy (PEG) is recommended, in which a feeding tube is passed through the anterior abdominal wall into the stomach (or in some instance duodenum). This procedure is carried out under sedation and involves an endoscopic procedure, with relatively little in the way of morbidity (Russell *et al.* 1984). Once in

*situ*, feeding is slowly increased through the PEG over a number of days. In most cases PEG feeding is done overnight.

Difficulties with the bulbar musculature also results in abnormalities of speech, dysarthria. This is often difficult to treat, and accurate assessment and advice from the speech therapist is helpful. However, in many cases speech eventually becomes unintelligible and then physical forms of communicator can be of benefit; most of these devices rely on reasonable limb power and co-ordination, and thus may not be of value to patients with widespread degenerative conditions of the CNS (DePippo 1994).

Finally, it is important to remember that in any chronic neurological disease, new unrelated disorders can arise and it is, therefore, essential that other compounding factors are excluded, such as ill fitting dentures, oral thrush, or pharyngeal pouches. In addition, other neurological disorders (e.g. myasthenia gravis) can occasionally develop in the context of pre-existing neurodegenerative conditions and one should almost be aware of such co-incidental pathology. The correct identification of the cause is important, as it obviously governs to a large extent the most appropriate management, and in these latter instances, therapy can often be curative.

## Spasticity

The mechanisms underlying the maintenance of normal muscle tone are unknown but it is thought that the monosynaptic reflex between the muscle spindle and the motor neurone innervating that same muscle is important (see Chapter 17). This reflex is heavily modulated by descending supraspinal inputs from a number of motor areas, including the cerebellum and brainstem. Interruption or damage to any of these structures or pathways will have a profound effects on muscle tone and mobility (Barker *et al.* in press) and in clinical practice the commonest symptom and sign from such a lesion is increased activity within the monosynaptic reflex, with movement of the limb causing spasticity. This is to be distinguished from other conditions in which there is continuous motor unit activity within the muscles; a situation that is rare and seen with the CNS disorders, such as the stiff man syndromes, and peripherally in Isaac's syndrome (reviewed in: Shaw 1999). Conditions that commonly cause spasticity by interfering with these descending pathways include spinal cord trauma and multiple sclerosis, as well as motor neurone disease and some of the complex extrapyramidal disorders. In all of these conditions, the lower limb is more often affected than the upper limb, with the patients complaining of stiffness, cramps, spasms, and decreased mobility, all of which tends to get worse with exercise.

There are two main approaches to the treatment of spasticity, which are complementary. One involves physical therapy, the other drug administration. It is important to mention, however, that early intervention with the spastic patient is recommended, especially in cases of acute CNS injury. For example, at the time of the injury, in the case of spinal cord trauma, it is important that active physiotherapy is pursued to prevent the development of contractures, as increased tone in the muscles will lead to fixed deformities of the limbs. Thus at a later point, when the patient is trying to be ambulant, their limbs will be fixed in abnormal postures, making it impossible to use the limb normally. In such a situation, anti-spastic therapy will be ineffective and surgical intervention aimed at lengthening or shortening tendons/muscles is required. It is therefore imperative that any patient at risk of developing spasticity should receive active physiotherapy in the immediate period following the original CNS insult.

Once established, either physical means and/or pharmacological intervention can treat spasticity. Physiotherapy is an extremely effective way of maintaining mobility in the face of spasticity. It is therefore strongly recommended that all patients who have a degree of spasticity and are noticing increasing problems of mobility, should be referred for physiotherapy. This can take the form of an assessment, with instructions on recommended daily exercises or, alternatively, may necessitate a time of intense inpatient/outpatient physiotherapy over a period of weeks (Gracies *et al.* 1997a).

An alternative, and often complimentary, way of treating spasticity is with the use of pharmacological agents designed to interfere with descending synaptic pathways mediating this motor phenomenon (Gracies *et al.* 1997b). The most commonly used drug is the GABA agonist baclofen, which enhances inhibitory synapses throughout the CNS. As a result, it suppresses the abnormal excitability within the spinal cord motor circuitry, although as one may suspect, it is not without effects at other sites within the CNS. It therefore has a number of side-effects, most notably hypotonia and sedation (see below), which can limit its use. Some of these effects are dose-dependent, and so it is important that this drug is started at low dose. If tolerated, the dose can then be increased and the beneficial effects of it titrated against the sedative and hypotonic side-effects. This side-effect of hypotonia may seem paradoxical, given that the drug is used for spasticity, but some patients remain able to stand, transfer, and ambulate, as a consequence of their increased muscle tone. Thus removing this excess tone can adversely affect the patient, such that the patient becomes less mobile despite less spasticity.

Baclofen, whilst being used in ambulate patients with spasticity, is also of value in some patients who have no useful function in their legs but who are greatly troubled by spontaneous extensor spasms, which can be so severe as to catapult them out of their chair. In these circumstances, the intrathecal administration of the drug may have greater efficacy (see below). The side-effects of baclofen when taken in the oral form, coupled to the identification of subgroups of patients with severe spasticity, has led to the intrathecal delivery of this drug into the lumbar region (Coffey *et al.* 1993). In these patients, inpatient admission is essential in order to start the medication. A catheter is inserted into the subarachnoid space and test doses of baclofen infused to see whether the spasticity can be affected without causing any adverse effect. Particular care has to be taken as, not only can an excessive dose induce a profound hypotonia, but in addition, it can diffuse up to the brainstem and cause significant respiratory depression. However, if an effective suitable dose of baclofen can be found, then the cannulae is fixed and internalised, and the patient is connected up to a baclofen pump and the drug delivered continuously. The use of these pumps has revolutionised the life of some patients (Middel *et al.* 1997) but does require a specialist unit with appropriate infrastructure. It has largely but not exclusively been used in patients with spinal cord trauma and MS.

An alternative drug to baclofen, which can be used synergistically with it, is dantrolene, which works peripherally at the level of the sarcoplasmic reticulum to reduce muscle tone. It is generally well-tolerated but regular monitoring of liver function tests is recommended, and overall it is less effective than baclofen for most patients.

An additional agent that has only recently come on the market for a treatment of spasticity, and which was originally trialed in MS, and spinal cord trauma, is tizanidine. This is an $\alpha_2$ adrenoreceptor agonist, which is thought to modulate the descending monoaminergic pathway input from the brainstem into the spinal cord motor circuitry. This drug can be affective in spasticity, especially in those patients who fail trials of baclofen or dantrolene (Brenner *et al.* 1998).

A further area that has recently been tried in spasticity is the local paralysis of muscles by the administration of botulinum toxin injected into spastic muscle, which blocks ACh release from the synapse (Simpson 1997). This is of limited value given the often widespread nature of the spasticity and the doses of botulinum toxin that are therefore required in order to paralyse them. However, it may be of value in the lower limb in those patients who have severe adductor spasm, where there are problems either of perineal hygiene (as the legs are pressed together) or performing intermittent self-catheterisation (see below). In the upper limb it can be used when there is severe spasticity or dystonia, with pain in the affected muscles or difficulties with injury and hygiene (e.g. the fingernails digging into the palm in some cases of dystonia). Botulinum toxin is therefore of value if the patients are carefully selected, although even then large doses of the toxin are required.

Finally a number of radical measures are available in the severely spastic patient. In the past, stimulation of cerebellar nuclei has been advocated due to the hypotonic effects of cerebellar efferent projections. In addition, actual destruction of the spinal cord has been advocated in some severe cases, although as one would expect this must be regarded as the last resort and is often only reserved for patients with severe painful spasticity with no useful movement.

In summary, there are a number of measures that can be used with spasticity. In the first instance the treatment is designed to increase the useful function of the muscle and thereby allow the patient to have increased activities of daily living. However, as the spasticity advances or is more severe, then the primary aim of treatment is to reduce or remove disabling spasms and/or pain which can be associated with severe spasticity.

## Flaccid paralysis

The development of weak, wasted muscles can cause profound problems, especially when the neck, respiratory, and upper limb musculature are involved. Such a problem arises in a number of neurological conditions, including motor neurone disease, some chronic neuropathies, and muscle diseases such as the muscular dystrophies. The resultant weakness can only be treated with supportive therapy and most conditions causing such problems are not amenable to drug therapy, with the obvious exception of some inflammatory neuropathies, such as multi-focal motor neuropathy with conduction block. In the case of a weak neck, supportive braces can be used to hold the head up, which not only improves the sensory outlook of the patient but makes feeding much easier. Indeed, even though many of these patients have a bulbar palsy making feeding hazardous, it nevertheless permits suctioning and caring for the patient much easier. In addition, it reduces any upper airway obstructive element to respiration, although the respiratory muscles themselves may be involved requiring ventilatory support (see below).

Physiotherapy is important in patients with weakness, to maintain any movement and avoid secondary joint dysfunction, and allows the patient to maximise their potential for using their muscles. The assessment of the patient by an occupational therapist is essential, as many modifications to everyday devices can be instigated with significant improvements in the quality of life (Langton-Hewer 1995).

## Bladder dysfunction

The normal functioning of the bladder relies on an intact sacral parasympathetic innervation, which in turn receives a descending input from the medial frontal cortex (reviewed in: Rushton 1996). Interruption of any of these pathways will produce abnormal bladder function, although the symptoms will vary depending on the site of the lesion. Destruction of the lower part of the spinal cord, including the sacral parasympathetic complex, will result in a neurogenic bladder, namely one that is completely unable to empty urine. In these circumstances there is no alternative to a long-term indwelling catheter to drain the urine, with all the inherent problems that this brings.

The more common clinical situation is that which

involves interruption of the descending pathways, producing an unstable bladder with symptoms of urinary urgency and frequency with nocturia and incontinence. The patient in this situation often experiences an urgent desire constantly to pass urine, although micturition itself only ever yields small volumes of urine and as a result urinary incontinence is not uncommon. The patient often has a feeling of persistent bladder irritation. Furthermore this disabling combination of symptoms can be associated with severe bladder pain.

The assessment of this situation requires, in the first instance, the exclusion of other possible causes, such as urinary tract infection and renal stones or bladder diverticuli, and in males prostatic hypertrophy. These having been excluded, the next important investigation is an estimation of the residual urine left in the bladder following bladder emptying. This can be done using ultrasound or alternatively a catheter can be inserted after the bladder has been 'emptied'. If the residual volume is greater than a 100 ml of urine, then the patient may be suitable for intermittent self-catheterisation (ISC; see below). However, if no large residual volume of urine is found, then the patient is best treated by pharmacological measures (Fowler 1997).

The mainstay of drug therapy is the use of anticholinergic agent, oxybutinin. This is often started at a low dose and helps stabilise the bladder, such that the degree of frequency and urgency can be reduced. However, the drug is not without systemic and local side-effects, and can result in the patient going into urinary retention. It can be used in combination with ISC, although the latter normally obviates the need for it (reviewed in: Fowler 1997).

An alternative drug therapy, especially for those who have severe nocturia, is the nocturnal administration of intranasal Desmopressin DDAVP, a peptide that mimics the anti-diuretic effect of ADH on the kidney (Hoverd and Fowler 1998). In addition, some patients with an unstable bladder benefit from this drug when it is used intermittently, at times when they find it difficult to get to the toilet, for example, when travelling. This is especially true for most patients with unstable bladders, as the descending motor pathways are also involved in the disease process, resulting in reduced mobility. However, it should be stressed that most patients can be managed with oxybutynin or ISC alone, as frequent use of DDAVP is not recommended because its anti-diuretic effect can cause excessive water retention and a secondary hyponatraemia.

An alternative non-pharmacological method of managing the unstable bladder with a large residual urinary volume is with ISC — the rationale being that draining the bladder completely of urine removes the sensory stimuli mediating the distressing symptoms of frequency and urgency. However in order to perform intermittent ISC, the patient or their carer must have good eyesight and upper limb function. In essence, the patient catheterises themselves two to three times a day, typically first thing in the morning and last thing at night. ISC is normally best taught by a nurse practitioner specialised in this particular technique, as proper education is required to prevent recurrent urinary tract infections, which can be a serious complication and may even lead to the abandonment of this approach in some patients (Sutton *et al.* 1991).

In summary, patients with bladder dysfunction in the context of chronic neurological disease need other causes excluding, most notably urinary tract infections and prostatism. Once this has been done, a detailed assessment of the actual bladder dysfunction needs to be undertaken, as the treatment options fall between the use pharmacological measures and ISC. The judicious use of these approaches can greatly ameliorate the patient's symptoms, which are often much underestimated by the clinician.

## Sexual dysfunction

Sexual dysfunction in neurological disease is probably a much underestimated problem. In the male this is relatively easy to quantify, as damage to the spinal cord or autonomic nerves mediating penile erection and ejaculation results in impotence and failure to ejaculate. In women it is more difficult to quantify.

Treatment of male impotence is a complex topic and psychological factors have to be taken into account, as in general this is the major cause of impotence for the male population. However, in the vast majority of patients with chronic neurological disorders there are obvious non-psychological reasons for their impotence. In these cases, pharmacological treatment can be of benefit including intracavernosal injections of papaverine, thymoxamine, or alprostadil. More recently, the orally administered drug, sildenafil (Viagra), has come onto the market although the prescribing of this drug is still controversial. However all of these treatments can be extremely useful, although they are not without side-effects, and counselling may be of benefit in some of these patients (reviewed in: Sharlip 1998).

# Bowel disturbance

Abnormalities in bowel function are extremely common in neurological disorders and typically take the form of constipation. The reason for this relates to a combination of factors, including disruption in the innervation of the bowel, altered dietary intake, and immobility. However it should be stressed that it is always important to exclude, in any patient presenting with constipation or an alteration in bowel habit, some other underlying process such as a colonic malignancy. In the vast majority of patients with neurological disorders there is often a very long history of bowel disturbance, which excludes the necessity to perform detailed bowel investigations.

Treatment of constipation is best done through the dietician and the general practitioner. In general, dietary advice coupled to the introduction of a laxative may be helpful, although the chronic use of laxatives is not always sufficient to cause regular complete bowel emptying. In these situations, suppositories or even enemas may be necessary, and often requires paramedical help such as the district nurse.

It is important to attend to this aspect of patient management as constipation is not only a disabling symptom in some patients, but can cause an apparent deterioration in their neurological capabilities. Furthermore, chronic constipation can cause secondary local problems, such as a sigmoid volvulus and bowel obstruction.

# Sensory symptoms

It is very common for patients with chronic neurological disorders of whatever aetiology to have a number of sensory symptoms. These can take their origin either from damage within the CNS or PNS, and broadly takes the form of either negative symptoms, such as the loss of feeling (i.e. numbness), or positive ones (paresthesiae or pain).

Negative sensory symptoms are more difficult to treat, and primarily require education of the patient to actively attend to the numb areas. This is particularly important in areas such as the feet, where accidental damage can easily take place, which in turn can lead on to secondary infection and tissue destruction. This is perhaps best seen in diabetic neuropathies, where damage can occur to such an extent that the patient can actually destroy their joints as a consequence (Charcot joints). It is therefore imperative that people who have

such problems regularly receive chiropody, as well as attention from the necessary medical personnel to ensure that no accidental damage or trauma goes unattended.

Positive sensory symptoms, such as paresthesiae, result from abnormal discharges along either central or peripheral sensory pathways (see Chapter 13). As a result, drug therapy for these symptoms relies on agents that primarily affect neuronal firing and includes carbamazepine, gabapentin, amitriptyline, and mexilitine. All of these agents are typically used in other neurological conditions but have all been shown to be effective for neurogenic sensory symptoms.

Of course it is important in all these cases to consider other pathologies, especially when the sensory symptoms are localised. For example, patients who complain of tingling and sensory phenomena in their hands must have a carpal tunnel syndrome or ulnar entrapment at the elbow excluded, especially as patients using crutches are at a greater risk of developing such entrapment neuropathies. Indeed, some patients may develop a treatable neuropathy that is unrelated to their underlying neurological condition, e.g. Guillain-Barré syndrome.

In some cases the sensory symptoms take the form of pain, which again can take its origin from either within the CNS or PNS. In general, pure pain syndromes are rare in neurodegenerative disorders, although they may occur in the context of severe spasticity, dystonia, or bladder instability. For example, patients with Parkinson's disease may develop painful dystonia in the 'off' period, which may respond to increasing doses of levodopa or in some instances lithium (Lang and Lozano 1998). In addition, certain pure pain syndromes are well described, including trigeminal neuralgia with multiple sclerosis. In cases of well-recognised pain syndromes, standard therapies apply and so, for example, with trigeminal neuralgia, carbamazepine and/or phenytoin are the drugs of choice with surgical intervention considered for refractory cases (Tenser 1998).

Thus the treatment of pain in the context of neurodegenerative disorders is no different to that seen in other situations. Simple analgesic agents are the typical first line of therapy, whilst compounding factors are excluded such as a secondary depression or other disease processes. If simple analgesic preparations are ineffective, then stronger drug therapy may be indicated, although non-pharmacological therapies need exploring including transcutaneous electronic nerve stimulation and acupuncture. Furthermore, drugs used in the amelioration of paresthesia also have a role to play (carbamazapine, amitriptyline, mexilitine) and some patients will benefit from local nerve blocks and epidural injections (reviewed in: Adams and Victor 1993).

## Psychiatric problems

It is important to remember that many patients with chronic neurodegenerative conditions will have psychiatric problems, which may either be part of the disease process (e.g. HD) or secondary to it (e.g. MS). This can take many forms, and on occasions will result in a functional deterioration of the patient in the absence of worsening objective neurological deficits. It is therefore important to exclude psychiatric problems, especially depression, in any patients who apparently deteriorate suddenly. The treatment of such psychiatric problems lies beyond the scope of this chapter, but a list of major therapeutic agents is presented in Table 20.3.

## Breathing

Some neurodegenerative conditions can affect either the central respiratory centres in the lower brainstem (e.g. dystrophia myotonica); the patency of the upper airways (e.g. multisyptem atrophys MSA) or the integrity of the respiratory muscles (e.g. MND). Therefore patients may present with respiratory symptoms of breathlessness or stridor, or alternatively may develop chronic right ventricular failure. It is therefore important to be alert to these symptoms and arrange for assessment using respiratory function tests and overnight sleep studies in patients at risk.

The identification of problems in such patients can lead to interventions with nocturnal ventilatory support, with or without the need for a tracheostomy, depending on the nature of the respiratory problem (reviewed in: Schneerson 1996).

In patients with high spinal injuries it may be necessary to perform artificial ventilation via a tracheostomy. However, if the phrenic motor neurones are preserved a phrenic nerve stimulator can be used.

## Cardiovascular

Patients with neurodegenerative conditions, especially those with autonomic involvement and wheelchair confinement, can develop significant orthostatic hypotension. Treatment for this condition (reviewed in; Mathias and Kimber 1999) involves:

**Table 20.3** Commonly used drugs in neurology and their indications, and major side-effects

| Drug | Other uses | Side-effects* | Comments |
|---|---|---|---|
| **Epilepsy** | | | |
| Phenytoin | • Trigeminal neuralgia<br>• ? Nystagmus | Hirsutism<br>Gum hypertrophy | Used in generalised epilepsy |
| Sodium Valproate | • Mood stabiliser | Tremor<br>Weight gain | Used in all forms of epilepsy |
| Carbamazepine | • Trigeminal neuralgia<br>• Neuropathic pain | Rash | Used in all forms of epilepsy |
| Phenobarbitone | | Sedation | Rarely used nowadays |
| Primidone | • Tremor | | Rarely used nowadays |
| Vigabatrin | | Behavioural<br>Abnormalities | Mainly used as add on therapy in refractory epilepsy |
| Lamotrigine | | Rash | Mainly used as add on therapy in refractory epilepsy |
| Gabapentin | • Neuropathic pain<br>• ? nystagmus<br>• ? spasticity | | Mainly used as add on therapy in refractory epilepsy |
| Topirimate | | Abdominal pain<br>Weight loss | Mainly used as add on therapy in refractory epilepsy |
| Ethosuximide | | | Used primarily in "petit mal" epilepsy in childhood |
| Diamox | • Glaucoma<br>• Benign intracranial hypertension (BIH) | Paresthesiae | Rarely used with questionable efficacy |

**Table 20.3** *Continued*

| Drug | Other uses | Side-effects* | Comments |
|------|-----------|---------------|----------|
| Clobazam | | Sedation | Used short term only due to tolerance |
| Clonazepam | • Tremor | Sedation | Mainly used with in myoclonic epilepsy |
| **Parkinson's disease** | | | |
| L-DOPA (Sinemet ©; Madopar ©) | • Dystonia in childhood | Nausea/vomiting Postural hypotension Drug induced Dyskinesias | Gold standard of treatment |
| Dopamine agonists (Bromocriptine; Pergolide; Lisuride; Ropinirole; Apomorphine; Pramipexole; cabergoline) | • ?Neglect | Nausea/vomiting Hallucinations | Used as first line therapy in young onset PD |
| Anti-cholinergics (Benzhexol; Orphenadrine) | • Dystonia | Confusion Dry mouth Constipation Urinary retention Nervousness | ?more efficacious than L-DOPA for tremor |
| Amantadine | • Cerebellar ataxia | | |
| Selegiline | | | Monoamine Oxidase Inhibitor (MAOI): Prolongs action of L-DOPA |
| Entacopone | | | COMT-inhibitor: Prolongs action of L-DOPA |
| Propanolol | • Essential tremor | Depression Asthma Cold hands/feet | Useful in sweats with PD and ?tremor |
| Lithium | • Mood stabiliser | Tremor Polyuria/polydipsia | Useful for painful dystonias |
| Atypical Antipsychotics (Olanzepine; clozapine) | • Schizophrenia | Bone marrow Suppression | Useful in confusion/hallucinations without aggravating PD |
| **Tremor** | | | |
| Propanolol | • PD | SEE ABOVE | First line treatment in essential tremor |
| Primidone | • Epilepsy | SEE ABOVE | Second line treatment in essential tremor |
| L-DOPA | • PD  • Dystonia | SEE ABOVE | PD tremor ?orthostatic tremor |
| Clonazepam | • Epilepsy | SEE ABOVE | |
| **Chorea** | | | |
| Tetrabenazine | • Dystonia  • Tics | Drowsiness Depression | Often not effective long-term |
| Neuroleptics (Sulpiride; pimozide haloperidol) | • Tics  • Dystonia | Parkinsonism | Can make underlying condition worse |
| **Dystonia** | | | |
| Tetrabenazine | • Chorea  • Tics | SEE ABOVE | Often used as a combination of therapies: |
| Neuroleptics (Sulpiride; haloperidol) | • Chorea  • Tics | SEE ABOVE | i.e. dopamine blocker with benzodiazepine with anti-cholinergic |

**Table 20.3** *Continued*

| Drug | Other uses | Side-effects* | Comments |
|---|---|---|---|
| Benzodiazepines (diazepam) | • Epilepsy<br>• Spasticity | Sedation | |
| Anti-cholinergics | • PD | SEE ABOVE | |
| L-DOPA | | SEE ABOVE | Primarily used in:<br>Dopa responsive dystonia of childhood or dystonia in PD |
| Botulinum toxin | • ? Spasticity<br>• ?Tremor | Local paralysis of muscles which can give problems e.g. dysphagia in cases of spasmodic torticollis. | Useful in focal dystonias |
| **Myoclonus** | | | |
| Sodium valproate | • Epilepsy | SEE ABOVE | Especially when associated with seizures |
| Benzodiazepines (Clonazepam) | • Epilepsy<br>• Tremor | SEE ABOVE | Especially when associated with seizures |
| Piracetam | | GI disturbances | Especially in myoclonus is of cortical origin |
| **Tics** | | | |
| Tetrabenazine | • Chorea<br>• Dystonia | SEE ABOVE | |
| Neuroleptics | • Chorea<br>• Dystonia | SEE ABOVE | |
| **Spasticity** | | | |
| Baclofen | • Trigeminal neuralgia<br>• ?nystagmus | Hypotonia<br>Sedation | First line treatment |
| Dantrolene | | Diarrhoea<br>Sedation | Rarely effective |
| Benzodiazepines (Diazepam) | • Epilepsy<br>• Myoclonus | SEE ABOVE | Rarely effective on their own |
| Tizanidine | | Sedation<br>GI disturbances | |
| **Urinary symptoms** | | | |
| Oxybutynin | | Dry mouth<br>Constipation<br>Blurred vision | First line therapy for an unstable bladder |
| Desmopressin | • Orthostatic hypotension | Hyponatraemia | Especially helpful for:<br>Nocturia<br>Daytime frequency |
| **Sexual dysfunction** | | | |
| Intracavernosal injections: (Papaverine Thymoxamine Alprostadil) Sidenafil | | Priapism<br>Penile pain | |
| **Sensory symptoms** | | | |
| Carbamazepine | • Epilepsy<br>Trigeminal neuralgia | SEE ABOVE | |
| Amitritylene | • Depression | Dry mouth<br>Constipation<br>Sedation | |
| Gabapentin | • Epilepsy<br>• ?nystagmus<br>• ?spasticity | SEE ABOVE | |

**Table 20.3**  *Continued*

| Drug | Other uses | Side-effects* | Comments |
|---|---|---|---|
| **Psychiatric** | | | |
| **Anti-depressants:** | | | |
| Tricyclic anti-depressants (TCAs): | | | |
| e.g. amitriptylene | • Sensory symptoms | SEE ABOVE | |
| Selective serotonin Reuptake blockers (SSRIs) | | | |
| e.g. fluoxetine | • ?pain syndrome | GI disturbances Dry mouth Hypersensitivity | |
| **Anti-psychotics:** | | | |
| Neuroleptics | • Chorea <br> • Tics | SEE ABOVE | |
| **Mood stabilisers:** | | | |
| Lithium | • Pain in PD due to dystonia | SEE ABOVE | |
| Carbamazepine | • Epilepsy <br> • Trigeminal neuralgia <br> • Sensory symptoms | SEE ABOVE | |
| Sodium valproate | • Epilepsy | SEE ABOVE | |
| **Others** | | | |
| **Drugs used in Dementia:** | | | |
| Donezepil | | GI disturbances | Useful only in mild to moderate Alzheimer's Disease. |
| Rivastigmine | ?advanced PD with confusion | | |

For full information on all of these drugs see British National Formulary, published by British Medical association twice a year.
*all these drugs can cause sedation, with nausea and signs of cerebellar dysfunction at toxic levels.

- the withdrawal of any medication that may be contributing to the symptomatology, e.g. L-DOPA in MSA may exacerbate the autonomic failure without producing any significant anti-parkinsonian action;

- head up tilt of about 15° of the bed at night — resets the renin–angiotensin system;

- the introduction of either non-steroidal anti-inflammatories (e.g. indomethacin), causing some fluid retention, desmopressin (DDAVP) spray, fludrocortisone, or ephedrine, which also causes vasoconstriction and some increase in cardiac output.

Finally, some patients with certain neurodegenerative conditions are predisposed to develop cardiac arrhythmias. In such individual the insertion of a permanent pacemaker may be indicated.

## Conclusions

Management of patients with chronic neurological diseases is complex and requires a multidisciplinary approach. It is important that these patients are assessed in all domains so that every effort is made to treat the problems symptomatically. In addition, secondary pathology either related or even independent to the primary pathological process, needs to be considered in any patient who develop new dysfunction in the context of their disorder.

## Further reading

Oxford Textbook of Pharmacology, Oxford University Press.

# 21 | *Neuropsychological rehabilitation*

## *By Ian H. Robertson and Barbara A. Wilson*

An alternative approach to the management of patients with brain damage is the rehabilitation of behavioural and psychological skills. Rehabilitative approaches have been developed in particular in the context of treatment and recovery of non-progressive brain damage, as for example occurs in stroke and trauma, rather than for progressive neurodegenerative disorders. This chapter reviews such approaches. Recall that the adult mammalian CNS exhibits a certain capacity for both anatomical and biochemical reorganisation, but the plasticity is limited. Rehabilitation addresses both the development of behavioural and cognitive strategies that can allow patients to develop alternative strategies to achieve their goals, and the fact that behavioural experience and training can alter the course of the structural reorganisation itself.

Acquired non-progressive brain damage in adulthood commonly leads to relatively rapid recovery in the early weeks and months post-injury, followed by a slower recovery, which can continue for many years after the original lesion; considerable recovery has been demonstrated following various types of brain injury for language deficits (Zangwill 1975; Kertesz 1979), perceptual deficits (Wilson and Davidoff 1993), unilateral neglect (Stone *et al.* 1991, 1992), motor functions (Lindmark 1988; Chollet *et al.* 1991), memory disorders (Wilson 1991), attention deficits (van Zomeren and van der Burg 1985), and general intellectual functions (Milner 1975).

One prevailing view within rehabilitation research is that espoused by Luria (Luria 1963; Luria *et al.* 1975), who argued strongly that compensatory processes underpin recovery. According to this view, given the fact that central nervous system neurones do not regenerate, recovery of neuropsychological functions is achieved largely by the reorganisation of surviving neural circuits to achieve the given behaviour in a different way (see Chapters 13 and 14). Compensation is indeed a key factor in rehabilitation and recovery, and we will discuss this at length later in this chapter.

While there is clear evidence that compensation is one important type of mechanism underlying recovery of function, more fundamental behaviour-dependent recovery of the impaired neuropsychological processes themselves appears to be possible, in some circumstances, and for some neuropsychological functions. This conclusion is in part based on evidence for greater plasticity of the adult central nervous system than has hitherto been acknowledged (Kolb and Whishaw 1989; Kaas 1991, 1995; Ramachandran *et al.* 1992a; Stein and Glasier 1992). In other words, brain-damaged individuals may not only learn to do things in different ways via compensation, but they may also show partial restitution of the impaired function (Robertson and Murre, in press). Before considering these two classes of mechanism, however, what is the evidence that rehabilitation can actually improve recovery following brain damage?

## Evidence for the effectiveness of rehabilitation

Reviews of animal research suggest that environmental enrichment and stimulation improves both functional recovery following lesion (Gentile *et al.* 1978; Kolb 1992; Stein and Glasier 1992; Will and Kelche 1992), as well as actual cortical structure (Greenough *et al.* 1985; Black *et al.* 1987; York *et al.* 1989; Mayer *et al.* 1992; Wallace *et al.* 1992). Furthermore, Mayer *et al.* (1992) showed that rats given striatal neural transplants only benefited from the transplants when they were given the opportunity for learning. In short, the experience arising from behavioural interactions with the environment appear not only to mitigate behavioural losses arising from lesions compared to animals in impoverished environments, but also appear in some cases to be able to modify underlying neural structures and, in particular, dendritic branching (Greenough *et al.* 1985; Wallace *et al.* 1992). However, compensatory learning underlies some of these effects (Gentile *et al.* 1978; Held *et al.* 1985; Rose *et al.* 1993).

Robertson and Murre (1999) have developed a connectionist model of recovery of function, which predicts that while restitution of function in lesioned circuits may be possible after relatively small lesions,

compensatory processes are more likely to underlie recovery from larger lesions. Kolb describes research evidence in support of such a prediction (Kolb 1996). It was found that small lesions may result in 'restitution' of the behaviours, through utilisation of spared tissue in the original tissue, while large lesions that remove most of the underlying circuit result in partial recovery, which is mediated by compensatory adjustments based on separate, intact, circuits. Human PET studies of recovered motor function in patients having suffered a cerebrovascular accident (CVA), suggest that a considerable plasticity of cortical function underpins recovered motor responses, with recovery being mediated by:

- recruitment of cortical areas in the undamaged hemisphere; and

- extension of specialised areas adjacent to the lesioned site (see Chapter 13; Chollet *et al.* 1991; Chollet and Weiller 1994).

More direct evidence that specific stimulation or forced use can aid recovery comes from Nudo and Grenda (1992) who stimulated the motor cortex of squirrel monkeys and mapped the location of digits, wrist, and forearm. The digit and wrist representations in the cortex were then lesioned, and 4 months later Nudo re-examined the representation of the digit, wrist, and forearm, and found that electrical stimulation no longer produced movements of any of the hand areas. It seemed that the loss of cortical representation of movement had spread beyond the original lesion. To see whether he could prevent such loss, Nudo forced another group of monkeys to use their affected limb after surgery. When he replotted the cortex in these animals, they still had an extensive region from which he could elicit movement of the digits, hand, and wrists. In other words, the rehabilitation had prevented loss of function by maintaining connectivity in the threatened networks.

Several human studies have attempted to force usage of the hemiparetic (paralysed) limb following stroke and, in general, improvements in function have been obtained long after the hemiparesis has plateaued (Ince 1969; Halberstam *et al.* 1971; Wolf *et al.* 1989). One small controlled study found improvements lasting up to 2 years in everyday usage of the hemiparetic upper limb after a 2-week period of immobilisation of the non-affected upper limb (Taub *et al.* 1993), along with encouragement to use the affected limb.

What is the evidence for more general effects of reha-

bilitation on recovery of function? A recent well-conducted review of stroke rehabilitation studies, which evaluated treatments of motor, cognitive, language, and visuo-perceptual functions, concluded that rehabilitation may improve functional performance in some patients (Öttenbacher and Jannel 1993). A meta-analysis was carried out of 36 trials of stroke rehabilitation aimed at language, visuo-perceptual, and motor processes, functional daily activity, and general cognitive processes. The analysis concluded that the average patient receiving a program of focused stroke rehabilitation performed better than approximately 65% of patients in comparison groups.

Benedict (1989) reviewed the literature on cognitive rehabilitation programmes for closed head injury. These mainly cover attention problems, self-regulation difficulties, and memory problems. Benedict concludes that there may be some evidence for improvement in self-regulation and attention skills, though the research has lacked methodological rigour, which limits this conclusion.

McGlynn (1990) reviewed the literature on behavioural approaches to neuropsychological rehabilitation, and concluded that, 'There is considerable evidence suggesting that behavioural techniques can be successfully applied to a variety of problems following neurological impairment'. These problems included inappropriate social behaviour, attention, and motivation, lack of awareness of deficits, memory, language, and speech and motor disturbance.

In short, though only preliminary in nature, studies of the effectiveness of rehabilitation support experimental human and animal research suggesting that behavioural improvement (and in some cases more specific neuronal change) may follow from rehabilitation in certain conditions. It is likely that a combination of restitution-based recovery and more indirect compensatory processes underpin the observed improvements, and that whether such restitution does happen may depend on a residual surviving connectivity in the lesioned circuits (Robertson and Murre, in press). Given the importance of attentional deficits in recovery of function, as mentioned above, it is important to note that some evidence exists that attentional deficits themselves can be improved through rehabilitation (Sturm *et al.* 1983; Sohlberg and Mateer 1987; Gray *et al.* 1992). Furthermore, one study of training that was aimed specifically at sustained attention (Robertson *et al.* 1995) found not only effects on sustained attention tasks, but also yielded a predicted effect on unilateral neglect, supporting the view that attentional processes

may have a wide importance in a range of different functions.

To summarise, there is evidence to support the view that behavioural and environmental manipulations can alter function of the brain following acquired brain damage in adults. We will now return to the question of restitution and compensation as vehicles for this improved function.

## Restitution of function

We have cited evidence that has shown that experience could produce behavioural, as well as dendritic, changes in lesioned animals, and we have shown also that rehabilitation of humans could produce behavioural changes following brain damage. Synaptic remodelling (as discussed anatomically in Chapter 13) appears to be a major mechanism of these experience-dependent changes. Thus, as discussed by Kolb (1996), not only does the brain change experience, but experience changes the brain. Evidence comes from various sources, in particular from studies in non-brain damaged animals and humans.

Tactile stimulation in the owl monkey has also been shown to change mapping in the primary somatosensory cortex (Jenkins *et al.* 1990). Experience-dependent plasticity in humans and animals has been demonstrated using a large number of different paradigms, too extensive to review comprehensively here. For instance, using somatosensory evoked potentials and transcranial magnetic stimulation, Pascual-Leone and Torres (1993) demonstrated that the right index finger of Braille readers had a larger somatosensory representational field in the cortex than the left index finger; compared to controls, this representational field was also larger. The authors conclude that reading Braille is associated with expansion of the sensorimotor cortical representation of the reading finger. These results are compatible with those on sensory reorganisation following amputation by Ramachandran (Ramachandran *et al.* 1992a, b).

In summary, synapses can be remodelled (in some cases via increases in dendritic arborization—Greenough *et al.* 1985; Jones and Schallert 1992; Wallace *et al.* 1992) as a result of experience in the normal mammalian brain. But what, more precisely, are the mechanisms of this learning with its associated synaptic changes? Candidates for this include the Hebbian co-activation of pre- and post-synaptic neurones (Hebb 1949), and Hebbian learning mechanisms may in part underlie the positive

effects of stimulation, forced use and rehabilitation which were reviewed above.

Another possible candidate mechanism for restitution is the manipulation of the inhibitory dynamics among circuits linked to the lesioned circuits. Damaged circuits in the brain suffer further loss of function because of inhibitory competition from undamaged circuits, particularly—but not uniquely—interhemispherically across the corpus callosum. Sprague (1966), for instance, demonstrated that hemianopia in cats could be ameliorated by destroying the superior colliculus on the side opposite to initial visual input, thereby freeing the lesioned hemisphere from the collicular inhibition of the intact hemisphere and allowing ipsilesional circuits to operate; this effect was confirmed using electrophysiological measures in rats (Goodale 1973). Wallace *et al.* (1990) demonstrated that cats with unilateral lesions of striate cortex show a severe contralateral neglect. He found substantial reductions in the neglect following a lesion of the substantia nigra in the opposite hemisphere, thereby reducing the competitive inhibition on the contralateral superior colliculus in the lesioned hemisphere. Monkeys with unilateral lesions of the posterior parietal cortex tend to make voluntary eye movements into the ipsilesional field when presented with bilateral stimuli. Lynch and McLaren (1989), however, showed that this bias is corrected when an additional lesion is subsequently made in the posterior parietal cortex of the opposite hemisphere. Again, the mechanism proposed to explain this is that the damaged hemisphere was freed from competitive inhibition from the undamaged hemisphere.

As an alternative to reducing activation in the undamaged hemisphere, the competitive strength of the damaged hemisphere may be improved by activating it. Robertson and North (1992, 1993) showed that unilateral left neglect following right hemisphere stroke could be improved if patients were required to make minimal movements with left limbs in left hemispace. This caused activation of interlinked spatial circuits for the left side of the body and for the left side of extrapersonal space. This combined activation, we argued, was sufficient to overcome the competitive inhibition from the equivalent circuits in the undamaged left hemisphere. When however these left hemisphere circuits were simultaneously activated through identical movements made with both hands, this effect disappeared (Robertson and North 1994). We argued that this was because the activation of the intact hemisphere overshadowed or extinguished the activation of the damaged hemisphere, the implication being that bilateral limb use may prevent under-utilised potential from being realised in the damaged hemisphere. These principles can be put into effective clinical practice, producing real gains in everyday functioning of stroke patients suffering from unilateral neglect (Robertson *et al.* 1992).

Another example of fostering activation in a lesioned circuit is based on a demonstrated relationship between two different types of attention—sustained attention and spatial orientation, respectively. Activation of a putatively right-frontal-parietal based sustained attention system was shown to result in significant improvements in unilateral neglect in eight patients. This study was based on Posner's (1993) hypothesis that the posterior spatial orientation system—implicated in unilateral neglect—was modulated by a separate right hemisphere sustained attention system. His prediction was that changes in alertness should cause changes in the ability to orient attention in space. This hypothesis was bolstered by evidence that non-lateralised auditory sustained attention impairment is a marker of unilateral neglect (Robertson *et al.* 1997).

Consequently, eight patients were trained to periodically improve their level of alertness using a self-instructional procedure. This not only improved the ability to sustain attention, but also had highly specific effects on spatial orientation with a consequent reduction in unilateral neglect (Robertson *et al.* 1995). Furthermore, these effects were confined to measures of sustained attention and unilateral neglect—no improvements on spatial orientation judgement were found. In a subsequent experimental study, it was shown that brief (300–1100 ms prior to presentation of visual stimuli) non-lateralised auditory alerting stimuli could—on average—temporarily abolish the spatial bias in a group of people with unilateral neglect (Robertson *et al.* 1998). In short, while there is as yet relatively little evidence that attentional processes can be harnessed therapeutically to enhance plastic reorganisation of more posterior circuits following brain damage, there are very strong grounds indeed to predict that this may be the case. Fig. 21.1 shows the effects on spatial bias of this phasic alerting.

A third and related candidate mechanism for restitution of function is attentional modulation of lesioned circuits. The receptive field sizes for stimuli in visual cortex area V4 can be rapidly tuned by directed attention (Desimone and Duncan 1995). Cells in V4 have large receptive fields but, under certain circumstances, the responsive area of the receptive field can be greatly restricted (Moran and Desimone 1985). For instance, if the monkey does not attend to a stimulus in a given

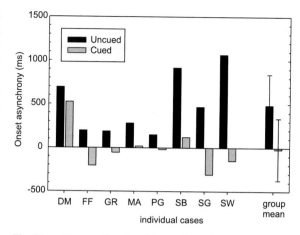

**Fig. 21.1** Degree of neglect (bias to the right) in uncued condition (*black bars*) reduced in all cases following presentation of non-lateralised auditory warning immediately prior to presentation of visual stimuli (*unfilled bars*).

location, the response of the cell is greatly reduced compared to when the monkey attends to the stimuli. As the monkey moves its focus of attention to different parts of the receptive field, the site at which one can elicit the most vigorous neural response moves along with the attentional focus, suggesting the presence of a 'roving activation' of basic receptor cells via what is probably a frontal-lobe mediated attentional system. Attentional effects on early sensory components of auditory processing have also been demonstrated (Woldorff *et al.* 1993), and this is also true of somatosensory processing (Drevets *et al.* 1995).

Such attention-dependent changes in the cortex may have implications for recovery and rehabilitation following brain damage. Desimone and Duncan (1995) argue that the top-down selection templates for both location and object selection in vision are likely to be derived from neural circuits mediating working memory, perhaps especially in the prefrontal cortex. It seems likely that attentional modulation mechanisms of this kind will apply to other sensory, motor, and higher cognitive processes, and that such input from 'attentional templates' may be crucial for the re-establishing of damaged and incomplete patterns of synaptic connections in lesioned circuits. This view would be strongly compatible with the evidence that integrity of attentional processes is crucially predictive of good general recovery following brain damage (Kinsella and Ford 1980; Sterzi *et al.* 1993; Blanc-Garin 1994; Vilkki *et al.* 1994; Robertson *et al.* 1997). This is also compatible with the finding that experience-dependent changes in the brain only occur when attention is paid to the stimulative experience in question (Recanzone *et al.* 1993).

Having argued that restitution of function may be possible following some types of brain damage, we now turn to the question of rehabilitation based on compensatory process training.

# Compensation and recovery of function

Zangwill (1947) was the first to categorise approaches to cognitive rehabilitation in this way. Zangwill worked to a large extent with aphasic patients, although he also addressed problems with attention, memory, and initiative. His important (1947) paper is well worth reading over 50 years later. The problem he addressed when he wrote, 'We wish to know, in particular, how far the brain injured patient may be expected to compensate for his disabilities and the extent to which the injured brain is capable of reeducation' (p. 62) is as pertinent now as it was then. He defines compensation as a '... reorganisation of psychological function so as to minimise or circumvent a particular disability' (p. 63). He believed that compensation for the most part took place spontaneously, without explicit intention by the patient, although in some cases it could occur by the patient's own efforts or as a result of instruction and guidance from the psychologist.

By substitution Zangwill meant, '... the building up of a new method of response to replace one damaged irreparably by a cerebral lesion' (p. 64). He recognised that this was a form of compensation, but taken much further, where the end result was obtained by other than normal means through re-education. Lip-reading for deaf people and Braille for blind people would be examples of substitution. Zangwill used the tactile sense as substitution during the rehabilitation of an aphasic patient who could no longer read through a visual route. Initially, by getting the man to trace the letters, then pretend to write them with his fingertip on his knee, and eventually to manage without the tactile sense except when faced with difficult words.

The third method mentioned by Zangwill (1947), which he considered to be training at its highest level, was direct retraining. Whereas compensation and substitution were the methods of choice for functions '... which do not genuinely recover' (p. 65), Zangwill thought it possible that some damaged functions could

be restored through training, and he clearly had in mind the notion of restitution discussed above.

Wilson (1995b) has examined the development of compensatory behaviour in brain-injured people in more detail and uses a theoretical framework provided by Bäckman and Dixon (1992) to understand compensatory behaviour. Bäckman and Dixon distinguish four basic steps in the progression of compensatory behaviour:

(1) origins;

(2) mechanisms;

(3) forms; and

(4) consequences.

Wilson (1995b) applies this framework to the development of compensatory behaviour in brain-injured people with severe memory impairment.

The origins of compensatory behaviour arise when there is either:

(1) a decrease in a given skill without an accompanying decrease in the environmental demands placed on a person; or

(2) an increase in environmental demands without an increase in the skills required for successful performance.

The former is typically seen following organic memory impairment. Any kind of brain injury or disease is likely to cause a decrease in cognitive functioning. Consequently if a brain-injured person tries to return to a former lifestyle, there is likely to be a mismatch between the present impoverished level of cognitive functioning and the demands of everyday life.

Even when environmental demands are reduced, the mismatch may still be there as compensatory mechanisms are not employed. A reduction in environmental demands without accompanying employment of compensatory strategies will be insufficient to overcome difficulties experienced by people with severe cognitive deficits.

Bäckman and Dixon also consider the severity of any given deficit to be important in the development of compensatory behaviour. Severity is believed to affect the extent to which compensation occurs. They suggest that the likelihood of using compensatory behaviour follows a U-shaped curve, with moderately impaired people being more likely to compensate, mildly impaired people being unaware of the need to compensate, and those with severe impairment lacking the skills required to implement compensatory behaviour. This is probably only partly true in brain-injured people as, for example, people with a very severe amnesia but no additional cognitive deficits may compensate very well (Wilson 1995a), whereas those with a moderately severe amnesia but additional deficits may be unable to learn compensatory behaviour.

The mechanisms by which a match is achieved between the level of skill and the everyday demands may occur through:

(1)   an increase in time and effort;

(2)   employment of a substitute skill; and

(3)   adjustment or adaptation to the new situation by changing expectations, selecting new tasks, or relaxing the criteria for success.

Examples can be found for each of these mechanisms being employed by brain-injured people (Wilson 1995b).

When discussing the forms of compensatory behaviour, Bäckman and Dixon (1992) suggest classification in a manner dependent on the extent to which the behaviour differs from the behaviour of a normal person in a given situation. The difference may be quantifiable, in that the person needing to compensate uses the same skills as those used by the normal population, but more time and effort are needed to achieve results. Alternatively, the difference may be qualitative in which case substitutable skills are used. These substitutable skills may be ones that normal people possess but typically do not use, or they may be completely new skills. One may observe brain-injured patients making heroic efforts to succeed by spending more time and effort at the task in hand through, for example, focusing on material to be remembered or giving self-instructions. Such attempts may be effective for some cognitive deficits, such as attentional problems, but not for others, for example, in a severe organic amnesia. Repetition is another method used by normal people and patients to remember something new. Although it is a widely used method for acquiring skills, repetition on its own is likely to be an inefficient or ineffective method when used by people with significant memory deficits. There are ways in which repetition or repetitive practice can be made more efficient, and this applies both to normal and brain-injured people. One of these is dis-

tributed practice, rather than massed practice (Harris 1992). In the former, practice is distributed over time, thus encouraging more effective learning than when the same amount of practice is fitted into a short space of time.

So far we have discussed compensatory strategies that are used both by those with and without memory deficits. Are there any skills developed by brain-injured people that are not normally used by people without brain injury? The examples given by Bäckman and Dixon include the Braille system used by people with visual impairments, or the implementation of higher order cognitive systems used by older typists (Salthouse 1984). In the latter case, however, it is hard to see how these are genuinely new skills rather than latent skills that are brought into play more and more as the component skills (such as tapping rate or reaction time) deteriorate.

Similarly, various compensatory strategies used by brain-injured people are typically the same as those used by people without brain injury. It is true that some brain-injured people will use certain cognitive strategies to compensate. For example, a patient with an immediate memory deficit known to us would say, 'Please can you repeat that?', or 'Please go slower', or 'Let me make sure I have understood that correctly'. The frequency with which he did this may be unusual, but the actual behaviour is seen in normal populations.

There are a few compensatory aids or strategies specifically designed for brain-injured people, and these perhaps come closest to new techniques not normally used by the general population. The use of computers as prosthetic memories, for example, is one such development. As Glisky (1995) pointed out, computers have great power for storing and producing on demand all kinds of information relevant to an individual's functioning in everyday life. Some have used computers as aids for activities of daily living (Kirsch et al. 1987). Computers here were used as 'interactive task guidance systems', which provided a series of cues to guide patients through a series of steps needed to perform practical tasks, such as baking and janitorial activities. The computer acts as a compensatory device by providing step-by-step instructions to complete a task. The user needs little knowledge of computer operation and responds by pressing a single key to indicate the instruction has been followed. However, even here we could argue that the component skills are no different from those normal people would use.

The consequences of compensatory behaviour can be

classified as successful or unsuccessful with the former being those that are functional or adaptive. However, as Bäckman and Dixon (1992) pointed out, we do not know whether successful or unsuccessful consequences are more frequent. In the case of brain-injured people, this probably depends on a number of factors including:

(1) the age of the person;

(2) the degree of impairment;

(3) the presence or absence of other impairments; and

(4) the type of rehabilitation offered.

Wilson and Watson (1996) provide evidence for the influence of these factors for people with a severe memory impairment.

Successful development of compensatory behaviour for people with neuropsychological deficits is a complex process. Patients seem to do better if they recognise that they have problems, and have good executive skills to enable them to cope with their difficulties. It helps to be young and intelligent. It probably helps to have received good rehabilitation and to have made use of compensatory strategies prior to the neurological insult.

## Other approaches to neuropsychological rehabilitation

In this final section of the chapter, we will consider other approaches to rehabilitation, which are related neither to compensatory or restitution-type processes. These are: bypassing or avoiding problems; functional adaptations or finding another way to achieve a goal; using residual skills more efficiently and improving learning.

### Bypassing or avoiding problems

One of the simplest ways to help people with cognitive problems is to arrange the environment so as to reduce the need for cognition. Norman (1988), discussing environmental designs for those who are cognitively and neurologically intact, argues for knowledge to be in the world rather than in the head. By this he means that the correct use of any object should be so obvious that it is almost impossible to make a mistake. How to open doors, turn on showers, and use the correct knob for each hot plate on the cooker are just some of the

many examples provided by Norman in his thought-provoking book. We could extend Norman's ideas to help those people with impaired cognitive functioning. For example, Wilkins, Plant, and Huddy (1989) describe how some environmental adjustments helped a stroke patient with visual perceptual difficulties. The woman had difficulty discriminating the inside from the outside of a cup. She also had problems walking, partly because she couldn't tell where her legs ended and her feet began. Wilkins *et al.* provided her with cups that were brightly coloured on the outside and white inside. This contrast enabled her to manage her drinking better. The same principle was used with the second problem. She was encouraged to wear dark trousers with light coloured socks (or vice versa).

Stroke patients with unilateral neglect are often helped if a bright red stripe is placed to the left of the telephone or reading material and other equipment, which may be neglected. People with planning problems may be helped by arranging the environment so the planning is done for them; if they cannot, for example, sort their clothes out for dressing, then garments could be put out one at a time.

Brain-injured patients with impaired judgement might be helped by organising rooms to reduce risks, by removing, for example, all medicines from the bathroom cupboard, locking up cleaning fluids, car keys, and important papers.

For people with very severe intellectual handicap or those with progressive deterioration, environmental adaptations may be the best we can do to enable people to cope with and reduce some of their confusion and frustration. Few studies have discussed ways in which environments can be designed to help people with severe cognitive impairment, although it would seem a fruitful area for therapists, psychologists, engineers, architects, and designers to join forces.

### Finding another way to achieve a goal

Just as occupational therapists provide equipment for people with physical disability to enable them to cope with activities of daily living, so we can use similar methods to help people with cognitive disability. Providing a long-handled picking-up stick or replacing buttons with Velcro for people with rheumatoid arthritis are analogous to the provision of 'talking books' for people who are blind or electronic personal organisers for those unable to remember without help. The general principle adopted here is to look for another way if the original way is no longer possible. In practice this is compensatory behaviour as discussed earlier.

## Using residual skills more efficiently

Whatever the degree of cognitive impairment, there is usually some residual, albeit malfunctioning, ability remaining. The most densely amnesic person will have some memory skills and the most perceptually impaired person will retain a certain level of perceptual ability.

Some rehabilitation programmes attempt to capitalise on these residual skills and help people to use them more efficiently. Von Cramon *et al.* (1991), for example, taught people with problem-solving deficits to deal with practical situations through applying specific problem-solving techniques. Alderman and Ward (1991) also described a treatment for helping a behaviourally and cognitively disturbed woman control her own behaviour. Berg *et al.* (1991) taught memory impaired people how to make better use of their residual memory functioning through a number of principles including:

(1)   acceptance of the problem;

(2)   use of external aids;

(3)   focusing attention;

(4)   allowing extra time;

(5)   repeating information;

(6)   making associations or links with other known material;

(7)   organising;

(8)   anticipating;

(9)   being systematic.

These general principles are similar to those described in Wilson (1992) when she described ways to improve encoding, storage. and retrieval.

Many of the programmes described for the treatment of patients with unilateral neglect are based on the principle of encouraging better use of residual abilities through, for example, self-instruction (Meichenbaum 1977) and finding an anchor point before scanning (Weinberg *et al.* 1979).

## Improving learning

Baddeley and Wilson (1994), and Wilson *et al.* (1994) demonstrated that people with severe memory disorders

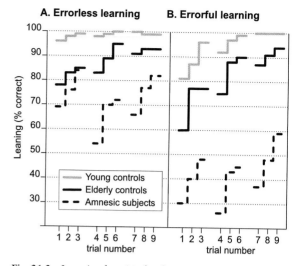

Fig. 21.2   Learning function for three groups of subjects tested using errorless or errorful learning procedures. (Adapted from Baddeley and Wilson 1994.)

learn better when trial and error methods are avoided during learning (see Fig. 21.2). Influenced by errorless discrimination learning from behavioural psychology (Terrace 1963, 1966), and by implicit learning in cognitive psychology (Tulving and Schacter 1990), errorless learning is a teaching technique whereby people are prevented as far as possible from making mistakes while they are learning a new skill or new information. Instead of teaching by demonstration, which may involve trial and error, the correct information or procedure is presented in ways that minimise the possibility of erroneous responses. Errors are likely to be reinforced by people with poor episodic memory because of their reliance on implicit memory, which is inefficient at error elimination. Errorless learning has proved effective over a range of tasks, including learning names, new information, identification of line drawings, and programming an electronic aid. It is also effective for a range of diagnostic groups including head injury, stroke, encephalitis, and Korsakoff's syndrome; and a range of times post-insult from post-traumatic amnesia to 12 years post-infection (Wilson *et al.* 1994).

We do not yet know whether errorless learning is superior for other brain-injured patients without significant memory impairment, such as those with language or perceptual disorders, nor do we know its value for non-brain-injured populations such as normal elderly people or children with development dyslexia.

# General guidelines

The problems faced by brain-injured people are not limited to the cognitive domain. They also have emotional, physical, and social problems that need to be addressed. Anxiety, for example, is common and may interfere with or limit cognitive progress if not dealt with appropriately. Wilson (1995a) discusses this issue in more detail and includes descriptions of groups that can be very effective in reducing anxiety and depression. Wearing (1992) provides a wealth of information about self-help groups that carers and relatives might find useful.

Information in counselling for patients and their families is an important part of therapy. Explanations about why patients are unable to remember, or why they experience difficulty in reading, or fail to recognise objects can make the problems easier to manage. Harder to deal with is the information patients and relatives demand concerning future expectations. Answers to their questions will depend to some extent on the cause of the brain injury. Head-injured patients, for example, tend to continue improving for longer than patients with encephalitis. Patients with degenerative diseases will not improve, although it might be possible to slow down the rate of decline (Arkin 1991, 1992). Prognosis also depends on time post-insult; progress will be different for a head-injured patient in the first few days following an accident, than it will for a similarly injured patient 12 months post-injury. Other factors determining progress include severity and extent of brain injury, personality characteristics, and so forth.

# Further reading

Robertson, I.H. and Murre, J.M.J. (1999). Rehabilitation of brain damage: Brain plasticity and principles of guided recovery. *Psychological Bulletin*, **125**, 544–575.

# Section VI
## Structural repair

In Chapter 12 the reasons for the failure of axon regeneration in the central nerous system (CNS) have been explored. In summary, these are:

(1) the non-permissive nature of the CNS environment, due to the ability of astrocytes, oligodendrocyte progenitors and oligodendrocytes to block axon growth; and

(2) factors intrinsic to the axons themselves, particularly the reduced vigour of regenerative axon growth as compared to developmental growth, and a mismatch between the cell surface adhesion molecules on the axons and those present in the environment.

However, despite these factors that inhibit axon regeneration in the CNS, significant amounts of regenerative growth have been induced experimentally using several different strategies. This chapter describes the efforts that have been made to date to persuade axons in the CNS to regrow, and the resulting re-innervation of terminal structures and behavioural recovery.

## Strategies to overcome the inhibitory effects of the CNS environment

The success or failure of axon regeneration depends on a balance of positive and negative factors. On the one hand, the CNS environment produces several molecules that are inhibitory to growth, many of which increase following injury, and on the other hand, CNS axons are attempting with variable vigour to regrow through this inhibitory environment. It follows that if one wishes to encourage axon regeneration, one might do so either by making the CNS environment less inhibitory, or by making the axons better able to regrow. The best chance of success must be if both these approaches are tried simultaneously, although experiments that have been designed simply to remove inhibitory molecules in the

CNS environment have demonstrated some regeneration. It is important to point out at this stage, however, that none of the experiments described below are as simple as they sound. While it is easy to plan in principle to remove a single inhibitory component from the CNS environment, inevitably the results of the intervention will be much more complex. For instance, removing a single cell type by injecting an antibody specific to that cell, together with complement into the CNS, will certainly kill the cell. However, the presence of dead cells will activate microglia, the presence of antibody and complement will also activate microglia and other cell types, and the end result will be a CNS environment that is modified not only by the removal of the targeted cell type, but also by the secretion of many different cytokines and growth factors by astrocytes and microglia. Most interventions in the CNS will break down the blood–brain barrier for a time, so simply injecting an antibody into the CNS will usually mean that the antibody will bind and activate serum complement. The reader should therefore remember, while reading the experiments we describe below, that they may be more complicated than they appear.

## Replacement of the CNS environment with peripheral nerve grafts or Schwann cells

If CNS glial cells are inhibitory, an obvious strategy is to replace them altogether with cells that have been shown to encourage regeneration. In adult mammals, axon growth or regeneration is only seen routinely in two situations: in damaged peripheral nerves, and in the olfactory pathway. In damaged peripheral nerves, regeneration only occurs in the presence of Schwann cells, and the axons regenerate in contact with Schwann cells (see Chapter 11). Schwann cells are therefore known to be a successful substrate for the regeneration of at least one type of axon, and are therefore an obvious choice if one wishes to replace CNS glia with glial cells able to promote regeneration; these cells have the added advantage that they are able to remyelinate axons in both the PNS and CNS. Olfactory ensheathing cells provide the environment through which the newly born olfactory neurones, which are created throughout life, grow their axons into the CNS to make contact with neurones in the olfactory bulb, and these are therefore another possible candidate for providing a substrate for regeneration (see below).

The first indications that CNS axons could be induced to regenerate in peripheral nerve came from the experiments of Tello and Cajal at the turn of the century. However, these experiments were done without the benefit of modern axon tracing techniques, and their interpretation was therefore open to some question. The idea was revived by Aguayo and his colleagues in 1981 (David and Aguayo 1981). They inserted lengths of peripheral nerve into the spinal cord, and then placed horseradish peroxidase (HRP) into the graft as a nerve tracer to demonstrate regenerating axons and trace their neurones of origin (Fig. 22.1). The basic finding was that large numbers of axons would regenerate into peripheral nerve grafts, many from CNS neurones. However even in these first landmark experiments, it was clear that not all CNS axons had equal powers of regeneration. Most of the axons that had grown into the peripheral nerve grafts came from neurones that were close to the grafts, and very few axons that had been cut far from their cell bodies would regenerate. Moreover, some axons, such as

those from dorsal root ganglion sensory neurones, were over-represented, while some other neurones showed little regenerative potential.

Peripheral nerve grafts have now been inserted into a large number of locations in the CNS, and some general principles have come out from the results. In general, axon regeneration is more likely to occur if the axon is cut close to the neurone, but not so close as to lead to neuronal death. For instance, in the optic nerve, grafts placed in the mid part of the nerve produce little regeneration, while grafts placed close to or in the retina attract many axons. Similarly in the spinal cord the majority of axons growing into peripheral nerve grafts originate from neurones close to the site of graft insertion, only few longer axons, such as those of the corticospinal tract, having regrown. One tract that has been very completely studied from this point of view is the rubrospinal tract. Here, axons in the rat will regenerate into a peripheral nerve graft placed in the cervical cord, but not into the thoracic cord (Tetzlaff *et al.* 1994). Not all neurones are equally good at regenerating their axons, regardless of where they are cut. Thus grafts inserted into the rat thalamus attract many regenerating axons, but the majority come from one type of neurone, in the thalamic reticular nucleus. Similarly, in the cerebellum the majority of axons growing in to peripheral nerve grafts are from the olivary nuclei, but the Purkinje cells stand out as neurones that will not regenerate their axons into a Schwann cell-containing graft wherever it is placed, nor will they regrow their axons into grafts of embryonic CNS tissue (Rossi *et al.* 1995).

A problematic feature of peripheral nerve and Schwann cell grafts into the CNS is that while axons grow in fairly large numbers from the CNS environment into the Schwann cell environment, there is generally little or no growth of axons from the peripheral nerve graft back into the CNS. This is clearly a major difficulty if Schwann cell-containing grafts are to be used for practical CNS repair. If regenerating axons are to have any useful effect on the damaged CNS they must be able to re-enter the CNS environment from the graft and synapse with host neurones. Regenerating axons meet a similar barrier when they try to regenerate down a dorsal root and back into the CNS (see Chapter 11). Here again, the regenerating axons are unable to make the transition of leaving a Schwann cell-containing environment to grow through a CNS glial environment.

However, there are experiments in which some growth of axons from a Schwann cell environment into CNS tissue has been achieved, and in which the axons

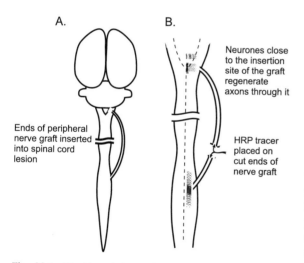

**Fig. 22.1** David and Aguayo's experiment to demonstrate that CNS axons can regenerate in a permissive environment. Two lesions in the spinal cord were made, and a length of peripheral nerve was inserted into them. Later, horseradish peroxidase (HRP) was placed in the nerve graft, so as to trace axons and their neurones that had regenerated into the graft. Most grafts contained many axons, but most of their neurones were close to the graft site.

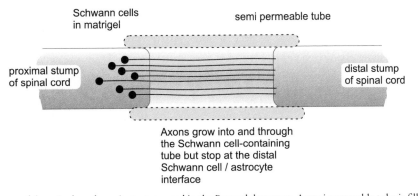

**Fig. 22.2** A diagram of the spinal cord repair strategy used in the Bunge laboratory. A semi-permeable tube is filled with Schwann cells embedded in matrigel, and the cut ends of the spinal cord are inserted into either end. Schwann cells do not migrate out of the tube into the host cord, rather a sharp Schwann cell/astrocyte interface forms. Axons are recruited into the Schwann cell containing tube, and many grow through it to the distal astrocyte interface, but they will not cross into the host CNS tissue.

have been shown to make functional connections with CNS neurones. It is clearly important to try to understand what factors make this possible. In one example, peripheral nerve grafts to the optic nerve have been shown to induce regeneration of a small proportion of retinal ganglion cell axons. If the distal end of the graft is inserted into the normal target of these retinal ganglion cell axons, the superior colliculus, a few of these axons have been shown to grow into the CNS tissue and make functional synapses there with collicular neurones (Carter *et al.* 1994). In a different pathway, axons of the nigro-striatal pathway were mechanically lesioned, and a bridge graft of Schwannoma cells placed between the lesion and the target in the striatum. Again, axons regenerating through the Schwann cell graft were able to exit it and make functional connections with the host CNS, to the extent of partially restoring the motor functions of the tract (Brecknell *et al.* 1996). The common feature in both these models may be that target neurones were directly adjacent to the margin of the graft, and therefore axons did not have to grow for significant distances through the inhibitory CNS environment before finding synaptic targets. However, there has also been a recent, very encouraging, experiment from Lars Olson's laboratory, taking a different approach. In these experiments the most difficult objective has been achieved, namely persuading some long tract spinally projecting axons to regenerate to produce a functional effect distal to a complete spinal cord transection. In this experimental paradigm, several parallel peripheral nerve grafts embedded in a fibrin gel containing FGF-1 were used to bridge a completely transected rat spinal cord (Cheng *et al.* 1996). Axons from as far up as the brainstem and

cortex were able to regenerate through the grafts and into the distal cord, and there was quite substantial behavioural recovery in several tests. The FGF-1 was a necessary component of this reconstructive surgery, and it may have been this that made it easier for axons to grow in the astrocytic environment of the cord by modifying the glial environment (see below), and thus made it possible for axons to leave the Schwann cell environment of the nerve graft. Two features, therefore, appear to be important in those experiments that have been successful in getting axons from a Schwann cell bridge back into the CNS, one is probably the proximity of suitable target neurones, and the other is probably the manipulation of the host glial environment with cytokines.

What is it about Schwann cells that makes them able to support CNS axon regeneration? As in peripheral nerve regeneration, CNS axons regenerate in direct association with Schwann cells. Patrick Anderson, Bob Lieberman and their colleagues have looked directly at the molecules upregulated on Schwann cells and regenerating axons when peripheral nerve grafts are inserted into the CNS (Anderson *et al.* 1998). The molecules involved are similar to those involved in peripheral nerve regeneration (see Chapter 11). *In vitro* studies of axon growth over Schwann cells showed that the critical molecular interactions involve laminin and the adhesion molecules L1 and N-cadherin. Regenerating CNS axons growing into peripheral nerve grafts upregulate L1 and N-CAM on their surface, and may also express the polysialyated form of N-CAM. L1 and N-CAM are also upregulated on Schwann cells. In addition, there is widespread expression of tenascin-C on CNS glia and

Schwann cells. The fact that some CNS neurones mount a much more vigorous regenerative response than others allowed Anderson and his colleagues to make correlations between regenerative response and upregulation of molecules. The general rule is that neurones that are successful at regenerating their axons into peripheral nerve grafts upregulate L1, GAP-43, and c-jun, while non-regenerating neurones do not. It is also possible that the secretion of diffusible trophic factors by Schwann cells may be a mechanism by which they can promote regeneration of CNS axons. Certainly, in lesioned peripheral nerves, Schwann cells start to secrete a variety of trophic factors, particularly nerve growth factor (NGF), ciliary neurotrophic factor (CNTF), brain-derived neurotrophic factor (BDNF), and glial cell line-derived neurotrophic factor (GDNF). However, in peripheral nerve, the production of these trophic factors depends partly on exogenous factors, for instance, IL-1 and other factors secreted by macrophages (Meyer *et al.* 1992). Some of these factors are largely absent, or much reduced, when Schwann cells are grafted into the CNS, where the macrophage response to injury is tiny when compared to peripheral nerve. It may be therefore, that Schwann cells placed in the CNS do not undergo some of the changes that occur after peripheral nerve damage that make them so attractive to regenerating axons, and are therefore less effective in promoting axon growth than those in peripheral nerves. The only indirect evidence on this point is that Schwann cells in damaged peripheral nerve greatly upregulate the immediate early gene c-jun, but Schwann cells grafted into the CNS do not, indicating that they are not in the same activated state (Vaudano *et al.* 1996). For this reason there is a rationale for adding additional exogenous neurotrophins to Schwann cells grafted into the CNS to try and make them more effective in attracting regenerating axons and promoting their growth. This strategy has been effective in one experimental model. Mary Bunge and her colleagues have developed a Schwann cell transplant model in which a semi-permeable tube containing Schwann cells is implanted into the dorsal columns of the spinal cord (Fig. 22.2). These transplants induce plentiful axon growth into the Schwann cell graft, but the number of axons is greatly increased if neurotrophin-3 (NT-3) or BDNF is infused into one end of the graft (Xu *et al.* 1995).

## Use of olfactory ensheathing cells to promote axon regeneration

Other than Schwann cells, the other cell type that promotes axon growth in mammals is the olfactory ensheathing cell. During life new sensory neurones are constantly generated in the olfactory epithelium to replace those that are lost. In order to carry olfactory sensations to the brain, these new neurones must grow axons into the olfactory bulb, to make connections with CNS neurones. The cells that provide the substrate for these regenerating axons are the olfactory ensheathing cells, which have many of the properties of Schwann cells. However, these cells achieve something that Schwann cells in the adult CNS do not, namely axons can grow from ensheathing cells into the CNS to make connections with CNS neurones. One might argue, therefore, that ensheathing cells would be preferable to Schwann cells for CNS repair. This argument has led to a number of trials of their use in regeneration models. The first transplant experiments were done in the spinal cord by Ramon-Cueto and Nieto-Sampedro, who implanted cells into the dorsal root entry zone area (Ramon-Cueto and Nieto-Sampedro 1994). This work suggested two important conclusions. First, following dorsal root re-attachment, axons were seen to regenerate into the spinal cord past the dorsal root entry zone in association with the ensheathing cells. Moreover, unlike Schwann cells, the ensheathing cells appeared to migrate for significant distances from their point of transplantation. This has led to several trials of ensheathing cells in various lesion models. Most recent and successful have been two trials in spinal cord lesions. In the first of these experiments, Li and Raisman (Li *et al.* 1997) transplanted olfactory cells (not purified ensheathing cells) into cervical lesions of the rat corticospinal tract (Fig. 22.3). When corticospinal axons were traced they had regenerated for considerable distances through the lesion and on into the spinal cord. Moreover, animals in which these axons had regenerated showed return of function in a skilled paw-reaching task, which has been shown to require corticospinal function. When the transplanted ensheathing cells were visualised, they had migrated for considerable distances from their point of insertion — much further than Schwann cells would have migrated. However, it appeared that the axons had regenerated further than the front of olfactory cell migration, suggesting that axons had not simply been towed behind migrating cells, but were able to leave the ensheathing cell environment and re-enter the CNS glial environment. Ensheathing cells have also recently been used in a composite strategy in combination with Schwann cells. In the previous section we described the Bunge spinal repair model, in which a semi-permeable tube containing Schwann cells embedded in matrigel is placed between the stumps of a complete cord section. We

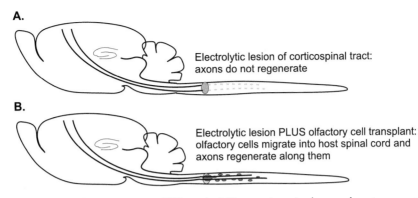

**Fig. 22.3** Ensheathing cell transplants to promote CNS repair. A Host corticostriatal axons do not regenerate through an electrolytic lesion in the spinal cord. B After transplantation of olfactory glia into the lesion, the ensheathing cells migrated widely in the cord and were accompanied by regenerating corticospinal axons. The axons appeared to regenerate beyond the migration range of the ensheathing cells and mediated recovery of a skilled paw reaching task. (Based on Li *et al.* 1997.)

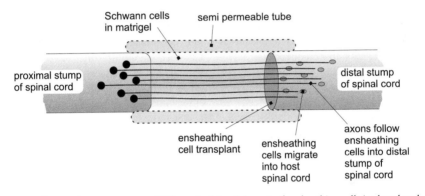

**Fig. 22.4** Ensheathing cell transplants to promote CNS repair. A local deposit of ensheathing cells is placed at the border between a Schwann cell-containing matrigel tube and the distal host spinal cord after complete transection. Instead of axon regeneration being blocked at the Schwann cell graft/host astrocyte interface (as in Fig. 22.2), the ensheathing cells migrated widely, and regenerating axons were seen to progress beyond the Schwann cells and into the host CNS, accompanying the migrating ensheathing cells. (Based on Ramon-Cueto *et al.* 1998.)

described how axons would grow into these tubes and through the Schwann cells, but were unable to exit the Schwann cell environment to re-enter the CNS glial environment. In order to try and persuade axons to grow on from the Schwann cell-containing tube into the host cord, a small deposit of ensheathing cells was placed by Ramon-Cueto and her collaborators at the graft/host interface (Fig. 22.4 Ramon-Cueto *et al.* 1998). The result was dramatic: the ensheathing cells migrated widely into the distal stump of the host cord, unlike Schwann cells, which completely fail to migrate. In the regions containing ensheathing cells there was a profuse outgrowth of regenerating axons that could be traced back to the proximal cord, up to the hindbrain. In general, there was a good correlation between the position of ensheathing cells and of regenerating axons, so in this case the presence of the ensheathing cells may

have been necessary for the axons to grow into CNS tissue, and there was less evidence for axons growing on beyond the migrating cells.

These studies have indicated that ensheathing cells may have important advantages over Schwann cells for use in CNS repair. The most important advantage may be the ability of the cells to migrate in a CNS environment (see Chapter 24). Schwann cells will only migrate into areas of damaged CNS that are relatively depleted of astrocytes and, in general, a Schwann cell transplant becomes encapsulated by astrocytes, with the formation of a sharp astrocyte/Schwann cell boundary, which axons are only able to cross in one direction — from astrocytes to Schwann cells. Ensheathing cells, however, do not seem to be constrained in the same way. Axons are probably able to follow the migrating ensheathing cells, which may be able to carry them out of the area of the CNS tissue that has reacted to injury by upregulating inhibitory molecules. Why might ensheathing cells be able to migrate while Schwann cells fail? Cell migration requires three main factors: cell motility, appropriate adhesion molecules, and secretion of proteases. If one compares the different cell types, Schwann cells and ensheathing cells are both extremely motile *in vitro*, and Schwann cells are also highly migratory following peripheral nerve injuries. Schwann cells are known to secrete at least some of the proteases that are associated with cell migration, but there is no data on ensheathing cells. Yet Schwann cell migration is strongly inhibited by astrocytes. Wilby and colleagues (1999) examined Schwann cell migration in association with astrocytes, and found that migration was inhibited not by a classical growth cone collapse-related inhibitory mechanism, but by the formation of very long-lived adhesive contacts between Schwann cells and astrocytes. The main shared adhesion molecule between the two cell types is N-cadherin. Wilby was able to show that N-cadherin-blocking reagents that reduced astrocyte-Schwann cell adhesion also promoted Schwann cell migration on astrocyte surfaces. Whether the different abilities of Schwann cells and ensheathing cells to migrate in CNS environments can be explained on the basis of N-cadherin remains to be seen. Both Schwann and ensheathing cells have L1, cadherins, integrins, and N-CAM on their surfaces, but intracellular mechanisms can vary the degree of adhesion due to these cell surface molecules. One molecule that has been shown to promote migration within the CNS is polysialyated N-CAM (PSA-N-CAM). The stem cells that migrate rapidly from the subventricular zone to the olfactory lobes express PSA-N-CAM on their surface, and Urs Rutishauser and his colleagues (Hu *et al.* 1996) were able to show that removing the PSA rendered the cells non-migratory in the CNS. The presence of multiple sialic acid side-chains on N-CAM can prevent the binding of not only N-CAM but also other adhesion molecules, reducing the adhesiveness of the cells, and therefore probably making it easier for them to migrate. One of the types of olfactory glia expresses PSA-N-CAM, but its role in the migration of these cells in the CNS has not been investigated.

## Use of embryonic grafts to promote axon regeneration

While adult CNS tissue is non-permissive to axon growth and regeneration, embryonic tissue is clearly able to promote growth during development. There

have therefore been attempts to use embryonic tissue to induce axon regeneration and functional repair in the damaged CNS, and particularly in the spinal cord. The general behaviour of embryonic neuronal grafts is well established, and discussed in the next chapter. In general, transplanted embryonic neurones can grow processes into the host CNS for limited distances, and make functional synaptic connections with host neurones. Similarly, host neuronal processes can sprout or regenerate into the transplant and make synapses with the grafted embryonic neurones. The limitation, however, is that axons from the graft will not grow for appreciable distances into the host CNS unless there are target neurones immediately adjacent to the graft. The extent of the connections made by grafts is very dependent on the age of the host. Grafts placed into newborn hosts, whose CNS has not yet become inhibitory to axon growth, grow axons extensively, and also receive a profuse axonal projection from the host neurones. However, as animals age, the glial environment of their CNS becomes inhibitory to axon growth, and the regenerative ability of their neurones decreases, and this is reflected in fewer connections to and from a graft of embryonic CNS tissue (Fig. 22.5).

Neural transplantation has been under investigation for some years as a possible therapy for spinal-cord injury, and there have recently been some encouraging results in animal models of the condition involving both transection and contusion injuries. A wide range of transplants into various lesion models in newborn and adult cord have been made, many of the experiments coming from the laboratories of Barbara Bregman and Paul Reier. As one would predict from the general biology of neural transplantation, the effects of spinal cord transplantation are very dependent on the age of the host. The most complete repair is seen when embryonic cord is transplanted into newborn animals. Embryonic spinal cord grafts are able to induce the regeneration of host axons into the graft, but only in newborn animals is there any evidence that they can act as a bridge, enabling axons to grow through the graft, and then on into the host CNS to form normal spinal cord tracts and normal anatomical connections. In fact, a newborn animal injured at birth and repaired with an embryonic spinal cord graft can have a very normal appearing cord, and almost normal behaviour (Diener and Bregman 1998). However, it is important to realise that the newborn spinal cord is still a developing structure, with axons still growing from brain to cord in the corticospinal tract. In adult animals, spinal cord transplants still have beneficial effects, but the mechanism by

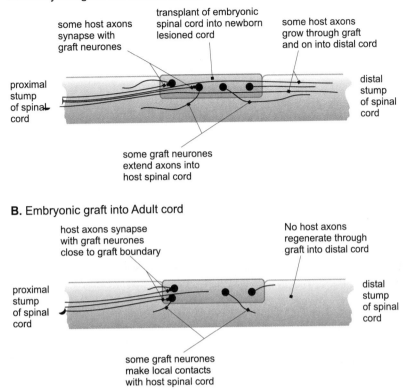

**A. Embryonic graft into Newborn cord**

some host axons
synapse with
graft neurones

transplant of embryonic
spinal cord into newborn
lesioned cord

some host axons
grow through graft
and on into distal cord

proximal
stump
of spinal
cord

distal
stump
of spinal
cord

some graft neurones
extend axons into
host spinal cord

**B. Embryonic graft into Adult cord**

host axons synapse
with graft neurones
close to graft boundary

No host axons
regenerate through
graft into distal cord

proximal
stump
of spinal
cord

distal
stump
of spinal
cord

some graft neurones
make local contacts
with host spinal cord

**Fig. 22.5** The results of transplanting embryonic spinal cord tissue into a lesion in either newborn or adult cord. In both cases graft neurones send out processes into the host tissue to make connections, although these are more plentiful and over a wider area in newborn hosts. In newborn hosts the graft can act as a bridge, enabling host axons to grow though the bridge and on into host tissue, with almost complete restitution of the normal neuroanatomy. Some host axons synapse with graft neurones, which have the potential to relay their information on into host cord. When transplants are made into adult spinal cord the host axons will only regenerate for a short distance into the graft, where they can synapse on graft neurones. No axons regenerate through the graft and on into the distal part of the cord. Such recovery as is mediated by these grafts must either be due to the relay of information from host axons via graft neurones which have made connections in the host cord, or due to local effects of the graft tissue on the injury response of the host tissue.

which they work is less clear. Host axon regeneration is much less impressive than in newborn animals, and the regenerating axons are restricted to the grafts, often only the part of the graft closest to the host interface. The graft neurones also grow axons: these make most of their connections within the graft itself, but some grow out into the host spinal cord, and make connections with host neurones. This outgrowth, however, is only restricted to a few millimetres surrounding the graft, and certainly does not extend more than a spinal segment or so. Yet despite this very limited connectivity, and lack of long distance regeneration of host axons through the graft bridge, there can be considerable return of lost function in a number of behavioural tests, some of which

are thought to require descending control from the cortex (Bregman *et al.* 1993). It is likely that in these circumstances the graft is acting as a relay. Host axons are able to grow into the graft and form connections with graft neurones, and the graft neurones in turn are able to grow axons into the host cord and form connections there. The graft may also be able to affect local injury responses and healing. For instance, when transplanted into contusion injuries in the cat spinal cord, foetal transplants modified the local injury response, and transplanted animals suffered less behavioural loss than controls (Stokes and Reier 1992). In addition, the graft may be acting as a source of neurotrophins and as a source of oligodendrocyte precursors.

# *Removal of inhibitory glial cells and inhibitory molecules*

## Removal of CNS glial cells

If, as we have described in Chapter 12, CNS glial cells produce inhibitory molecules, the question arises as to what would happen to axon regeneration in the CNS if the CNS glia were removed. There is commonly extensive sprouting around large CNS lesions for a few days, until the normal CNS injury response creates a glial scar, and the sprouting stops or retracts. It is possible, however, to make rather more specific lesions. Ethidium bromide binds to nucleic acid, and particularly to DNA, and in sufficient amount kills cells by damaging their nucleus. In low concentration it does not, however, kill axons whose cell body is some distance away, and blood vessels may also be spared. Recently Moon and colleagues (1999) have examined axon regeneration in a tract cleared of glia by injections of ethidium bromide delivered along the length of the tract. The axons of the nigro-striatal tract were cut mechanically, then ethidium bromide was injected along their pathway. The initial result was a large cylindrical lesion in which there were no oligodendrocytes, astrocytes, or oligodendrocyte precursors, and in this lesion there was robust regeneration of nigro-striatal axons. However, regeneration appeared to stop after about 4 days. During the stages when axons were regenerating, the main cell type present was microglia. By the time regeneration ceased, the lesion had recruited oligodendrocyte precursors, and the astrocytes in the lesion wall had started to organise into a traditional scar. This experiment demonstrates two important principles. First, it shows that removal of oligodendrocytes and astrocytes is in itself sufficient to allow some axons to regenerate. Second, it shows that lesion experiments must be interpreted with great care, since simply creating a glial-depleted lesion can produce axon regeneration. This is particularly important, since attempts to deplete one type of cell selectively may often affect other cell types as well.

## Removal of oligodendrocytes

Since oligodendrocytes have molecules on their surface that can inhibit axon growth, the removal of these cells from regions where axon regeneration is required is an obvious step. Axon regeneration has been achieved in animals in which oligodendrocytes have been depleted by a variety of methods. Schwab and his colleagues were the first to do this by irradiating the spinal cord of newborn rats before myelination. The blockage of cell division brought on by irradiation prevented the proliferation of oligodendrocytes, and thus myelination. Two weeks after birth, the dorsal two-thirds of the spinal cord of these animals was sectioned, and then 2–4 weeks later an injection of the nerve tracer HRP was made into the motor cortex. After 24 h delay to allow HRP transport, the spinal cord was examined. Some regeneration of corticospinal axons was visible for up to 1 cm below the lesion, while in control animals regenerated axons had only penetrated 1.5 mm beyond the lesion. In the optic nerve of irradiated animals, regeneration over similar distances was observed, but only if trophic factors were injected into the orbit to support the axotomised retinal ganglion cells (Schwab 1990).

A similar experiment was performed by Keirstead and Steeves in the chick. Axons in the chick CNS will regenerate up to the 16th day of embryonic life, but after that time regeneration fails. The onset of regenerative failure is co-incident with the appearance of oligodendrocytes and myelin. By injecting into the cord the oligodendrocyte cell surface antibody, anti-galactocerebroside, Steeves and his colleagues were able to delay for 3 days the appearance of oligodendrocytes, and during this period the ability of axons to regenerate in the cord persisted (Keirstead *et al.* 1995). These two experiments were not designed to effect a repair of function in the spinal cord, but rather to test the hypothesis that oligodendrocytes are inhibitory to axon regeneration, and therefore no functional testing of the experimental animals was done to see whether the regenerated axons had made functional connections. However, in a later study, Steeves used infusions of the anti-galactocerebroside antibody together with complement to remove the oligodendrocytes from a region of the spinal cord in adult chicks in a more direct attempt to see whether oligodendrocyte depletion might form part of a strategy for repair of the injured spinal cord. As with the embryonic animals it was possible to render a region of cord free of myelin, and within this region there was some axon regeneration following lesioning. Functional recovery was tested electrophysiologically, by stimulating the brainstem and using electromyograms to test for motor re-innervation. Clear but small electromyogram responses were recorded, which were almost certainly attributable to regenerating axons having formed appropriate connections with post-synaptic neurones. However, there were no behavioural signs of recovery from the lesions, indicating that the number of regenerating axons was probably small.

The previous experiments involved the active removal of oligodendrocytes from otherwise normal animals. There are, however mutants in which oligodendrocytes die during development, and which are therefore naturally demyelinated. These animals have a very limited lifespan before they succumb to the problems with their nervous systems, but before then it is possible to make lesions and test for axon regeneration. Experiments of this type were performed by Berry and his colleagues using the optic nerve (Berry *et al.* 1992). The results of these experiments were rather different to those in which the demyelination was caused by experimental intervention, in that axon regeneration was very limited, although measurably increased over control animals.

## Depletion of astrocytes

At present there is no technique for selectively depleting astrocytes in the CNS. Moreover, because astrocytes play such a key structural and metabolic role in the CNS, one suspects that removing all the astrocytes would have serious consequences for the integrity of the remaining structures. However, removing both astrocytes and oligodendrocytes with ethidium bromide does not kill those axons left behind. The nearest to astrocyte depletion that has been achieved are the ethidium bromide experiments mentioned above, and the experiments of Sims and Gilmore in which irradiation was used to create glial-depleted regions (Sims and Gilmore 1994). In both these experiments, axon regeneration was observed in those regions that were depleted of astrocytes, but also of oligodendrocytes and oligodendrocyte precursors. One can only speculate about the degree to which axon regeneration was due to astrocyte depletion, and to what extent it was due to removal or invasion of the other cell types.

## Counteracting the inhibitory effects of oligodendrocytes

Oligodendrocytes have on their surface two main axon growth inhibitory molecules, Nogo A (originally called NI-250) and MAG. They also secrete into their matrix tenascin-R and versican, both of which have inhibitory properties (see Chapter 12). There may be other molecules as well, since, when oligodendrocyte cell surface molecules are fractionated, there are inhibitory fractions that are neither MAG nor Nogo. Most of the experiments designed to counteract inhibitory molecules have been aimed at Nogo. The molecule has recently been cloned and sequenced and it will therefore soon be pos-

sible to prevent its expression, and to develop specific inhibitors based on a knowledge of molecular structure. However Schwab and his colleagues have developed a monoclonal antibody IN-1, which prevents the inhibition of axon growth by oligodendrocytes and by purified Nogo A in tissue culture models, probably by binding to the molecule and neutralising its effects. When this antibody is applied to oligodendrocytes or purified myelin *in vitro*, axons will grow over them readily, while in the absence of the antibody growth is inhibited by both oligodendrocytes and myelin extract (Schwab 1990). This antibody has been used for a variety of *in vivo* studies. The basic experiment has been to introduce the antibody into the CNS in high concentrations, at the same time as making a lesion in an axonal pathway. Such lesions with IN-1 treatment have been made in the spinal cord, the optic nerve, and in the fimbria-fornix input to the hippocampus. In the optic nerve, which contains the axons of retinal ganglion cells projecting to the visual structures of the brain, anatomical studies showed considerably more axon regeneration than normal, but only if the retina was treated with basic fibroblast growth factor (FGF-2) or brain derived neurotrophic factor (BDNF) to minimise retinal ganglion cell death and axonal retraction. Similarly, there was increased regeneration of septal axons into the hippocampus when animals were treated with the IN-1 antibody.

The majority of experiments, however, have been performed in the spinal cord, and have been designed to demonstrate both anatomical and functional recovery of the corticospinal tract. These experiments have been very encouraging, particularly since the main practical application of treatments to induce axon regeneration is likely to be in spinal cord injury. The basic experimental paradigm has been to inject a nerve tracer into the motor cortex, which is taken up by neurones and can be used to visualise the axons of the corticospinal tract. Either before or after the tracer injection, the spinal cord is lesioned mechanically so as to cut the cortico-spinal tract. The first studies showed that in antibody treated animals, but not in controls, a small number of axons could regenerate for distances of up to 1 cm (Fig. 22.6; Schnell and Schwab 1990). However, this was not sufficient to produce gross functional recovery — the animals were not able to walk with their hind legs. Nevertheless, more sensitive functional tests, designed specifically to pick up partial recovery of corticospinal function, have in some cases shown a significant degree of functional return in antibody treated animals, while other tests show no improvement over controls. While the precise synaptic arrangements underlying these functional improvements have yet to be elucidated, these experiments seem to provide further evidence that a very small number of axons can underlie a surprisingly large behavioural effect (Bregman *et al.* 1995).

MAG is inhibitory to the growth of several types of axon *in vitro*. Since this molecule has been sequenced it has been possible to use a rather more direct approach to see whether it is an important factor in preventing regeneration. The gene has been knocked out in two independent transgenic mouse lines. The MAG knockout mice do not show dramatic increases in axon regeneration in the CNS, although there may be subtle increases. There are, however, very significant changes that can be detected in tissue culture in MAG knockout tissue and through other manipulations (McKerracher *et al.* 1994; Mukhopadhyay *et al.* 1994). MAG is also produced in peripheral nerves, and the MAG knockouts show some increase in axon regeneration in peripheral nerves (Schäfer *et al.* 1996).

## Counteracting the inhibitory effects of astrocytes and oligodendrocyte precursors

Inhibition of axon growth by astrocytes and oligodendrocyte precursors is largely by the production of chondroitin sulphate proteoglycans (CSPGs) (Fawcett and Asher 1999). *In vivo* studies trying to promote regeneration by reducing inhibition due to CSPGs are less advanced that those on oligodendrocyte-mediated mechanisms. The simplest type of experiment is simply to reduce the number of astrocytes and oligodendrocyte precursors. As described above, this can be done in young animals by irradiation: irradiation of the spinal cord reduces the density of astrocytes and other cell types around the dorsal root entry zones, and allows Schwann cell migration and some axon regeneration (Sims and Gilmore 1994). Tissue culture studies have shown that interfering with proteoglycan synthesis can make astrocytes more permissive (see Chapter 12), but these approaches are only beginning to be translated into *in vivo* experiments. An experiment by Lawrence Moon has shown that axon regeneration in the axotomised nigrostriatal tract can be stimulated by injections of chondroitinase, which removes the glycosaminoglycan chains from CSPGs (Moon *et al.* 1999). Both FGF-1 and -2 make astrocytes less inhibitory, and FGF-1 is a necessary component of the complicated spinal cord transection operations of Olson, described above under Schwann cell

grafting. Some inflammatory cytokines, together with FGF, also make astrocytes less inhibitory (Fok-Seang *et al.* 1998), and some repair experiments may turn out to have had a beneficial effect as much because they have caused inflammation as for any other reason.

# Treatments that act on the neurone to enhance regeneration

As explained in previous sections, neurones differ greatly in their ability to regenerate their axons. Embryonic neurones can grow axons through terrain that would stop the growth of regenerating axons, and even adult neurones differ considerably in their ability to regrow their axons. An obvious strategy for enhancing regeneration is therefore to try and find treatments that will increase the regenerative potential of axons. In general, the regenerative potential correlates well with the expression of GAP-43 in neurones: those neurones whose axons regenerate always express GAP-43 or CAP-23, which probably has a similar function, but expression of GAP-43 will not by itself cause axons to regenerate. Thus, GAP-43 is necessary but not in itself sufficient. As described earlier in this chapter, CNS axons will regenerate into peripheral nerve or Schwann cell grafts, but only if they are cut near the cell body. In the example studied by Tetzlaff, axons from red nucleus neurones will regenerate into peripheral nerve grafts that are placed in the cervical cord, but not grafts that are placed further down the cord. This correlates with GAP-43 expression, which is induced by cutting the axons in the cervical cord, but not in the thoracic cord. These findings were illustrated in Chapter 2 (Figure 2.3; Tetzlaff *et al.* 1994). Similarly, in the optic nerve, if peripheral nerve grafts are joined onto the nerve just behind the orbit, many retinal axons will grow through the Schwann cells of the graft. If the nerve graft is placed more distally, there is little axon regeneration, and this again correlates with GAP-43 expression in the retinal ganglion cells (Doster *et al.* 1991).

An obvious strategy to try and increase the regenerative potential of neurones is to treat them with neurotrophic factors. This is certainly a strategy that works in tissue culture models, and there are now several examples where it has been used with success *in vivo*. In the red nucleus model described above, infusing BDNF on the neurones themselves makes them express GAP-43 when their axons are cut distally in the thoracic cord, while normally GAP-43 is only upregulated by proximal axotomy in the cervical cord. More importantly, these

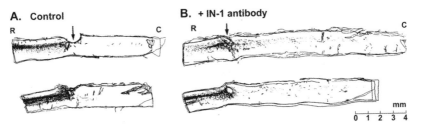

**Fig. 22.6** A diagram from the study by Schnell and Schwab (1990), demonstrating the regeneration of axons in rat corticospinal tract following a lesion in the cord. In the top two diagrams the animal has received the IN-1 antibody following the lesion, and some axons have regenerated beyond the lesion and into the distal cord. The lower diagram shows a control lesion, in which the animal did not receive the antibody, showing that there is no regeneration past the lesion.

distally cut axons are now able to regenerate their axons into peripheral nerve grafts placed in the thoracic cord, which would otherwise not attract any regenerating axons (Kobayashi *et al.* 1997). Neurotrophins have been successful in promoting the regeneration of sensory axons in the dorsal columns of the spinal cord, and across the dorsal root entry zones. Stephen McMahon and his co-workers have infused large doses of NT-3 into the lesioned rat spinal cord, and found sensory axon regeneration after lesioning in the dorsal columns, and also through the dorsal root entry zone after dorsal root crushes (Bradbury *et al.* 1998). Impressive increases in regeneration following trophic manipulation have been seen in optic nerve axons. One experimental strategy has been to graft peripheral nerve to a cut optic nerve just behind the eye. Most retinal ganglion cells die after the nerve is cut, but of those that survive a proportion regenerate their axons into the peripheral nerve graft. In order to try and increase the number of axons, BDNF and NT-4/5, both of which are active on retinal ganglion cells *in vitro*, were injected into the eye. The result was a considerable increase in the number of axons growing within the retina itself, but little increase in the number entering the nerve graft. Presumably the cut axons die back to within the retina and are then unable to penetrate the astrocytic plug at the retinal end of the optic nerve, despite their increased regenerative potential (Sawai *et al.* 1996). Very dramatic results have come from another model, in which the optic nerve is simply crushed. Normally the crushed nerve does not regenerate. However, if lengths of peripheral nerve are placed in the eye, there is a large amount of axon regeneration through the crush, and into an optic nerve that is full of degenerating myelin (Berry *et al.* 1996). The function of the peripheral nerve lengths is presumably to secrete trophic factors that can then diffuse to the retina, and act on the ganglion cells. However, inflammation in the eye, cause either puncturing the lews or inducing inflammation can also promote regeneration, so inflammation-related cytokines may be the key. Neurotrophins have also been successfully used as an adjunct to treatments to block oligodendrocyte-mediated inhibition. Schnell and Schwab investigated the effects of BDNF and NT-3 on regeneration of corticospinal axons. They found that NT-3, and to a lesser extent BDNF, injections into the cord caused a considerable increase in the sprouting of the cut axons proximal to the lesion. This treatment was then coupled with the antibody IN-1, which, as described above, by itself induces some axons to regenerate after they are cut. The combination of IN-1 and NT-3 increased the density of regenerating fibres, and the maximum distance of regeneration. The conclusion of these various experiments is that a combination of trophic factor treatment together with other manoeuvres designed to promote regeneration will have additive effects.

## Microglia and regeneration

Microglia accumulate in and around CNS damage, and if there is damage to blood vessels there may be blood-derived macrophages as well. Are these cells helpful or harmful to CNS repair? There is evidence that they may be both. When the optic nerve is cut, many retinal ganglion cells die, which means that there are few remaining axons able to regenerate into peripheral nerve grafts attached to the cut optic nerve. The dying ganglion cells are surrounded by microglia, so Solon Thanos asked whether inhibiting microglial activity might decrease the number of dying ganglion cells. This was done with a peptide, macrophage inhibitory factor (MIF). Putting MIF in the eye decreased the number of ganglion cells that died when their axons were cut. It also increased the number of axons that regenerated into peripheral nerve grafts (Moore and Thanos 1996). In this instance, microglia were unhelpful. However, in other experiments, macrophages have been placed directly into the lesion area, and here they have enhanced regeneration. Streit placed semi-permeable tubes containing microglia, or astrocytes mixed with microglia, in the spinal cord and found many axons regenerating in the microglia-rich regions. He also found that microglia made astrocytes more permissive to regeneration (Rabchevsky and Streit 1997). Activated macrophages have also been placed around optic nerve lesions, and have increased the regeneration of axons. It is likely that the macrophages are secreting cytokines that are acting on astrocytes and perhaps oligodendrocytes to make them more permissive.

## Conclusion

Only a few years ago the general view was that CNS axons could not be made to regenerate in the CNS, and that it was therefore hopeless to think of, for instance, repairing spinal-cord injuries. Now, as detailed in this chapter, there is not just one but several treatments that have induced significant amounts of regeneration in animal models. Whether these treatments, if added together, will produce additive effects has only been tested in an experiment where NT-3 and the IN-1 antibody together produced greater effects than either

singly. The question that arises from these studies is, 'When is it appropriate to start treating human patients with spinal cord injuries?'. The answer to this question depends on the answer to the next question, which is, 'How many axons will have to regenerate over how great a distance to produce useful return of function?'. Many patients are injured at spinal levels C4–5 or C5–6, which leaves some upper arm function, but no finger control. Regeneration over two spinal segments should bring back some finger movement control, and greatly improve the ability of patients to lead an independent life. Similarly, for patients with very high lesions, regeneration over one or two spinal segments could bring back spontaneous respiration. The amount of axon regeneration that has been demonstrated in the experiments described above could, therefore, be of benefit now in human pateints.

## Further reading

Brecknell, J.E., Du, J., Muir, E., Fidler, P.S., Hlavin, M., Dunnett, S.B., and Fawcett, J.W. (1996). Bridge grafts of FGF-4 secreting Schwannoma cells promote functional axonal regeneration in the nigrostriatal pathway of the adult rat. *Neuroscience*, **74**, 775–784.

Schwab, M.E., Kapfhammer, J.P., and Bandtlow, C.E. (1993). Inhibitors of neurite growth. *Annual Review of Neuroscience*, **16**, 565–595.

Even though in a few situations we can now induce the damaged brain to repair itself by spontaneous re-organisation and regeneration, there still remain many circumstances where intrinsic repair processes are inef-fective. The most obvious situation is where there is pro-gressive or complete loss of some one or other essential population of neurones that cannot be substituted by another (spared) set of neurones.

For example, we have seen that dopamine neurones have a remarkable capacity to undergo biochemical plasticity. Following partial damage of some neurones, the remaining dopamine neurones are upregulated and compensate for the biochemical and functional loss (see Chapter 14). In Parkinson's disease, such plastic processes can retard the development of symptoms early in the disease, and pharmacological replacement strate-gies (e.g. with l-dopa) are clearly effective in the middle stages of the disease. However, as Parkinson's disease progresses, the drug response becomes dominated by devastating side-effects. It was in trying to resolve the issues of dopamine system repair that neuronal grafts were first found to be functionally effective. This problem will guide the selection of examples and provide the main focus of our discussion in the present chapter.

## Effective transplantation in the adult mammalian brain

Let us start by looking at the basic methods necessary to achieve successful transplantation of nerve tissues in the adult mammalian brain. As we have seen, the regen-erative capacity of the adult brain is markedly reduced in comparison to early development, and the same applies to the survival of neurones following transplan-tation. Adult mammalian neurones survive transplanta-tion into the living brain no better than they survive in tissue culture. However, if they are handled correctly, developing neurones can survive transplantation well. This was first demonstrated by Elizabeth Dunn in 1917.

Dunn described the outcome of a series of experiments spanning more than 10 years in which she grafted wedge-shaped pieces of neonatal rat cortex into cortical cavities in the brains of 9–10-day-old rat pups. Only four out of a total of 44 cases showed any evidence of graft survival. However, in the course of these experi-ment she not only identified the necessity of using young donor tissues but she also identified the other main factors necessary to yield good survival. With remark-able insight she summarised her findings (Dunn 1917, p. 572):

The two points of chief importance in successful cerebral trans-plantation are first, the retention in place of the material trans-ferred, and second, the furnishing to it of an adequate blood supply . . . . In my own successful operations the transplanted portions have remained adherent to the denuded portions of the cortex but have taken some position near the choroid plexus of the lateral ventricle and have apparently received their blood supply from that source. Dr Ranson permits me to mention that in carrying on some further (unreported) studies in the transplantation of nerve ganglia into the brain he found the most nearly normal conditions in those ganglia which were within or adjacent to the choroid plexus.

Remarkably, in subsequent decades these observa-tions did not receive the attention we might now con-sider they deserve. Rather, the *Zeitgeist* of the age was that regeneration does not (indeed, cannot) take place in the mammalian CNS and evidence to the contrary was effectively ignored. This was true, even in spite of subsequent reports from well-respected anatomists of the period, such as William Le Gros Clark (1940), that they too had been able to achieve even better survival of neuronal tissues when using foetal donor tissue. It took developments in a different area, most notably those of Geoff Raisman, using the electron microscope to demonstrate unequivocally that spontaneous regen-eration can and does take place under appropriate cir-cumstances even in the adult brain (see Chapter 13; Raisman 1969), to prepare a sceptical audience for the prospect that neural transplants may be more than just a curious anomaly.

Dunn's studies highlighted two factors that have turned out to be critical in achieving effective graft survival: the age and identity of suitable donor tissues, and the selection of a technique/placement that can provide effective vascularisation of the grafts.

## Intraocular grafts as a model transplantation site

Since the early 1970s, Lars Olson and colleagues have developed the use of the anterior eye chamber as an effective site for studying the survival and growth of neural transplants (Olson and Malmfors 1970; Olson and Seiger 1972). Placement of small pieces of neural (or indeed other) tissues into the eye chamber is a rapid and simple operation that causes minimal distress to the host animal (see Fig. 23.1), and the grafted tissues survive well on the rich vascular bed provided by the iris. A distinct advantage of the intraocular model is that the survival and growth of the grafts can be easily monitored day after day, by simple inspection through the transparent cornea while the rat is under light anaesthesia.

Olson and colleagues have used the intraocular model to provide a systematic evaluation of the survival of different donor tissues at different developmental ages. For example, this was studied for grafts of locus coeruleus (the brain area containing the neurones that provide the major noradrenergic innervation of the cortex and hippocampus). Locus grafts survive and grow well if taken from embryonic donors at the stage of development when the cells are just born, but the volume to which grafts will grow declines rapidly once the tissue is dissected from donors at progressively later stages of development (Fig. 23.2; Olson *et al.* 1983).

Comparison of the survival and growth of grafts from different areas of the brain indicates that the critical developmental age differs from one area to another, and peak viability is obtained when the tissue is collected within a couple of days after the birth dates of each particular population of neurones of experimental interest (Olson *et al.* 1983). Consequently, neurones that undergo final mitosis relatively early, such as brainstem dopamine or noradrenaline neurones, survive better when collected from relatively young embryos (e.g. E14–15 days of embryonic age in rats), whereas neurones that are formed relatively late in development, such as the granule cells of the dentate gyrus or cells of the neocortex, can survive transplantation well even when taken from neonatal donors.

The iris has a rich cholinergic and noradrenergic innervation from ciliary and superior cervical ganglia, respectively. The intraocular model also provided one of the first demonstrations for axon growth and the reformation of connections from neural grafts into host targets. In an important experiment, Olson and Seiger (1972) first extirpated the superior cervical ganglion in order to remove the intrinsic noradrenergic innervation of the iris, followed by implantation of embryonic locus coeruleus into the anterior eye chamber. They used the catecholamine fluorescence technique to visualise noradrenaline neurones and fibres histochemically in iris whole mounts. The grafts were seen to give rise to an extensive network of noradrenergic fibres growing back to re-innervate wide areas of the iris with a pattern of organisation remarkably similar to the plexus observed

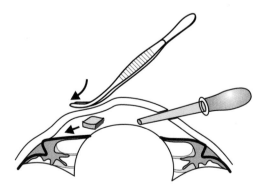

**Fig. 23.1** Schematic illustration of the intraocular transplantation technique. (Redrawn from Olson *et al.* 1984.)

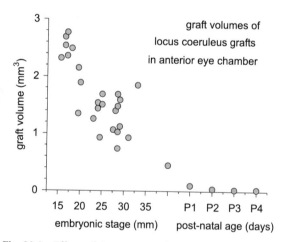

**Fig. 23.2** Effects of donor age on the survival and growth of grafts in the intraocular model. The points represent mean volumes of grafts of locus coeruleus dissected from the dorsal pons of donor embryos and neonates of different developmental ages. (Data from Olson *et al.* 1983.)

in the normal iris (Fig. 23.3). These studies demonstrate that neurones can be transplanted from the developing brain into adult hosts and can establish connection into and from the nervous system of the host.

## Intracerebral grafts

Similar principles apply within the brain itself, so long as a suitable transplantation site can be identified. Earlier studies, like those of Dunn and LeGros Clark, had found that tissues implanted into cortical cavities would occasionally survive, in particular if the grafted tissue made contact with ventricular surfaces, although survival was typically neither reliable nor good. Consequently, in 1976, Stenevi, Björklund, and Svendgaard (1976) undertook a systematic study of alternative strategies for implanting pieces of catecholamine-rich peripheral ganglia and embryonic CNS tissues into the forebrains of adult rats. Of the several alternative implantation sites that were used, only one was reliable: the choroidal fissure (Fig. 23.4).

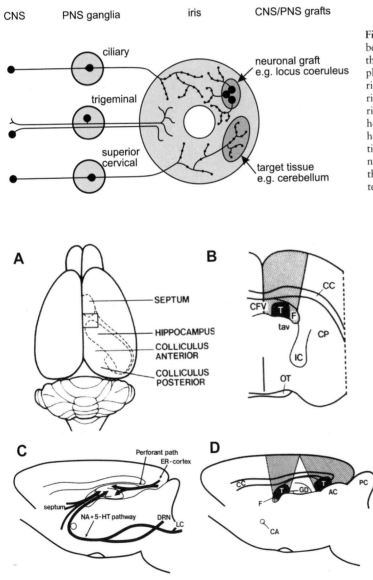

**Fig. 23.3** Afferent and efferent connections between grafts and the host nervous system in the intraocular model. The noradrenergic fibre plexus in the intact iris originates from the superior cervical ganglion. A locus coeruleus graft, rich in central noradrenergic neurones, can give rise to a new noradrenergic innervation of the host iris, in particular following lesion of the host innervation. Conversely, a central target tissue, such as the cerebellum, will receive a new noradrenergic innervation when grafted onto the iris by sprouting of the local host PNS terminals. (Redrawn from Olson *et al.* 1983.)

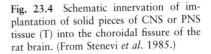

**Fig. 23.4** Schematic innervation of implantation of solid pieces of CNS or PNS tissue (T) into the choroidal fissure of the rat brain. (From Stenevi *et al.* 1985.)

## Naturally vascularised surfaces of the brain

Several different graft tissues were investigated, including adult and newborn superior cervical ganglia, dopamine-rich grafts from embryonic ventral mesencephalon, and noradrenaline-rich grafts from embryonic dorsal pons. When implanted onto the choroidal fissure, all graft tissues survived well and contained many fluorescent catecholaminergic neurones. Healthy neurones were seen not only after a relatively short (2–4 weeks) period, but also after protracted survival times up to 6 months after transplantation. Moreover, similar to the observations of Olson and Seiger in the anterior eye chamber, the grafts gave rise to a rich outgrowth of fluorescent fibres that grew extensively into the adult host brain, above all the hippocampus (Fig. 23.5). The catecholaminergic nature of the fibres was confirmed by showing that they could be destroyed by the specific toxin 6-hydroxydopamine.

By contrast, grafts implanted by embedding directly into the brain parenchyma (either in the caudal diencephalon or in the caudate nucleus) or by laying in a cortical cavity onto the dorsal surface of the caudate nucleus survived rather poorly. In each of these cases, the grafts were either totally necrotic or contained at most a few scattered catecholamine neurones, which were only visible after short (2–4 week) survival times.

As first suggested by Dun 60 years before, Stenevi and colleagues hypothesised at the critical difference between the choroidal fissure and other transplantation sites related to the effectiveness of revascularisation of the transplanted tissues (Stenevi *et al.* 1976, p.16). Thus:

Only those areas of the transplant that become revascularised from the brain will survive transplantation. The rich vascular supply of the pia in the choroidal fissure seems to make this structure an ideal support for the 'culturing' of the graft. From here the graft will become rapidly vascularised, the larger the contact surface the better the survival. In this respect the pia will thus serve the same purpose as does the richly vascularised iris, which support transplants placed in the anterior eye chamber.

## Artificial vascular beds

If grafts in the brain were only going to survive when placed in a limited number of highly vascularised sites (such as in the choroidal fissure or on a ventricular surface), then the application of the techniques would of necessity be rather limited. Stenevi and colleagues themselves speculated about alternative strategies that might broaden the range of effective placements. One approach was to consider a two-stage operation. In the first stage, a cavity is created in the brain linking the choroidal fissure to a preferred but remote target, such as the caudate nucleus. A piece of suitable tissue (such as the iris) is implanted as a bed in the cavity, which itself becomes vascularised over a period of weeks. Then, in a second operation, the embryonic tissue is placed at the target site in the cavity, and can now survive with vascularisation from the artificial bed.

Stenevi *et al.* showed that this rather complex chained transplantation procedure would indeed work (Stenevi *et al.* 1976). However, in the process, they discovered that simply making the cavity and transplant in a two-stage operation was equally effective. Thus, when an aspiration cavity is made in the neocortex to expose

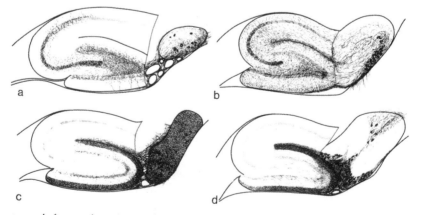

**Fig. 23.5** Fibre outgrowth from embryonic neural grafts of different neurotransmitter phenotype into the deafferented hippocampus in the adult rat: (a) noradrenergic fibres from a superior cervical ganglion graft, (b) noradrenergic fibres from a locus coeruleus graft, (c) serotonin fibres from a dorsal raphé graft, and (d) dopamine fibres from a nigral graft. (From Björklund *et al.* 1976.)

the dorsal surface of the caudate nucleus, followed by simply plugging the wound with sterile gel foam, a new pial membrane reforms to cover the floor and walls of the cavity over a period of 3–6 weeks. This newly formed pia is itself highly-vascularised and provides an effective bed onto which pieces of embryonic tissue can be grafted (Stenevi *et al.* 1980). This two-stage cavity technique first provided the basis for a systematic evaluation of the functional effects of embryonic nigral grafts (see below).

## Cell-suspension transplants

A further major technical development arose in the early 1980s, by applying the techniques of cell culture to the problem of intracerebral transplantation. In essence, dissociated cell suspensions of embryonic CNS can survive transplantation by injection directly into the parenchyma in adult brain. In particular, when made as cell suspensions, the grafts do not require any special provision for rapid revascularisation that is required by donor tissue when implanted in chunks.

The cell-suspension technique was introduced by Björklund, Schmidt, and Stenevi (1980a), using a procedure for preparing the cells that had previously been found to be effective for dissociating hippocampal cells prior to their growth in cell culture (Fig. 23.6). In essence, the procedure involves using an enzyme such as trypsin to provide mild digestion of the dissected pieces of embryonic tissue in order to break down inter-cell adhesion. The tissue is then washed prior to mechanical dissociation, achieved by sucking the pieces back and forth through the smoothed glass tip of a fire-polished Pasteur pipette. The cell suspension can then be drawn up into a glass microsyringe for stereotaxic placement and injection into the brain of the anaesthetised host.

In that first study, dopamine cells of the embryonic ventral mesencephalon were implanted into the dopamine denervated neostriatum of rats. Grafted dopamine cells survive well in suspension transplants, and give rise to a good fibre outgrowth re-innervating the host striatum (Fig. 23.7). Moreover, as would be expected from the previous studies of graft survival in the anterior eye chamber, cell suspensions derived from E15 embryos survived better and contained more dopamine neurones than suspensions derived from older E17 embryos.

The basic dissociated suspension method of cell transplantation is highly flexible and remains widely used. Although there have been numerous modifications of this procedure, they differ only in minor detail. Not only do cell suspensions have the advantage that they can be placed virtually at will into any site in the brain, the stereotaxic implantation procedure is relatively less traumatic than involved in making cavities for implantation of chunks or solid pieces of tissue into the brain, and multiple deposits on one or more tissues can readily be positioned at multiple sites in a single brain, providing the possibility of developing additive or combination grafts treatments.

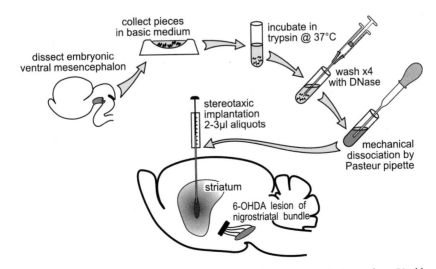

**Fig. 23.6** Schematic illustration of the dissociated cell-suspension graft procedure. (Redrawn form Björklund *et al.* 1983a.)

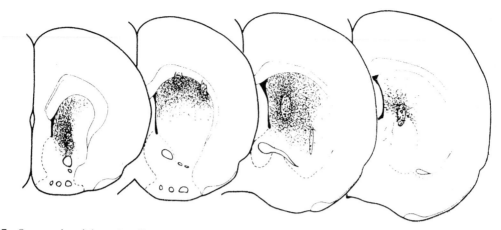

**Fig. 23.7** Outgrowths of dopamine fibres from nigral suspension grafts implanted into the dopamine-depleted neostriatum. (From Björklund *et al.* 1983b.)

## The nigral graft model in rats

The first (and still most extensive) studies of the functional capacity of neural grafts have been conducted in the dopamine-depleted rat. As already described in the section on biochemical and pharmacological strategies for compensation and recovery (Chapter 14), the toxin 6-hydroxydopamine was used to deplete forebrain dopamine. Similar to the symptoms seen in Parkinson's disease, 6-hydroxydopamine treated rats have profound impairments in their abilities to initiate and sequence voluntary movement. Of course, if the lesions are only partial, the residual population of surviving dopamine neurones exhibit a considerable degree of plasticity allowing for a substantial or even complete recovery of symptoms over a period of weeks (see Chapter 19). As such, the partial lesion model is unsuitable for evaluating the effects of transplants, since it is difficult to separate the functional effects of the grafts from the functional recovery attributable to upregulation of intrinsic biochemical parameters.

The only way to ensure that spontaneous recovery does not take place is to ensure that the lesions are relatively complete, which in practice means inducing dopamine depletion by at least 97–99%. With such a selective and potent toxin as 6-hydroxydopamine, this is relatively easy to achieve but is associated with a second problem: rats with such profound bilateral dopamine depletions are severely akinetic, and fail to initiate any voluntary, goal-directed behaviours. In particular, they do not spontaneously eat or drink and will die within a few days unless maintained by tube feeding several times per day. Such a degree of debilitation and

ill health does not make for a convenient model to test the effects of grafts. However, a simple alternative is to make the lesions unilaterally. This leaves one side of the brain intact to sustain normal motivational and regulatory functions, but still produces profound lateralised motor impairments on the contralateral side of the body. It is this unilateral lesion model that has been very widely used for assessing the functional effects of grafts, not least because of the clear, quantifiable motor deficits that result.

The Swedish pharmacologist Urban Ungerstedt (1971a, 1971b) first described in detail the motoric effects produced by unilateral 6-hydroxydopamine lesions of the ascending forebrain dopamine system. The rats have a marked postural bias to the side of the lesion. More dramatically, if the animals are activated either by stress or by a stimulant drug (e.g. amphetamine), the bias and locomotor activation combine to produce head-to-tail turning in circles (see Fig. 23.8). This response is known as 'rotation', and is widely used to monitor the effects of unilateral dopamine dysfunction. Rotation is both easy to quantify and correlates closely with the degree of dopamine depletion induced by the lesion.

Indirect agonist drugs, such as amphetamine, induce ipsilateral rotation by providing a dopaminergic activation of the neostriatum only at dopamine terminals on the intact side of the brain. By contrast, a direct agonist, such as apomorphine (which acts at the post-synaptic receptor), induces rotation in the opposite, contralateral direction. This is due to the development of supersensitivity of the dopamine receptors on striatal neurones following deafferentation of their dopamine inputs on the lesion side (Fig. 23.8). Indeed it was this behavioural

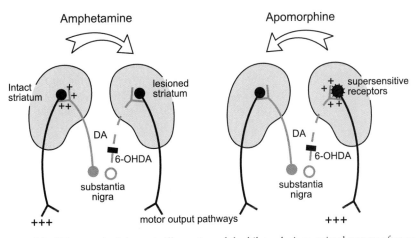

**Fig. 23.8** Rotation model of Ungerstedt. Schematic illustration of the bilateral nigro-striatal system after unilateral nigro-striatal lesion on the right side in rats, viewed from above, and indicating: (*left*) the postural asymmetry, side bias, and ipsilateral direction of turning after systemic injection of a stimulant drug such as amphetamine; and (*right*) the contralateral direction of turning after injection of a direct agonist such as apomorphine, which acts preferentially at supersensitive dopamine receptors on striatal neurones on the lesioned side. (Based on Ungerstedt 1971a, 1971b.)

observation that provided the first experimental evidence for the development of dopamine receptor supersensitivity in this system, and the phenomenon has now been well validated by direct receptor binding studies (see below).

## Recovery of drug-induced rotation

Nigral grafts reverse rotation deficits induced by nigro-striatal lesions (Fig. 23.9). This effect was first reported by two separate groups almost simultaneously. Mark Perlow and colleagues implanted pieces of embryonic substantia nigra into the lateral ventricle adjacent to the dopamine-depleted neostriatum and found a partial reduction in contralateral apomorphine rotation (Perlow *et al.* 1979). In subsequent studies this was shown autoradiographically to be accompanied by a reduction of receptor supersensitivity in the medial parts of the neostriatum adjacent to the grafts. At the same time, Björklund and Stenevi used the two-stage transplantation procedure to implant solid grafts of embryonic substantia nigra into cortical cavities overlying the head of the caudate nucleus, and found a complete compensation of amphetamine-induced rotation (Björklund and Stenevi 1979). Histological analyses not only demonstrated good survival of dopamine cells within the grafts but indicated that the degree of functional compensation was correlated with the extent of fibre re-innervation of the denervated host brain (Björklund *et al.* 1980b). Recovery from both amphetamine and apomorphine rotation may be achieved even more rapidly

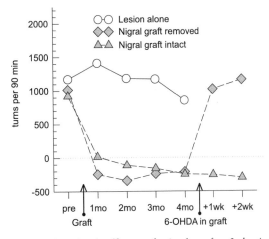

**Fig. 23.9** Functional efficacy of nigral grafts. Induction of amphetamine-induced rotation after unilateral 6-OHDA lesions ('pre-graft' test), recovery over approximately 1 month in two subgroups receiving nigral grafts, and reinstatement of the initial asymmetry after graft removal in one subgroup of grafted rats. (Data from Dunnett *et al.* 1988.)

and effectively by cell suspension grafts implanted into the dopamine denervated neostriatum (Dunnett *et al.* 1983).

Subsequent studies have added considerable information to the selectivity and specificity of these effects.

First, placement of the grafts is important. The grafts must be in a location where they can re-innervate dorsal areas of the neostriatum in order to ameliorate deficits in rotation, whereas grafts implanted in a more lateral location, which re-innervated ventral and lateral segments of the neostriatum, are without effect on this particular measure (Dunnett *et al.* 1981a, 1981b, 1983). This does not imply that laterally placed grafts are without effect altogether. Rather the neostriatum is a topographically organised structure, with function of each segment determined by its connections, including the topography of inputs from discrete areas of neocortex. The ventral and lateral neostriatum receives denser inputs from somatosensory areas of neocortex, and grafts in these areas are associated with recovery on tests of sensorimotor neglect (see Fig. 23.10).

Second, recovery is dependent upon the use of specific embryonic nigral tissues — other non-dopaminergic grafts have no effect. Thus, Dunnett *et al.* (1988) compared the effects of grafts of embryonic nigral tissue rich in dopamine neurones, grafts of embryonic raphé tissue rich in an alternative group of brainstem monoaminergic neurones using serotonin as neurotransmitter, and grafts of embryonic striatal eminence, which may be richest in growth factors promoting

striatal development and reorganisation. Only the nigral grafts compensated the amphetamine and apomorphine rotation asymmetries of the rats, whereas the other two graft types had no detectable effects whatsoever.

Third, recovery is not simply due to the grafts stimulating non-specific recovery processes, but rather is specifically dependent upon survival of the graft. As shown in Fig. 23.9, removal of the graft from recovered rats immediately re-instates the initial levels of motor asymmetry induced by the lesions. This was first demonstrated by aspirative removal of solid grafts (Björklund *et al.* 1980b), but similar re-instatement of functional deficits has been replicated both by using local injections of 6-hydroxydopamine to lesion the dopamine neurones alone within the grafts (Dunnett *et al.* 1988), and by immunological rejection of nigral xenografts that had been sustained up to that point by immunosuppression (Brundin *et al.* 1989).

## Nigral grafts in Parkinson's disease

Based on the positive outcome in many experimental studies using rats, several hundred patients with Parkinson's disease have now (by 2000) received implants into the caudate nucleus and/or putamen. Similar basic experimental techniques have been employed as used in animals, involving either implanting pieces of embryonic ventral mesencephalon into ventricular cavities or by stereotaxic injection of small tissue fragments or dissociated cell suspensions directly into the patient's basal ganglia.

In the best cases quite dramatic recovery has been achieved. For example Olle Lindvall has described progress in several patients operated in Lund, Sweden (Lindvall *et al.* 1990, 1992; Wenning *et al.* 1997). Many of these patients have shown a pronounced and sustained recovery, as demonstrated by the following tests and illustrated in Fig. 23.11.

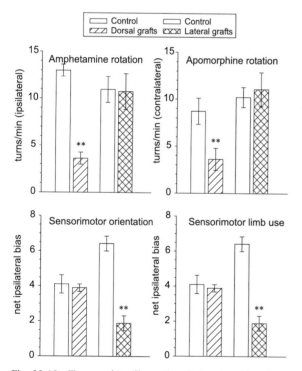

Fig. 23.10 Topographic effects of graft function. The placement of nigral grafts in the host striatum influences the pattern of graft function: dorsal re-innervation allows recovery of rotation asymmetry but not sensorimotor neglect, whereas a lateral re-innervation produces the converse pattern of recovery. (Data from Dunnett *et al.* 1981a, 1981b.)

- A marked improvement in symptoms of akinesia or rigidity, although there is generally little detectable improvement in tremor.

- A marked improvement in standardised motor tests (e.g. the time to make a series of 20 pronation/supination movements, or to stand, walk a fixed distance, return, and sit back down). These tests are conducted both during defined periods when ongoing drug treatment is withdrawn overnight (see Fig. 23.11B), as well as in periods when the patient is well medicated.

## A. patient 4: drug responses

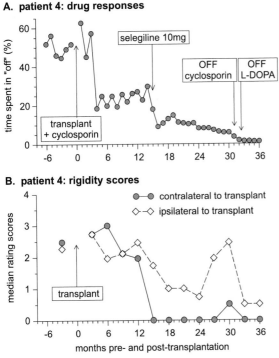

## B. patient 4: rigidity scores

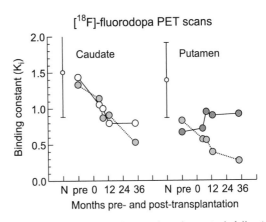

**Fig. 23.12** PET scan evidence of graft survival following clinical transplantation of embryonic nigral tissues into the right putamen in a patient with Parkinson's disease. The fluorodopa uptake constant is restored into the normal range over 3–6 years after surgery in the transplanted putamen, whereas the PET signal continued to decline as the underlying disease progressed in the non-transplanted putamen and caudate bilaterally. (Data from Lindvall 1997.)

**Fig. 23.11** Neurological recovery after clinical nigral transplantation in a patient with Parkinson's disease. A. progressive recovery in the period in the 'on' state of l-dopa response, and progressive reduction in the requirement for additional drug treatment over 36 months after transplantation. B. Progressive recovery in rigidity scores in defined 'off' state, over the same period after transplantation. (Data from Lindvall 1997.)

- An improved response to ongoing l-dopa therapy, as manifested by a prolonged positive response to each drug dose, a reduced number of 'off' periods and a longer time spent in the 'on' state each day (see Fig. 23.11A).

- Gradual and progressive rather than immediate recovery. The first signs of benefit typically do not appear for approximately 6 months after the operation and then improve progressively. In several patients, the need for high-maintenance doses of l-dopa to maintain an optimal drug response has declined. Indeed, in one patient, parallel l-dopa treatment has been withdrawn completely, while the patient remains in a functional state of permanent 'on'.

One strength of the Lund studies is that each patient has been followed by regular brain scans to monitor the survival and growth of the grafts. The ligand [$^{18}$F]-

fluorodopa has been used in positron emission tomography (PET) to visualise the location of graft placements and to provide quantitative measurements of the changes in fluorodopa uptake. This is illustrated for one of the cases (Fig. 23.12).

The disease is visualised as a marked loss of fluorodopa signal in the caudate and putamen bilaterally, and its progress is monitored by a progressive decline in the residual signal (in the ungrafted striatum) in successive scans at approximately yearly intervals.

The implantation of the graft unilaterally into the right putamen is seen as a progressive increase in fluorodopa signal in that one structure, and a quantitative increase in the associated binding potential.

Like the recovery of symptoms, the restitution of functional dopamine uptake in the brain as measured by PET is not a rapid change, but involves a slow and progressive change over a period of months or years.

There are now available two cases that have come to post-mortem, in which there is a clear correlation between positive PET scans, functional recovery and clear survival of large healthy grafts, containing many thousands of surviving dopamine neurones and which give rise to a rich fibre re-innervation of the host brain (Kordower *et al.* 1995). The anatomical and morphological similarity between the grafts in these individual cases and that observed in the best of the animal studies gives increased confidence about the validity of the PET data in the many patients still alive, and that the

## Box 23.1   The ethics of foetal tissue transplantation

The use of foetal tissue for research and transplantation is controversial, in large part because tissue is procured through elective abortions, the morality of which is controversial. It may be argued that if abortion is legal, permitting termination of foetal life under certain regulated and approved conditions, then the subsequent use of resulting tissues imposes no additional fundamental moral issue. Conversely, those who oppose abortion under any circumstances argue that putting the foetal tissue to a perceived beneficial use may reduce individual or public opposition and so help to legitimise abortion itself.

Many different countries have now undertaken national, independent, or governmental enquiries on the use of foetal tissues for transplantation. Whereas such practice is precluded in some countries, such as Italy or Ireland, many others, including Sweden, UK, USA, France, the Netherlands, and Canada, have concluded that using foetal tissues for research or therapy is not in principle unethical providing appropriate steps are followed to protect the mother, to ensure proper consent, and to prevent abuse. Guidelines and legislation are generally similar from country to country in overall scope although they do of course vary in detail. The central principle in each case is to ensure full separation of the decision on whether, when, and how to undertake an abortion, and the subsequent information, decision, and consent to collect tissue for research and/or therapy. By way of illustration, the NECTAR (the Network for European CNS Transplantation And Restoration) guidelines adopted by all participating transplantation centres in Europe impose the following restrictions:

Clinical and experimental groups or institutions that are members of NECTAR will obey the present ethical guidelines, irrespective of the fact that national legislation may permit them to deviate from these guidelines and provided national legislation allows them to follow these guidelines.

1. Tissue for transplantation or research may be obtained from dead embryos or foetuses, their death resulting from legally induced or spontaneous abortion. Death of an intact embryo or foetus is defined as absence of respiration and heart beats.

2. It is not allowed to keep intact embryos or foetuses alive artificially for the purpose of removing usable material.

3. The decision to terminate pregnancy must under no circumstances be influenced by the possible or desired subsequent use of the embryo or foetus, and must therefore precede any introduction of the possible use of the embryonic or fetal tissue. There should be no link between the donor and the recipient, nor designation of the recipient by the donor.

4. The procedure of abortion, or the timing, must not be influenced by the requirements of the transplantation activity when this would be in conflict with the woman's interests or would increase embryonic or fetal distress.

5. No material can be used without informed consent of the woman involved. This informed consent should, whenever possible, be obtained prior to abortion.

6. Screening of the woman for transmissible diseases requires informed consent.

7. Nervous tissue may be used for transplantation as suspended cell preparations or tissue fragments.

8. All members of the hospital or research staff directly involved in any of the procedures must be fully informed.

9. The procurement of embryos, foetuses, or their tissue must not involve profit or remuneration.

10. Every transplantation or research project involving the use of embryonic or fetal tissue must be approved by the local ethical committee.

From Boer, G.J. (1994) Ethical guidelines for the use of human embryonic or fetal tissue for experimental and clinical transplantation and research. *Journal of Neurology*, 242, 1–13.

recovery seen in these patients is attributable to surviving dopamine-rich implants.

Thus, in the best cases, neural transplantation can provide a dramatic alleviation in symptoms of Parkinson's disease. However, in only a few cases is the degree of recovery as clear-cut as this (e.g. see also Peschanski *et al.* 1994; Freeman *et al.* 1995; Kopyov *et al.* 1996, 1998; Wenning *et al.* 1997). The results obtained at other centres have often been more limited in extent or of only rather transitory benefit. At the time of writing, embryonic cell transplantation in Parkinson's disease is still an experimental technique. Several reasons can be offered for the variability in results obtained by different centres:

- differences in operative technique;

- use of tissues from embryonic donors of inappropriate developmental age;

- lack of standardisation or objective measures for neurological evaluation.

Given the level of interest in these clinical trials, rapid progress is expected in the next few years to identify the critical parameters necessary for neural transplantation in order for it to provide a reliable therapeutic option. Nevertheless, for many people, the collection and use of human foetal tissues is controversial (see Box 23.1), and the use of human foetal tissues for research or therapy is prohibited in some societies, and heavily regulated in most others. Advances in cell clinical transplantation will require, in the short-term, substantial improvements in the viability and use of foetal tissue itself and, in the longer term, identification of a suitable alternative to replace completely the present dependence on this source of donor tissue.

## Improving the viability of transplanted cells

Although several centres have now demonstrated clear functional benefit associated with transplanting embryonic ventral mesencephalon for transplantation in Parkinson's disease, the procedure is at present highly inefficient. Graft survival is poor, so that even the best nigral grafts in rats typically contain no more than 2–10% of the numbers of dopamine cells that were initially implanted. The situation is likely to be even worse in the clinical applications since other factors associated with handling the tissues and delays to implantation are sub-optimal. As a consequence, in order to achieve effective graft survival (as measured in PET) and clear

functional recovery, all successful trials are based on implanting tissue from multiple donors (up to seven embryonic nigra per putamen) in order to achieve effective engraftment in each recipient (Olanow *et al.* 1996). Thus, although neural transplantation of primary embryonic or foetal tissues can demonstrate the feasibility of transplantation repair, it is not likely, with present technology, to offer a practical basis for developing a widely-available clinical therapy. Consequently, there is now an active investigation of alternative sources of cells, tissues, or other molecular delivery system that can replace primary foetal tissue for transplantation. We can consider technical developments at several different levels.

One set of approaches involves improved use of available foetal tissues:

- we can seek to enhance the survival of neurones, so that limited amounts of donor tissue can be used more efficiently in more patients;

- we can seek to preserve cells for prolonged periods after harvest, so that the limited amounts of tissue can be screened more effectively, and the tissue donation can be separated in time and space from neurosurgical implantation to allow better preparation and care of the recipient patient;

- we can seek to grow and expand cells in culture to increase the source of supply from a limited number of donors.

A second set of approaches involves finding alternative sources of tissue for transplantation that avoid the problems associated with human foetal tissues. This can include taking more readily available human cells, such as autografts from the adult peripheral nervous system. We can consider using non-neuronal cells that would then need to be engineered to exhibit critical neuronal or neurosecretory features. We can consider cell lines with appropriate characteristics. Or we can consider using the correct populations of embryonic cells, but derived from non human donors as xenografts.

As alternative sources of cells are developed, raising novel problems for genetic engineering or delivery, new technologies then offer novel strategies and combinations for repair. Thus, the development of techniques for gene manipulation and transfer of cells for transplantation *in vitro*, has led to new strategies for '*in vivo* gene transfer' by delivery of the gene construct in appropriate vectors directly into target cells within the host nervous system. Alternatively, as one approach to protecting xenografts from rejection, cells have been encapsulated within semi-permeable polymer tubes that have turned out to offer a number of other technological and safety advantages for delivering and protecting implanted cells.

Each of these main approaches will be addressed in turn in the following sections and chapters.

## The technology of graft preparation

Stereotaxic transplantation of grafts into deep brain sites requires first preparing the cells for implantation. This involves dissection and dissociation of the tissues to an extent that allows aspiration and injection via the stereotaxic implantation needle. The embryonic stage at which cells are harvested (and hence the degree of neurite outgrowth they exhibit), the enzymes and media used to dissociate the cells, the method of dissociation by drawing cells back and forth through the aperture of a narrow pipette, and the degree of fragmentation can all influence the amount of damage the cells sustain and consequently how well they survive subsequent transplantation. Improvements in cell preparation techniques are guided primarily by common sense backed up by empirical confirmation (Brundin 1992; Barker *et al.* 1995).

## Growth factor treatments

We have seen in an earlier chapter that all neurones are dependent on a variety of neurotropic and neurotrophic factors for regulating their differentiation, growth, and survival during development, and that the neurotrophic environment is important in maintaining neuronal health and plasticity throughout life. So could the reason for poor survival of transplanted embryonic dopamine cells be that the adult brain is deficient in some critical survival factor molecule on which these neurones are dependent in their early post-mitotic phase of active neurite growth and formation of connections?

This hypothesis was first proposed by Harry Steinbusch and supported in a series of studies in which he showed that central injections of basic fibroblast growth factor (FGF-2) into the vicinity of a nigral graft in the standard rat model enhanced survival of the embryonic dopamine neurones in the grafts. Subsequent studies have shown that a variety of growth factor molecules, which enhance survival of dopamine neurones in culture, also enhance survival of dopamine neurones in nigral grafts, including the neurotrophins BDNF, NT-3, NT-4/5, as well as PDGF and GDNF. Of these, GDNF, which can increase yields of surviving dopamine cells by up to ten-fold, appears to be the most potent (see Fig. 23.13; Sinclair *et al.* 1996).

The biggest problem associated with using growth factors to enhance graft survival, is that these molecules are large and do not cross the blood–brain barrier. Consequently they cannot be given by peripheral injection (indeed if they are they can cause marked side-effects due to actions at both neuronal and non-neuronal peripheral targets), and require some form of central administration. This can be achieved experimentally by central injections either into the ventricles (which works for relatively stable factors) or directly into the brain parenchyma proximal to the neuronal graft, as was required in the experiments on neuroprotection of dopamine cells, above.

The alternative strategy for delivery is via co-transplantation of cells that exhibit endogenous secretion of the relevant factor, or are engineered *ex vivo* for its production (see Chapter 26). The first of these approaches has been employed by co-transplantation of peripheral nerve tissue, which manufactures high levels of nerve growth factor (NGF), with adrenal medulla chromaffin cells, a catecholamine-secretory population that is dependent on NGF for long-term survival, with apparent benefit. The second approach is illustrated by engineering of NGF-secreting fibroblasts which are then co-grafted with embryonic cholinergic cells into the neocortex. The secreted NGF has a protective effect on the co-grafted embryonic cells which exhibit an improved rate of survival. The logical development of this strategy is to engineer the embryonic dopamine cells themselves to enable them to generate autologously directed factors with a neuroprotective effect. Although this may prove difficult if primary neurones are to be not only transfected but also selected and screened prior to implantation, this strategy is less fanciful, at least in an experimental context, if the donor cells can be taken from either cell lines or transgenic donors that are manipulated to express the relevant growth factors, in particular if linked to promoters for the particular cell phenotype (e.g. tyrosine hydroxylase promoter to specify cells of dopaminergic phenotype) of target interest.

## Neuroprotection of implanted cells

In recent years a third factor influencing nigral graft survival has come to the fore: the fact that factors released in the injured host environment may not be conducive, or are actually toxic, to graft survival. The act of lowering an implantation cannula and injecting cells in the host brain induce a cascade of changes:

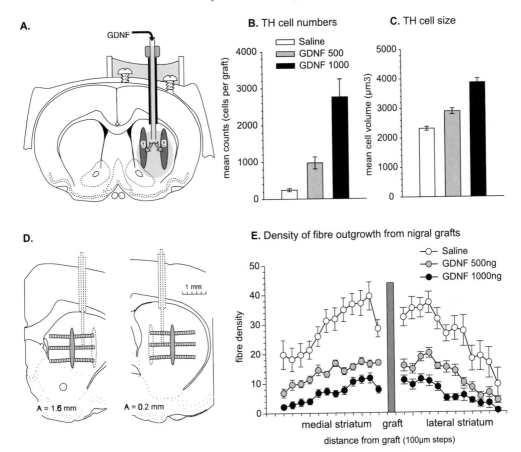

**Fig. 23.13** Growth factors can enhance graft survival. Dopamine cell survival and fibre outgrowth are both markedly increased in embryonic nigral grafts in the rat striatum following treatment with glial cell line-derived neurotrophic factor (GDNF). (From Sinclair *et al.* 1996.)

- potassium, calcium, and other ions that change the ionic and pH balance of cells;

- excitatory amino acids, such as glutamate, that are known to be neurotoxic;

- free radicals and other compounds that disrupt metabolic balance and induce oxidative stress, to which dopamine neurones in particular are sensitive.

A variety of antioxidative treatments that scavenge free radicals and promote glutathione and superoxide metabolism have been shown to promote dopamine cell survival *in vitro*, and to enhance survival and functional efficacy of nigral grafts. There is now accumulating evidence that alternative strategies to block production of oxygen radicals, or to promote free-radical scavenging, can promote nigral graft survival, including treatment of the host with n-acetylcysteine or lazaroids, or promoting glutathione peroxidase and superoxide dismu-

tase activity, can all enhance graft viability (Nakao *et al.* 1994; Barkats *et al.* 1996). Moreover, since lazaroids have passed the relevant safety evaluations and are already approved for clinical application in stroke, the first clinical trial of adding lazaroids to the graft preparation is now underway in Parkinson's disease patients in Sweden. In addition, as described in Chapter 7, a variety of anti-apoptotic agents can also reduce cell death *in vitro*, and recent attention has been given to the use of caspase inhibitors also for the protection of nigral grafts (Schierle *et al.* 1999).

## The search for alternative graft tissues

Even if the techniques of embryonic neural tissue transplantation in patients are developed to the point of being completely reliable, there remains the substantial problem of their practicability. The use of primary foetal donor tissues is ethically controversial in many quarters, and is likely to remain so for the foreseeable future. Indeed, in some countries the development of neural transplantation therapies is illegal while they remain dependent upon use of human foetal tissues. There has consequently been considerable interest in the identification of alternative sources of viable donor tissues.

## Adrenal grafts

Embryonic nigral grafts were not the first tissues transplanted in Parkinson's disease. Bill Freed and Mark Perlow first suggested that the catecholamine secreting cells of the adrenal medulla might provide a suitable alternative source. In addition to avoiding the ethical controversy surrounding foetal tissues, it is possible that adrenal tissues could be collected from the patients themselves and transplanted as 'autografts', circumventing any possibility of immune rejection. Freed implanted adrenal chromaffin cells into the lateral ventricle in the 6-hydroxydopamine lesioned rat model, and found that this significantly reduced the rate of turning in the apomorphine rotation test (Freed *et al.* 1981). This effect has been replicated in many subsequent studies and is due at least in part to a down-regulation of supersensitive dopamine receptors in the lesioned striatum (Curran *et al.* 1993).

On the basis of these preliminary results, in 1982 Olaf Backlund in Stockholm made the first attempt to transplant adrenal medulla in Parkinson's disease (Backlund *et al.* 1985). These first trials were without any great success, and were not actively pursued further. However, the issue was raised again when a team from Mexico City led by Ignacio Madrazo reported, in 1987, dramatic recovery in two further patients.

The Madrazo technique involved a two-stage operation, the first to collect tissue from one adrenal gland, and the second to implant the dissected adrenal medulla into the patient's own brain. In these first two patients and a series of over 50 subsequent patients, the Mexican team has claimed rather sustained and dramatic improvements in many of their patients (Madrazo *et al.* 1990). These claims naturally led to widespread interest and excitement in patient groups and neurosurgical centres, and resulted in many other groups world-wide trying similar procedures. Many of these trials were rather poorly organised and lacked systematic data collection, so that it is difficult to evaluate their outcomes objectively. However, in North America in particular,

a neurosurgical registry was established to provide systematic collection of comparative data (Bakay *et al.* 1990), and the American neurologists undertook a multicentre trial involving standardised assessment procedures to compare outcomes (Goetz *et al.* 1991). By and large, the results of those more rigorous trials was disappointing and did not support the initial enthusiasm. In summary:

- adrenal medulla grafts can yield detectable experimentally measurable changes in a minority (40–50%) of patients;

- the changes are small and generally not of great clinical benefit;

- the dual abdominal–brain operation is associated with considerable risks: there is a substantial morbidity and marked side-effects in many patients and a mortality rate of approximately 5–10% (Quinn *et al.* 1990).

The outstanding conclusion is that the risks associated with the present procedures outweigh the limited benefits. Whilst this strategy has not been completely abandoned, there is a general consensus that substantial improvements must be achieved in both efficacy and safety before reconsideration.

## Xenografts

If what works best is the correct population of cells at the correct stage of development, when phenotype is specified and growth capacity is optimal, then an alternative strategy to overcome the limited availability of human foetal tissues is to harvest the graft tissue from non-human embryos.

First attempts to graft mouse substantia nigra into the parkinsonian rat brain yielded very poor survival (Björklund *et al.* 1982). Although a few dopamine cells were seen to survive, the grafts were to a large extent rejected.

The intervening years have seen considerable advances in our understanding of the immunology of neural transplantation, although the limits of this complex field are still not well understood. Medawar (1948) introduced the concept of the brain as an 'immunologically privileged site' on the basis of his classic studies of skin grafting into alternative sites in the body, and it is certainly the case that allografts (i.e. between unrelated individuals of the same species) will survive readily in the brain, whereas similar grafts are rapidly rejected when placed into most other sites in the body. Indeed, the whole field of neural tissue transplantation based on foetal allografts, as outlined throughout this chapter, relies on the relative privilege of the brain for reliable survival of the grafted tissue without the need for special immunoprotection.

The relative immune privilege of the brain appears to be attributable to several factors.

- The blood–brain barrier excludes circulating antibodies and cells (e.g. lymphocytes) of the immune system entering the brain, necessary to encounter and react to foreign antigens. This suggests that grafts into sites in the brain where the blood–brain barrier is relatively permeable, will survive less well than grafts into the depths of the brain parenchyma.

- Neurones express very low levels of histocompatibility molecules on their surface, so neural tissue exhibits a rather low level of antigenicity, although astrocytes (particularly when activated) express MHCs at much higher levels.

- The lymphatic drainage system is sparse in the brain so that the afferent arm of the immune system, the specialised component to channel activated cells back to the lymph glands to raise a response, is itself restricted.

Nevertheless, once there is greater disparity between donor and host, when grafting between species (and occasionally also when grafting between strains of rats or mice that differ markedly in both major and minor histocompatibility loci), the grafts become susceptible to raising an active immune response and survive poorly (Mason *et al.* 1986; Finsen *et al.* 1988).

However, a variety of strategies are available to further reduce immunological reactions in the brain and thereby protect graft tissues from rejection (Lund and Bannerjee 1992).

- *Neonatal grafts.* During development, the immune systems learns to distinguish 'self' from 'non-self', which takes place during the first week of life in rodents. Consequently, if xenografts are implanted into neonatal animals, the graft tissues are not recognised as foreign, and the immune system comes to recognise histocompatibility molecules on the grafted cells as much 'self' as any other cell in the body.

- *Cell sorting.* Since neurones are far less antigenic than astrocytes, Bartlett and colleagues (1990) have found that sorting xenograft cell suspensions to exclude the astrocytes reduces the major immune response precipitated by these cells and allows substantially improved survival of grafts comprising purified neurones.

- *Cyclosporin A*: the major anti-rejection drug for organ transplantation also works well in the brain. Cyclosporin works by blocking components of complement necessary in raising the immune response by T cells. Thus, mouse, pig, or human foetal substantia nigra, will all show extended survival after transplantation into the rat brain, if the hosts are treated daily with cyclosporin (Brundin *et al.* 1985a, 1986; Huffaker *et al.* 1989). For xenografts, it is necessary to maintain the animals on cyclosporin long-term, since subsequent cessation of treatment even after 3–6 months leads to rapid rejection of the grafted tissue and relapse of the functional recovery it had provided. Cyclosporin treatment is now widely used to immunosuppress host animals in a variety of xenograft paradigms, and indeed it is typically included in most human clinical trials as a prophylactic treatment even for allografts.

- *Antibody treatments.* An alternative immune suppression strategy is to treat host animals with antibodies against critical components of the immune system in order to block the complement cascade at a critical stage. The first effective demonstration of this strategy was that treatment of rats with antibodies against the interleukin IL-2 blocked T-cell recognition of murine neural tissue as foreign and thereby prevented its rejection (Honey *et al.* 1990). The impressive advance over conventional cyclosporin treatment is that only a single treatment over 1–2 weeks at the time of transplantation is required to block the response, and the animals do not require chronic maintenance therapy thereafter. Although this strategy has now been demonstrated to work well in several model systems, it is technically more complicated than cyclosporin. Effective antibodies are not yet widely available, although this may be expected to be a growing strategy in the future.

- *Transgenic donors.* The alternative to protecting the host is to reduce the immunogenicity of the donor. Following the earlier lead of sorting out antigenic glial cells, there is recent interest in modifying surface molecules on donor cells to reduce their recognition as foreign. A major component of normal xenograft rejection is the 'hyperacute' rejection induced by preformed host antibodies binding to carbohydrate epitopes (such as galactose-alpha-(1,3)-galactose, GAL) on endothelial cells. One approach has been to generate a transgenic pig that makes human fucosyl transferases, which will convert the pig alpha-galactose into an antigen similar to that of human blood group antigens (Koike *et al.* 1996). Such tissue will then not be recognised by human anti-pig antibodies and hyper-acute rejection will be blocked. A related strategy is to block the complement cascade involved in hyper-acute rejection. The complement cascade is controlled by a number of regulators, including the decay-accelerating factor (DAF), which inhibit C3 to C5 conversion and hence block formation of membrane attack complexes. Since human complement is not effectively inhibited by porcine DAF, David White and colleagues have generated a line of transgenic pigs that express human DAF, and they have shown that this is effective in inhibiting the complement cascade, reducing hyperacute responses and delaying rejection of peripheral organ transplants (van den Bogaerde and White 1997).

On the basis of these alternative strategies for immunoprotection, there is now active consideration of whether cross-species transplantation may provide a more readily available source of foetal nigral cells for transplantation in Parkinson's and other diseases of the CNS. Indeed, the first trials of xenotransplantation from porcine embryonic donors has now been undertaken by a team in Boston, evaluating both nigral transplants in Parkinson's disease and striatal transplants in Huntington's disease (Schumacher and Isacson 1997), although it is too early to conclude how well the grafts are surviving and functioning in these patients. Although concern has been expressed about whether an optimal immunosuppression therapy has been adopted in these trials, the first post-mortem of a porcine nigral xenograft shows many surviving dopamine neurones 6 months after implantation (Deacon *et al.* 1997), even though the numbers do not approach what would be expected from an allograft of similar amounts of implanted tissue (Kordower *et al.* 1995).

## Cultured cells

Ultimately, the optimal solution to problems of limited availability of cells for transplantation will be to develop

the means to generate cells with precise characteristics designed for each particular application. Several different strategies have been considered.

- *Hibernated or cryopreserved cells.* One strategy is to make the cells more readily available simply by separating the time of collection from the time at when they are implanted. Embryonic neurones can survive freezing, rethawing, and subsequent implantation, but the viability of grafts subject to cryopreservation falls substantially below that achieved with fresh tissues (Redmond *et al.* 1988; Frodl *et al.* 1994; Sautter *et al.* 1996). More effective is 'hibernation', maintaining the cells at 4–8°C in a non-physiological medium that slows cell metabolism. Embryonic ventral mesencephalon can be maintained in hibernation media for up to seven days without loss of viability when subsequently implanted into host rats (Saue and Brundin 1991; Grasbon-Frodl *et al.* 1996). Thus, hibernation of cells can overcome some of the practical clinical constraints of co-ordinating uncertain availability of suitable donor tissues with preparation of the host patient for neurosurgery. However, this approach cannot overcome either the practical problems of the large volumes of human foetal tissue that would need to be implanted or the more fundamental ethical concerns that restrict availability of human foetal tissues in the first place.

- *Cell cultures.* Primary embryonic neurones can be grown in culture. This can both promote their availability for transplantation over a period of several weeks, and provide opportunities for cellular selection and manipulation. However, grafts of primary cells that have been maintained in culture do not survive as well as if the cells were implanted immediately after initial dissection (Brundin *et al.* 1985b).

- *Cell lines.* Much higher yields can be obtained from cell lines that proliferate in culture, such as those derived form various neuronal or glial tumours. One widely studied cell line is the phaeochromocytoma PC12 line. Originally derived from an adrenal tumour, PC12 cells synthesise and secrete high levels of catecholamines, including dopamine. When PC12 cells are implanted into hemi-parkinsonian rats, they survive well if immunosuppressed with cyclosporin, release dopamine into the dopamine depleted striatum, and reverse the hosts' motor deficits in tests of apomorphine rotation (Bing *et al.* 1988; Okuda *et* al. 1991). However, the major problem with this strategy is that cells derived from tumours can retain their tumourigenicity, the cells continue to proliferate after transplantation, and kill the host animals within a few weeks (Bing *et al.* 1988; Hori *et al.* 1993).

- *Expanded precursor cells.* One strategy to overcome the tumourigenicity of proliferating cell lines may be to identify and isolate self-replicating precursor cells (or 'stem' cells) in the developing embryo, and then expand these cells in culture before differentiation into particular neuronal or glial cell populations for implantation. There have been several advances in culturing technique that may make this approach more flexible, such as the use of roller culture systems (Spenger *et al.* 1996), in particular with the prospect of extending the viability of primary cultures. The use of expanded precursor cells for transplantation is explored further in Chapter 25.

- *Engineered cells.* A final strategy is to engineer cells *de novo*, using the powerful new tools of gene therapy. One strategy is to undertake a conditional immortalisation of cells for grafting, engineering them to proliferate under some circumstances (e.g. at a temperature of 33°C) but not under others (e.g. at body temperature of 37–39°C). This can be achieved by engineering the cells with specific temperature-sensitive proto-oncogenes. However, these new tools now allow a much greater range of manipulations: not simply controlling cell proliferation but changing any or all features of a cells phenotype. The possibilities for designing and engineering cells *de novo* for many different applications, including transplantation, are elaborated further in Chapter 26.

# *Mechanisms of graft function*

The search for alternative sources of cells for transplantation and the identification of different patterns of recovery in different experimental and clinical circumstances has highlighted the fundamental importance of the question, 'How do grafts work?'. If we can answer this question, then there is a chance of developing new strategies of repair more efficiently, based on a rational understanding of the fundamental processes involved and not just an empirical approach with serendipity as the outcome. It turns out however that there is no simple

answer. Rather, different grafts are seen to work by different mechanisms in different model systems (see Table 23.1). Each particular set of circumstances requires individual analysis to identify the alternative mechanisms that can apply, and consequently each will impose very different demands on the requirements for true functional repair.

## Non-specific mechanisms

Not all effects of neural transplants need necessarily be due to specific replacement of damaged connections or deficient neurochemicals. A variety of non-specific mechanisms must be considered and excluded (or not, as the case may be).

- *Placebo effects.* Trials of neural transplantation are as susceptible to placebo effects as any other clinical treatment and can only be excluded if evaluated using appropriate standardised and well-controlled assessment procedures.

- *Negative side-effects.* The neurosurgical procedures themselves cause unintended damage; the growth of grafts can cause additional 'space occupying' lesions.

- *'Noise'.* Spontaneous electrical activity in grafted cells and their associated fibre outgrowth may introduce 'noise' rather than patterned information into connected host systems.

## The neuro-endocrine model

The simplest way in which a graft might provide a specific functional influence is for it to provide a chronic replacement of a deficient neurochemical or neurohormone by diffuse secretion or release, either within the host brain or into the circulation. In support of this mechanism, neural grafts have been found to be effective in a number of model systems involving discrete forms of neuro-endocrine disturbance in the hypothalamic–pituitary system.

One of the clearest examples involves disturbance in sexual development and function following damage in the basal hypothalamus. This line of research gained particular impetus with the development of a selective and sensitive animal model within which to evaluate graft function — the *hpg* (hypogonadal) mouse. The *hpg* strain involves a single gene mutation leading to a total absence of synthesis of gondadotrophin releasing hormone (GnRH) by the relevant population of hypothalamic neurones. As a consequence, homozygotes

**Table 23.1**    Potential mechanisms of graft function

| Mechanism | Explanation |
| --- | --- |
| *Non-specific* | Grafts exert placebo effects, adverse effects of the neurosurgery or graft-derived 'noise' into host brain. |
| *Hormonal and neuro-endocrine* | Grafts secrete diffusible neurohormones circulating to distant targets |
| *Diffuse neurotransmitter release* | Grafts secrete deficient neurotransmitters at physiological levels and acting at local receptor sites |
| *Neurotrophic influences* | Grafts secrete neurotrophic molecules that retard ongoing degeneration or promote compensatory plasticity in the host brain |
| *Graft–host connections* | The grafts provide a local re-innervation for transmitter release at synaptic sites |
| *Circuit reconstruction* | The grafts establish reciprocal connections with the host brain and become integrated into the host neuronal circuitry |

manifest a total failure of gonadal development and of sexual function in adulthood.

Krieger *et al.* (1982) found that implants of embryonic hypothalamus from normal mice would survive and restore GnRH release following implantation into the third ventricle of mice. This not only restored circulating levels of gonadotrophin, but if implanted early in life would also restore proper development of the testes in males and the ovaries in females. Most dramatically, grafts in homozygote *hpg* mice have restored sexual activity to the level where mutant mothers have conceived and given birth to viable litters (Fig. 23.14).

These and other studies indicate that neuro-endocrine deficiencies can be restored by neural grafts. It would appear sufficient for the grafts to restore circulating concentrations of the deficient neurohormones, which could be achieved simply by diffuse release of the relevant substances. However, in each case where this has been investigated in detail, a more complex level of reorganisation appears to be the norm. In the particular case of the *hpg* mice, the grafted GnRH-secreting cells give rise to rich axonal outgrowth into the median eminence of the host brain where the axon terminals establish specialised contacts with the fenestrated capillaries. Thus, even though a diffuse release mechanisms may theoretically be sufficient for functional efficacy, in fact the grafts reconstruct the specialised apparatus for regulated neurohormonal release directly into the portal capillaries, similar to that observed in the intact brain.

## Grafts as pharmacological 'minipumps'

The rationale that initially underlay both embryonic nigral grafts and adrenal grafts was to provide a replace-

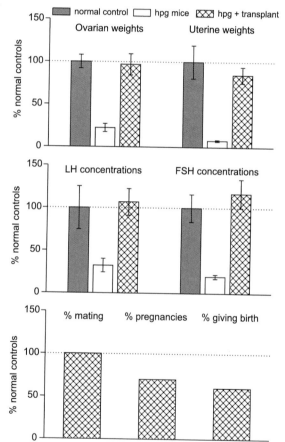

**Fig. 23.14**   Restoration of sex hormone secretion, sex organ development, and functional sexual behaviours in female gonadotrophic releasing hormone (GnRH) deficient hypogonadal *hpg* mice following transplantation of GnRH-secreting hypothalamic cells into the hypothalamus. (Data from Wood and Charlton 1994.)

ment of the catecholaminergic activation of the neostriatum lost as a consequence of degeneration of the intrinsic projections. Although nigral grafts do give rise to an axonal re-innervation of the host brain and establish new synaptic connections with the appropriate striatal targets, it is not at all clear that this is either necessary or sufficient for their functional activity. Since even peripheral pharmacological replacement, using l-dopa and related agents, is effective in early stages of the disease, it is quite plausible that nigral grafts exert their effect via a similar pharmacological mechanism. Grafts may be more effective than other drugs in advanced stages of the disease by virtue of providing a stable rather than phasic delivery of dopamine, at physiological concentrations, at just the selected loci in the brain, rather than throughout the body, reducing side-effects. However, none of these advantages preclude an essentially pharmacological mode of action.

Support for a pharmacological perspective on graft action comes from the recent development of alternative dopamine delivery systems in the brain, all of which have been found to be effective in reducing at least apomorphine-induced rotation following implantation into the neostriatum of dopamine depleted rats:

- direct infusion of dopamine into the denervated neostriatum via implanted cannulae (Hargraves and Freed 1987);

- slow release polymers encapsulating dopamine (Becker *et al.* 1990);

- non-neuronal cells engineered to secrete dopamine or its precursors (Horellou *et al.* 1991);

- dopamine secreting cell lines encapsulated in semipermeable polymer tubes (Winn *et al.* 1989).

The main argument against a simple pharmacological interpretation of the action of nigral grafts is that it does not account for the full range of functional recovery observed (Dunnett and Björklund 1994b). Whereas each of these different treatments has been found to be effective in down-regulating receptor supersensitivity and reversing apomorphine rotation, none of the dopamine-delivery treatments, with the exception of nigral grafts, is effective in alleviating amphetamine-induced rotation or sensory neglect. The broader range of recovery achieved by nigral grafts suggests that they exert their action via some mechanisms over and above simple pharmacological reactivation of the denervated striatum. The most plausible hypothesis remains that

dopaminergic re-innervation and the reformation of new synaptic connections play an important role in the functional recovery.

## Trophic mechanisms of recovery

Although they did not yield great clinical benefit, the trials of adrenal grafts in patients with Parkinson's disease gave rise to a number of surprising observations that raised substantial theoretical doubts about how those grafts actually work. In particular, three separate lines of evidence suggest that any benefit of the implantation was unrelated to the ability of the grafts to restore catecholamine function lost in the disease.

- Biochemical studies of the adrenal glands collected from patients post-mortem, suggest that there can be as great a loss of catecholamines from the adrenal gland in Parkinson's disease as is lost from the brain (Stoddard *et al.* 1989).

- All attempts to identify restoration of secreted catecholamines in adrenal grafted patients *in vivo*, e.g. by biochemical analysis of cerebrospinal fluid or by positron emission tomography, have been without success.

- A few patients with adrenal grafts have now died. In most cases, post-mortem histology has found either a complete necrosis of the grafts or, at best, very few surviving chromaffin cells, even in patients that were reported to show measurable recovery.

When taken together, these observations suggest that any positive effects of adrenal grafts may in large part not be attributable to catecholamine replacement. The most plausible alternative is that the adrenal grafts induce recovery by trophic stimulation of a reorganisation and regeneration of intrinsic systems in the host brain. The trophic model has now gained substantial experimental support, in particular arising out of further experimental studies on the mechanisms of adrenal graft function.

Martha Bohn and colleagues were the first to emphasise the trophic response induced by adrenal grafts in mice (Bohn *et al.* 1987). They used tyrosine hydroxylase (TH) immunostaining to study the possibilities of fibre production from adrenal grafts, and noted a marked stimulation of TH-positive fibres surrounding the grafts, even in cases in which the grafts contained few or even no TH-positive cells. Rather, the grafts appeared to stimulate sprouting from nigro-striatal axon terminals that were incompletely lesioned. Thus, the grafts were exerting a trophic influence on the damaged host brain to enable the partially lesioned intrinsic system to regenerate with apparent functional consequences.

Why should there be such a difference in the interpretation of results between these observations in mice and the earlier studies in rats? The earlier studies all used the toxin 6-hydroxydopamine, which produces relatively complete lesions of the ascending nigro-striatal pathways, leaving little of the system spared and available for intrinsic regeneration. Consequently, a trophic response was never seen in rats with nigro-striatal bundle lesions, although has subsequently been replicated by making partial lesions into the substantia nigra itself. The Bohn study in mice used the alternative toxin MPTP (which is not effective in rats, see Chapter 6). While producing good nigro-striatal lesions and extensive striatal dopamine depletion, MPTP substantially spares the meso-corticolimbic dopamine system innervating more ventral striatal areas, such as the nucleus accumbens. The sprouting observed by Bohn originated from (and was dependent on the survival of) this spared ventral pathway.

Similar trophic effects have subsequently been observed both in MPTP-lesioned monkeys and in several of the human post-mortem studies. These studies highlight how the selection of a particular animal model can influence the outcome of experiments. In this particular context, 6-hydroxydopamine may provide a convenient tool to produce stable and complete forebrain dopamine depletion, but it does not fully replicate the slow, progressive, and partial nature of the degeneration that is the basis for the clinical disease. Consequently, whereas animal models may be helpful early in development, the validity of any new treatment strategy has ultimately to be evaluated clinically.

## Functional connections: retino-tectal system

The retino-tectal system provides a clear example of one system in which graft function is clearly dependent upon the formation of its connections with the host brain. Lund and colleagues first showed that the embryonic retinae can be implanted over the superior colliculus of newborn rats so as to form new retinal projections into the host brain. The grafted retinae project to many, but not all, of the normal targets within the host brain. This

has provided a powerful model system within which to study developmental axon guidance in mammalian central nervous system.

The functional nature of the retino-tectal projections formed from the grafts has been studied in two main paradigms. First, the simple transduction of sensory stimuli has been shown by demonstrating restitution of the pupillary reflex. The pupil contracts when a bright light is shone on the intact retina, a reflex mediated through a well-established circuit linking the retinal ganglion cells to the pupilloconstrictor muscles via the olivary pretectal nucleus, Edinger-Westphal nucleus, oculomotor nerve, and ciliary ganglion (see Fig. 23.15). Klassen and Lund (1987) showed that retinal grafts projecting to the tectum restored the reflex in rats when the transplanted retina was illuminated through a bone hole in the skull.

Of course the pupillary reflex may demonstrate restitution of a hard-wired reflex, but it does not indicate whether the grafts in any way restore the rats' ability actually to 'see'. In the second series of studies, Coffey and Lund have trained rats to use light as a discriminative stimulus to control their ongoing behaviour (Coffey *et al.* 1989). Rats with one intact eye and a retinal graft were trained to press a lever in a test chamber to receive food pellet rewards. In this situation, if rats are given a warning signal, such as a light or a tone, before a brief foot shock, they will freeze in anticipation of the coming shock. This freezing is apparent as a cessation of ongoing lever pressing for food — a phenomenon known in animal learning theory as 'conditioned suppression'. Coffey and Lund trained rats to suppress lever pressing for food in a series of daily test sessions, with a light stimulus to provide an accurate warning of forthcoming foot shock and a tone as a much longer (and hence less accurate) warning. Not surprisingly, normal animals and animals trained while having the intact eye open, learned to suppress lever pressing only during the light stimulus. Other rats were trained while viewing the world only through the transplant. This was achieved by placing a clear Perspex window in the skull over the graft and by placing a patch over the intact eye. These rats were also able to learn to suppress responding only when the light was switched on, just like normal rats (see Fig. 23.16).

From these experiments, we can conclude that grafts not only make axonal connections with the host brain but they do so in such a way that the host animal can use those connections functionally to transduce and relay useful information in the control of adaptive behaviour.

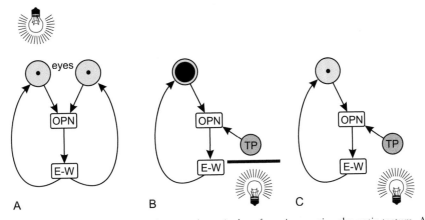

**Fig. 23.15** Functional reconstruction of the visual system by retinal grafts re-innervating the optic tectum. A Schematic illustration of the normal pupillary reflex: light detected in the retina is relayed via the retinal ganglion cells, the olivary pretectal nucleus, and the Ehringer-Westphal nucleus to the ciliary ganglion that provides autonomic control over pupillary constriction. B One eye is removed and a retinal transplant grafted to the tectum. When both the intact eye and the transplant are screened from light, the pupil remains dilated. C Selective illumination of the transplant results in pupil constriction in the intact eye, indicating restitution of the functional circuit controlling this visual reflex. (Redrawn from Klassen and Lund 1987.)

## Circuit reconstruction: striatal grafts

The retino-tectal system provides clear evidence of the capacity of grafts to process neuronal information in a functionally meaningful way. A remaining level of complexity is whether grafts can become established with reciprocal connections to and from the host brain, so as to replace lost cells within damaged complex networks.

Perhaps the best evidence for circuit reconstruction is provided with striatal grafts. The neostriatum provides a primary projection of the neocortex and is involved in the selection and initiation of cortical plans of action. In addition to the well-known motor consequences of striatal damage, striatal lesions in rats and monkeys also disrupt performance in a variety of cognitive and learning tasks. These include classical 'prefrontal' tasks such as spatial delayed response and delayed alternation, and result from disruption of the major outflows from prefrontal cortex. Striatal grafts can restore performance in rats with striatal lesions not only on simple motor tests but also in these more complex cognitive tasks (Isacson *et al.* 1986; Dunnett *et al.* 1988; Döbrössy and Dunnett 1998).

Several lines of evidence suggest that this recovery is due to the striatal grafts providing a reconstruction of the damaged cortical-striatal-pallidal circuitry.

- Performance of delayed alternation and related cognitive tasks is dependent upon the integrity of cortical-striatal-pallidal projections.

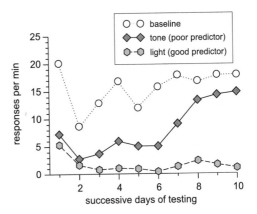

**Fig. 23.16** Retinal transplants can restore usable visual information. Rats can learn to detect a visual stimulus as viewed through a Perspex window over a retinal transplant on the tectum when the light predicts foot shock, as measured in a conditioned suppression test. (Data from Coffey and Lund 1989.)

- Cognitive deficits cannot be restored by drugs or other diffuse strategies of remediation, either in animals with experimental striatal lesions or in patients with Huntington's disease.

- The grafts establish appropriate efferent projections to host globus pallidus and (in some cases) to the substantia nigra and receive appropriate afferent projections from host neocortex, thalamus, substantia nigra, and raphé nucleus (Wictorin 1992).

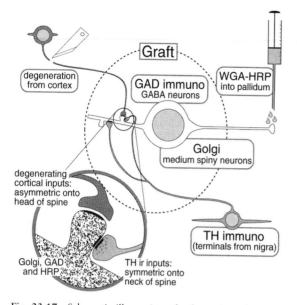

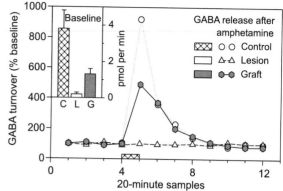

**Fig. 23.17** Schematic illustration of reformation of synaptic input and output connections of striatal grafts, evaluated at the electron microscopic level. Neurones within the grafts are indentified as having a medium spiny morphology by Golgi impregnation, as being GABAergic by GAD immunohistochemical staining, and as projecting to the globus pallidus by retrograde transport of WGA-HRP into the target area. These GABAergic medium spiny projection neurones within the grafts receive synaptic inputs from the neocortex, as demonstrated by undercutting the corticostriatal axons to reveal degenerating terminals making asymmetric synapses on the heads of dendritic spines, and by immunohistochemistry to visualise dopaminergic terminals making symmetric synaptic contacts onto the necks of the same population of spines. (Based on data from Clarke and Dunnett 1993.)

- The thalamic and nigral inputs make appropriate synaptic contacts with GABAergic medium spiny output neurones within the grafts (see Fig. 23.17; Clarke and Dunnett 1993).

- Activation of host nigral inputs to striatal grafts induces a surge of GABA release from striato-pallidal terminals in the globus pallidus with the same temporal characteristics as release from intact striato-pallidal neurones (see Fig. 23.18; Sirinathsinghj *et al.* 1988).

Taken together these studies indicate that (at least in some circumstances) grafts can make reciprocal axonal connections with the brain to reconstruct damaged functional networks in the host brain.

**Fig. 23.18** Striatal grafts restore functional circuitry in the host brain, as detected by push-pull perfusion analysis of GABA turnover in the host pallidum. Striatal lesions result in approximately 97% depletions of pallidal GABA turnover, which is restored to about a third of normal levels after re-innervation by striatal grafts. Activation of dopamine inputs to the striatum by injection of amphetamine causes a 9-fold surge in GABA release, which is completely abolished after striatal lesions and largely restored after striatal grafts. These data suggest a reconstruction of a functional nigral-striatal-pallidal circuit via striatal grafts. (Based on Sirinathsinghji *et al.* 1988.)

## Summary

Just because grafts can provide a remarkable degree of recovery in certain experimental situations, it must not be taken to imply that extensive reconstruction is always (or even normally) the case. Rather, the preceding examples indicate that grafts can (and do) work by a variety of different mechanisms. Although they can be beneficial, they can also produce abnormal or deleterious effects. Moreover, more than one mechanism can apply in a given situation, and the effects of each can be partial or incomplete. Consequently, there is no simple answer to the questions, 'Do grafts work?' and, 'How do they work?' — each particular case needs to be analysed in its own right.

## Further reading

Barker, R.A. and Dunnett, S.B. (1999). *Neural Repair, Transplantation and Rehabilitation*, The Psychology Press, Hove.

Freeman, T.B. and Widner, H. (1998). *Cell Transplantation for Neurological Disorders*. Humana Press, Totowa, New Jersey.

# 24 | *Glial transplantation*

### *Robin J.M. Franklin*

## *Why does spontaneous remyelination fail?*

The variable nature of remyelination has been documented in an earlier section (Chapter 15) in a variety of clinical situations and experimental models. In addition to the decline in remyelination that occurs in progressive demyelinating diseases that has already been described, there are many other factors such as age, sex, species, and strain that have a bearing on the efficiency of spontaneous remyelination. As shown in Fig. 24.1, young rats remyelinate more rapidly than old rats, female rats remyelinate more rapidly than male rats, and rats remyelinate better than rabbits following lysolecithin-induced demyelination (Gilson and Blakemore 1993). Since there is an incomplete understanding of how remyelination occurs, it is unsurprising that, for the most part, there are still incomplete explanations for why remyelination fails. Clearly, for such a complex, multi-process event as remyelination, there are a variety of ways in which the process can be impaired.

One possible explanation is that there is a shortage of cells with remyelinating potential. If the source is oligodendrocytes, then this would seem an unlikely explanation — where there is intact white matter there will always be an abundance of these cells.[1] Conversely, if the adult oligodendrocyte progenitor is the principal source of remyelinating cells, as seems increasingly likely, then we can envisage a situation in which the fluctuations in the size of this population would be reflected in the efficiency of remyelination. For example, the gradual depletion of these cell with age might account for the age-related changes in remyelination. It is certainly the case that fewer of these cells are harvested in tissue culture with increasing age of the donor tissue. The notion that local depletion of oligodendrocyte progenitors will decrease the ability of the tissue to support

remyelination has been discussed in an earlier section (see Chapter 15).

Changes in the ability of the environment of a demyelinating lesion to initiate and sustain remyelination are also likely to have a profound bearing on the extent of repair. In this regard, the cellular composition of the lesion (particularly astrocytes, microglia/macrophages, and demyelinated axons) has attracted much interest. There is a long-standing suggestion that the astrocytosis associated with chronic, non-remyelinating multiple sclerosis plaques may be an impediment to remyelination. There is certainly *in vitro* evidence that some types of astrocyte discourage oligodendrocyte progenitor migration and differentiation. On the other hand, other types of astrocyte may well be beneficial to remyelination by providing growth factors. Astrocytes are cells capable of showing such a diversity of properties that in different guises they could both help and hinder remyelination. There is clear evidence emerging of the importance of the inflammatory response that

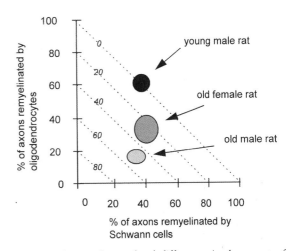

**Fig. 24.1** Age- and sex-related differences in the extent of spontaneous remyelination 3 weeks after lysolecithin-induced demyelination. The dotted lines and numbers in italics indicate the percentages of axons that remain demyelinated. (Adapted from Gilson and Blakemore 1993.)

---

[1] Note that it is not just the white matter but grey matter also that contains oligodendrocytes, particularly the satellite oligodendrocytes that surround neuronal cell bodies.

accompanies demyelination (see Chapter 4) in initiating remyelination. A robust microglia/macrophage response leads to rapid clearance of myelin debris, which alone is a beneficial function, and increased expression of remyelination-enhancing growth factors, either directly or via activation of astrocytes. It is somewhat paradoxical that attempts to prevent immune-mediated demyelination by damping down the inflammatory response may concurrently inhibit remyelination from occurring. An earlier suggestion that chronically demyelinated axons are incapable of being remyelinated no longer seems tenable.

## Promoting endogenous remyelination

A conceptually attractive approach to enhancing remyelination is the administration of remyelination-associated growth factors. The development of this approach is still very much in its infancy, although Henry Webster's group at the NIH have shown that systemic delivery of a growth factor they had previously demonstrated to be associated with remyelination, IGF-I, promotes remyelination after experimental allergic encephalomyelitis (EAE) lesions (Yao *et al.* 1995). Although it is assumed that these effects relate to the well-documented effects of IGF-I on the oligodendrocyte lineage, it now seems likely that some of the effects of IGF-I in EAE are due to its systemic effects on the immune system. Testing the direct effects of putative remyelination-enhancing growth factors on demyelinating lesions is handicapped partly by an incomplete knowledge of the dynamics of growth factor expression during remyelination, and partly by the technical challenges of direct delivery of growth factors. However, as described in Chapter 26, the rapid advances that are being made in indirect protein delivery via *ex vivo* or *in vivo* gene transfer (e.g. transplantation of transfected cells or injection of replication-defective viral vectors, respectively) offers exciting prospects. A potential problem in developing these approaches for the treatment of human disease is the emerging differences between rodents and humans in the responsiveness of oligodendrocyte lineage cells to growth factors. Thus, it cannot be assumed that the growth factors that are shown to work in the rodent will necessarily do so in the patient.

An alternative approach to enhancing inherent remyelination using immunoglobulins has been pio-

neered by Moses Rodriguez and his colleagues at the Mayo Clinic. Systemic delivery of a number of immunoglobulins, such as polyclonal immunoglobulins against myelin basic protein (MBP) or against a partially characterised oligodendrocyte surface antigen, results in more extensive remyelination of areas of demyelination induced in the mouse CNS by infection with Theiler's virus (Rodriguez *et al.* 1996). Although the basis of this effect is not fully understood, the results in experimental models have been sufficiently encouraging to warrant the setting up of clinical trials in multiple sclerosis patients.

## Experimental models for glial cell transplantation

In parallel with the development of neuronal transplantation, glial cell transplantation has rapidly evolved as an experimental technique to study cellular interactions during glial development, and as a potential strategy for repair to remyelinate areas of persistent demyelination in clinical conditions.

An important feature of all glial cell transplantation models is that the host environment into which cells are transplanted must contain non-myelinated axons of an appropriate diameter for myelination (see Table 24.1). Such environments can arise for a variety of reasons, and many have been used as host environments in transplantation studies, such as the non-myelinated axons of the retina or during development before myelination is complete. However, the majority of transplantation studies have been undertaken using one of two models.

### Myelin-deficient mutants

The first of type of model system comprises the so-called 'myelin-mutants', i.e. strains of animal in which the CNS never becomes fully myelinated due to defects in genes encoding one of the major myelin-proteins. Of these, the hypomyelinated shiverer mouse (an MBP mutant) has been widely used since the pioneering studies of Madeleine Gumpel and her co-workers. The mutation not only results in there being axons available for myelination by the transplanted cells but also provides the basis for identification of transplant-derived myelin sheaths, which are MBP-positive and, in contrast to the mutant, contain a major-dense line. The shaking pup and, particularly, the myelin-deficient rat (Fig. 24.2)

**Table 24.1** Experimental models used to study transplant-mediated myelination and remyelination

| | Experimental model | Availability of axons for interactions with transplanted cells | Basis of identification of transplanted cells |
|---|---|---|---|
| *Gliotoxic lesions* | Focal injection of EB | Temporarily demyelinated axons available due to destruction of local glia | Transplant cell marker, and/or behaviour inferred by alteration of inherent repair response |
| | Focal inject of lysolecithin | *ditto* | *ditto* |
| | Focal injection of EB into X-irradiated white matter | Persistently demyelinated axons available due to destruction of local glia | Suppression of local glial response |
| *Genetic myelin mutants* | *Shiverer mouse*: hypomyelinated, MBP gene deletion | Axons available during development or by injection of gliotoxin | Transplant cell marker, and/or immunocytochemical or ultrastructural detection of myelin sheaths containing MBP |
| | *Myelin-deficient rat*: severe myelin deficiency, oligodendrocyte degeneration, PLP gene mutation | Axons available due to degeneration of myelinating oligodendrocytes | Absence of host myelin, and/or transplant cell marker, immuno- cytochemical detection of myelin sheaths containing normal PLP |
| | *Shaking Pup*: severe myelin deficiency, oligodendrocyte degeneration, PLP gene mutation | *ditto* | *ditto* |
| *Myelin-deficiency in normal animals* | Retina | Intra-retinal axons of many species are unmyelinated | Absence of host myelin |
| | Development | Axons available prior to myelination by host cells | Transplant cell marker |

*Abbreviations:* EB, ethidium bromide; MBP, myelin basic protein; PLP, proteolipid protein.

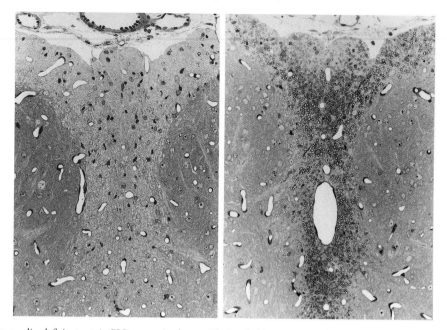

**Fig. 24.2**  The myelin-deficient rat (a PLP mutant), along with the shaking pup (another PLP mutant) and the shiverer mouse (an MBP mutant), have each proved to be useful models for studying the behaviour of transplanted myelinogenic cells on account of the deficiency of the host oligodendrocytes. (*Left*) The spinal cord of the untransplanted myelin-deficient rat contains no myelinated axons. (*Right*) At 12 days following the transplantation of a mixed glial cell culture prepared from normal neonatal rats, regions of transplant-derived oligodendrocyte myelination are found. (Micrographs kindly provided by Drs Ian Duncan and David Archer.)

(both involving X-linked mutations of the proteolipid protein gene) have also been used for transplantation studies by Ian Duncan and others on account of their profound hypomyelination (Archer *et al.* 1997).

## Focal toxic demyelination

The second model involves the creation of focal areas of demyelination in adult white matter by direct injection of ethidium bromide or lysolecithin, both of which are agents toxic to oligodendrocytes (Fig. 24.3). Since gliotoxin-induced demyelination undergoes spontaneous remyelination to a greater or lesser degree, these models provide a situation where transplanted cells interact with host-derived cells during repair. A particularly useful variant of the gliotoxin model developed by William Blakemore and colleagues involves creating demyelination in tissue exposed to 40 Grays of X-irradiation. This dose of X-irradiation has the effect of suppressing the spontaneous repair response resulting in a demyelination lesion that is never repopulated by host glia and which fails to remyelinate (Fig. 24.4). Such a lesion provides an excellent environment with which to

ask questions about the behaviour and particularly the myelinogenic properties of transplanted glia.

Although none of these models accurately mimic the chronic demyelinated plaques of multiple sclerosis, they have nevertheless provided valuable information from which one can assess the likely suitability of a range of transplanted cell populations.

## *Transplants of glia and glial precursor cells*

A suitable cell for transplantation must fulfil several requirements:

- *Remyelination.* The principle requirement is the ability to generate new myelin sheaths capable of restoring saltatory conduction to demyelinated axons.

- *Proliferation.* The cell should be able to undergo controlled proliferation. This would then enable the transplanted population to generate sufficient cells

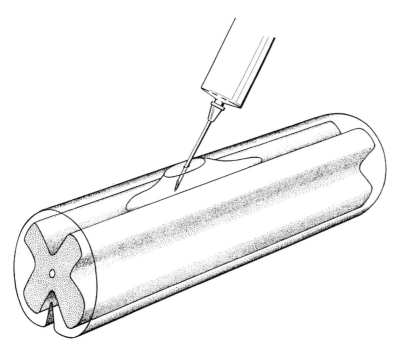

**Fig. 24.3** A useful model for studying both spontaneous and transplanted-mediated remyelination involves injecting gliotoxins (usually ethidium bromide or lysolecithin) into the dorsal funiculus of the adult spinal cord. This creates a discrete fusiform lesion confined to the white matter. The lesion can be easily re-located for transplantation studies in which cells are injected into the tissue using a similar procedure for that used for injecting toxins.

appropriate to the extent of the area needing repair in response to local mitogens.

- *Local migration.* Although proliferation alone may constitute a means by which transplanted cells can fill a lesion, the ability of the transplanted cells to migrate is likely to assist this process. In a multifocal condition, such as multiple sclerosis, it would also be beneficial if cells were not only able to migrate within but also between areas of demyelination. If this were the case, then multiple injections of cells, in which each clinically-relevant plaque is targeted separately, might not be necessary.

With these three requirements for myelination, proliferation and migration in mind, we can examine the suitability of the available types of myelinogenic cell.

## Cells of the oligodendrocyte lineage

The oligodendrocyte lineage has been well characterised in tissue culture studies and as a result it has been possible to isolate populations of cells enriched for a particular phenotypic stage, which can then be transplanted into one of the available transplantation models. It is clear from such studies that all *in vitro* stages of the oligodendrocyte lineage, from the polysialyated N-CAM (PSA-N-CAM)-expressing preprogenitor to O1-positive oligodendrocyte (see Chapters 15 and 25) are able to myelinate axons following transplantation. The ability of mature myelinating oligodendrocytes isolated from adult tissue to myelinate axons for a second time following transplantation is more controversial. However, the various stages of the lineage differ in their proliferative and migratory capacity when transplanted into myelin-deficient mutant models, where it is apparent that earlier stages generate more myelin over a wider area than do later stages (Groves *et al.* 1993; Warrington *et al.* 1993). This lineage variability following transplantation reflects well-documented differences between the biology of the motile, proliferative oligodendrocyte progenitor and the non-motile, non-dividing differentiated oligodendrocyte (see Box 15.1). Thus, according to the criteria outlined above, the oligodendrocyte progenitor seems a particularly suitable candidate. A further advantage of the oligodendrocyte progenitor is that it also exhibits greater plasticity than the mature oligodendrocytes. Thus, *in vitro*, this cell can give rise to an astrocyte as well as a myelinating oligodendrocyte, although such bipotentiality appears not to occur to any great extent during normal development (Franklin and Blakemore 1995).

The ability of the transplanted oligodendrocyte progenitor to migrate through normal, intact adult CNS has been a matter of some controversy. It is clear that these cells can migrate following transplantation into

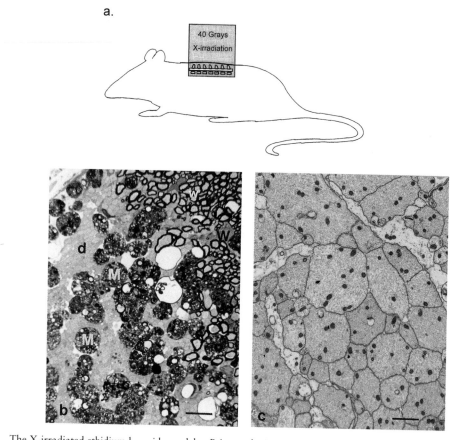

**Fig. 24.4** The X-irradiated ethidium bromide model. a Prior to the injection of ethidium bromide into spinal cord white matter (see Fig. 24.3) the spinal cord is locally exposed to 40 Grays of X-irradiation. b This creates a demyelinating lesion in which the spontaneous repair response is suppressed. The lesion, which has a distinct border separating it from normal white matter (W), consists of demyelinated axons (d) and macrophages (M). Scale bar = 25 μm. c At the ultrastructural level, the demyelinated axons can be seen to reside in an environment that contains no glial cells, although degenerating astrocyte process can sometimes be seen. Scale bar = 1.4 μm. This environment has proved useful in understanding the interactions between demyelinated axons and transplanted glial cells.

developing normal or myelin-deficient CNS, where they presumably join the endogenous population of migrating cells. A number of studies in the mouse have reported not only that transplanted oligodendrocyte progenitors can migrate through normal adult tissue, but also that they migrate preferentially towards areas of demyelination (Baron-Van Evercooren *et al.* 1996). However, when similar studies are undertaken in the rat, extremely limited migration is seen in the adult CNS, and the transplanted cells survive very poorly (Franklin *et al.* 1996a). Only when the cells are placed close to active areas of demyelination (within an area of comparable dimensions to the area from which endogenous remyelinating cells are recruited) are cells able to enter the lesion. The distance over which endogenous oligo-

dendrocyte precursors can migrate towards an area of demyelination was tested by irradiating the lesioned spinal cord, and therefore killing the endogenous precursors, for increasing distances surrounding the lesion. The conclusion was that cells will only migrate for 2 mm or less towards a lesion, and the same figure would presumably apply to implanted cells (Franklin *et al.* 1997). This also correlates with *in vitro* studies showing that astrocytes are inhibitory to the migration of oligodendrocyte precursors (Fok-Seang *et al.* 1995).

The reason for the poor survival of transplanted oligodendrocyte progenitors in normal adult rat CNS is not known. The most plausible hypothesis is that they succumb to a shortage of survival factors, the levels of which are tightly regulated during development and

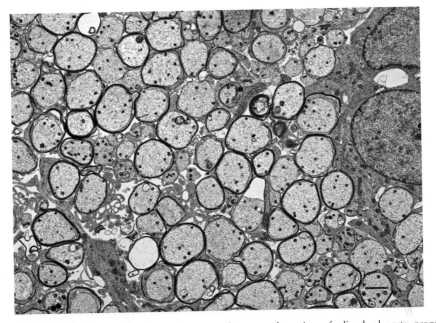

**Fig. 24.5** Extensive oligodendrocyte remyelination 21 days after transplantation of oligodendrocyte progenitors into an X-irradiated ethidium bromide lesion (see Fig. 24.4). Scale bar = 2 μm.

adulthood to match the number of oligodendrocyte lineage cells, initially generated in excess, to the number of axons requiring myelination. Presumably, the levels of survival factor are elevated within active areas of demyelination, since when oligodendrocyte progenitors are transplanted directly into such an environment they survive and are able to remyelinate demyelinated axons. Since cells appear to survive when present at the edges of a demyelinating lesion, we can imagine a scenario in which survival factors present within the lesion are also present as a diminishing gradient around the lesion. The presence of penumbral effects around a lesion, may account for the apparent discrepancy between the observations in the rat and those in the mouse, where the relative extent of the penumbra and the precise position of the transplant with respect to the lesions borders may lead to apparently opposite effects on the behaviour of transplanted oligodendrocyte progenitor cells.

If oligodendrocyte progenitors transplanted into normal tissue fail to survive, then the prospects for remyelinating widespread multifocal areas of demyelination by transplantation of a supposedly migratory population of cells are greatly diminished. To overcome this problem it will be necessary to change the properties (or identity) of the transplanted cell and modify the environment in such a way that it supports survival and migration. To this end, the non-permissive adult CNS

can be made supportive of oligodendrocyte progenitor survival, proliferation, and migration by prior exposure to 40 Grays of X-irradiation. Indeed, if the tissue is treated in this way then transplanted, cells not only survive and migrate but also enter remote areas of demyelination which they proceed to remyelinate (Fig. 24.5). The nature of the changes in permissiveness brought about by X-irradiation is not known, but clearly if one could identify these factors, then we can devise alternative means of altering the ability of adult CNS to support transplanted oligodendrocyte progenitors that do not carry the potentially hazardous side effects of high dose X-irradiation.

## Sources of oligodendrocyte progenitors for human transplantation

Non-histocompatible glial transplants undergo rejection, although this problem could be side-stepped if one were to use cells obtained from the patient. The small size of the sub-ventricular zone in adult humans, in contrast to the adult rat, means that it is unlikely to be as rich a source of uncommitted progenitor cells. Whereas a number of recent studies have shown that oligodendrocyte progenitors can be isolated from adult human brain (Fig. 24.6), the yields that can be obtained by present techniques are not yet sufficient to envisage their

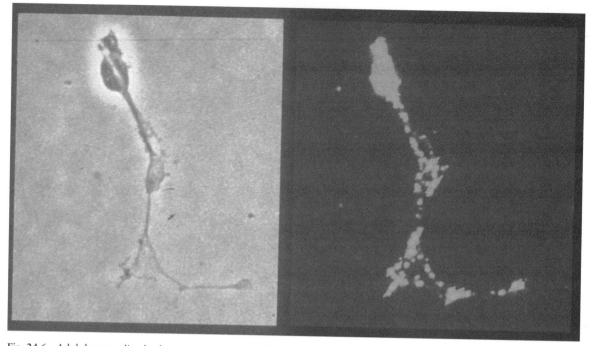

**Fig. 24.6**  Adult human oligodendrocyte progenitors in cell culture. These progenitors have been stained using indirect immuno-fluorescence with an antibody (A2B5) directed against cell-specific gangliosides. (Reproduced with the kind permission of Dr Neil Scolding.)

transplantation (Scolding *et al.* 1995). It might, however, be possible to expand these cells *in vitro* with appropriate combinations of growth factors, as has already been achieved using oligodendrocyte progenitors from the neonatal rat. Although these cells are capable of division, the identity of the mitogens remains elusive and it seems likely that the mitogens required by human progenitors differ from those that are effective in the rat. Until it is possible to expand oligodendrocyte progenitors from adult human brain one must be cautious about the prospects of autologous transplantation.

## Oligospheres

Because of the difficulties in obtaining sufficient numbers of oligodendrocyte progenitors from the adult human brain, other potential sources of oligodendrocyte lineage cells suitable for transplantation are being investigated, such as multipotential stem cells from foetal tissue that can been propagated *in vitro* as 'neurospheres' (see Chapter 25). A promising variation of the neurosphere approach is that developed by Annik

Baron-Van Evercooren and co-workers who are able to generate large numbers of oligodendrocyte lineage cell as 'oligospheres' in tissue obtained from post-natal brain (Avellana-Adalid *et al.* 1996).

## Schwann cells

Since cells of the oligodendrocyte lineage fail at present to fulfil all requirements, we might look to the other myelinating cell of the nervous system, the Schwann cell. At first glance the case for the Schwann cell looks promising:

- they myelinate demyelinated CNS axons, either following transplantation or when recruited from endogenous sources, and thereby restore saltatory conduction (Blakemore 1977; Honmou *et al.* 1996);

- they can be grown and expanded from autologous biopsy material;

- unlike oligodendrocytes, they are not targets of auto-immune injury that underlies the genesis of the demyelinating lesions of multiple sclerosis.

However, in spite of this impressive list of credentials, the interactions that occur between astrocytes and Schwann cells impose limitations on their suitability. There is a large body of evidence from developmental, pathological, and *in vitro* studies, which indicates that Schwann cells will only occupy regions of the nervous system from which astrocytes are absent. They do not appear to migrate through astrocyte-defined territories, nor will they myelinate axons surrounded by astrocytic processes such as would occur in chronic multiple sclerosis plaques. It will be necessary to devise ways of overcoming the mutual exclusivity between Schwann cells and astrocytes based on a better understanding of its molecular basis before Schwann cell transplantation for multiple sclerosis becomes a feasible proposition. An *in vitro* study by Wilby has shown that one of the mechanisms by which Schwann cell migration is inhibited by astrocytes is through excessive adhesion mediated by N-cadherin, and that reagents that block this interaction can enhance migration (Wilby *et al.* 1999). There are probably other types of interaction between these cell types, but it seems probable that they can be modified so as to make the Schwann cell useful for remyelination.

## Olfactory glia

An alternative to the Schwann cell may be provided by the glia of the olfactory system. The olfactory bulb-ensheathing cells are a distinct group of glia that ensheath the small-diameter axons of the olfactory nerve as it enters the olfactory bulb. Although found within the CNS, they share properties with both Schwann cells and astrocytes. It has recently been shown that the Schwann cell-like properties of these cells can be pushed to the extent that they will attain a myelinating phenotype when confronted with demyelinated large-diameter axons, following transplantation into an X-irradiated ethidium bromide lesion in the adult rat spinal cord (Franklin *et al.* 1996b). This myelinating phenotype resembles a myelinating Schwann cell both ultrastructurally and in synthesising myelin containing P0. Moreover, these myelin sheaths will restore con-

duction similar to that achieved by Schwann cells (Imaizumi *et al.* 1998). The current interest in these cells is that, unlike Schwann cells, they co-exist with astrocytes in their normal environment and may therefore not be subject to the restrictions that a CNS glial environment imposes on the behaviour of Schwann cells.

## *Future directions*

Because remyelination can occur as a spontaneous process, we can be optimistic that clinical benefits will accrue from an improved understanding of basic developmental and regenerative mechanisms. The challenge is to reactivate and prolong a process that already occurs. It may be possible to do this by enhancing remyelination by the endogenous oligodendrocyte precursors and Schwann cells of the CNS. However, if it transpires that the number of these becomes depleted following repeated remyelination, it will be necessary to add cells by transplantation. The problem confronting neuronal repair, where the relative absence of spontaneous regeneration after neuronal or axonal pathology in the CNS offers a different challenge: how to initiate developmental processes that are otherwise non-existent or dormant in the adult brain.

## *Further reading*

Blakemore, W.F. and Franklin, R.J.M. (2000). Transplantation options for therapeutic CNS remyelination. *Cell Transplantation* 9, 289–294.

Blakemore, W.F., Crang, A.J., and Franklin, R.J.M. (1995). Transplantation of glial cells. In *Neuroglia* (ed. H. Kettenman, and B. Ransom), pp 869–882. Oxford University Press, London.

Duncan, I.D., Grever, W.E., and Zhang, S.C. (1997). Repair of myelin disease: strategies and progress in animal models. *Molecular Medicine Today* 3, 554–561.

Franklin, R.J.M. and ffrench-Constant, C. (1996) Transplantation and repair in multiple sclerosis. In *The Molecular Biology of Multiple Sclerosis* (ed. W.C. Russell), pp. 231–242. John Wiley & Sons, New York.

# 25 | *Stem cells*

Until fairly recently, interest in stem cells was restricted within neurobiology to studies on the fundamental principles of neural development, although in other fields (such as oncology) they have been a topic of major investigation for understanding the principles surrounding control of cell proliferation, in particular as it relates to the haematopoietic system and leukaemia. However this situation has changed rapidly in the last decade, not least because of the realisation that if we can understand the lineages of cell birth during normal development, then maybe we can manipulate neural precursors *in vitro*, allowing for potentially unlimited expansion and controlled differentiation of different populations of neuronal cells both *in vitro* and *in vivo*. This then would offer the potential of providing unlimited supplies of precisely specified cells for transplantation, and open up other, completely new, strategies for repair.

## Cell birth and cell replacement

Unlike in the nervous system, in most tissues of the body a continuous turnover of cells by death and replacement is the norm rather than the exception. Cell replacement can be achieved in two ways (Gage *et al.* 1995a).

- *Division of differentiated cells.* Following damage in the skin, dead epithelial cells are replaced by division of adjacent healthy cells, each mature cell dividing to produce two similar copies.

- *Differentiation from precursor cells.* In other tissues, most notably the white blood cells of the haematopoietic system, a resting population of precursor cells divides, one of the progeny then differentiates into a mature white blood cell, and the other remains as a precursor cell replacing its parent. The detailed lineages of the different cells and the factors regulating each stage of differentiation have now been worked out in considerable detail for the haematopoietic system.

Similarly, from a single embryonic stem (ES) cell precursor, the nervous system develops by a process of progressive division, differentiation, migration and specification down complex lineages to yield the wide diversity of cell types that make up the adult nervous system. During development, then, there is a process of cell division and specialisation with the early cells in the developmental lineage having a multipotential capacity. At successive stages of the process, however, the cells become progressively more committed to a certain phenotype (see Fig. 25.1).

Some of these precursors are 'progenitor cells' in that they are committed to a particular lineage and as they divide they form new cells further down the lineage. Conversely, other cells have a self-renewing and proliferative capacity. These are 'stem cells'. Precise usage varies, but the following features may be taken to define the concept of a neural stem cell, even though in many situations not all critical features of particular cell types have been identified:

- they are *pre-differentiated* cells — i.e. they have the potential to divide, they are not in a final stage of differentiation, and may continue to divide throughout life;

- they are *self-renewing* — i.e. they can divide to form multiple copies of themselves, allowing expansion in stem cell numbers, as well as other cells of more restricted fate; under appropriate conditions, division and self replication can potentially carry on indefinitely, in principle allowing infinite exponential expansion;

- they are *multipotential* — i.e. they have the capacity to differentiate in response to different signals down a variety of different committed lineages or into a variety of different cell types.

As they progress down the developmental lineage, precursor cells pass through a number of progenitor cell stages leading to progressively more-restricted terminal phenotypes. At the final stages of differentiation, the

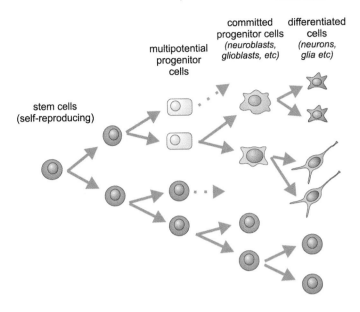

multipotential
progenitor
cells

committed
progenitor cells
*(neuroblasts,
glioblasts, etc)*

differentiated
cells
*(neurons,
glia etc)*

stem cells
(self-reproducing)

**Fig. 25.1** Conceptual replication and differentiation of stem and progenitor cells in the nervous system.

precursors are committed to restricted neuronal or glial lineages ('neuroblasts' or 'glioblasts') before finally undergoing terminal cell division into cells, not only with a committed neuronal (or glial) fate, but also a particular phenotype. Although there is not yet a consensus on definition, the term 'stem cells' is generally retained for cells earlier in the lineage, with an emphasis on self-replication and multipotentiality, whereas 'progenitor cells' are later in the lineage, and although also not terminally differentiated have a more restricted fate. The term 'precursor cell' can apply more generally to any cell before the final stage of differentiation into its final phenotype.

## Stem and progenitor cells in the CNS

The lineages of cells in the nervous system have been well worked out in a number of simple organisms and for a number of particular cell types. This is best illustrated for *C. elegans* in which the precise lineage of each of the 302 cells in the mature nervous system has been precisely mapped (White *et al.* 1986) (Fig. 25.2). This enterprise has revealed fundamental features of nervous system development, including the genetic programming and molecules involved in cell death, and provides a model within which the signals that trigger each stage in differentiation can be precisely identified.

By contrast, the lineages of cells in the mammalian

(and more generally the vertebrate) CNS are still poorly understood and the topic of active current investigation. In particular, whereas the fate of some neurones may be determined by the cell's lineage, in many situations multiple cell types are derived within a single lineage, and the precise differentiation may be determined by a variety of local signalling factors. Some of the best worked examples are provided by the lineage of oligodendroglia in the rat optic nerve, and the differentiation and migration of developing neurones in the neural crest and floor plate in the developing chick.

## Specification of nerve cells in development

In normal development, multiple different cell types derive from single multipotential progenitors. This is illustrated in a series of studies by Christine Holt and colleagues on the developing retina of frogs (Holt *et al.* 1988). Labelling of a single progenitor cell and following its subsequent divisions indicated that all major cell types of the retina — photoreceptors, amacrine, ganglion and bipolar cells — are all from the same precursor (Fig. 25.3). Thus, it is not the lineage of the precursor itself that determines cell fate but presumably local signals that allow the precursor cell to divide into multiple different cell types.

Restrictions in the phenotype of progenitor cells are not necessarily correlated with their potential for mitotic expansion. Thus, in some circumstances, a very great clonal expansion can be obtained from progenitor

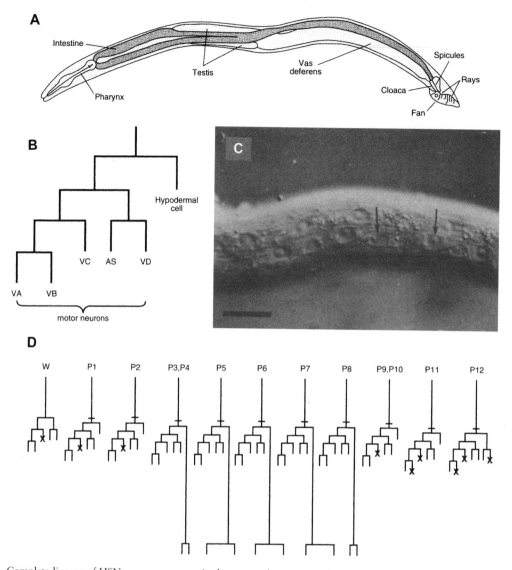

**Fig 25.2**  Complete lineage of HSN motor neuronees in the nematode worm *C. elegans* (A). The genes that regulate each stage of cell division are being progressively mapped. B Individual motor neuronees can be visualised in the newly hatched nematode by phase contrast microscopy. C Cell lineage of the five motor neuronees at each segment of the body arises from a line of single progenitor cells. D The lineage of the motor neuronees at each segment follows a relatively invariant pattern. The *crosses* indicate programmed cell death. The lineage of every other neurone in the *C. elegans* nervous system can be mapped similarly. (Reproduced from Kandell *et al.* 1995.)

cells that are restricted to neuronal lineages (Mayer-Proschel *et al.* 1997). On the other hand, there are progenitor cells with limited capacity for further divisions but which can divide into many different cell types (Turner and Cepko 1987). What we need, and what is only beginning to be achieved, is to identify those factors that regulate continued mitotic expansion, from

other factors that regulate differentiation, and provide markers for different cells in the lineage.

## The O-2A lineage

The best characterised restricted lineage in the mammalian nervous system is the O-2A precursor cell

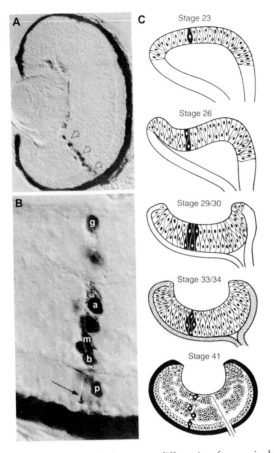

**Fig 25.3** Multiple cell phenotypes differentiate from a single-labelled precursor in the developing *xenopus* retina. Abbreviations of cell types: a, amacrine; b, bipolar; g, ganglion; p, photoreceptor. (Reproduced from Holt *et al.* 1988, with permission.)

derived from the perinatal rat optic nerve (Fig. 25.4; see also Chapter 15). The O2A cell was first identified as a progenitor cell that differentiates into either an oligodendrocyte or a type 2 astrocyte under different culture conditions. (Raff *et al.* 1983). This can be expanded *in vitro* retaining its bipotential status (ffrench-Constant and Raff 1986). Detailed analysis has identified a variety of different immunohisto-chemical markers to characterise each stage of the cell lineage and the growth factors that will induce the cells to differentiate down different pathways (see Fig. 25.4).

## Progenitor cells in the adult CNS

Until recently, the pervading view was that neuronal differentiation was absolutely complete in early development: our full complement of neurones are formed in the pre- or early post-natal period and then remain throughout life. Nevertheless, although birth of new neurones in adulthood has been well established in a variety of non-mammalian species, for example, in the vocalisation centres in songbirds (Nottebohm *et al.* 1986), the appearance of similar patterns of neurogenesis in the adult mammalian brain has proved much more controversial. Certainly neurogenesis in adult animals is extremely limited and restricted to a few specific locations, notably the dentate gyrus and the olfactory bulb of adult rats (Altman 1963; Bayer 1982, 1983), others have argued that a similar phenomenon cannot be replicated in monkeys (Rakic 1985).

The precursor cells that give rise to these 'new'

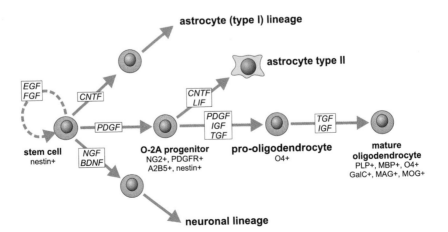

**Fig. 25.4** The lineage of oligodendrocytes and type-2 astrocytes derived from a single O-2A precursor cell, indicating the primary markers of each cell type and the growth factors regulating the transitions.

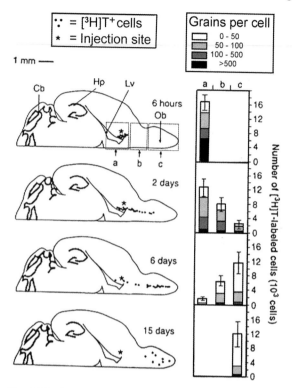

**Fig. 25.5** Stem cells in the adult CNS: rostral migratory stream. A Cells from the subventricular zone (SVZ) of a donor mouse that carried a neurone-specific marker transgene were implanted into the SVZ of adult hosts. B Two weeks later donor cells were identified by staining with the X-gal reaction. Some remained in the SVZ, whereas others had migrated to the olfactory bulb. C Alternatively, dividing cells were labelled with ($^3$H)-thymidine and sections cut at serial time points to reveal migratory stream of cells from the SVZ to the olfactory bulb. (Reproduced from Lois, and Alvarez-Buylla 1994, with permission.)

but also in some cases the formation of new neurones. Indeed, Gage and colleagues have recently shown that the numbers of new neurones labelled in the hippocampus is influenced by experience Kemperman *et al.* (1998).

Until recently, there has been considerable debate about whether the continuous presence of precursor cells into adulthood was a predominant feature of rodent brain but absent from higher primates and humans. However, taking advantage of the therapeutic use of the cell division marker bromodeoxyuridine in terminal cancer patients, Erikson and colleagues have recently demonstrated neurogenesis by the presence of labelled, newly divided neurones in the adult human hippocampus Ellksson *et al.* (1998). This then opens at least the theoretical possibility of isolating adult human progenitor cells that may be divided, expanded and differentiated *in vitro* to yield new sources of cells for transplantation.

## *Precursor cell expansion* in vitro

### 'Neurospheres'

Reynolds and Weiss (1992; Reynolds *et al.* 1992) first described a reliable method for isolating and expanding stem cells from the mouse brain *in vitro*. When embryonic brain tissue is harvested and grown in specific culture conditions, then the tissue can be maintained in a dividing state, allowing for the expansion of large numbers of neuronal precursors. These specific culture conditions are as flollows.

- *The absence of a substrate for the cells to settle.* Normal differentiation requires the cells have a suitable substrate on which to divide and grow, so if this is absent they remain in a pre-differentiated state.

- *A suitable neurotrophic factor cocktail.* The capacity of precursor cell to self-replicate and the lineage down which cells differentiate is regulated by their trophic environment. Specific neurotrophic factors can maintain stem or precursor cells in a proliferative rather than differentiating state. For cultures derived from embryonic rat or mouse brain, the two main mitogenic factors are EGF and FGF.

Consequently, the critical conditions for proliferation and expansion of stem cells are to grow the cells free floating in a medium containing high doses of EGF and/or FGF. When this is provided, differentiated neurones and glia rapidly die, whereas stem and progenitor

neurones are not themselves resident in the areas in which the neurones end up but rather in a 'subventricular zone' (SVZ) in the lining of the brain ventricles and a subgranular zone in the dentate gyrus (Luskin 1993). From there the cells migrate in a rostral migratory stream down to the olfactory bulb (Fig. 25.5; Lois and Alvarez-Buylla 1994), and over shorter distances within the hippocampus (Kuhn *et al.* 1997).

It is intriguing that the two areas in which adult-dividing neurones take up residence, the dentate gyrus and the olfactory bulb, are both implicated in fundamental processes of learning. This has stimulated speculation that representations of new memories may involve not only the modification of synaptic connections (as characterised by LTP and related phenomena)

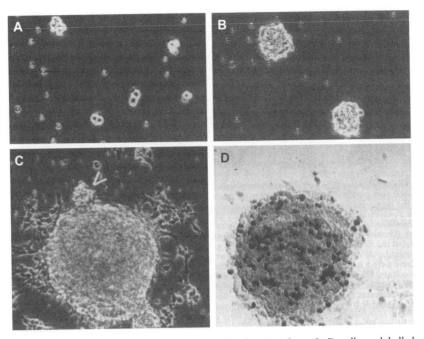

**Fig. 25.6** Expansion of EGF-generated neurospheres over successive days in culture. In D, cells are labelled with Brdu to indicate continuing cell division at 1 week after seeding. (Reproduced from Svendsen *et al.* 1995, with permission.)

cells aggregate into free-floating spheres of proliferating cells (see Fig. 25.6), termed 'neurospheres' by Weiss.

Over the course of 7 days growth, neurospheres expand from single cells to clusters of several thousand cells. They can then be 'passaged' by dissociation, dividing into multiple wells to re-seed new cultures. Such a protocol results in rapid (theoretically exponential) proliferation of culture dishes, some of which are taken for analysis, others are retained to maintain or expand the colony, and yet others can be frozen for later use.

Whereas the principle of long-term expansion of precursor cells is now established for the mouse brain, there may be distinct species differences. A variety of both technical and theoretical issues arise regarding the specificity and utility of the neurosphere technology.

- Are the cells true stem cells with indefinite capacity for self-replication, or are there intrinsic limits (e.g. relating to the cellular basis of ageing) to the numbers of divisions through which cells can be passaged?

- Are the cells truly pluripotential, with the capacity to generate all the differentiated phenotypes of the nervous system (under the control of appropriate

signals), or are the cells progenitors with a restricted fate?

- How can we in practice control the differentiation of expanded populations of cells derived from neurospheres into distinct phenotypes of mature cells as required for different experimental or therapeutic purposes?

- Can neurospheres provide a functional replacement for primary neurones whose differentiation is controlled in the natural embryonic environment?

## Are the expanded cells multipotential?

When grown under these conditions, the stem/progenitor cells will proliferate exponentially to form growing spheres of dividing cells: 'neurospheres'. If the culture conditions are subsequently changed back to those favouring differentiation and development, the cells differentiate into neurones and glia but not other cell types (Fig. 25.7). Although originally developed with mouse neural tissue, subsequent studies have shown that similar cells can be grown from rat, pig, monkey, and human embryonic tissues, and that altering the culture conditions can affect the proportion of neurones or glia that ultimately develop. However many of the critical

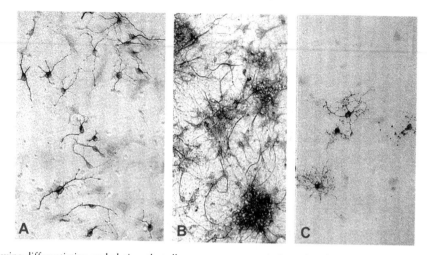

**Fig. 25.7** Following differentiation and plating, the cells can generate morphological and histochemical features of different cell types of the nervous system. A Neurones, stained with MAP1. B Astrocytes, stained with GFAP. C Oligodendrocytes, stained wit gal-C. (Reproduced from Svendsen *et al.* 1995, with permission.)

stages in the developmental process for these cells are not known, although there is a hope and expectation that it should be possible to differentiate neurospheres into distinct populations of specific cell types suitable for transplantation, for example dopamine, striatal or hippocampal neurones or oligodendrocytes.

## Clonal lines

Ultimately the question of whether expanded numbers of progenitor cells retain multipotentiality can only be answered by demonstration of different cell phenotypes developing from clones of a single precursor cell. This is a difficult question to address technically, because at the early stage of culture cells grow better when grown at a moderate density so that each cell can benefit by support from factors released by its partners.

In an early attempt to demonstrate multipotentiality from clonal lines McKay and colleagues generated cell lines from the developing rat cerebellum on the basis of their expression of the precursor cell marker, nestin, and showed that the immortalised cells could be induced to differentiate into both neurones and glia. Although highly suggestive of multipotentiality, the clonal analysis on which this study was based employed seeding several cells into each culture well. A cleaner demonstration of clonal analysis was provided by Reynolds and Weiss (1996) based on testing the differentiation potential of cells derived from EGF-expanded neurospheres. This was done three ways (see Fig. 25.8). First, the spheres were simply dissociated and plated,

and the proportions of astrocytes, oligodendrocytes, and neurones that developed were counted. Alternatively, the spheres were passaged up to 10 successive times, on the basis that at each passage each neurosphere develops as a clone from single dissociated cells of the previous passage. Third, after dissociation, individual cells from an expanded sphere were grown starting with a single cell in each well of multi-well plates. Not only do the progenitors expanded from each passage of the spheres retain a similar capacity to generate neurone, astrocyte and oligodendrocyte precursors in approximately equal ratios through the generations, but similar proportions were also generated from spheres derived from single progenitor cell clones. On this basis, Reynolds and Weiss concluded that the precursor cell populations expanded (up to $10^7$-fold) in neurospheres exhibit the clonal multipotentiality required to demonstrate that they comprise true stem cells.

## *Can they be expanded indefinitely?*

There continues to be some debate about whether neurospheres comprise true stem cells with unlimited capacity for pluripotential and clonal expansion, or represent progenitor cells with an already restricted fate and limited proliferative capacity. Nevertheless, it is possible to generate large numbers of neurones from a small starting population using this technique. There seems to be some species variation in the extent to which these populations can be expanded, mouse cells being more

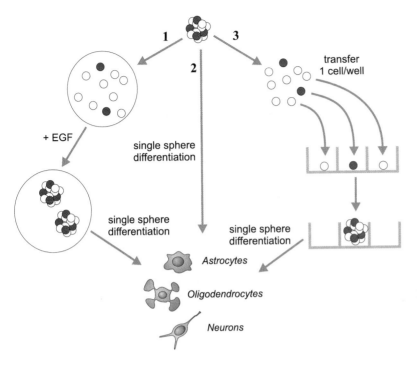

**Fig 25.8** Clonal analysis of multipotentiality of stem cells derived from neurospheres. (Reproduced from Reynolds and Weiss 1996, with permission.)

or less indefinitely expandable, while those from human and rat will only divide for a limited number of divisions (Svendsen *et al*. 1997b).

## Can phenotypic differentiation be controlled at will?

Although expanded cells retain a multipotentiality to differentiate into both neurones and glial cells, their application will require control over the final differentiated phenotype. The problem arises when attempts are made to differentiate the expanded neurones into particular phenotypes of experimental interest. This issue has been addressed in the context of seeking to obtain large numbers of cells of a specific phenotype, in particular dopaminergic neurones.

When progenitor cells are expanded long term *in vitro* as neurospheres and then differentiated by plating in serum-rich media onto standard poly-L-lysine coated plates, as in other studies they readily differentiate into neurones and glia, but very few of these neurones express a dopamine phenotype as determined by immunohistochemical staining for tyrosine hydroxylase (Ptak *et al*. 1995; Svendsen *et al*. 1995; Ling *et al*. 1998; Santa-Olalla and Covarrubias 1998). In particular, Santa-Olalla and Covarrubias (1998) tried a variety of

growth factors to trigger enhanced differentiation of a dopaminergic phenotype without great success. Similarly, following description of the role of sonic hedgehog in the differentiation of dopaminergic neurones from the developing floor plate (Hynes *et al*. 1995), Svendsen (unpublished studies) has tried using this developmental gene as a differentiation switch, again without great success. However Lin *et al*. (1998) recently screened 18 different cytokines for their specification capacity and report that one particular interleukin, IL-1, is highly effective. The effectiveness of IL-1 was further enhanced by combination treatment with IL-II, LIF and GDNF, although these latter factors were without effect on their own. With these combinations of treatment, a mature dopaminergic phenotype (based on immunoreactivity against tyrosine hydroxylase, DOPA-decarboxylase, the dopamine transporter and dopamine itself) was expressed in 20–25% of all expanded cells and 50% of the neurones within the cultures.

It is clear that the way forward will most likely involve a judicious selection and empirical screening of developmentally-relevant signals identified from fundamental developmental studies to yield the parameters necessary to generate the specific phenotypes required for each particular purpose. Alternatively, it may be that the issue of phenotype requires a variety of triggering signals that remain poorly understood but which may nevertheless be available *in vitro*. For this reason, we will return to the phenotypic specification of precursor cells *in vivo* after first considering the basic phenomena associated with their transplantation into the brain of neonatal and adult hosts.

## Transplantation of expanded precursor cells

The use of progenitor cells for transplantation has already been touched on in the preceding chapter on glial cell replacement, where it was found that implants of O-2A progenitor cells had a greater capacity for remyelination than implants of differentiated oligodendrocytes. This advantage relates primarily to the greater phenotypic plasticity of the precursor cells. By contrast, when considering implants of neuronal precursors the interest has rather been in the possibility of precursor cell expansion, yielding greater numbers of cells for implantation. The controlled plasticity of the cells to adopt particular phenotypes then becomes one of the major technical hurdles to be overcome.

### Grafting immortalised stem/progenitor cells

Several studies have now reported a remarkable plasticity of transplanted stem cell precursors to adopt a phenotype appropriate to the area of brain into which they are implanted. For example, McKay and colleagues have developed the HiB5 cell line, which is a stem cell line derived from the embryonic hippocampus that has been conditionally-immortalised with the temperature-sensitive Sv40T proto-oncogene. When implanted into the developing hippocampus, the cells adopted a phenotype appropriate to this forebrain location, they migrated into the dentate gyrus becoming aligned with the host cell layer, and they adopted a morphological phenotype with orientation of cell body and dendrites appropriate for dentate granule cells. Conversely, when implanted into the cerebellum, the cells adopted a location, orientation and morphology appropriate to cerebellar granule neurones (Renfranz *et al.* 1998). This plasticity is not dependent either on the selection of immortalised cells nor on their particular source from the hippocampus. Thus, precursor cells derived from the early embryonic cerebellum prior to their final differentiation will adopt a hippocampal phenotype if implanted into the hippocampus (Vicario-Abejón *et al.* 1995).

A variety of other cell lines show similar features, in adult as well as in the developing brain. Thus, for example, Whittemore and colleagues have used the immortalised RN33B cell line derived originally from the embryonic raphé nucleus. This cell line also differentiates into hippocampal-like neurones upon implantation into the adult hippocampus (Onifer *et al.* 1993), but the phenotype depends on the location into which

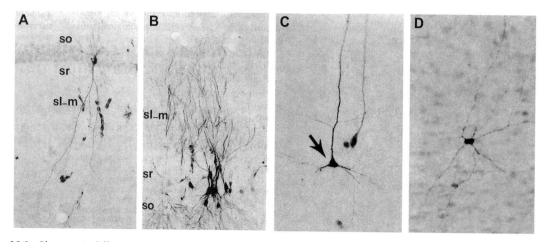

**Fig. 25.9** Phenotypic differentiation of grafted immortalised stem cells from the RN33B cell line. The cells differentiate into neurones with characteristic hippocampal-like pyramidal morphologies when implanted in to the CA1 or CA3 regions of the hippocampus (A, B), but into cortical-like neurones when implanted into the neocortex (C, D). Implanted cells labelled with β-galactosidase. (Reproduced from Shihabuddin *et al.* 1995, with permission.)

the cells are placed. Thus, RN33B cells adopt appropriate granule or pyramidal cell morphologies when located in the dentate gyrus or CA1–3 regions, respectively (Fig. 25.9; Shihabuddin *et al.* 1996a). Conversely, if implanted into the striatum, the same cell line will again differentiate into neurones, many of which exhibit morphological features of medium-sized spiny striatal neurones, and perhaps most remarkably develop long-distance axon projections to normal striatal targets in the globus pallidus (Lundberg *et al.* 1996a).

However, the integrity of the host brain has been seen influence the phenotypic differentiation of immortalised stem cells. If the host neuronal phenotype is destroyed then the implanted cells no longer differentiate appropriately. Thus, in the above study in which RN33B cells adopted appropriate cell phenotypes dependent upon their hippocampal location (Shihabuddin *et al.* 1996b), in some hosts the dentate gyrus and CA1–3 regions were lesioned with colchicine and kainic acid, respectively. When implanted into the host neurone-depleted environment, the implanted cells no longer adopted granule or pyramidal phenotypes, as would have been appropriate to their locations, but rather they took on immature bipolar morphologies. This indicates that, at least in the adult brain, the differentiation of implanted precursor cells into cell types that are specific and appropriate to their sites of implantation is dependent upon the presence of some surviving endogenous neurones along with an at least partially conserved cytoarchitecural organisation. These results may indicate potential problems with achieving an appropriate differentiation of expanded precursor cell implants if the goal is to replace lost neurones (see further below, with respect to functional repair of damaged dopamine systems).

## Grafting expanded neurospheres

In contrast to implants of immortalised stem cell lines, expansion of primary stem cells as neurospheres has not always proved so reliable. Thus, when EGF-expanded stem cells are grown as neurospheres and passaged several times (so as to ensure that the grafts are derived entirely from expanded precursor cells and do not contain primary neurones that were already differentiated when harvested from the embryonic brain) prior to implantation into the adult striatum, only small grafts are seen. This is in part because of extensive migration away from the site of implantation, in part because most of the cells differentiate into astrocytes rather than neurones (see Fig. 25.10), but also because the cells may not survive well either (Svendsen *et al.* 1996; Svendsen *et al.* 1997a; Winkler *et al.* 1998).

A somewhat different pattern of results was reported by Gage and colleagues when they used precursor cells expanded with FGF from adult rat hippocampus for transplantation. These cells did differentiate into neurones upon implantation back into the host hippocampus (Gage *et al.* 1995b). Although there are several features that differ between these two sets of experiments, including the source of the cells, the age of the donors, and the mitogen used, the most likely reason for the observed differences in differentiation of the expanded precursors into neurones may lie in the selection of the hippocampal target site in the latter studies. When similar cells were implanted into the cerebellum they did not yield any differentiated neurones whatsoever, whereas when they were implanted into the rostral migratory pathway the cells migrated into the olfactory bulb and differentiated into neurones that expressed calbindin and tyrosine hydroxylase immunoreactivity, characteristic of two populations of olfactory neurones (Suhonen *et al.* 1996).

Thus it appears that the implantation site will determine the fate of the cells. There are only a limited number of sites in the adult mammalian brain that support spontaneous neurogenesis, and it seems that it is only when implanted into these restricted areas that expanded stem or progenitor cells differentiate into neurones. Otherwise and elsewhere, it seems that the signals necessary to regulate the differentiation of precursor cells down particular neuronal lineages are extremely limited if not absent. This is of course not to conclude that neuronal differentiation cannot be achieved if the appropriate signals are provided, but that may require predifferentiaton *in vitro* rather than relying on local signals in the host brain to control appropriate differentiation after implantation.

## Functional repair

A major rationale for grafting expanded and immortalised precursor cells is not just to study the signals of development and plasticity but for functional repair of brain damage (Martinez-Serrano and Björklund 1997; Svendsen 1997). Studies of functional repair remain extremely limited, but preliminary results are now available for grafts both of immortalised cells and of neurosphere-expanded stem cells. The present discussion excludes those studies in which these cells are further engineered to express trophic factors, which will

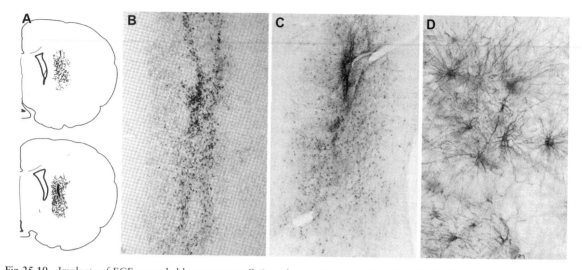

**Fig 25.10** Implants of EGF-expanded human stem cells into the rat striatum. A Injection sites in the striatum. B Injected cells labelled with bromodeoxyuridine. The majority of cells adopt an astrocytic phenotype as visualised using a human specific astrocyte antibody, viewed at low (C) and high magnification (D). (Reproduced from Svendsen *et al.* 1997a, with permission. )

be considered in the next chapter in the context of gene therapy.

The first reports of functional effects following implantation of immortalised stem cell lines have been in a rodent model of ischaemia. Sinden and colleagues (1997) developed the MHP36 cell line from the embryonic hippocampus of a transgenic mouse carrying the temperature-sensitive Sv40T gene (so that the cells proliferated at 33°C *in vitro* but changed to a differentiation phase at body temperature) and the lacZ gene so that the cells could be tracked by $\beta$-galactosidase staining. MHP36 cells were implanted into the hippocampus of rats 2–3 weeks after reversible 15 min 4-vessel occlusion ischaemia. This level of ischaemia induces selective death of the CA1 field of the hippocampus and a marked deficit in spatial learning as tested in the Morris water maze. The implanted cells were visualised by $\beta$-galactosidase histochemistry and seen to repopulate the zone of cell loss in the CA1 field of the ischaemic hippocampus. More dramatically, in two separate experiments, the implanted rats exhibited a dramatic improvement in spatial learning that did not differ from non-ischaemic controls (Fig. 25.11). This result clearly suggests that implanted progenitor cells can differentiate and exert functional effects in brain-damaged animals. Needless to say, the specificity of the recovery still requires further validation, not least because excitotoxic lesions in this area producing similar maze learning deficits have been reported to be alleviated by glial as well as by primary neuronal grafts (Bradbury *et al.* 1995).

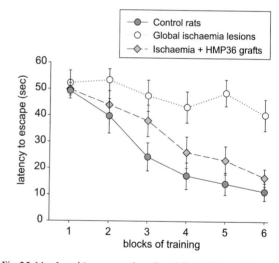

**Fig 25.11** Intrahippocampal grafts of the MHP36 cell grafts alleviate deficits of ischaemic rats in spatial learning in the Morris water maze. (Reproduced from Sinden *et al.* 1997, with permission.)

The second area in which functional repair has been sought is in the parkinsonian (dopamine-depleted) rat striatum. Here, most studies have been with expanded neurospheres. Initial studies on implanting EGF-expanded neurospheres into the 6-OHDA lesioned striatum yielded very small grafts, very few surviving dopamine neurones and no clear functional recovery (Svendsen *et al.* 1996). In a subsequent study a combination of EGF and FGF was used to expand human cells for transplantation into immunosuppressed rats and several dozen neurones were seen to survive in many cases (Svendsen *et al.* 1997a). Indeed, a significant reduction of amphetamine-induced rotation was seen in the two animals with more than 100 surviving TH neurones (170 and 240, respectively). Nevertheless, in these two studies the numbers of dopaminergic neurones surviving and differentiating within the striata of the host animals (typically just a few dozen from approximately 600,000 cells implanted) was not impressive. Studer and colleagues therefore tried differentiating the cells *in vitro* prior to their implantation (1998). FGF-expanded spheres were first predifferentiated in roller tube cultures before implantation as cell aggregates. Higher yields of dopamine cells were obtained *in vitro*, higher numbers were then seen to survive following transplantation *in vivo* ((Fig. 25.12) an average of 1221 cells per graft), and the grafts were associated with a significant group effect on reducing amphetamine rotation.

These studies have now demonstrated in principle the essential feasibility of expanding and transplanting precursor cells. However, the present techniques are still constrained by the relatively small numbers of neurones that express a dopaminergic phenotype in the grafts. and a correspondingly poor alleviation of the motor deficits in the host animals with parkinsonian lesions. The problems still to be solved with expanded neural progenitor populations are therefore largely problems of developmental biology: what influences are needed during the final stages of differentiation to turn a progenitor into a particular type of mature neurone. A combination of gene transfer and/or trophic factor treatment of the dividing cells prior to transplantation may eventually overcome these initial problems.

## Grafting adult stem cells

The discovery that precursor cells can be identified in the adult brain, opens the way to seeking their expansion *in vitro*. Although the numbers of multipotent

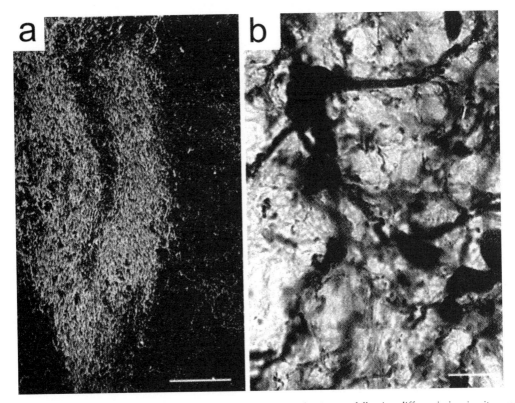

**Fig 25.12** Grafts of expanded neurospheres into the dopamine depleted striatum, following differentiation *in vitro*, results in numerous TH-immunoreactive cells in the grafts. (Reproduced from Studer *et al.* 1998, with permission.)

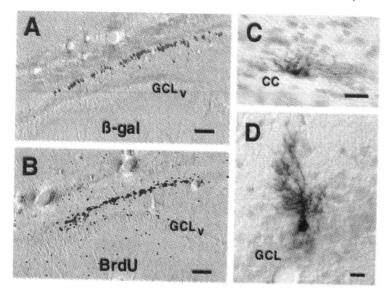

**Fig. 25.13** Grafts of adult expanded precursor cells. A Expanded adult FGF-sensitive cells were labelled with β-galactosidase and ($^{3}$H)-thymidine before implantation into the hippocampus. Labelled cells migrated to the dentate granule cell layer (A, B). At higher magnification (C, D), β-galactosidase-labelled cells are seen to adopt a neuronal morphology. (Reproduced from Gage *et al.* (1995b), with permission.)

precursor cells are much lower than in the embryonic brain, precursor cells from the ventricular zone of adult rats and mice brains can similarly be expanded *in vitro* by treatment with high concentrations of EGF and/or FGF (Reynolds and Weiss 1992; Richards *et al.* 1992). Furthermore these expanded adult precursor cells can not only be induced to differentiate into mature neurones and astrocytes *in vitro*, but they have also been successfully transplanted into the brains of adult hosts. For example, Gage and colleagues (1995b) expanded FGF-sensitive progenitor cells from the hippocampus of adult rats and maintained them through multiple passages for over 1 year *in vitro*. In culture, these cells could be stained both with markers of precursor cells, such as nestin, but also markers of mature neurones and astrocytes. Moreover, they went on to transplant expanded cells into the adult host brain, specifically the hippocampus. Before implantation the cells were labelled with the marker gene for β-galactosidase that stains the cells blue and enables the fate of graft cells to be followed in the host brain. Several months after implantation the cells had migrated to take up residence in the granule cell layer of the host dentate gyrus, where they differentiated into neurones.

Thus, adult progenitor cells retain the capacity to differentiate into neurones when transplanted after even long term isolation and expansion *in vitro*, but significantly they showed no evidence of tumour formation These cells may therefore offer another source of generating large supplies of phenotypically appropriate neurones for transplantation and indeed even raises the theoretical prospect for generating neuronal autografts by biopsy from the recipient's own brain. However, at this stage caution is warranted. The technology is at an early stage, and functional differentiation and incorporation of these cells is not yet demonstrated.

## Further reading

Gage, F.H., Ray, J., and Fisher, L.J. (1995). Isolation, characterization, and use of stem cells from the CNS. *Annual Review of Neuroscience*, **18**, 159–192.

McKay, R. (1998). Stem cells in the central nervous system. *Science*, **276**, 66–71.

Genetic engineering may be defined as the development of techniques to manipulate the genotype of cells or organisms in order to modify their phenotype. Gene therapy is the use of those techniques to alleviate injury, repair damage, or change the course of a disease. These techniques are potentially applicable to all living cells, not just cells of the nervous system, and indeed much of what we presently know about genetic engineering and gene therapy comes from the study of other cells, organs, and systems of the body, such as identifying and manipulating genes that predispose to cell proliferation and cause cancer ('oncogenes').

Gene therapy can have various goals. The two major ones are the correction of genetic disease, and the delivery of genes to the nervous system to alter a disease process.

For the correction of inherited disease, such as the mutations involved in cystic fibrosis or Huntington's disease there are two goals.

1.  To treat the affected individual to eliminate or replace the defective gene, e.g. to block expression of a faulty dominant gene or to insert a functional allele of a defective gene.

2.  When the disease gene is dominant, a second potential goal may not only be to correct the faulty expression of the gene in the affected individual, but also to manipulate the germ line so as to prevent the disease being passed on. Alterations of the germ line are highly controversial, not least because of fears about potentials for misuse of this potent technology. At present genetic manipulation of the germ line is prohibited in most Western countries and since there are few anticipated applications in the CNS, this strategy will not be considered further here.

Gene therapy is also potentially useful in diseases that do not have primarily a genetic basis. In these conditions, the goal for gene therapy is to provide new tools to deliver specific molecules and cells into targeted sites in the nervous system. As such the rationale is akin to conventional pharmacological and transplantation strategies but the tools of gene therapy can enhance the regulated delivery of selected molecules to targeted sites in the CNS, bypassing many of the present problems of delivering large molecules, such as growth factors, into the brain, and enable the design and manipulation of novel cells with specific phenotypes for transplantation.

Although this is not primarily a molecular or genetic textbook, it is necessary to start with a consideration of the basic techniques for transfer of genes into living cells *in vitro*, because that provides the basis and sets the limitations on the manipulation of cells for subsequent replacement into the nervous system by transplantation (so called '*ex vivo* gene therapy') and the direct manipulation of cells in the living animal (so called '*in vivo* gene therapy').

## Gene transfer into cells

The ability to deliver genes efficiently to target cells in a manner that results in stable retention and expression of a therapeutic gene product, represents a major challenge in the developing field of gene therapy. DNA can be introduced directly to cells or in combination with agents, such as polylysine or cationic lipids that enhance cellular uptake. However, the efficiency of such systems is often low and, unless the delivered DNA is integrated into the host genome, degradation of the transduced DNA will result in transient gene expression. For this reason most strategies for gene therapy employ modified viruses as vectors for gene delivery.

Viruses have evolved efficient mechanisms for the delivery of nucleic acids into recipient cells. Thus the basic principle behind the use of viruses as vectors is to disable them, such that they are no longer pathogenic or immunogenic, but in a manner that does not influence their ability to efficiently transduce the target cells of interest. The major types of virus vectors currently in use or under development are listed in Table 26.1. Of

**Table 26.1**   Comparison of viruses used for *in vivo* gene transfer in the CNS (based on During, and Ashenden 1998)

|  | Infects non-dividing cells | Targets neurones | Efficiency of infection | Expression | Insert size | Titres | Cytotoxic/ immunological problems |
|---|---|---|---|---|---|---|---|
| Retrovirus | No | No | Dividing cells only | Short-term | Moderate | Low | Little |
| Herpes simplex (HSV) | Yes | Yes | Good | Short-term | Large | Moderate | Yes |
| Adenovirus (AV) | Yes | No | Good | Moderate | <8 kb <30 kb[1] | Large >10$^{12}$ | Yes |
| Adeno-associated virus (AAV) | Yes | No | Modest | Long-term | <5 kb | Low | Limited |
| Lentivirus (LV) | Yes | No | Modest | Long-term | moderate | Low | Limited |

[1] Third generation gutless vectors.

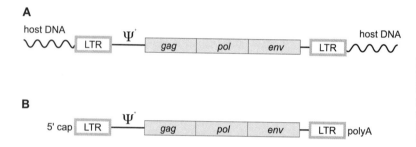

Fig. 26.1   A Structure of an integrated DNA intermediate of Moloney murine leukaemia virus (MMLV). B DNA genome of MMLV encoding group-specific antigens (gag), polymerase (pol) and envelope (env) genes. $\Psi^+$ (Psi) denotes the packaging signal sequence.

these vectors, the most widely employed are those based on recombinant murine C-type retroviruses.

## Retrovirus vectors

The interest in the use of retroviruses as vectors for gene delivery stems from the fact that these viruses exhibit a high efficiency of gene transfer into target cells, and the fact that transferred genes are stabley integrated into the host genome and are therefore maintained in a dividing cell population (Vile and Russell 1995).

Retroviruses consist of an enveloped capsid, which contains two copies of a positive sense viral mRNA genome including 5' cap and 3' poly(A) structures (Fig. 26.1). The capsid also contains a number of proteins critical for viral replication, such as the protease, integrase, and reverse transcriptase enzymes. The long terminal repeats (LTRs) flanking the internal coding regions contain cis acting sequences required for transcription, genome packaging, and integration into the host genome. It is the property of virus genome integration following reverse transcription that enables the stable introduction of foreign gene sequences into dividing cell populations by retroviruses.

The single most important advance in the development of retrovirus vectors was the development of packaging cell lines that could be used to propagate replication defective vectors (Miller 1990) (Fig. 26.2). Such vectors lack the coding sequences, gag, pol, and env, and thus contain only the LTR sequences that flank the coding sequence of interest. The LTRs and adjacent packaging sequence provide the essential cis-acting functions necessary for reverse transcription, integration, expression, and packaging of defective virus genomes. With all coding sequences deleted, such vectors can accommodate approximately 7 kilobase pairs (kbp) of heterologous coding sequences. Above this size limit, RNA transcripts are too large to be packaged efficiently into retroviral particles. The retroviral packaging cell line provides the helper functions, gag, pol, and env, in trans to facilitate replication and the formation of infectious retroviral vector virions. First-generation packaging cell lines were constructed using plasmid clones of retroviruses, which lacked a packaging sequence (Mann *et al.* 1983). Such cell lines stably expressed the necessary helper functions, and the helper-derived RNAs produced were inefficiently packaged into virions. Using such cell lines, greater than 99% of progeny virions were replication-defective. However, the low level of helper-derived RNA that

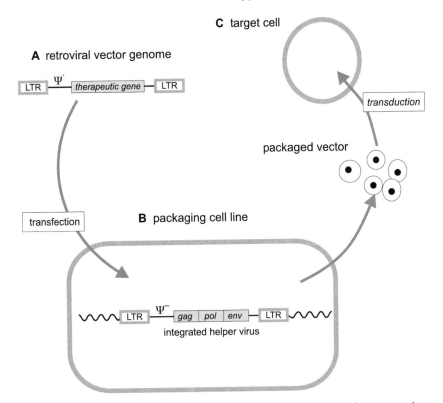

**Fig 26.2** A A cloned DNA copy of the retroviral vector genome, shown as a linear molecule, carries a therapeutic gene, functional packaging sequence ($\Psi^+$), and is flanked by viral long-terminal repeats. B Following transfection and integration of this vector DNA into a packaging cell line, the gag, pol, and env proteins produced from an integrated packaging deficient ($\Psi^-$) helper virus, results in the non-cytolytic production of retrovirus particles containing only the $\Psi^+$ vector RNA. C The packaged vector RNA can then be used to transduce the target cell of interest.

was packaged represented a considerable safety concern due to the possibility of generating replication-competent virus, leading to the risk of vector-induced target cell transformation as a consequence of insertional mutagenesis.

In order to reduce the probability of recombination between helper- and vector-derived nucleic acids to generate replication-competent virus, second-generation packaging cell lines were developed using extensively deleted helper plasmids with minimal sequence homology with the vector genome or by using multiple helper plasmids (Miller and Buttermore 1986). Such packaging cell lines offer considerable safety advantages, since multiple recombination events would be required to generate replication-competent contaminating retrovirus. Nonetheless, despite the inherent safety built in to such systems, all stocks of retroviral vectors intended for clinical use must be subjected to screening to exclude the possibility of replication-competent virus contaminating vector stocks. There is still a theoretical risk of

insertional mutagenesis resulting from the integration of a replication-defective vector, although this is in reality highly unlikely. Replication-competent viruses, such as murine leukaemia virus (MLV), are associated with leukaemia many months after infection due to retrovirus integration adjacent to genes involved in growth regulation. For this to occur at a detectable frequency, continued viral production and numerous random integration events are necessary (Donahue *et al.* 1992). In contrast, the single integration event resulting from infection with a replication-defective retroviral vector is unlikely to result in such deregulation of cellular gene expression. In addition, since tumour formation is a multistep process involving a number of gene mutations, multiple retroviral integration events are necessary to initiate tumour progression. On a theoretical basis it would appear that the risk of insertional mutagenesis with replication-defective vectors is minimal, a view strengthened by the fact that cell transformation has not been observed in animal models and human gene therapy trials that have utilised replication-competent free vectors.

A major problem associated with many viral vector systems is the ability to produce high titre purified stocks. In the case of retroviruses, titres of approximately $10^7$ pfu/ml can be readily achieved. However, the instability of retrovirus particles has made the further concentration of stocks difficult to achieve. Many of these problems have been overcome by the production of pseuedotyped vectors incorporating the vesicular stomatitis virus (VSV) G-protein (Burns *et al.* 1993). Replacement of the retroviral surface glycoprotein with the VSV G-protein results in stable particles, which can then be purified to high titre ($>10^9$ pfu/ml) by ultra centrifugation. Furthermore, these VSV G-protein pseudotyped vectors have a wider host range, increasing the range of cell types that can be transduced by retrovirus-based vectors.

The commonly used amphotropic murine retrovirus vectors can only infect dividing cells, as the capsid of type C retroviruses lack a nuclear targeting signal and can only enter the nucleus during disruption of the nuclear membrane during mitosis (Miller *et al.* 1990). This limitation precludes the use of such vectors for the transduction of post-mitotic cells. For this reason, considerable interest in recent years has focused on the development on lentivirus-based vectors, such as the human immunodeficiency virus (HIV). These complex retroviruses contain nuclear targeting signals on their capsid, which allow their transport through intact nuclear membranes. This property allows lentiviruses to efficiently infect post-mitotic cells, such as neurones, and recent data has shown that replication-defective HIV-based vectors offer considerable promise for the *in vivo* transduction of CNS tissue (Naldini *et al.* 1996; Blomer *et al.* 1997).

Areas of further development of retrovirus-based vectors include targeted retrovirus attachment (Cosset and Russell 1996), whereby the tropism of the vector is enhanced or altered and the utilisation of promoter strategies, which can sustain prolonged, regulatable, and targeted transgene expression *in vivo* (Miller and Whelan 1997). Further basic research into these areas will undoubtedly increase the utility of retroviruses as vectors for therapeutic gene delivery.

## Adenovirus vectors

Adenoviruses have been proposed as attractive candidates for use as vectors for gene therapy, as they can be readily propagated and purified to high titre

($10^{11}$ pfu/ml), are well understood at the molecular level, and can be easily manipulated (Smith *et al.* 1995b). Furthermore, they can efficiently transduce both dividing and non-dividing cells and, most importantly, they have a history of safe medical use. Millions of American and Canadian military recruits have been vaccinated orally using live adenovirus without any major ill effects. Human adenovirus types 2 and 5, which are not tumourigenic in mice, have been chosen for vector development.

Adenoviruses comprise a non-enveloped capsid, which contains a double-stranded genome of approximately 36 kb (Fig. 26.3). The genome is functionally divided into two major regions encoding early and late gene products (Shenk 1996). The early region encodes genes that are transcribed before the onset of DNA replication. Of significance to the development of replication-defective adenovirus-based vectors, is that entry into a susceptible cell transcription from the E1A region occurs without the aid of viral-encoded trans-activators. Thus the E1A region represents a classical immediate early gene region, whose expression is necessary for initiation of the lytic cascade of gene expression. The E1A proteins activate transcription from other viral promoters by binding to, and modifying the function of, a variety of cellular proteins including genes important for the control of cell growth. The E1A protein induces expression of the adenovirus E1B gene, which, like E1A, modulates cell-cycle progression. As the infected cell enters S phase, viral DNA replication is initiated from the terminal repeats of the virus genome, which precipitates late gene expression and the formation of structural proteins. These structural proteins aggregate to form empty capsids, which then package newly replicated progeny genomes. Crucial to the packaging event is a cis-acting packaging sequence located at the left genomic terminus.

Given this detailed understanding of the adenovirus replication cycle, the first generation of vectors were

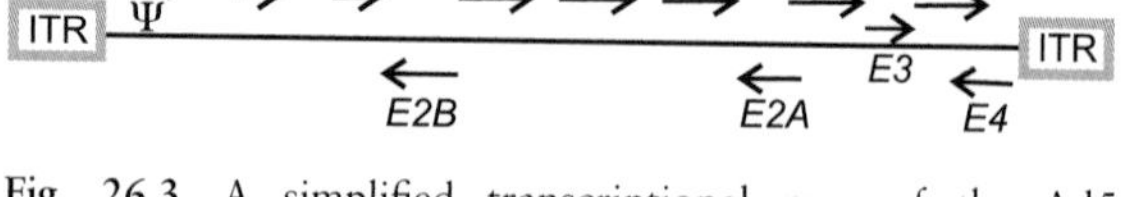

**Fig. 26.3** A simplified transcriptional map of the Ad5 genome. The early transcription units (E1–E4) each encode multiple gene products. The late gene products (L1–L5) are under the control of the major late promoter. The 36 Kb genome is flanked by inverted terminal repeats (ITRs) and the cis-acting packaging sequence Ψ is located at the left end of the genome.

constructed to lack the E1A and E1B regions. Deletion of these genes rendered the resultant virus defective for growth in non-complementing cells. Propagation of such defective vectors is only possible on cell lines that express the products of the E1 region (Graham *et al.* 1977). Using such a replication-defective vector as a backbone, it is possible to clone a heterologous gene of up to 3.2 kbp into the deleted E1A region. However, this limited insert capacity can be further increased by deleting other non-essential genes from the viral vector. For example, second-generation vectors were constructed to lack the non-essential E3 gene, allowing a maximum insert size of approximately 7.5 kbp. A problem with deleting the E3 region lies in the fact that the E3 gene product is involved in adenovirus immune evasion by blocking MHC class I migration to the cell surface (Wold and Gooding 1991). Thus deleting the E3 gene results in an enhanced immune response to the virus.

A fundamental problem associated with first-generation adenovirus vectors is the development of inflammatory immune responses at the *in vivo* site of delivery. At least part of the problem is likely to be due to the reliance of a single immediate early gene block. Should an E1A-like cellular function be produced in transduced cells, initiation of the lytic cycle would ensue. In addition, it is possible that low-level expression of other intact genes in the replication-defective backbone, following high multiplicity infection, would induce an immune reaction to virus-transduced cells. In order to overcome these potential problems, a second-generation adenovirus vector containing a temperature-sensitive mutation or deletion in the essential E2A gene, which encodes a DNA-binding protein and is required for viral DNA replication, has been constructed (Yang *et al.* 1994a; Zhou *et al.* 1996). Such vectors, incorporating a defective E2A gene on an E1-deleted backbone, result in a decreased inflammatory response and prolonged transgene expression in transduced liver cells *in vivo* (Engelhardt *et al.* 1994). Nonetheless, the ideal adenovirus vector would lack all genes capable of being transcribed and inducing immune responses, and in recent years much effort has been focused on generating such vectors, which have been termed 'gutless'. The 'gutless' vector requires all adenovirus genes to be provided for vector propagation and, since this cannot yet be achieved using a packaging cell line, they must be provided using a helper virus (Fisher *et al.* 1996).

One approach has involved flanking the packaging sequence with lox P sites derived from bacteriophage P1 (Fig. 26.4). These 33 base pair (bp) sequences result

in the removal of the packaging sequence via recombination in the presence of the phage-encoded cre recombinase (Parks *et al.* 1996; Hardy *et al.* 1997). An essential component of this system is the construction of modified E1 expressing complementing cells, which also express the cre recombinase. Thus propagation of a modified vector containing a lox P flanked packaging signal, will occur at normal efficiency on standard E1 complementing cell lines. However, a single passage of this vector on an E1/cre cell line results in a 90% reduction in viral yield. Such a helper system can be used to propagate 'gutless' adenovirus vectors consisting of inverted terminal repeats flanking the the transgene and an intact packaging sequence. These vector systems offer considerable promise in the generation of adenovirus vectors of low toxicity and immunogenicity, and considerably increased coding capacity of up to 30 kbp. The major challenge ahead lies in the utilisation of such novel systems for the reproducible production of high-titre stocks, which can then be assessed in animal models. In this way it should be possible to address more fundamental questions regarding the fate of the viral DNA following transduction, and assess the longevity of gene expression following vector administration to tissues *in vivo*. Since adenovirus does not integrate into the host genome as part of its normal life cycle, and has not evolved a mechanism for the stable maintenance of 'latent' viral DNA, it will inevitably be diluted out with each cycle of cell division, and the fate of transduced DNA in post-mitotic cells remains uncertain. For these reasons adenovirus vectors are likely to be best suited for therapies requiring short-term expression such as cancer therapy.

## Adeno-associated viral vectors

Adeno-associated virus (AAV) is a naturally occurring defective parvovirus with no known association with human disease. It exists as five serotypes but the most extensively characterised is AAV-2. It is the smallest known DNA virus, which comprises a single-stranded genome of 4.6 kbp flanked by 145 bp inverted terminal repeats (Muzyczka 1992). The genome is packaged in plus or minus polarity into a non-enveloped icosahedral capsid following co-infection of cells with either a herpes simplex virus or adenovirus helper. These helper viruses provide proteins necessary for AAV replication and packaging. Interest in AAV-derived vectors stems from the fact that these viruses are stable and can efficiently infect many cell types — both mitotic and post-mitotic. Furthermore, in the absence of a helper virus,

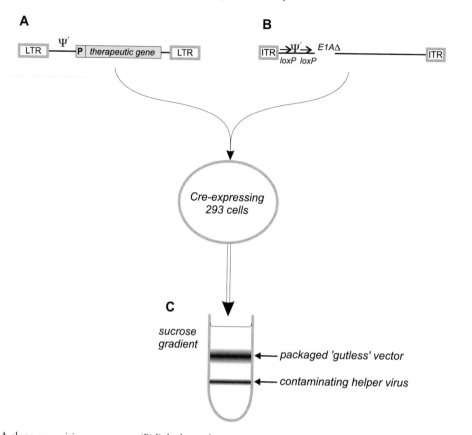

**Fig. 26.4**   A A clone comprising a promoter (P) linked to a therapeutic gene, flanked by the adenovirus inverted terminal repeats (ITRs) and an intact packaging sequence ($\Psi^-$), is transfected into the complementary E1 and cre recombinase expressing 293 cells. B Introduction of a defective E1 deleted helper virus, which has a packaging sequence flanked by loxP sites, results in efficient replication and packaging of the 'gutless' vector and inefficient packaging of the cre recombinase generated $\Psi^-$ helper virus. C Further purification of the 'gutless' vector is achieved by sucrose gradient centrifugation.

and in its wild type state, the viral genome integrates into the host cell genome specifically into chromosome 19 and can therefore be stably maintained in a dividing cell population (Samulski *et al.* 1991). This latent AAV provirus is stable, although it should be remembered that AAV can be reactivated following super-infection of cells with a wild-type helper virus. A significant disadvantage of this vector is a consequence of its small genomic size, which restricts the amount of foreign DNA that can be carried by the vector to approximately 4.5 kilobases (kb).

Of critical importance to the development of AAV vectors was the demonstration that a cloned double-stranded version of the virus could be used to generate wild-type AAV virus (Samulski *et al.* 1983). Thus a plasmid containing the entire AAV genome can be transfected into cells, and following super-infection with an adenovirus helper, infectious AAV is generated. The next major advance in the development of AAV vectors was the demonstration that a foreign gene sequence could be cloned into a plasmid copy of the AAV genome, substituting the virus capsid genes of the virus. This recombinant vector could be propagated by providing the capsid genes in trans on a second plasmid, such that, following super-infection with helper virus, a replication-defective virus harbouring the gene of interest could be propagated and could be used to stably transduce cells in culture. The minimal sequences necessary for AAV DNA replication, packaging, integration, and rescue from latency, reside within the 145 bp repeats flanking the replication (Rep) and capsid (Cap) genes (Samulski *et al.* 1989). Thus a minimal AAV vector comprises these repeat sequences flanking the promoter-gene construct of interest. In most protocols utilised to date,

AAV vectors are propagated by co-transfection of the vector plasmid together with plasmids containing the Rep and Cap genes (Fig. 26.5). Since there is no sequence homology between vector and helper sequences, this protocol prevents the generation of wild-type AAV. Following transfection into E1 complementing cell lines with such plasmids, a replication defective E1 deleted adenovirus is used to super-infect the transfected cells and provide helper functions necessary for AAV replication. The resultant progeny are a mixture of the replication-defective adenovirus helper and AAV vector. The recombinant AAV is then purified from the contaminating adenovirus by sucrose density centrifugation. This is a complex and cumbersome procedure relying heavily on high-transfection efficiencies and is difficult to perform on a large scale. As a consequence, the resulting AAV titres are generally low — rarely exceeding $10^5$ infectious units (iu)/ml. A point of note here is that in the absence of Rep gene products, AAV looses its property for site-specific integration into chromosome 19 and integration becomes a random event raising the inevitable concerns of site specific mutagenesis.

It is generally perceived that the failure to produce high-titre AAV stocks using the procedure outlined above is due to the relatively low amounts of Cap gene

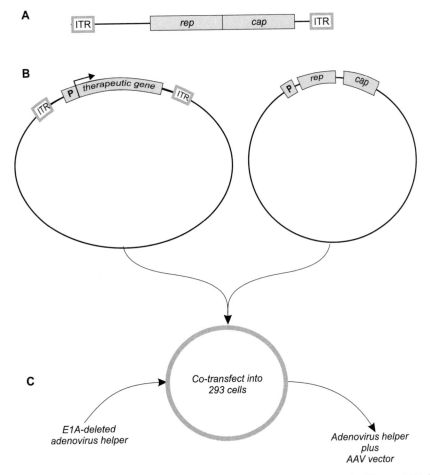

**Fig. 26.5** Adeno-associated virus (AAV) vector propagation. A Schematic representation of wild-type AAV showing the replication (rep) and capsid (cap) genes flanked by 145 bp inverted terminal repeats. B A plasmid comprising a gene of interest flanked by the AAV ITRs is transfected into 293 cells along with a second plasmid carrying the AAV rep and cap genes under control of a heterologous promoter. C The transfected cells are then infected with a replication-defective E1A deleted adenovirus as a helper. The recombinant AAV is replicated and packaged using the rep and cap gene products. AAV and the helper adenovirus released from the 293 cells are separated by centrifugation since these viruses have different buoyant densities.

*Brain Damage, Brain Repair*

product produced from transfected plasmid templates (Vincent *et al.* 1997). For this reason considerable effort is underway into the development of novel methods for high-titre vector propagation involving hybrid vectors (Conway *et al.* 1997). An example of such a recently developed system involves the construction of a mini adenovirus helper plasmid and an optimised expression vector for Rep and Cap production. The adenovirus helper gene products necessary for AAV propagation have been defined and comprise the E1A, E1B, E2A, E4 genes and the VA RNAs. In order to circumvent problems associated with contamination of AAV stocks with helper adenovirus, and prevent helper virus associated interference of AAV replication, these essential helper functions are transfected into cells in conjunction with a defective AAV vector and a plasmid supplying the Rep and Cap functions under control of two copies of the AAV P5 promoter. Using this approach it has been possible to increase recombinant AAV vector yields 40-fold, in comparison to more conventional transfection-based approaches resulting in the production of up to $10^5$ particles per cell (Xiao *et al.* 1998).

Considerable effort is underway to develop recombinant AAV packaging cell lines that incorporate both vector and packaging elements into the same cell in order to eliminate the need for plasmid transfection. The development of such cell lines would undoubtedly facilitate large-scale vector production, however, currently available systems (Clark *et al.* 1996; Tamayose *et al.* 1996), do not appear to be as efficient as the conventional transfection-based methods. The problem in constructing efficient packaging cell lines stems largely from the toxicity of the Rep gene products, which makes it difficult to construct cell lines permanently expressing the Rep and Cap genes. For this reason, research into the utilisation of inducible promoters and systems, which will result in an increase in both the Rep and Cap gene copy number following helper virus superinfection, is in progress.

The recent demonstration that recombinant AAV expressing factor IX achieved long-term partial correction of haemophilia B in a canine model of the disease, clearly demonstrated that this vector is an efficient non-immunogenic vector capable of mediating therapeutic gene delivery (Herzog *et al.* 1999; Snyder *et al.* 1999) The ability of AAV vectors to mediate sustained gene expression following integration into the host genome is of critical importance. It is known that AAV integrates as a concatamer consisting of multiple copies arranged in a head-to-tail configuration. It is possible that such a configuration prevents the silencing of promoters, a

problem frequently observed with many other vector systems, and/or that integration occurs within 'open' chromatin regions which remain responsive to transcriptional activation over prolonged periods.

## Herpes simplex virus

Herpes simplex virus (HSV) type 1 is a natural pathogen of humans causing recurrent oropharyngeal cold sores. The virus is transmitted through close personal contact, establishing a productive infection in epithelial cells from where it gains access to sensory nerve endings supplying the infected area and travels by retrograde axonal flow to neuronal cell bodies within the respective dorsal root ganglia (Wagner and Bloom 1997). Lytic virus replication in the nervous system is generally limited and the virus establishes life-long latency within sensory neurones. During latency the virus genome persists in an episomal state, in the absence of any detectable viral protein synthesis. The ability of HSV to establish life-long latent infection within neurones has stimulated considerable interest in the development of this virus as a vector for gene delivery to the nervous system (Lachmann and Efstathiou 1997).

The lytic cycle pathway of HSV infection in the nervous system is well understood. Following virus entry into a susceptible cell, the 152 kb double-stranded viral DNA genome enters the nucleus and a cascade of gene expression is initiated (Roizman and Sears 1996). The first genes to be expressed are the immediate early (IE) genes, whose transcription is activated by the action of a structural component of the virus particle known as VP16, in conjunction with the cellular proteins Oct-1 and HCF. Once IE gene expression is underway, virus encoded early and late genes are expressed leading to the production of progeny virions and death of the infected cell. In contrast to the initiation of lytic infection in permissive cells, no viral gene expression is required for the establishment or maintenance of virus latency. However once latency has been established, a family of nuclear RNAs, termed latency associated transcripts (LATs), are expressed (Stevens *et al.* 1987). These RNAs are transcribed from a diploid region of the virus genome, which is located within the viral terminal repeats flanking UL (Fig. 26.6). The precise function of the virus encoded LATs remains unclear. Studies with virus mutants unable to synthesise these RNAs during latency, have revealed that they play no essential role in the establishment or maintenance of latent infection. However there is increasing evidence that expression of

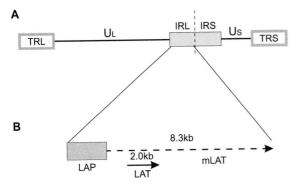

**Fig. 26.6** A Schematic representation of the 152 kb herpes simplex virus type 1 genome. The viral DNA consists of two unique regions, designated unique long ($U_L$) and unique short ($U_S$), each flanked by terminal and internal repeats. B The internal repeat long IRL is expanded to show the location of the latency associated transcripts (LATs). During latency, LATs are transcribed from the latency associated promoter (LAP). The high abundance 2.0 kb major LAT is a stable intron spliced from the low abundant minor LAT (mLAT).

LATs influences the efficiency of both latency establishment and reactivation (Wagner and Bloom 1997).

Critical to the development of HSV vectors has been the development of non-cytotoxic replication defective viruses and the need to develop strategies for the prolonged stable expression of transgene products from the latent genome. Since the virus can establish latency without the expression of virus gene products, the strategy adopted for the creation of non-cytotoxic vectors has been to delete or inactivate genes responsible for initiation of the lytic cascade. To this end viruses have been generated that carry mutations in either VP16 (Ace *et al.* 1989) or the essential IE gene, IE3 (De Luca *et al.* 1985). Such mutants can establish neuronal latency and can be administered by direct intracranial inoculation although considerable cytotoxicity has been observed *in vivo* (Ho *et al.* 1995). In order to overcome such cytotoxicity, viruses deleted for more than one IE gene have been generated and their toxicity evaluated in tissue culture systems. Mutants defective in VP16 or IE3 are toxic to cells in culture as a consequence of even low-level expression of the intact IE genes (Wu *et al.* 1996). However if virus mutants containing a defective VP16 gene, in addition to defects in IE1 and IE3, are evaluated in tissue culture cells, no toxicity is observed (Preston and Nicholl 1997). To this end there has been considerable progress in the generation of complementing cell lines for the propagation of replication defective vectors lacking all IE genes.

An alternative approach to gene delivery using HSV vectors has been the development of amplicon-based systems. An amplicon is a plasmid that can be propagated in both prokaryotic and eukaryotic cells (Ho 1994). Thus a bacterial plasmid is engineered to contain an HSV origin of replication and packaging signal. If such a plasmid is transfected into eukaryotic cells that are then super-infected with a replication-defective HSV helper virus, the amplicon will be replicated and packaged along with the helper virus (Fig. 26.7). The virus progeny therefore consist of a mixture of both helper virus and packaged amplicons, which cannot be physically separated. The limitation of amplicon-based systems largely revolve around optimisation of the transfection/super-infection protocols to generate high amplicon to helper virus ratios. In addition, since amplicons cannot be separated from the helper virus, the toxicity of vector stocks is dictated by the toxicity of the helper virus used in amplicon propagation. A recent advance in this area has been the development of a helper free amplicon system (Fraefel *et al.* 1996). This system involves co-transfection of the amplicon plasmid with a set of cosmids that encompass the entire HSV-1 sequence but lack a packaging signal. In this case, the cosmids provide all necessary transacting functions for the replication and propagation of infectious progeny carrying the packaged amplicon DNA. Since the overlapping cosmids lack a packaging signal, any helper virus generated will not be incorporated into virions, resulting in the generation of non-cytotoxic 'pure' amplicon stocks.

A more perplexing problem in the development of HSV vectors for neuronal gene delivery has centred around difficulties in obtaining long-term gene expression from the latent genomes. In the context of the latent genome, all viral promoters, except for the latency associated promoted (LAP), are transcriptionally silenced (Fraser *et al.* 1991). In order to overcome this silencing, two approaches have been adopted. The first has centred around the insertion of strong heterologous promoters into the virus genome and the second to utilise the virus LAP to drive transgene expression. The insertion of strong heterologous promoters, such as the HCMV IE promoter, into the virus genome generally results in only transient gene expression from the latent genome indicating that such promoters do not escape the transcriptional silencing of the virus genome (Ecob-Prince *et al.* 1995). Long-term expression using neurone specific promoters, such as the neurone-specific enolase or pre-proenkaphalin promoters, have been reported but this is associated with a decrease in transgene

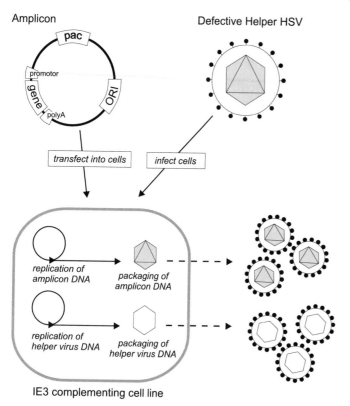

**Fig. 26.7** The principle underlying the generation of amplicon virus vectors. The amplicon vector contains an origin of virus DNA replication (ORI), packaging signal (Pac) and the gene of interest. The amplicon is transfected into cells, which are then super-infected with a defective helper virus lacking the essential immediate early 3 (IE3) transactivator. The IE3 gene product is produced in trans in the complementing cell line to initiate the cascade of lytic gene expression from the defective virus genome. These gene products replicate and package both amplicon and defective virus DNA, resulting in the release of a mixed virus population. Subsequent infection of a target cell will result in delivery of both amplicon and defective helper virus DNA but the lytic cycle will not be initiated due to the absence of a functional IE3 gene product.

expressing cells with time (Andersen *et al.* 1992; Kaplitt *et al.* 1994). More promising results have emerged from the insertion of large regulatory domains encompassing the tyrosine hydroxylase promoter in the context of amplicons (Song *et al.* 1997) and the observation that promoter silencing may not equally apply to all regions of the virus genome. For example, a number of groups have shown that if the Moloney murine leukaemia virus (MMLV) LTR is inserted within the LAT region, it is possible to obtain long-term gene expression (Dobson *et al.* 1990; Carpenter and Stevens 1996). These results indicate that the LAT region remains accessible to the transcriptional apparatus during neuronal latency.

Since the LATs are transcribed during latency, there have been several attempts to utilise the HSV LAP to drive transgene expression. The regulatory regions of this promoter, which mediate long-term gene expression during latency, remain poorly understood. However it would appear that efficient long-term expression from the HSV LAP requires elements located both upstream and downstream from transcription start site (Margolis *et al.* 1993; Lokensgard *et al.* 1994). Long-term reporter gene expression has been obtained from

this promoter in both peripheral and central nervous system neurones by insertion of a reporter gene 1.5 kbp downstream of the LAT transcription start site (Lachmann and Efstathiou 1997). Such data indicate that it is possible to utilise the endogenous LAP region of the virus to drive long-term gene expression in the nervous system, opening the way for the experimental evaluation of disabled HSV vectors expressing therapeutic genes.

# Ex vivo *gene transfer*

Once cells can be manipulated *in vitro* to express particular phenotypes, then we can consider using those manipulated cells as vectors for gene transfer into the nervous system. It is immediately obvious that the same techniques can be used in two different ways. On the one hand, our goal may be to deliver a particular gene product at targeted sites into the nervous system. Thus, for example, there is considerable interest in the use of gene therapy to provide targeted delivery of neurotrophic factors into discrete sites within the CNS, where the growth factor will be transcribed and secreted at stable physiological levels over a long-term period. On the other hand, we may be using gene therapy to modify the phenotype of cells for transplantation. Thus, for example, we may want to improve the availability of particular types of cells by immortalising them with a temperature-sensitive proto-oncogene so that they will proliferate *in vitro* but then differentiate and develop along a neuronal lineage following implantation into the brain. Alternatively, survival and growth of the implanted cells may be promoted by inserting genes to express anti-apoptotic or growth-promoting factors.

The design of suitable cells for gene therapy for any particular experimental model or clinical disorder will therefore require attention to several fundamental choices.

- Which cells should be selected for engineering?

- Which genes are to be transferred?

- What method(s) are available for transfer of this gene to these cells?

- Is it necessary to regulate gene expression, and if so what methods are available?

We can draw up a list of features that will be exhibited by an ideal cell for *ex vivo* gene transfer.

- It will be readily available, it will grow well in tissue culture, and it will be robust to the various manipulations involved in most gene transfer approaches.

- It may be easily hibernated or stored frozen, and then at a later date thawed, grown, and expanded in tissue culture to generate large numbers of cells at will.

- At the same time as being readily grown in culture, it will have no tendency to form tumours after implantation in the adult brain.

- It will reliably survive transplantation into the adult nervous system.

- It will be relatively inert with little tendency to induce inflammatory, glial, or immunological reactions in the host brain.

Safety considerations may require selection of a cell or implantation technique that allows the implanted cells to be removed in the case of any adverse reaction.

The essence of *ex vivo* gene transfer is to engineer the cell *in vitro* (e.g. by infection with a viral vector carrying the gene), to select infected cells (e.g. by killing all cells not carrying a second gene that confers antibiotic resistance), to expand the selected cells by growth *in vitro*, to characterise the phenotype of engineered cells, and finally to implant the engineered cells into the host brain (see Fig. 26.8).

## Primary non-neuronal cells

With these considerations in mind, one of the most widely used cell types from the very first for gene transfer into the nervous system has been fibroblasts. Fibroblasts have the potential advantage that they can be harvested from the skin of the to-be-transplanted host (thereby bypassing any immunological complications) and they can be expanded readily in culture prior to engineering. *In vitro*, fibroblasts will expand to fill available space but then stop further expansion once they become confluent, suggesting that they should not exhibit uncontrolled tumour formation (Fisher 1995). Following this logic, Gage and colleagues first engineered fibroblasts with a retrovirus carrying the marker gene, *lacZ* (see Box 26.1), along with a neomycin resistance selector gene, and then implanted the infected cells into the striatum and hippocampus of host rats (Gage *et al.* 1987). The engineered cells were visualised in the hippocampus and striatum post-mortem by X-Gal histochemical staining. Although the initial reports were potentially confounded by the appearance of endogenous X-Gal staining even in control brains, subsequent studies used selective immunohistochemical staining with antibodies specific for the *E. coli* form of β-galactosidase to confirm effective transfer and expression of the transgene in the host rat brain (Fig. 26.9; Shimohama *et al.* 1989).

Whereas engineered fibroblasts can exhibit long-term survival without tumour formation for up to two years following implantation in the rat brain, maintaining long-term expression of the transgenes has proved more problematic (Fisher 1995). Gene expression has been reported for up to two months after implantation but thereafter appears to decline in several different model systems (Doering and Chang 1991; Fisher *et al.* 1991). Instability of gene expression appears to be attributable to a variety of intrinsic and extracellular factors, in particular when associated with retroviral gene transfer, and may be addressed by adaptation both of the vectors and the promoters used to regulate expression in different target cells (see above; Schinstine *et al.* 1992; Fisher 1995).

## Box 26.1　Reporter genes

An essential requirement for the development of effective gene transfer methods is the availability of suitable reporter genes that can be used to identify cells that carry the transferred gene and to monitor the expression of those genes, whether in cells manipulated *in vitro*, after transplantation of cells engineered *ex vivo*, or after direct *in vivo* delivery. Interest lies not in the functional effect of the reporter gene but in the ability to identify its presence and expression by *in situ* hybridisation or immunohistochemistry. The two most widely used reporter genes are the *E. coli* β-galactosidase gene, *lacZ*, and more recently the gene for green fluorescent protein, GFP.

The *lacZ* gene encodes the enzyme β-galactosidase, which can be visualised using the X-gal histochemical reaction to produce a dense blue labelling of cells expressing β-galactosidase activity. Although endogenous cells also express lysosomal β-galactosidase activity, endogenous activity can be distinguished from activity of the transferred gene by virtue of the fact that histochemical reaction against endogenous rat brain activity is optimum at pH 3.5, whereas *E. coli*-derived enzyme is optimally active at pH 7.3. Consequently the X-gal reaction can be used to easily identify successfully transfected cells, e.g. in grafts of engineered fibroblasts (Shimohama *et al.* 1989; Gage *et al.* 1987). Nevertheless, separation by pH alone is not optimal, and even control grafts and control brain can exhibit some false-positive staining (Shimohama *et al.* 1989; Rosenberg *et al.* 1992). Consequently, it is preferable to complement histochemical staining with immunohistochemical visualisation of the gene product, since selective antibodies

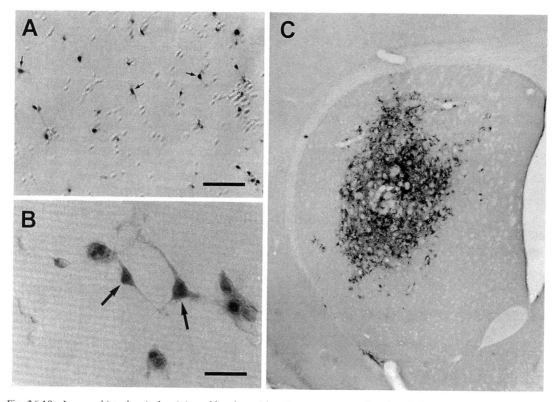

Fig. 26.18　Immunohistochemical staining of b-galactosidase in neurones transfected with the lacZ gene A, B. Cortical neurones transfected in vitro using an adenovirus vetor. C. Transfection of the rat striatum by direct injection in vivo, using a herpes simplex virus vector. Scale bars = 100 μm in A, 20 μm in B. (A, B, Reproduced with permission from Lowenstein et al., 1994. C, by courtesy of E.M. Torres.)

*Continued*

are now available that are specific to *E. coli* β-galactosidase and do not cross-react with the rat brain form of the enzyme. The *lacZ* gene has been widely used over the last decade for determining the efficacy of alternative gene transfer technologies.

Although *lacZ* is the most widely used reporter gene, others have been used in various studies according to requirements for different staining and expression characteristics, including chloramphenicol acetyltransferase (CAT) and the fluorescent molecule luciferase. Recently, the green fluorescent protein (GFP) has come into favour as an alternative reporter gene (Chalfie *et al.* 1994). GFP is the protein in bioluminescent jellyfish *Aequorea victoria* responsible for spontaneous green fluorescence under blue light illumination. Because GFP requires no exoge-

nous substrate or cofactor, it is particularly suitable as a marker for successful gene transfer, since it can be used to visualise gene expression directly, without further histological processing, in living cells. Under appropriate illumination, the activity is stable and subject to very little photobleaching. First tested for effective gene transfer in *E. coli* (Chalfie *et al.* 1994), GFP is increasingly widely used as a reporter gene for *in vivo* and *ex vivo* gene transfer into mammalian neurons. For example, Aboody-Guterman *et al.* (1997) used HSV-1 amplicon vectors to transfer *gfp* both into dividing multipotent precursor cells derived from rat gliomas in culture, and into post-mitotic neurones in the rat frontal cortex following direct intracerebral injection of the viral constructs.

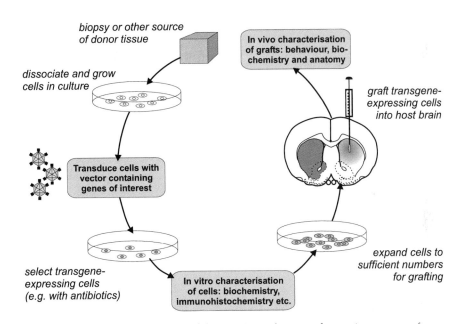

**Fig. 26.8** Schematic illustration of the experimental strategy for *ex vivo* gene transfer.

An alternative cell type that has attracted attention because of its apparent capacity to sustain longer term gene expression is muscle cells or their precursors (myoblasts), a cell type that normally turns over rather slowly. Jiao first showed β-galactosidase staining of *lacZ* transfected myoblasts implanted into the rat caudate nucleus and cortex over 2 months (Jiao *et al.* 1992) and extended this to 4 months in a subsequent study in which the TH enzyme was transferred in muscle cells

into hemiparkinsonian rats (Jiao *et al.* 1993). However, in other hands, there has been concern that myoblasts themselves may survive only rather poorly in the brain, and that the grafts become encapsulated in a glial scar with the individual myoblast cells ensheathed by a local glial limitans that will serve to isolate the implants and their gene products from effective interaction with the host (Lisovski *et al.* 1997).

A third naturally occurring cell type that has been

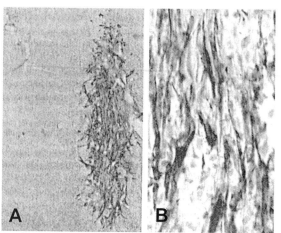

**Fig. 26.9** LacZ expressing fibroblasts implanted into the host brain, stained by β-galactosidase immunohistochemistry at A low (×40) and B high (×200) magnifications (Reproduced with permission from Shimohama *et al.* 1989.)

widely used is astrocytes. Astrocytes may have an advantage in being the primary glial cell type in the CNS, so they are, in one sense, 'natural' for transfer back into the brain. Ridoux and colleagues (1994) have shown effective engineering of primary astrocyte cultures with the *lacZ* gene using an adenoviral vector prior to implantation into the hippocampus and substantia nigra. They argue in favour of this particular combination because of the capacity of the adenovirus to infect large numbers of cells with high efficiency *in vitro*, and the long-term survival of the implanted astrocytes and expression of the *lacZ* gene product over at least 5 months. Other studies have replicated these basic observations and raised other advantages of astrocytes including their secretory nature and ready expansion *in vitro* (La Gamma *et al.* 1994; Lundberg *et al.* 1996). Nevertheless, the issue of long-term expression of the primary transgene remains an issue, and although long-term survival appears reliable, as with fibroblasts and myoblasts, so also astrocytes are more frequently seen to shut down gene expression within a few weeks of implantation (Lundberg *et al.* 1996).

## Primary neuronal cells

Other cell types have also attracted attention for gene transfer. As well as non-neuronal primary cells, as exemplified by fibroblasts, myoblasts. and astrocytes, the two other major classes of cells that have been used for *ex vivo* gene transfer are cell lines of various types and neu-

ronal cells, both primary and precursor (see Chapter 25).

A number of studies have engineered primary embryonic neurones prior to their implantation. For example, primary cerebellar cells were transfected with the marker gene chloramphenicol acetyltransferase (CAT) prior to implantation into the adult host cerebellum, and were seen to survive well at least for 3 weeks, although CAT-positive cells were no longer detectable at 3 months (Tsuda *et al.* 1990). Other studies have however been more successful in achieving long-term expression of *lacZ* as a reporter gene transfected into primary suprachiasmatic nucleus neurones transplanted into the adult hypothalamus over at least 7 months (van Esseveldt *et al.* 1998). In addition to reporter genes, others have transfected brainstem dopamine neurones with the anti-apoptotic gene *bcl-2* as a strategy to promote graft survival (Anton *et al.* 1995). The major limitation of gene transfer in primary neurones relates to the fact that they are essentially post-mitotic. It is not therefore possible (with the exception of transfection of immortalising genes, *q.v.*) to select and then expand *in vitro* subpopulations of cells that have been successfully infected. Transfection can only be achieved with viral vectors that can cause expression in post-mitotic cells, i.e. herpes, adeno, adeno-associated and lentiviruses. This then implies that each experiment is unique — it is not possible to characterise some cells *in vitro* for efficiency and specificity of phenotype, implant a second portion of the cells, and retain a third portion for future use by freezing and/or further expansion.

## Cell lines, immortalised cells, and 'conditional immortalisation'

A variety of cell lines, such as PC12 cells, at first appeared attractive because of their ease of growth *in vitro* and their existing expression of a number of neuronal features. However, most spontaneously generated cell lines have originated from neuronal, glial, or neuroendocrine tumours, and although a variety of tumour suppression strategies have been attempted with some success, e.g. by treating with the anti-mitotic drug mitomycin C (Okuda *et al.* 1991) or retinoic acid (Trojanowski *et al.* 1997), there remain major safety concerns relating to using cell lines for gene transfer in any therapeutic context.

A related but potentially safer strategy is the conditional immortalisation of cells for gene transfer. An immortalised cell is one that, rather than progressing through its normal developmental programme of differentiation and maturation, instead remains in continuous division. Conditional immortalisation then means that there are procedures for terminating division and allowing the cell to then develop normally. Several different strategies are available for cell immortalisation, the most common of which involves the insertion of an oncogene, such as myc, p53, neu, or Sv40T. For example, a mutated form (tsA58) of the Sv40 large T antigen is a gene derived from simian virus that confers a temperature-sensitive regulation on cell division. Cells expressing Sv40T will continue to undergo cell division when maintained at a temperature of 33 °C but differentiate and develop a mature phenotype (the nature of which is determined both by the cells original lineage and by its site of implantation) at 37–39 °C. Since this latter value reflects mammalian body temperature, Sv40T-expressing cells are 'immortal' in that they will proliferate indefinitely in tissue culture at a warm room temperature but then transform and develop into mature cells that do not divide further following transplantation into the brain.

There are now active programmes developing a variety of conditionally immortalised cell lines that can be used either for direct transplantation or for subsequent engineering to express particular further modifications of phenotype. Several of these lines are derived from the embryonic nervous system to yield immortalised neuronal precursors that will then differentiate into mature neurones following transplantation. Of particular interest in this regard are cells that appear to retain a degree of pluripotentiality, such that their phenotype is regulated by the site into which they are implanted and the specific patterns of cell loss that have been sustained by the host brain (Renfranz *et al.* 1998; McKay *et al.* 1993; Onifer *et al.* 1993; Shihabuddin *et al.* 1995; Vicario-Abejón *et al.* 1995; Lundberg *et al.* 1996). Thus, for example, Onifer, Whittemore and colleagues (1993) implanted a cell line derived by Sv40T immortalisation of primary embryonic raphé neurones (RN33B cells) into the brainstem or hippocampus of adult host rats. The cells also carried the *lacZ* transgene so that graft-derived cells could be visualised immunohistochemically with primary antibodies both against β-galactosidase and against the Sv40T antigen itself. The development of the cells into bipolar or multipolar neuronal morphologies differed depending on where the cells were implanted, suggesting that local cues regulated the phenotypic differentiation of the immortalised neurones. In a subsequent study from the same group (Shihabuddin *et al.* 1996a), RN33B cells were implanted into the neocortex or hippocampus. Cells implanted in

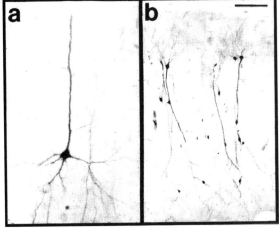

**Fig. 26.10** Immortalised brainstem precursor cells differentiate into typical cortical (a) or CA1 (b) pyramidal morphologies when implanted into the neocortex or hippocampus, respectively. The immortalised graft cells are visualised by β-galactosidase immunohistochemistry. (Reproduced with permission from Shihabuddin *et al.* 1996.)

the neocortex adopted characteristic morphologies of cortical pyramidal neurones, whereas those implanted into the CA1 region of the hippocampus showed extensive apical and basal dendrites typical of hippocampal pyramidal neurones (Fig. 26.10). Moreover these cells also exhibited both ultrastructural and immunohistochemical features characteristic of normal cortical and hippocampal neurones, respectively, indicating remarkable specificity in their differentiation and expression of a phenotype appropriate to their site of integration.

## Encapsulation

One of the major issues surrounding gene transfer turns out to be compatibility of the engineered cells with the host brain. On the one hand, ideal cells may be grown and expanded indefinitely *in vitro* but must not then form tumours when implanted into the host brain. On the other hand, the cells must be relatively inert and not induce host inflammatory or immunological reactions. 'Encapsulation' provides a way of addressing both of these issues, with the potential of dramatically enhancing the options for using a broader range of engineered cells, including from other species, for transplantation.

The essential feature of encapsulation technology is that cells for implantation are packaged into a capsule

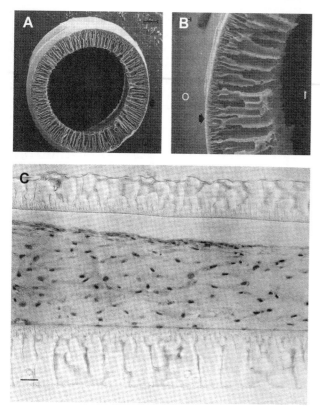

**Fig. 26.11** Encapsulation of cellular grafts in semi-permeable polymer tubes for implantation in the CNS. A, B Cross-section scanning electron micrograph of the porous tube walls. C Longitudinal histological section of surviving chromaffin cells in a capsule. (Reproduced with permission from Tan and Aebischer 1996.)

or tube made of a semi-permeable membrane that at one and the same time isolates the graft cells from direct physical contact with the host brain, and allows free exchange of molecules to diffuse across the capsule membrane into and out of the graft (see Fig. 26.11; Tan and Aebischer 1996). The pore size of the capsule membrane is selected to allow passage of essential nutrients in to nourish the grafted cells, and to allow the secreted target products of the graft (transmitters, growth factors, hormones, drugs, etc.) to pass freely back out to the host brain, while excluding passage of larger molecules (e.g. antibodies) or cells (e.g. of the immune system) that may be immunoreactive against the graft or toxic to the host.

The safety features are clearly illustrated in the case of encapsulation of cross-species grafts. Whereas a major problem for direct implantation of xenografts is how to overcome the efficient immunological mechanisms for their rejection, encapsulation protects the foreign cells both from recognition by circulating host antibodies and from the rejection response precipitated by host lymphocytes, macrophages, and microglia. In case of an adverse reaction by the host to the graft, a capsule is easily removed. Moreover, if in spite of all care in capsule preparation it were to rupture, then the implanted cells would themselves be exposed to the host immune system and be rejected.

The second safety feature of the capsules is that they can prevent the overgrowth of cell lines that would otherwise develop into tumours. For example, PC12 cells that can release dopamine and alleviate rotation deficits but have limited effectiveness because of their tumourigenic potential when implanted directly into the brain, can provide more sustained effectiveness for long-term delivery of dopamine into the brain when encapsulated (Aebischer *et al.* 1991, 1994; Emerich *et al.* 1994). In this context, using cell lines from a different species is advantageous, again because of the added safety that the grafted cell will be rejected in the case of any failure in the capsule integrity.

By overcoming the problems of xenograft rejection and tumour formation, the optimal cells can then be selected for encapsulation. For example, in developing cells that will secrete trophic factors, baby hamster kidney (BHK) cells have been well characterised *in vitro* and exhibit several distinctive features that make them particularly suitable for engineering, but would require massive immunosuppression if implanted directly into the adult rodent or primate brain. Encapsulated CNTF-expressing BHK cells have been implanted both intrathecally in the spinal cord and into the basal ganglia in the forebrain in not only experimental models (as described in the next section) but also in initial clinical trials of ALS and Huntington's disease, respectively (Emerich *et al.* 1996; Aebischer *et al.* 1996).

# Gene transfer of neurotrophic molecules

The most straightforward functional models of gene therapy in the central nervous system relate to the transfer of genes for trophic factors. Here the primary goal is to obtain stable transcription and expression of the growth factor gene, synthesis of the protein, and diffuse secretion of the growth factor into the host neuropil at chronic and stable physiological levels. Unlike neuronal grafting, the implants do not need to replace lost neurones or lost connections, or to reform synaptic contacts between cells. Rather, the criterion for functional efficacy will be manifest in the survival and/or growth of host neurones dependent upon the factors released by the grafts. Neurotrophic factor release can be expected to be effective so long as a stable physiological level of secretion is restored, and will not require temporal or local regulation of turnover, although the ability to turn the gene on and off may have clear relevance in terms of both therapeutics and safety.

## NGF protection of central cholinergic neurones

The first functional studies of gene transfer in the CNS related to the classic neurotrophic factor NGF. As we have outlined in earlier chapters, the septal cholinergic cells that project via the fimbria-fornix bundle to the hippocampus are dependent for their survival upon support by target-derived NGF throughout life. When NGF is blocked or the target is removed the cells undergo atrophy, loss of cholinergic phenotype, and in some circumstances (dependent upon the nature of the insult) cell death. Rosenberg and colleagues (1988) exploited the well-established protocol of central administration of NGF to protect septal cholinergic neurones following transection of the fimbria-fornix (see Chapter 9) to evaluate *ex vivo* gene therapy as an

improved method of trophic factor delivery. Instead of administering NGF by cannulation and infusion, fibroblasts were engineered to secrete NGF and implanted directly into the fimbria-fornix cavity rats. The grafts of NGF-secreting fibroblasts protected the septal cholinergic neurones against retrograde cell death, whereas control fibroblasts engineered with a marker gene were without effect (Fig. 26.12). This basic observation has been replicated many times, using different methods of gene transfer into cells of different types, including implantation of encapsulated BHK cells, as well as engineered primary fibroblasts, fibroblast cell lines, immortalised cells, and progenitor/stem cells (Senut *et al.* 1998). Moreover, a similar pattern of protection extends to primates (Emerich *et al.* 1994), as well as to other central cholinergic systems such as the cortical cholinergic projection following excitotoxic lesions in the basal forebrain (Piccardo *et al.* 1992).

Since then there have been numerous reports with a variety of cell types engineered with NGF showing survival after transplantation into the CNS, modification of the course of a variety of lesions in the CNS, and a beneficial impact on the behavioural deficits in such animals. Some of the most impressive of these have been the studies by Martinez-Serrano and colleagues (Martinez-Serrano *et al.* 1995a,b, 1996; Martinez-Serrano and Björklund 1997). These studies are based

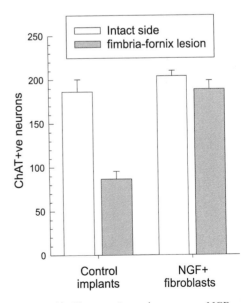

**Fig. 26.12** Fibroblasts engineered to secrete NGF protect septal cholinergic neurones against retrograde degeneration following axotomy, made by transection of the fimbria-fornix. (Data from Rosenberg *et al.* 1988.)

on the HiB5 cell line, which is derived from multipotent neural stem cells that have been immortalised using the temperature-sensitive Sv40 large T proto-oncogene. The cell line was then engineered with the mouse NGF gene and clones that expressed high levels of NGF activity *in vitro* were selected. The engineered cells could then be maintained *in vitro* or frozen until required for transplantation. Following demonstration that the implants block the atrophy of septal neurones in response to axotomy, these authors have undertaken a series of studies to evaluate whether grafts of NGF-secreting cells can protect or reverse cholinergic deficits in ageing. As illustrated in Fig. 26.13. both strategies worked. Grafts implanted acutely into the basal forebrain or septum of aged rats reduced the age-related atrophy of cholinergic neurones and reversed the deficits in spatial navigation learning in the Morris water maze. Conversely, chronic treatments by implanting the cells in middle aged (16-month-old) rats before the onset of either cellular atrophy or behavioural dysfunction prevented the development of either class of deficit.

## Neurotrophic protection in the striatum

Several other trophic factors have more recently been explored with increasing interest, in particular CNTF and GDNF. As we have seen in earlier chapters, each of these molecules has been found to be neuroprotective within the basal ganglia, for intrinsic striatal neurones and nigral dopamine neurones, respectively. As with NGF, there are major technical problems in delivering these large molecules across the blood–brain barrier into deep brain target sites. The opportunity to implant cells engineered *ex vivo* to secrete the particular growth factor molecule might provide a simple resolution of this problem, with the cells first characterised and selected *in vitro* according to the particular properties required, and then implanted in defined numbers into circumscribed target areas giving control over both the site and levels of delivery.

Neuroprotection against excitotoxic lesions of the striatum, as a model for gene therapy in Huntington's disease, has been one of the main themes investigated

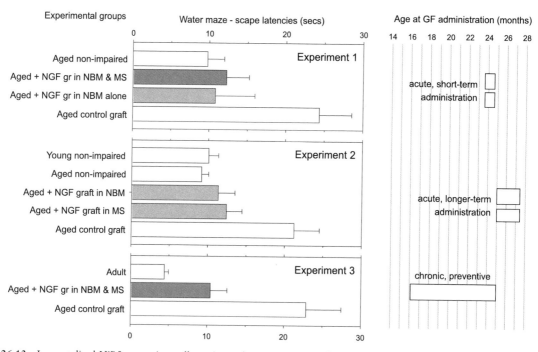

**Fig. 26.13**  Immortalised HiB5 progenitor cells engineered to secrete NGF alleviate spatial navigation deficits in aged animals. Each bar indicates escape latencies in the Morris water maze of each group of young, adult, or aged rats. The three experiments differ in the timing and duration of NGF administration as shown in the *right* panel. (Redrawn from Martinez-Serrano and Björklund 1997.)

here. Thus, for example, implantation of the striatum with NGF-secreting fibroblasts protected striatal neurones and, in particular, the large cholinergic interneurones, against quinolinic acid lesions (Schumacher *et al.* 1991). In a subsequent study from the same lab, three different trophic factors were compared: implants of fibroblasts engineered to secrete NGF and FGF were both successful in reducing the lesion areas, although BDNF-secreting cells were not effective (Frim *et al.* 1993). More recently, attention has turned to CNTF as perhaps the most potent single factor for striatal neuroprotection (Anderson *et al.* 1996). Although studies with CNTF are still rather few in number, Emerich and colleagues have delivered CNTF to the

striatum using encapsulated engineered BHK cells, and shown substantial protection against quinolinic acid lesions in both rats (Fig. 26.14; Emerich *et al.* 1996, 1997a) and primates (Emerich *et al.* 1997b). Indeed, the second of these rat studies is notable for providing a far fuller profile of behavioural analyses than is usual, and recovery was shown on tests as diverse as reduced mortality, improved body weight gain after lesion, lesion-induced impairments in locomotor activity, a range of neurological tests of sensorimotor function, skilled reaching, learning abilities in the Morris water maze, and an operant delayed matching tests of short-term memory (Fig. 26.14; Emerich *et al.* 1997a).

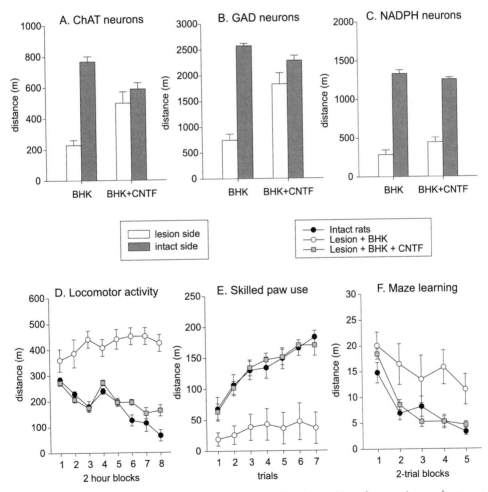

**Fig. 26.14** CNTF delivery from engineered and encapsulated BHK cells implanted into the neostriatum of rats protects striatal neurones against striatal quinolinic acid lesions. A–C. Neuroprotection of ChAT, GAD, and NADPH diaphorase neurones after unilateral lesions and CNTF-secreting capsules (from Emerich *et al.* 1996). D–F. Sparing of deficits in hyperactivity, skilled paw reaching, and spatial navigation after bilateral lesions and CNTF-secreting capsules. (Data from Emerich *et al.* 1997a.)

# Gene therapy to promote axon regeneration

Three main methods have emerged to promote axon regeneration (see Chapter 22). The first is to provide the axons with permissive surfaces on which to grow, the second is to neutralise inhibitory molecules, and the third is to enhance the regenerative response of the axon by applying trophic factors. In principle all three methods could be applied by the techniques of gene therapy.

## Trophic factors

Repairing a spinal-cord injury will require the grafting of material that can promote axon regeneration into the injury site, and practical experiments to enhance CNS regeneration have therefore focussed on grafting growth-promoting cells or tissues into the CNS. The successful grafts have consisted of peripheral nerve grafts, Schwann cells, or olfactory ensheathing cells (see Chapter 22). However, these techniques have important limitations. Schwann cell grafts are able to recruit regenerating axons in moderate quantities to grow into the graft, but very few axons are able to leave the grafts and re-enter the host CNS. There have therefore been efforts to produce more successful grafts. Trophic factors *in vitro* can promote the regenerative response of axons, and are chemotactic towards axons. In addition, Schwann cells in damaged peripheral nerves can secrete a range of trophic factors, including NGF, BDNF, NT-3, and CNTF, which may be one of the reasons for their ability to promote axon regeneration when grafted into the CNS. There have therefore been attempts to promote regeneration by transfecting cells to secrete trophic factors, then graft them into CNS injuries. The first experiments of this type have been done with fibroblasts. While these are not particularly favourable cells for promoting axon growth, they are particularly suitable as cells for transplantation since they are easy to transfect, and can be grown in large quantities from adult animals and grafted back into the same animal. The first experiment of this type was performed by Kawaja *et al.* (Kawaja and Gage 1991), who transfected fibroblasts to secrete NGF and transplanted these and control fibroblasts into the striatum. The finding was that many axons grew into the NGF-transfected grafts, but not into the control grafts. Since then, fibroblasts transfected with NGF, NT-3, BDNF, and LIF have been transplanted into spinal-cord injuries. All have

promoted regeneration of axons to a much greater extent than control fibroblasts. The results have differed between trophic factors. Thus the NGF-secreting grafts attracted large numbers of axons into the grafts, but few axons grew on into the host CNS. However, the BDNF and NT-3 grafts promoted regeneration over longer distances, with axons regenerating for several spinal segments beyond the grafts (Grill *et al.* 1997; Liu *et al.* 1999). NT-3 grafts had the unexpected effect of not promoting growth of corticospinal axons into the graft, but instead the axons grew around the graft, and on past it. It is particularly interesting that in the case of the BDNF and NT-3 grafts, axons regenerated for some distance beyond the trophic factor secreting grafts: from *in vitro* results it might have been predicted that axons would grow towards a source of trophic factor, but not away from it. Clearly axons have some ability to grow down a trophic factor concentration gradient.

Fibroblasts have limited ability to promote axon regeneration, while Schwann cells have many additional properties that can support axon growth. Moreover Schwann cells can be obtained from peripheral nerve explants in human patients, expanded *in vitro*, and potentially can be transfected during this time. Experiments to demonstrate the ability of transfected Schwann cells to promote regeneration were first done with immortalised Schwann cell lines in the nigro-striatal pathway. Grafts secreting FGF and GDNF have promoted axon regeneration, and functional recovery (Brecknell *et al.* 1996). Primary Schwann cells have been transfected to produce NGF, and these support more profuse regeneration than non-transfected cells. Alternative strategies could involve the use of viruses to transfect trophic factors into the glial and neuronal cells of the damaged CNS. This strategy has been used in various neuroprotection models, as described below, but not yet to promote axon regeneration.

## Cell surface adhesion molecules

Many *in vitro* experiments have shown that transfecting fibroblasts and other cells with cell surface adhesion molecules, particularly NCAM, L1, and N-cadherin, makes them better able to promote axon growth. A similar strategy could therefore work *in vivo*. However, only one of these experiments has been performed to date. This did not involve gene therapy in the sense used in this chapter, but instead used transgenic technology to transfer the L1 gene to mice under the control of a GFAP promoter, so that is was expressed in astrocytes, and particularly astrocytes in CNS injuries, where GFAP expression is upregulated. Astrocytes from these animals showed an increased ability to promote axon growth *in vitro*, but there was no measurable effect on regeneration *in vivo* after CNS lesions (Mohajeri *et al.* 1996).

# In vivo *gene therapy*

Whereas the advantage of an *ex vivo* strategy is that the engineered cells can be characterised and selected *in vitro* prior to implantation, an alternative strategy is simply to modify cells of the host brain *in situ*. If we can modify cells in a culture dish by using a virus to transfer a gene into the cells, we might equally be able to inject the virus directly into the brain to transfer the desired gene into the living tissue, so called *in vivo* gene therapy. The goal here, then, is to achieve safe and efficient gene transfer directly into cells in the brain. The main constraint is that mature neurones of the adult nervous system are not dividing, and so the most efficient viruses for gene transfer in culture — inserting genes into dividing cells using retroviruses — will not work for gene therapy in the mature CNS, at least not for targeting post-mitotic neurones. However, as outlined earlier, other classes of virus are available that will infect post-mitotic cells. The main classes currently under active investigation include attenuated forms of herpes simplex virus, adenovirus, adeno-associated virus, and lentiviruses, all of which have now been used for *in vivo* gene transfer directly into the adult brain (Wilkinson *et al.* 1994; Verma and Somia 1997).

Taking adenoviruses as an example, Le Gal La Salle and colleagues (1993) used a replication-defective adenovirus containing the *lacZ* marker gene under the control of the Rous sarcoma virus long-terminal repeat promoter. An advantage of adenovirus is that it can package relatively large gene constructs and it can be produced in high titres. Rats received injections of 1–5 µl medium containing the virus at a concentration of $10^{10}$ pfu/ml into either the hippocampus or the substantia nigra. High levels of β-galactosidase staining was seen in neurones expressing the transgene as early as 24 h after injection, with labelling lasting up to 2 months in the hippocampus (Fig. 26.15).

Efficient transfer into non-dividing neurones in the adult brain has been seen using other vectors and marker genes also. For example, Kaplitt *et al.* (1994) packaged the *lacZ* marker into adeno-associated virus under control of a cytomegalovirus immediate early promoter and showed labelling of numerous neurones

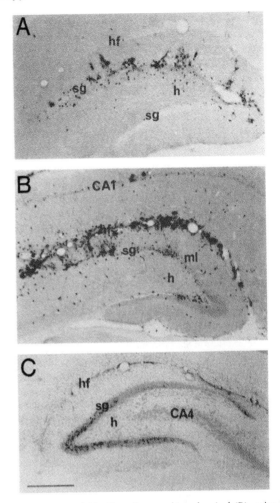

**Fig. 26.15**  Xgal (A, C) or immunohistochemical (B) stained sections of β-galactosidase expression in the hippocampus (A) 1 day, (B) 1 week, or (C) 1 month after *in vivo* gene transfer using an adenoviral vector containing the *lacZ* gene under control of an RSV–LTR promoter. Marker bar = . (Reproduced with permission from Le Gal La Salle *et al.* 1993.)

and expression lasting up to 3 months after injection into the adult rat hippocampus, striatum, or neocortex. Similar effects have also been described using herpes simplex and lentiviruses as vectors (Maidment *et al.* 1996; Naldini *et al.* 1996).

Notwithstanding the apparent efficacy of all these vectors, a number of problems remain (see Table 26.1; During and Ashenden 1998).

- First, the viruses differ in their capacity to package large genes (herpes viruses being able to accommodate much larger genes than earlier generations of adenoviruses or adeno-associated viruses, for example).

- Second, the efficiency of transduction is often not high, and typically only a few dozen or a few hundred labelled cells are seen among the many thousand neurones within the vicinity of the injection. Consequently, the ability to generate viruses at sufficiently high titres from the packaging cell lines can be limiting. This may be particularly critical when the goal is to transfer a neuroprotective gene that acts intracellularly (such as bcl-2) since in this case all neurones in the target area will need to be infected to obtain effective protection. Conversely, if the gene product is for a secreted growth factor, neurotransmitter or other neuroactive molecule, it may be sufficient to infect only a small proportion of cells in the target area.

- Third, there is increasing evidence that many viruses can induce quite marked toxicity at the site of injection, which is believed to be due at least in part to the induction of immunological responses in the host brain. This has been claimed to be a problem in particular for adenoviruses. However, newer generations of viruses may be able to overcome this limitation, at least partially, by deleting the more antigenic components of the virus (Yang *et al.* 1994b).

- Fourth, there have been concerns, especially with earlier constructs, about long-term expression. Thus adenoviruses may show diminished expression within 2–4 weeks after implantation. This may be a particular advantage for some purposes (acute expression of a targeted cytotoxin or growth factor, for example) but may in other contexts be extremely limiting for the therapeutic utility of the vector.

The efficiency of labelling and duration of expression may in part be overcome by the selection of more appropriate promoters. Thus, whereas early constructs tended to use chronically expressing viral promoters, such as RSV and CMV, it may be possible to use more selective promoters to target the cells in which the transgene is expressed, such as by using promoters for neurone-specific (e.g. neurone-specific enolase, tyrosine hydroxylase) or glia-specific (e.g. myelin basic protein, GFAP) proteins (Reeves 1998). For example, Klein *et al.* (1998) have achieved both more efficient labelling of hippocampal neurones and longer term expression of the GFP marker gene packaged in an adeno-associated virus

vector by using a neurone-specific enolase promoter rather than the standard CMV promoter.

Second, new promoters may allow experimental or therapeutic regulation of gene expression. This has particular safety concerns because the side-effects of extended gene expression in different cells are not always predictable. To take an early example from outside the nervous system, it has been found possible to overcome the stunted growth in a mouse growth-deficiency model by gene therapy with a growth hormone gene. However, the deficiency was not only completely reversed but resulted in gigantism (Hammer *et al.* 1984).

In developing any gene delivery system, it is highly desirable to incorporate a means for regulating transgene expression (Reeves 1998). In its simplest form this would involve the ability to turn transgene expression on and off. Such a system would not only provide added safety in a clinical setting, but would also provide a powerful tool for cell biology applications, allowing the fate of presynthesised pulses of protein to be investigated. The tetracycline regulatable system (TRS) provides such a means of controlling the level of transgene expression using a simple and non-toxic pharmacological agent (Shockett and Schatz 1996). In its simplest form, the tet transactivator protein (tTA — a fusion of the tet repressor of *E. coli* with the transcriptional transactivation domain of HSV VP16) is used to regulate gene expression from an inducible promoter (tetP) consisting of seven copies of the tet resistance operator (tetO), which binds the tet repressor with high affinity, immediately upstream of a minimal HCMV 1E promoter (Gossen and Bujard 1992). When tetracycline is present, it binds the tTA and prevents its binding to tetP, and reduces transcription from tetP by up to six orders of magnitude. As well as being used in transgenic animals and various plasmid based transfection systems, the TRS has been used to give tetracycline controlled gene expression from retroviral vectors (Hofmann *et al.* 1966), adenoviral vectors (Neering *et al.* 1996), and HSV amplicon vectors (Ho *et al.* 1996; Fotaki *et al.* 1997).

Even better would be a promoter that allowed regulation of the level of expression by titrating the dosage of the effector drug. To achieve these goals, particular interest has focussed on the tetracycline-controlled transactivator responsive promoter (the so-called Tet system). The basic Tet system involves two components: response and regulator units. The target gene is linked to a minimal CMV promoter, which has an embedded *E. coli* derived *tet*O response gene. The target gene is only expressed when the *tet*O element is activated by binding of a transactivator hybrid protein (tTA or rtTA) secreted by a second regulator element. However, the antibiotic drug tetracycline will bind to the transactivator protein, causing it to dissociate from the *tet*O/minimal CMV promoter and shutting off transcription of the target gene (Reeves 1998). More recent developments of the basic Tet system, in which administration of drug switches off gene expression, allows the use of tetracycline or derivatives such as doxycycline to alternatively act to switch on gene transcription.

To enhance experimental and therapeutic applications, a number of groups have combined the response and regulator units into the backbones of a variety of different viral vectors (Reeves 1998), which have, however, been evaluated so far primarily *in vitro*. Applications for regulated delivery in the CNS remain extremely limited, and have focussed, on the one hand, on the expression of reporter genes in the CNS, and on the other, on application of cell death genes for the inducible regulation of tumour growth in the brain (Reeves 1998). Although still in its early days, the spatial and temporal regulation of transgene expression and activation will almost certainly be a major area of investigation in the coming decade.

# Gene transfer for Parkinson's disease

The model systems in which both *in vivo* and *ex vivo* gene therapy have been evaluated more than any other, relate to transfer of potentially therapeutic genes for Parkinson's disease. These attempts have involved two alternative targets for gene transfer: neurotransmitter-related genes to replace dopaminergic transmission in the dopamine-depleted striatum, and neurotrophic/neuroprotective molecules to reduce the neurodegenerative process in the nigrostriatal neurones.

The first attempts focused on strategies to replace the dopamine deficiency, selecting targeting in dopamine synthesis. Dopamine is synthesised by neurones from precursor amino acids, under the control of the enzymes tyrosine hydroxylase (TH) and aromatic amino acid decarboxylase (AADC) (see Fig. 6.6). AADC is widely expressed in the striatum even after nigro-striatal lesion. By contrast, TH is localised in the nigro-striatal terminals, is lost following nigro-striatal lesion, and is the rate-limiting enzyme in dopamine synthesis. Replacement in the striatum of cells that express TH may provide the basis for restoration of dopamine secretion

and thereby restore a functional dopaminergic activation of target striatal neurones. Consequently, transfer of the TH gene has provided one major target for gene therapy.

By way of *ex vivo* transfer, both fibroblasts and astrocytes have been engineered to express TH, resulting in measurable production of dopa and dopamine *in vitro* and recovery on simple rotation tests of function (in particular based on apomorphine, reflecting changes in the sensitivity of dopamine receptors located on post-synaptic striatal neurones) following implantation into the brain in the standard unilateral dopamine lesion model in rats (Wolff *et al.* 1989; Horellou *et al.* 1990; Lundberg *et al.* 1996).

In parallel, the nigro-striatal lesion model has been used for evaluating the functional effects of *in vivo* gene transfer of the TH transgene. Thus, for example, Horellou *et al.* (1994) used an adenoviral vector to transfer the human TH gene into the striatum of 6-OHDA lesioned rats. They found that the virus infected cells in the host striatum, both astrocytes and neurones, which incorporated the transgene. Expression of TH in the infected cells was demonstrated immunohistochemically, and a functional effect was suggested by an acute reduction in apomorphine rotation. The major problem here was the limited duration of the functional effect exhibited by the virus, which may have been due to down-regulation of expression, or to the virus having induced an inflammatory or immune response, thereby killing those striatal neurones that had been successfully transfected.

Longer-term expression and behavioural recovery have been obtained using both HSVs and AAVs (During *et al.* 1994; Kaplitt *et al.* 1994). Thus, for example, During *et al.* (1994) inserted the human TH gene into a replication-defective HSV type 1 vector and injected the resulting construct into the striatum of hemiparkinson rats. Apomorphine-induced rotation was then measured at one-month intervals and seen to be reduced by 60–70% on the first test after injection of the TH virus vector but not in control animals injected with saline or a control virus. Moreover, the recovery on this test lasted a full 12 months after treatment. Both *in vivo* microdialysis and histology were undertaken to determine the levels of TH activity and dopamine production. The microdialysis measured L-DOPA activity and the production of dopamine in the lesioned striatum 4–6 months after infection and both were shown to be substantially increased over the level in the lesion brain, but only partially back to control levels. At postmortem, a large number of neurones in the striatum, and a few in adjacent areas such as globus pallidus, were seen to express high levels of TH (see Fig. 26.16), indicative of their capacity to synthesise dopamine.

One constraint on the effectiveness of TH gene transfer relates to the fact that to be fully effective, TH requires the cofactor tetrahydrobiopterin (BH4). In culture, engineered cells only synthesis dopa in the presence of this cofactor (Horellou *et al.* 1990). Although BH4 is expressed in the host brain it occurs at only low levels in non-monoaminergic neurones, so that the levels

of DOPA and dopamine synthesised by non-dopamine cells transfected to express TH are almost certainly at suboptimal-levels. Uchida and colleagues (1990) used microdialysis probes to show that they could only measure a substantial restoration of L-DOPA and dopamine from TH-transfected fibroblasts implanted in the parkinsonian rat brain, when a supplemental supply of BH4 was infused via the probe. These observations led naturally to the use of a double-gene transfer strategy to transfer the gene for GTP cyclohydrolase I, an enzyme critical for BH4 synthesis, along with the TH gene into primary fibroblasts, which then were seen to secrete high levels of DOPA without the need for additional supplements both *in vitro* (Bencsics *et al.* 1996) and following transplantation into the brain (Leff *et al.* 1998). This double-gene transfer strategy has not yet been used for direct *in vivo* gene transfer with viral vectors that carry both genes.

An alternative strategy to replacing lost dopamine production from degenerated nigro-striatal terminals in Parkinson's disease would be to block the neurodegenerative process itself. Several growth factors, and in particular GDNF, have been shown to protect nigro-striatal dopamine neurones against degeneration, using knife-cut axotomy of the nigro-striatal tract, and neurotoxic lesions using MPTP or 6-OHDA (Hoffer *et al.* 1994, Sauer *et al.* 1995, Gash *et al.* 1996). In these first studies, GDNF was given by repeated central injections. However, several groups have recently shown the efficient and effective delivery of GDNF into the lesioned

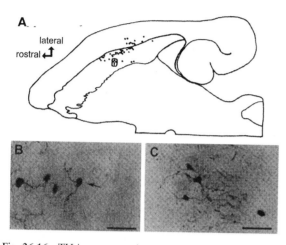

**Fig. 26.16** TH-immunoreactive neurones in the striatum (A, B) and globus pallidus (C) following transfection with a HSV-1 vector carrying the human TH gene. Scale bars 50 μm. (Reproduced with permission from During *et al.* 1994.)

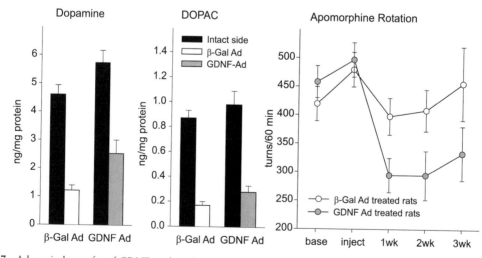

**Fig. 26.17** Adenoviral transfer of GDNF to the substantia nigra 10 weeks after partial nigro-striatal lesion increases production of dopamine by residual dopamine neurones and alleviates rotational asymmetry in the host rats. (Data from Lapchak *et al.* 1997a.)

substantia nigra or into the striatum by a single trans-fection using adenovirus and adeno-associated virus vectors (Bilang-Bleuel *et al.* 1997; Choi-Lundberg *et al.* 1997; Lapchak *et al.* 1997a,b; Mandel *et al.* 1997). In these model systems, GDNF appears to have both a pro-tective and a restorative effect. Thus, for example, if the virus is injected prior to the lesion, then it will protect nigral dopamine neurones against the effects of 6-OHDA lesions injected into the striatum (Bilang-Bleuel *et al.* 1997; Mandel *et al.* 1997). Conversely, in rats that have already received partial nigrostriatal lesions, GDNF transfection in the substantia nigra 6–10 weeks later can enhance production of dopamine and its metabolite DOPAC by the residual neurones spared in the chronic lesion (see Fig. 26.17; Choi-Lundberg *et al.* 1997; Lapchak *et al.* 1997).

## Conclusion

In summary, the new technologies for engineering cells both *in vitro* and in the living brain are not only pro-viding new tools for the analysis of the prinicples of degeneration and regeneration in the nervous system, but offer new opportunities for altering the course and progression of neurodegenerative disease that we are only now beginning to explore. In this chapter we have focussed on neuroprotection and replacement, drawing examples in particular from the basal ganglia disorders of Parkinson's and Huntington's disease, but many wider applications are now under active consideration from the control of malignant tumours, to a wide variety of acute and chronic neurodegenerative condi-tions including stroke, epilepsy, demyelination, and the dementias (Verma and Somia 1997; During and Ashenden 1998).

## Further reading

Chiocca, E.A. and Breakefield, X.O. (ed.) (1998). *Gene Therapy for Neurological Disorders and Brain Tumours.* Humana Press, Totowa, NJ.
During, M.J. and Ashenden, L.-M.AA. (1998). Towards gene therapy for the central nervous system. *Molecular Medicine Today*, 4, 485–493.

# Appendices
Important neurological diseases

# Appendix 1

# Alzheimer's disease

## History

1906 Alois Alzheimer describes pathological appearance of neuritic plaques and neurofibrillary tangles within the cortex of two patients dying of presenile dementia.

1910 Kraeplin introduces the term 'Alzheimer's disease' for patients dying with this form of presenile dementia.

1967 Sir Martin Roth provides evidence that decline in mental test scores in life correlates with plaque and tangle pathology at post-mortem.

1970 Tomlinson characterises the neuropathology in a large cohort of patients dying with senile dementia: approximately 50% exhibit plaque and tangle pathology (senile dementia of the Alzheimer type), 20% exhibit multi-infarct dementia, and the remainder exhibit mixed or other patterns of pathology.

1976 Several groups demonstrate decline in cholinergic enzymes in AD neocortex.

1981 Whitehouse demonstrates loss of cholinergic neurones in basal forebrain in AD.

1982 Bartus explicitly formulates the cholinergic hypothesis of geriatric memory dysfunction.

1984 Glenner and Wong isolate and sequence perivascular amyloid from AD brain.

1983 Masters and Beyreuther identify and sequence amyloid from AD and Down's brains.

1985 Crowther and Wischik describe the paired helical filament structure of neurofibrillary tangles.

1987 Kang et al. sequence the amyloid precursor protein.

1988 Goedert et al. clone and sequence tau, the main constituent of paired helical filaments.

1991 First reports of transgenic mice overexpressing amyloid precursor protein (APP).

1994 Presence of the ε4 allele of the ApoE gene increases risk of developing late-onset AD.

1996 Mutations in the presenilin gene associated with AD.

1997 Double transgenics with Swedish mutation APP and presenilin 1 transgenes show accelerated development of pathology.

## Senile dementia of the Alzheimer's type

The senile dementias, involving profound cognitive decline associated in a proportion of aged individuals has been recognised since antiquity. Dementing conditions can involve a broad range of symptoms including memory loss, impairments for learning new information, disorientation and confusion, and a variety of other cognitive impairments associated with all aspects of intellectual function. Although dementia can occasionally occur in young and middle age, it is typically associated with ageing and the incidence rises dramatically from 5% at age 65, to over 50% over the age of 90. With ageing of Western populations, dementia imposes a severe economic pressure on health services and society world-wide.

## Classical pathology

Dementias are associated with widespread cortical and subcortical dysfunction, degeneration, and atrophy.

This is not a unitary disease, but can be caused by a variety of disease processes — inherited, infectious, traumatic, and idiopathic. By far the commonest cause is Alzheimer's disease (AD), which accounts for approximately 50% of senile dementias and the majority of presenile cases. AD is defined and diagnosed by a particular pattern of neuropathology involving widespread extracellular neuritic plaques, which are a degenerating mass of neurites around an amyloid core, and intracellular neurofibrillary tangles, which are neurofilamentous inclusions within the cytoplasm of neurones, particularly large pyramidal cells of the cortex and hippocampus. AD can often only be diagnosed conclusively on the basis of neuropathology after death. Living subjects should receive a diagnosis of senile dementia of the Alzheimer type, based on the profile of symptoms, rate of progression, brain scanning and other data, pending post mortem verification.

## Cholinergic pathology

Aged subjects in general, and AD patients in particular exhibit progressive atrophy and loss of cholinergic neurones in the basal forebrain and a decline in associated markers of cholinergic activity in the neocortex and hippocampus. Mental test scores correlate with cholinergic decline (as they do also with classical pathology) giving rise to the 'cholinergic hypothesis' that geriatric memory dysfunctions are particularly attributable to cholinergic dysfunction. If true, this offers considerable opportunities for developing selective pharmacotherapeutics; and is still actively promoted. However, direct evidence that cholinergic dysfunction is a primary cause of AD is lacking, and the benefits offered by cholinomimetic therapies are, to date, modest. Nevertheless, secondary changes in forebrain cholinergic systems may exacerbate symptoms associated with primary cortical dysfunction and may reduce the plasticity of compensatory cortical responses to injury.

## Molecular biology

Advances in molecular biology have allowed identification of the proteins amyloid and tau that are the primary constituents of plaques and tangles, respectively. Mutations in the amyloid precursor protein underlie a number of pedigrees with rare familial AD, in particular characterised by early (pre-senile) onset. Mutations in other genes, in particular the presenilins, have been associated with other inherited forms of AD, and carriers of a particular ($\varepsilon$4) allele of apolipoprotein E have substantially increased risk of developing sporadic AD. The tau protein also exists in multiple isoforms, due to different splicings of the tau gene, the ratios of which change with age and disease. In spite of multiple theories, the causes of pathological development of plaque and tangle deposition, and the precise relationship between these two hallmarks of the disease remain unclear.

## Prospects for treatment

Notwithstanding many claims for the modest efficacy of a variety of pharmacological agents in alleviating particular aspects of cognitive disturbance and disease progression, AD is at present untreatable.

# *Appendix 2*

# *Amyotrophic lateral sclerosis (ALS)/Motor neurone disease*

## *History*

1850  Aran used the term *progressive muscular atrophy*, but attributed this to a muscle disorder.

1853  Bell and Cruveilhier noted the thinness of the anterior spinal roots in this condition and regarded it as a myelopathic condition.

1858  Description of *labioglossolaryngeal paralysis* by Duchenne.

1859  Term changed to *progressive bulbar palsy* by Wachsmuth.

1869  Charcot studied the pathological features, and noted the involvement of the corticospinal tracts, suggested the term Amyotrophic Lateral Sclerosis (ALS) and, with Joffroy, recognised relation ship to progressive bulbar palsy.

1882  Relationship of progressive bulbar palsy to ALS established by Déjerine.

1883  Brain introduced the term *motor neurone disease* in recognition of the relationship between ALS, progressive bulbar palsy, and progressive muscular atrophy, depending on the topography of anterior horn cell loss. Identification of familial cases.

1991  Linkage to chromosome 21 by Siddique *et al.*

1992  Identification of involvement of mutations in exon 2 and 4 of CuZn SOD gene by Rosen.

1993  Identification of other mutations within this gene by Deng *et al.*

## *Symptoms*

Motor neurone disease (MND) is a progressive disorder of motor neurones in the spinal cord, brainstem, and cortex — the precise clinical picture depending on whether all of these groups of motor neurones, or only a subset, are affected by the disease progress. In the most common type there is degeneration of both the lower motor neurones in the spinal cord and the descending corticospinal and corticobulbar tracts. This produces both hypotonia and muscle wasting due to the lower motor neurone lesion, and rigidity and hyper-reflexia due to the upper motor neurone lesion. This form is also termed amyotrophic lateral sclerosis (amyotrophy refers to the muscle weakness and wasting due to the dennervation of that muscle), and one of its hallmarks is a combination of both upper (rigidity and hyper-reflexia) and lower (weakness, wasting, and fasciculation) motor neurone signs in one body part. If the weakness and wasting predominates in the muscles innervated by the lower cranial nerve nuclei, the condition is often termed progressive bulbar palsy. In a much rarer form, the descending tracts are principally affected, and if there appears to be involvement of descending tracts only, over an extended period of time, the condition is known as primary lateral sclerosis, although there is not universal acceptance that this is definitely related to other forms of MND. As the disease progresses (usually over 2–5 years), there is progressive weakness and loss of muscle bulk until the patient is wheelchair or bed-bound, mute, and unable to swallow. Muscles controlling sphincter action are usually unaffected, even in the later stages, and sensory symptoms are essentially absent. Respiratory muscle weakness is common in the latter stages and frequently is the cause of death.

## Neuropathology

The principal pathology is loss of neuronal cells in the anterior horns of the spinal cord, lower cranial nerve nuclei, and Betz cells in the motor cortex. Many remaining neurones in these regions are shrunken and small, and filled with lipofuscin. There is also evidence of astrocytosis. Secondary to the loss of these cell bodies, there is thinning of the anterior spinal roots and degeneration in the corticospinal and corticobulbar tracts. There are a small number of cases associated with dementia, in which there is also neuronal loss and gliosis in the superior frontal gyri and inferolateral cortex of the temporal lobes.

## Genetics

Of MND cases, 5–10% are familial. Most of these familial cases show autosomal dominant inheritance, although a few are autosomal recessive. Apart from the family history, on the whole the condition is identical to the sporadic form, although some familial cases show degeneration of posterior columns and spinocerebellar tracts. The familial condition was linked to chromosome 21 and since then 10–20% of familial disease has been linked to a number of mutations in the gene encoding Cu, Zn superoxide. Genes responsible for the other familial forms have yet to be identified.

## Cellular pathology and pathogenesis

In common with a growing number of neurodegenerative diseases (see Huntington's disease and Alzheimer's disease), there is evidence of altered proteins in vulnerable neurones in the form of intracellular inclusions, although their role in the pathogenesis is as yet unclear, and the cellular and molecular steps leading to the neuroneal degeneration seen in MND are as yet unknown. In terms of familial MND due to the CuZn SOD mutation, it is thought likely that the mutation impairs the activity of the CuZn SOD enzyme leading to increased generation of superoxide radicals and that motor neurones are particularly sensitive to oxidative damage. It is not known whether cell death in sporadic MND is by similar mechanisms, and a number of theories have been put forward for the mechanism of cell including: environmental toxins; premature ageing, as motor neurone death also occurs with normal ageing; interruption of the endogenous production of trophic factors necessary for motor neurone maintenance; viral infection of motor neurones; metabolic abnormalities (a wide range of relatively minor metabolic abnormalities have been reported in ALS); and autoimmune destruction.

## Current treatments

Currently there is no specific treatment for this disease other than supportive measures. Riluzol has been shown to lengthen life-expectancy by a number of months, although it was not shown to improve quality of life in these studies, and insulin-like growth factor (IGF-1) also prolongs survival. A number of other experimental approaches are ongoing, for example, ciliary neurotrophic factor (CNTF) delivered by means of genetically-engineered cells housed within a semi-permeable polymer membrane in within the spinal canal have not proved helpful in small scale trials, but with modification may still prove to be useful.

# *Appendix 3*

# *Creutzfeldt–Jakob disease (CJD)*

## *History*

1920 Creutzfelt described a case of what is now thought to be CJD.

1921 Jacob described a similar case.

1922 Spielmeyer brought together the two cases and introduced the term Creutzfeldt–Jakob disease.

1936 Scrapie shown to be transmissible by Cuille and Chelle.

1966 Kuru shown to be transmissible by Gajusek *et al.*

1967 Griffith proposing that infective agent was some form of protein.

1968 CJD shown to be transmissible by Gibbs *et al.*

1974 First case of iatrogenic CJD in a woman receiving corneal graft from infected donor.

1981 Transmission of the familial form of CJD (Gerstmann–Sträussler disease, GSS) demonstrated by Masters *et al.*

1982 Prusiner introduced the term prion.

1989 Owen *et al.* identified the first mutation in GSS. in codon 144 of the human prion gene.

1989 Hsiao *et al.* found a second mutation in the 102 codon that has since been found in numerous other unrelated GSS kindred.

1990 Hsiao *et al.* demonstrated that transgenic mice over-expressing a prion protein with an analogous mutation to 102 developed spongiform degeneration spontaneously.

1991 Collinge *et al.* demonstrated predisposition to sporadic CJD in valine 129 homozygous geneotype.

1995 Britton *et al.* and Bateman *et al.* described two cases of CJD in teenagers in the UK, which were also unusual in having Kuru-type plaques, which occur only rarely in sporadic CJD.

1996 Will *et al.* suggest a link between new variant CJD affecting young adults with bovine spongiform encephalopathy.

## *Symptoms*

CJD usually occurs in the 45–75 year age group and most commonly presents as a rapidly evolving multifocal dementia with myoclonic jerks in the latter stages. The disease is usually of short duration with death within about 6 months, although there may be an extended prodrome with depression, weight loss, malaise, and subtle changes in cognition. Other neurological deficits may occur and include poor co-ordination, parkinsonian symptoms, and cortical blindness (i.e. blindness originating in damage to the cortex rather than the eye or the pathway to the cortex). Diagnosis can be difficult (until the latter stages when the clinical picture and specific changes on the EEG make a diagnosis of CJD overwhelmingly likely), particularly as there are no specific changes on CT or MRI and diagnosis at this stage would rely on a brain biopsy. New variant CJD, which has been strongly linked to infection from meat products of cows with BSE, tend to affect young patients and presents with behavioural and psychiatric disturbances progressing to inco-ordination and dementia with myoclonic jerks. In these cases tonsillar biopsy has been suggested to be a helpful diagnostic procedure. The course tends to be more prolonged than in sporadic CJD.

## *Neuropathology*

The prototypic prion disease is scrapie, an infection of sheep that has been recognised as an entity for over 200 years. Human prion diseases have traditionally been classified into CJD disease, GSS (an inherited disease similar to CJD), and Kuru, although the spectrum of prion diseases in humans is now known to be wider than this and includes disease due to transmission of bovine spongiform encephalopathy. Transmissibility of all of these diseases has now been demonstrated and they all share common histopathological features of spongiform vacuolation, astrocytic proliferation, and neuronal loss, which may be accompanied by the deposition of amyloid plaques.

## Genetics and pathogenesis

The prion is the infective agent and consists of an abnormal isoform of a host-encoded protein, the prion protein (PrP), which is designated PrP$^{sc}$. PrP$^{sc}$ appears to derive from the cellular form (PrP$^{C}$) by post-translational modifications and is not sensitive to proteolysis, whereas PrP$^{c}$ is. The human PrP gene is on chromosome 20 and is a single copy gene that contains mutations in the familial GSS. Recent work has lead to the idea that the infective form of protein interacts with the normal cellular form to produce more of the abnormal form, which then leads to a chain reaction with progressive conversion of the normal cellular form to the abnormal form. It is also postulated that in the familial form, there is production of a form of PrP that converts spontaneously to PrP$^{sc}$ explaining how the familial form can be both inherited and infectious at the same time. It has also been suggested that prion protein interaction occurs more readily in individuals with identical copies of the protein explaining why homozygotes for valine or methionine are more susceptible than heterozygotes. The aetiology of sporadic CJD remains unclear — it has been suggested that it may result from rare mutation of PrP$^{c}$ to PrP$^{sc}$, or by unrecognised exposure to a human or animal source of prions.

## Current treatments

There are no treatments for CJD, other than supportive measures and nursing care as appropriate.

# *Appendix 4*

# *Epilepsy*

## *History*

Epilepsy is the tendency towards seizures and thus, an individual must have had more than one event to qualify for this diagnosis. The condition has been recognised since ancient time, the word epilepsy being derived from the Greek word meaning to 'seize upon'. Over the centuries epilepsy has frequently been associated with the presence of demons or evil spirits and has carried with it unpleasant connotations. Hughlings Jackson, a British neurologist of the nineteenth century, is attributed with the first recognition of the association between likely disordered cerebral discharge and the clinical features. Over the twentieth century, treatment of epilepsy advanced enormously, first with the introduction of barbiturates, such as phenobarbitone, followed by the use of phenytoin, and then the introduction of newer drugs such as Carbamazepine, with its superior adverse effects profile, in the early 1960's. Since then an increasing number of new anti-epileptic drugs have become available.

## *Symptoms*

Epilepsy is an extremely heterogeneous disorder and can be defined as intermittent derangement of cerebral function due to a sudden and disorderly discharge of cerebral neurones. There is a large range of seizure types and a multitude of underlying causes. The most dramatic and best known type of seizure is generalised tonic clonic seizure, in which the subject loses consciousness, falls to the ground, becomes stiff and shakes violently, and may become blue in the lips and foam at the mouth. However, there are many other clinical presentations, for example: minor generalised seizure, in which there is simple alteration of consciousness without the motor features (such as in petit mal); partial or focal seizure without loss of consciousness, such as Jacksonian seizure in which there is onset of movement confined initially to one body part, but which may spread to

other parts of the body and simple sensory seizures; and complex partial seizure in which there is impaired consciousness, either at the start of the seizure or with its development. Most commonly patients have one stereotyped form of seizure, although partial seizure may progress to generalised tonic clonic seizure. There may be a warning of seizure onset, for example, an olfactory, visual, or auditory hallucination, or a sensation of pain or nausea, although seizures may strike out of the blue and some forms of seizure are very rarely preceded by a warning. For example, in petit mal there is often no warning and the loss of consciousness is so brief that the subject may be unaware of its occurrence. Generalised and complex partial seizures are frequently followed by drowsiness, which may last for several hours.

## *Cellular pathology and pathogenesis*

Typically a seizure arises from an assembly of abnormally excitable neurones. This collection may be associated with a visible lesion (see below), but may not be visible macroscopically or microscopically. This abnormal discharge may be recorded on an electroencephalogram (EEG) both during seizures and in-between seizures. Why neurones in or around a lesion discharge is not known. Such neurones seem to be hyper-excitable and appear to have increased membrane ion permeability. Epileptic foci are also known to be sensitive to acetylcholine and a deficiency in GABA, and changes in glycine glutamate and taurine have been reported in excised eleptogenic tissue.

## *Neuropathology*

Epilepsy may be divided into primary epilepsy, in which there is no gross pathology on post-mortem, and secondary epilepsy, in which a lesion can be identified and associated with the condition. Very many identified lesions have been associated with seizures including ischaemic strokes, vascular malformation, glial scars, tumours, and infections. The anatomical position of the lesion may influence the nature of the seizures, for example, lesions in the temporal lobes are associated with partial complex (or temporal lobe) epilepsy. However, with ever improving imaging and pathological techniques, an increasing proportion of so-called primary seizures can be seen to be secondary to subtle lesions. It has also become apparent that focal areas of abnormal cell migration during development (dysembryogenesis) may produce small focal lesions that are epileptogenic and are difficult to visualise in life.

## Genetics

Heritability is important in epilepsy and variable depending on the specific syndrome under consideration. Some types of epilepsy are clearly familial, such as petit mal, but in others the genetic component is less clear. For example, generalised tonic clonic epilepsy is under the influence of a genetic factor, suggested by a familial coincidence of about 5–10%. In partial and focal epilepsy's the inherited component is less clear.

## Current treatments

For the majority of patients, seizures can be well-controlled by one or a combination of medications, usually prescribed and monitored by a general practitioner or specialist. Some types of epilepsy, particularly certain types of childhood epilepsy, may remit with time. However, a substantial minority have epilepsy that is difficult to control and interferes severely with everyday living. For a carefully selected proportion of these subjects, excision of the lesion may lead to clinical improvement.

# *Appendix 5*

# *Huntington's disease*

## *History*

1872    George Huntington first described an inherited form of chorea as a discrete clinical entity.

1877    Meynert attributed chorea in Huntington's disease (HD) to lesions in the corpus striatum.

1908    Punnett proposed a dominant Mendelian pattern of inheritance in HD.

1983    The Hereditary Disease Foundation's Venezuela project launched into the unique population of Lake Maracaibo Indians with very high concentration of the disease, which has provided a fundamental resource to the subsequent genetic analysis of the disease.

1983    James Gusella and colleagues localise disease locus to tip of short arm of chromosome 4.

1985    Jean Paul Vonsattel described anatomical criteria of striatal atrophy that is still in widespread use for staging progression of the disease.

1992    First report from Czechoslovakia and Cuba of striatal transplantation in HD.

1993    Huntington's disease study group identify the expanded CAG repeat in the IT15 gene. The gene encodes a previously unknown protein, designated huntingtin, of unknown function.

1996    Publication of CAPIT-HD, the core assessment protocol for assessment of intracerebral transplantation and other reparative treatments

1996    Mangiarini, Bates and colleagues describe first HD transgenic mouse, which produces overt dyskinetic neurological phenotype.

1997    Nuclear intranuclear inclusions (NIIs) first described in a transgenic mouse model of HD and subsequently confirmed in the human disease.

## *Symptoms*

Huntington's disease involves a triad of symptoms: motor, cognitive, and psychiatric. The choreiform (dance-like) movements were emphasised by Huntington and early neurological studies, characterised by uncontrolled dyskinesias of the arms and legs, writhing of the body, difficulties in chewing and swallowing, and weight loss. The associated symptoms of bradykinesia, rigidity and loss of balance are equally disabling. In the last 20 years, cognitive deficits, in particular in spatial, planning, and executive functions of the frontal type, and psychiatric deficits, involving mood swings, irrational behaviours, affective changes and a high level of suicide, have received more widespread attention, leading to a change in terminology from 'Huntington's chorea' to 'Huntington's disease'.

Onset of overt symptoms is most commonly in early middle age, with a mean age of onset between 35 and 44 years in different studies. This is however typically past the age when most affected individuals have already had their families, with potential transmission of the affected gene. The first signs are often not the motor changes easily detected by neurological examination, but emotional swings in mood and changes in social behaviour that are more obvious to the families. Disease typically progresses from symptom onset to advanced disability and death due to infection, pneumonia, or inanition in approximately 15 years. The later the onset, the slower the progression. In approximately 5–10% of cases, onset is much younger (the 'Westphal' variant), and progresses to death much faster.

## *Neuropathology*

Huntington's disease is associated with progressive and profound degeneration of the striatum, measured in MRI or CAT scans as an enlarging of the lateral ventricles and widening of the intercaudate distance. The caudate nucleus is typically affected more extensively and earlier than the putamen, and atrophy and cell loss spreads in a dorsal medial to lateral ventral direction. At the cellular level, the medium spiny projection neurones are primarily affected with relative sparing of large and medium striatal interneurones, accompanied by moderate gliosis. In advanced disease, other brain nuclei are also affected, in particular those associated with the basal ganglia, such as atrophy of the cortical (especially frontal and other association areas) inputs and cell loss in the pallidial and substantia nigra pars reticulata outputs of the striatum. Recently abnormal inclusion bodies have been identified in affected striatal neurones that stain densely for both ubiquitin and huntingtin (NIIs).

## Genetics

HD is an autosomally dominant inherited disease passed from affected parent to 50% of their children, who will in turn all express the disease and pass on the gene with the same probability to their children. The critical gene has been identified on chromosome 4, encoding a protein of unknown function, huntingtin, which contains a polyglutamine (polyQ) repeat. This polyQ repeat is of 5–36 amino acids in length in unaffected individuals but is expanded (39–120 repeats) in length in individuals with HD. The age of disease onset is inversely correlated with repeat length. Inheritance of the gene repeat length is relatively stable when inherited from the mother but there is a tendency for slight increase in length when inherited from the father, accounting for the observation of paternal anticipation effects in families. The discovery of the gene now allows accurate premorbid, as well as diagnostic, testing both for family planning advice and in experimental and therapeutic studies for development of novel or neuroprotective treatments.

## Cellular pathology and pathogenesis

The mechanisms by which an expanded polyQ repeat in the huntingtin gene results in selective neuronal degeneration in the striatum is currently unknown. Nor is it known whether the NIIs observed in affected cells are a cause or only a degenerative consequence of cell death. Mitochondrial function is disturbed in the disease and toxins that disrupt the mitochondrial energy chain can yield similar patterns of pathology in animals and man, but again the relationship between this and cellular or molecular pathology is unknown. Clarification of these relationships in the coming decade are likely to open completely new avenues to prevention and treatment.

## Current treatments

There is no available treatment for HD and no way at present of blocking disease onset or progression. Tranquilising and neuroleptic drugs can suppress some of the more overt motor and psychiatric symptoms, whereas there are no means to alleviate cognitive symptoms. Three main strategies are under investigation for novel therapies. One is to investigate antioxidant, antiexcitotoxic and other neuroprotective drugs that may block hypothesised mechanisms of cell death. Second is to administer neurotrophic molecules that may promote neuronal survival in the striatum. Third is to replace striatal neurones by cell transplantation. Each of these approaches show some promise in experimental animal models but none have yet been demonstrated to be effective in patients.

# Appendix 6

# Multiple sclerosis

## Epidemiology

Multiple sclerosis (MS) is the commonest neurological disorder of young adults, and affects about 1:1000 of the population. It is commoner in women than in men, the ratio being 3:2. The age of onset is usually between 20 and 40 years old, the disease being rare in children. MS is commoner in countries further from the equator, above 40° latitude. If children move from one country to another before they are 15 years old, they acquire the risk associated with the new environment.

## Genetics

Close relatives of patients suffering from MS have a 10–20 times greater probability of developing the condition. Identical twins of patients with MS have a 1 in 3 chance of being affected. About 20 genetic locations have been identified that contribute to the risk of developing MS, but no single gene has been shown to have a major influence.

## Progression of the disease

MS can present with any neurological symptom or sign. The disease may follow various courses, but classically there are acute exacerbations followed by partial recovery. Four patterns of disease are generally recognised.

- *Benign MS* presents with one or more mild attacks, usually involving a sensory modality, followed by complete recovery. There is no permanent disability.

- *Relapsing–remitting MS*. Attacks with neurological dysfunction are followed by remissions. The relapses may involve pathways that have previously been affected, or may be in new areas. In the early stages of the disease there is almost complete return of function during remission, but with increasing numbers of relapses there is more and more residual dysfunction in between.

- *Secondary progressive MS*. This pattern of disease usually starts as relapsing–remitting MS, but after repeated attacks the remissions stop and the patient shows steadily progressive disease with no return of function.

- *Primary progressive MS*. In some patients the pattern of disease from the start is of steadily worsening symptoms and progressive disability.

## Diagnosis

MS can present with almost any neurological symptom or sign. Because it is a common condition it is high on the list of differential diagnoses for any neurological problem. The classical clinical diagnosis requires that there be at least two episodes of neurological dysfunction, involving at least two separate areas of the CNS, lasting at least 24 h, and occurring at least one month apart. However, a definite diagnosis rests on three main tests.

1. *Visual and auditory evoked potentials*. The optic nerve and auditory pathways are very commonly affected. Demyelination leads to a slowing of axonal conduction, and this can be detected by measuring the latency of cortical responses to auditory and visual stimuli.

2. *MRI scan*. An MRI scan may reveal areas of demyelination in affected areas. Regions in which the blood–brain barrier is leaking as a result of an MS lesion can be detected by imaging the leakage of gadolinium from the vasculature into the brain.

3. *Lumbar puncture*. The CSF will usually contain antibodies to myelin components, which may be present as oligoclonal bands on electrophoresis,

and may be shown to be reactive to myelin molecules.

## Pathology

The hallmark of the disease is the occurrence of localised regions of demyelination, usually less than 1 cm across. These can occur in any white matter area of the CNS, but are particularly common in the optic nerve. In the acute stage, these lesions show evidence of inflammation, containing large numbers of lymphocytes, and variable numbers of microglia/macrophages. During the inflammatory phase, there is breakdown of the blood–brain barrier, with extravasation of serum proteins. When the initial inflammatory event is finished, the MS plaque typically consists largely of naked axons surrounded by astrocytes, which may take the form of a classic glial scar, or may be more less dense with more extracellular space. A proportion of MS plaques show evidence of complete or partial remyelination. This is usually by oligodendrocytes, but in aggressive MS involving the spinal cord there may be Schwann cell remyelination. There is evidence from functional, pathological and imaging studies of progressive axonal loss within chronic MS plaques.

## Treatment

Exacerbations of the disease can be significantly shortened by high-dose steroids. Methylprednisolone, dexamethasone and ACTH are used. Three treatments are routinely available that have been shown to reduce the incidence of relapses.

1. Glatiramer acetate (salts of synthetic peptides that mimic myelin basic protein) has shown a 29% lowering of the number of relapses.

2. Interferon $\beta$-1a (Avonex) is a recombinant form of human interferon beta.

3. Interferon $\beta$-1b (Betaseron) is an alternative recombinant preparation.

Interferon treatment has been shown in trials to result in a roughly 30% reduction in exacerbation frequency and progression of disability. Other experimental immunosuppressive treatments are discussed in relevant chapters. The mainstay of treatment is symptomatic relief of the various symptoms affecting the patient. Foremost amongst these is pain, affecting all parts of the body, which may be very refractory to treatment. Treatment of spasticity, urological problems, and other conditions may also be necessary.

# *Appendix 7*

# *Parkinson's disease*

## *History*

1817 James Parkinson. First description in his *Essay on the Shaking Palsy*.

1905 Tretiakoff identifies loss of pigmented cells in the substantia nigra of Parkinson's disease (PD).

1912 Lewy describes 'Lewy body' inclusions in the basal forebrain of PD.

1960 Ehringer and Hornykiewicz identify dopamine loss in post-mortem PD brains.

1961 Birkmeyer and Hornykiewicz first treat PD patients with l-dopa.

1966 Cotzias *et al.* introduction of soluble l-dopa/carbidopa as PD therapy.

1981 Langston describes parkinsonian syndrome associated with MPTP.

1983 Backlund and Olson first report human neural transplantation in PD.

1987 DATAtop trials of deprenyl slowing progression of PD.

1990 Lindvall *et al.* Unequivocal therapeutic benefit of nigral grafts in PD.

## *Symptoms*

The cardinal symptoms of Parkinson's disease are a poverty of movement (akinesia or bradykinesia), muscular rigidity, and tremor. In particular the motor deficits involve impairment in the initiation and sequencing of voluntary movements and sequences of movement. The disease is also associated with other characteristic signs, including a waxy expression, stooped posture, shuffling gait, micrographia. Although the topic is of long dispute, there is now clear evidence

that a substantial minority of patients manifest cognitive impairments, in particular involving frontal-like symptoms and a slowing of thought ('bradyphrenia'). There are distinctive deficits in controlled motor tasks (serial choice reaction time) and the planning, initiation and sequencing of motor acts.

## *Diagnostic tests*

The motor symptoms are generally the earliest signs of the disease process. The presence of Parkinson's disease can be confirmed by a therapeutic response to L-DOPA (in contrast to other forms of striato-nigral degeneration, which are dopa-independent) and by PET scanning using the radioisotope $^{18}$F-DOPA to visualise loss of dopamine terminals in the neostriatum.

## *Progression*

PD is a slow progressive disease. It may rarely occur in young adults but onset is more typically in late middle age. Patients may live 20–30 years after diagnosis, and the symptoms can generally now be well contained for many years by L-DOPA or other drug treatments. However, in advance stages of the disease, the drugs have reduced effective dose-ranges, rapid wearing off, pronounced 'On-Off' swings, and severe dyskinetic side-effects. In the terminal stages, the patient is unable to execute any co-ordinated voluntary movements, and is bed-bound and dependent on total nursing care. Death is not usually due to PD itself, but to indirect consequences of terminal disease such as pneumonia.

## *Neuropathology*

PD involves a primary degeneration of the dopamine cells of the substantia nigra and associated depletion of forebrain dopamine content in terminal areas in the basal ganglia. Dopamine depletions occur earlier and to a greater extent in the putamen than in the caudate nucleus. Lewy body inclusions in degenerating neurones are a characteristic neuropathological feature of the disease and are seen not only in the substantia nigra but also in other melanin-containing cell groups of the brain, including the locus coeruleus and nucleus basalis. Although the dopamine loss is the earliest and most marked neurochemical feature of the disease, there are also less marked depletions in noradrenaline and acetylcholine, and more widespread neuronal degeneration can occur at late stages of the disease.

## Epidemiology, genetics, aetiology

PD occurs world-wide with an incidence of approximately 250 per 100,000, but there occur pockets of higher concentration both within and between countries. It is not associated with strong genetic linkage, and where it occurs in several members of a family, the different individuals are more likely to show similar time of onset rather than similar age of onset, suggesting an infectious or toxic causation. Although several specific toxic causes of parkinson-like syndromes have been identified (such as consumption of the cycad bean in Guam, self-administration of the heroin-substitute MPTP or manganese poisoning), specific attribution of idiopathic PD to an environmental toxin has not been established.

## Current treatment

The most widespread treatment for PD is administration of the dopamine-precursor drug L-DOPA to replete forebrain dopamine content. The peripheral sympathetic side-effects of L-DOPA are blocked by co-administration of the decarboxylase inhibitor carbidopa, which does not cross the blood–brain barrier. In the advanced stages of the disease, when L-DOPA may have declining efficacy, dopamine receptor agonists (e.g. bromocriptine, apomorphine) can be beneficial. Anticholinergics (e.g. amantadine) may also be beneficial at an early stage to delay start of L-DOPA or in patients for whom the L-DOPA response is poor.

Drug treatments are most effective against the akinetic and rigid symptoms. Tremor is not well treated by dopamine-replacement pharmacotherapies, but in the most sever cases may be controlled by neurosurgical lesions of the ventral thalamus.

PD has become the major focus of initial clinical trials of various forms of therapy based on neural transplantation and implantation of various central dopamine-delivery systems.

# *Appendix 8*

# *Spinal-cord injury*

## *Epidemiology*

The incidence of spinal-cord injury and its causes vary greatly from country to country. In the developed world the overall annual incidence is 25 injuries per million population, with around 11 000 new injuries per year in the USA, around 1000 per year in the UK. The largest group of patients are those injured in young adulthood, the mean age of injury in the USA being 33; of these, 70% are male, 30% female. Because of advances in the care of spinally injured patients, life-expectancy is not very much less that in the able-bodied population. There are therefore large numbers of people disabled by spinal-cord injury living in communities around the world, the estimate for the USA being 250 000 people affected with varying degrees of disability. Of these 55% are paraplegic, and 44% quadriplegic.

The causes of spinal-cord injury vary between countries. However, in all developed countries, vehicular accidents are the commonest cause, being responsible for 40% of injuries in the USA. Falls from various causes are responsible for up to 20% of cases. In most European countries, sporting injuries are the next most common cause. Diving, horseback riding, skiing, and climbing are common causes, with American football and rugby football as significant causes. Violence and gunshot injuries are the cause of around 25% of injuries in the USA, but for a much smaller proportion in Europe. Spinal injury is common amongst soldiers in wartime.

## *Symptoms and diagnosis*

Diagnosis is seldom difficult, since all patients will have been involved in some form of severe trauma. If conscious, the patient may well complain of paralysis and loss of sensation below a certain level. In patients with high injuries, breathing may be threatened and patients may need immediate assisted respiration. In most cases there will initially be a flaccid paralysis of the affected limbs, and an obvious lack of spontaneous movement.

The main methods of assessment are clinical signs and imaging of the cord. Examination early after the injury will show a flaccid paralysis in the affected limbs, and loss of sensation. Depending on the site of the lesion, autonomic outflow from the cord will be affected, which will affect vasomotor control and therefore skin colour. Control of the bladder is lost, and the patient is commonly in urinary retention. Many cord injuries are incomplete, with some surviving axonal projections, and it is important to map surviving function. As time progresses, the paralysis will change to a spastic paralysis with signs of loss of upper motor neurone control. Also, as the oedema and inflammation resulting from the injury resolves, considerable amounts of neurological function may return in patients with incomplete transections.

Imaging of the spine will usually show fracture and/or dislocation, often with narrowing or complete disruption of the spinal canal. However in some cases the spine appears surprisingly normal. The spinal cord can be imaged in some detail by MRI, although the surrounding bone affects resolution. In extreme cases, the cord may be completely transected, but often there is tissue in continuity across the lesion. Early after injury the cord is oedematous, and as time progresses varying degrees of cystic lesions appear. The correlation between the appearance of the cord by MRI and clinical signs is rather approximate, and an accurate prognosis cannot be made until some time after the initial injury.

The commonest levels of injury are above or just below the ribcage, since this structure to some extent braces the spine against injury. Commonest levels are from C4 to C7, and in the upper lumbar spine.

## *Progression*

Immediately after injury most patients will have symptoms and signs of complete spinal cord transection.

However in about one-third of patients, a proportion of the lost function will return in the following weeks. This is due the resolution of the oedema and inflammation affecting the surviving part of the partially transected cord, and to removal of compression. There may also be much slower and longer term return of function due to remyelination of demyelinated axons. In a further third of patients, imaging will show some cord remaining in continuity, but functionally the patient has a complete transection.

## Treatment

Immediately after injury the main concern is to transport the patient to hospital without exacerbating the injury. A significant proportion of disability results from damage to the cord sustained after the initial injury. The NASCIS (National acute spinal cord injury study) trial in the USA showed that there was a significant benefit in terms of neurological function from giving high dose methylprednisolone immediately after injury. This is done routinely in the USA, and variably in other countries. The immediate concern after admission to hospital is usually with the extensive injuries that have been suffered by many patients, and with establishment of ventilation, if this is necessary. It may be necessary to stabilise the spine. There is at present no treatment that can be applied to human patients to induce repair of spinal-cord injuries. The major thrust of treatment is therefore rehabilitation, and teaching the patient to function in society with whatever neurological function remains. A major concern is always bladder function: in many cases this has to be dealt with by regular catheterisation. Rigidity and spasticity may need to be treated with drugs.

# *Appendix 9*

# *Stroke*

## *Symptoms*

This group of syndromes represents the commonest neurological disorder, and the third-commonest medical condition in the developed world after heart attacks and cancer. Stroke usually presents as a sudden and abrupt onset of focal neurological deficit, which may be so severe as to render the patient comatose or lead to immediate death. In its mildest form the deficit may be so subtle as to go unnoticed. Although the vast majority of strokes are abrupt in onset, occasionally evolution may be slower or stuttering. The clinical features depend on the brain region supplied by the vessel or vessels involved. A commonly affected vessel is the middle cerebral artery, total occlusion of which produces contralateral hemiplegia, hemianaesthesia, and visual field defect, plus language deficit if the occlusion has occurred in the dominant hemisphere. This large stroke is often associated in the early stages with loss of consciousness or drowsiness and confusion. On the other hand, complete basilar artery occlusion may lead to the 'locked in syndrome' in which the patient is mute, quadraplegic, but conscious, due to interruption of motor pathways and sparing of the reticular activating system. Another extreme is the blockage of small penetrating arteries, which produces tiny lesions that in themselves produce little or no deficit, but with accumulation may lead to neurological deficits. Following a stroke, functional recovery ranges from none to complete, although improvement is the rule if the patient survives. However, although the bulk of the recovery occurs in the first few months following a stroke, maximal recovery may require a couple of years.

## *Neuropathology and pathogenesis*

The brain is exquisitely reliant on the minute to minute supply of oxygenated blood and the constancy of this system is regulated by a series of baroreceptors and vasomotor receptors under the control of centres in the lower brainstem. Brain tissue deprived of this blood supply undergoes ischaemic necrosis, also termed 'infarction'. The most common cause of interruption of this blood supply is obstruction of a cerebral artery by a thrombus or embolus, but other mechanisms may underlie the condition, such as circulatory failure following a heart attack. Stroke may also be caused by intracranial haemorrhage, which may be due to rupture of an arterial aneurysm or arteriovenous malformation. Additionally, a stroke syndrome may be the result of venous, rather than arterial blockage, which in turn causes abnormalities of blood flow and oxygenation of brain tissue. As can be seen from this discussion, the pathogenic mechanisms underlying stroke are many and varied. Well-known associated risk factors for arterial thrombotic stroke include cigarette smoking, hypertension, diabetes, and hyperlipidaemia, which are thought to influence the state of the arterial endothelium and coaguability of the blood. Following a recent infarction, there is an area of brain that is destined to die and a surrounding area (the penumbra) that is at risk, but theoretically rescuable. Interventions to reduce cell death in this population of cells have been the subject of recent research.

## *Genetics*

Although there are a small number of clearly defined genetic conditions associated with stroke, for example, 'cerebral autosomal dominant arteriopathy with subcortical infarcts and leukoencephalopathy' (CADASIL), for most stroke syndromes any genetic association is much less clear or absent. However, there may be a familial tendency in a significant proportion of ischaemic stroke cases, which may be related to the inheritable nature of risk factors.

## *Current treatments*

It could be said that some of the most important current interventions in stroke are to treat or remove risk factors and thus to prevent the occurrence of stroke where possible. Once a stroke has taken place the majority of patients require supportive management, minimisation of risk factors, rehabilitation, and treatment with aspirin, which has been shown to significantly reduce recurrence in the case of ischaemic stroke. Depending on the circumstances, other antiplatelet or anticoagulant drugs may be appropriate, and there are now ongoing a number of clinical studies to examine the efficacy of 'clot busting' drugs, such as streptokinase. There is also considerable interest in developing drugs to influence the survival of the neurones in the penumbra (see Chapter 7). Additionally, surgical measures may be appropriate in selected cases, for example, in the case of an accessible and significant stenosis, to remove a blood clot that is causing pressure symptoms, or to treat an arteriovenous malformation at risk of re-bleeding. However, for most patients surviving a stroke there will be a degree of natural recovery (see symptoms) and during this recovery period the rehabilitation services including physiotherapy, occupational therapy, and speech therapy play an important role.

# References

Aboody-Guterman, K.S., Pechan, P.A., Rainov, N.G., Sena-Esteves, M., Jacobs, A., Snyder, E.Y., Wild, P., Schraner, E., Tobler, K., Breakefield, X.O., and Fraefel, C. (1997). Green fluorescent protein as a reporter for retrovirus and helper virus-free HSV-1 amplicon vector-mediated gene transfer into neural cells in culture and *in vivo*. *NeuroReport*, **8**, 3801–3808.

Ace, C.I., McKee, T.A., Ryan, J.M., Cameron, J.M., and Preston, C.M. (1989). Construction and characterization of a herpes-simplex virus type-1 mutant unable to transinduce immediate-early gene-expression. *Journal of Virology*, **63**, 2260–2269.

Achiron, A., Gabbay, U., Gilad, R., Hassin-Baer, S., Barak, Y., Gornish, M., Elizur, A., Goldhammer, Y., and Sarova-Pinhas, I. (1998). Intravenous immunoglobulin treatment in multiple sclerosis — Effect on relapses. *Neurology*, **50**, 398–402.

Achte, K., Jahro, L., Kyykka, T., and Esterinen, E. (1991). Paranoid disorders following war brain damage: preliminary report. *Psychopathology*, **24**, 309–315.

Adams, R.D. and Victor, M. (1993). *Principles of Neurology*. McGraw-Hill, New York.

Adamson, D.C., Wildemann, B., Sasaki, M., Glass, J.D., McArthur, J.C., Christov, V.I., Dawson, T.M., and Dawson, V.L. (1996). Immunologic NO synthase: elevation in severe AIDS dementia and induction by HIV-1 go41. *Science*, **274**, 1917–1921.

Aebischer, P., Tresco, P.A., Winn, S.R., Greene, L.A., and Jaeger, C.B. (1991). Long-term cross-species brain transplantation of a polymer-encapsulated dopamine-secreting cell line. *Experimental Neurology*, **111**, 269–275.

Aebischer, P., Goddard, M., Signore, A.P., and Timpson, R.L. (1994). Functional recovery in hemiparkinsonian primates transplanted with polymer-encapsulated PC12 cells. *Experimental Neurology*, **126**, 151–158.

Aebischer, P., Schluep, M., Deglon, N., Joseph, J.M., Hirt, L., Heyd, B., Goddard, M., Hammang, J.P., Zurn, A.D., Kato, A.C., Regli, F., and Baetge, E.E. (1996). Intrathecal delivery of CNTF using encapsulated genetically-modified xenogeneic cells in amyotrophic lateral sclerosis patients. *Nature Medicine*, **2**, 696–699.

Agger, W., Case, K.L., Bryant, G.L., and Callister, S.M. (1991). Lyme disease: clinical features, classification and epidemiology in the Upper Midwest. *Medicine (Baltimore)*, **70**, 83–90.

Agrell, B. and Dehlin, O. (1989). Comparison of six depression rating scales in geriatric stroke patients. *Stroke*, **20**, 1190–1194.

Ahlberg, J., Norlen, L., Blomstrand, C., and Wikkelsö, C. (1988). Outcome of shunt operation on urinary incontinence in normal pressure hydrocephalus. *Journal of Neurology, Neurosurgery and Psychiatry*, **51**, 105–108.

Aigner, L., Arber, S., Kapfhammer, J.P., Laux, T., Schneider, C., Botteri, F., Brenner, H.R., and Caroni, P. (1995). Overexpression of the neural growth-associated protein GAP-43 induces nerve sprouting in the adult nervous-system of transgenic mice. *Cell*, **83**, 269–278.

Akwa, Y., Young, J., Kabbadj, K., Sancho, M.J., Zucman, D., Vourch, C. *et al.* (1991). Neurosteroids — biosynthesis, metabolism and function of pregnenolone and dehydroepiandrosterone in the brain. *Journal of Steroid Biochemistry and Molecular Biology*, **40**, 71–81.

Akwa, Y., Morfin, R.F., Robel, P., and Baulieu, E.E. (1992). Neurosteroid metabolism — 7-$\alpha$-hydroxylation of dehydroepiandrosterone and pregnenolone by rat brain microsomes. *Biochemical Journal*, **288**, 959–964.

Albert, E. (1987). On organically based hallucinatory-delusional pyschoses. *Psychopathology*, **20**, 144–154.

Albin, R.L. (1995). Selective neurodegeneration in Huntington's disease. *Annals of Neurology*, **38**, 835–836.

Albin, R.L., Young, A.B., and Penney, J.B. (1989). The functional anatomy of basal ganglia disorders. *Trends in Neurosciences*, **18**, 63–64.

Alderman, N. and Ward, A. (1991). Behavioural treatment of the dysexecutive syndrome: Reduction of repetitive speech using response cost and cognitive overlearning. *Neuropsychological Rehabilitation*, **1**, 65–80.

Alexander, G.E. and Crutcher, M.D. (1990). Functional architecture of basal ganglia circuits: neural substrates of parallel processing. *Trends in Neurosciences*, **13**, 266–271.

Alexi, T., Venero, J.L., and Hefti, F. (1997). Protective effects of neurotrophin-4/5 and transforming growth factor-$\alpha$ on striatal neuronal phenotypic degeneration after excitotoxic lesioning with quinolinic acid. *Neuroscience*, **78**, 73–86.

Allman, P. (1992). Drug treatment of emotionalism following brain damage. *Journal of the Royal Society of Medicine*, **85**, 423–424.

Allman, P., Hope, T., and Fairburn, C.G. (1992). Crying following stroke: a report of 30 cases. *General Hospital Psychiatry*, **14**, 315–321.

Alpers, M.P. (1987). Epidemiology and clinical aspects of kuru. In *Prions* (ed. S.B. Prusiner and M.P. McKinley), pp. 451–465. Academic Press, New York.

Alpert, E. and Seigerman, C. (1986). Steroid withdrawal psychosis in a patient with closed head injury. *Archives of Physical Medicine and Rehabilitation*, **67**, 766–769.

Altman, J. (1962). Are new neurons formed in the brains of adult mammals? *Science*, **135**, 1127–1128.

Altman, J. (1963). Autoradiographic investigation of cell proliferation in the brains of rats and cats. *Anatomical Record*, **145**, 573–592.

Altman, J. and Das, G.D. (1965). Autoradiographic and histological evidence of postnatal hippocampal neurogenesis in rats. *Journal of Comparative Neurology*, 124, 319–336.

Alzheimer, A. (1907). Über eine eigenartige Erkrankung der Hirnrinde. *Allgemeine Zeitschrift für die gesamte Neurologie und Psychiatrie*, 64, 146–148.

Ames, B.N., Shigenaga, M.K., and Hagen, T.M. (1993). Oxidants, antioxidants and the degenerative diseases of aging. *Proceedings of the National Academy of Sciences of the United States of America*, 90, 7915–7922.

Anderson, D.N. (1990). Koro: the genital retraction symptom in stroke. *British Journal of Psychiatry*, 157, 142–144.

Anderson, N.E. (1995). The immunobiology and clinical features of paraneoplastic syndromes. *Current Opinion In Neurology*, 8, 424–429.

Anderson, J.R. and Field, H.J. (1983). The distribution of herpes simplex type 1 antigen in mouse central nervous system after different routes of administration. *Journal of the Neurological Sciences*, 60, 181–195.

Anderson, N.E., Rosenblum, M.K., Graus, F., Wiley, R.G., and Posner, J.B. (1988). Autoantibodies in paraneoplastic syndromes associated with small-cell lung cancer. *Neurology*, 38, 1391–1398.

Andersen, J.K., Garber, D.A., Meaney, C.A., and Breakefield, X.O. (1992). Gene-transfer into mammalian central-nervous-system using herpes- virus vectors — extended expression of bacterial lacz in neurons using the neuron-specific enolase promoter. *Human Gene Therapy*, 3, 487–499.

Anderson, K.D., Panayotatos, N., Corcoran, T.L., Lindsay, R.M., and Wiegand, S.J. (1996a). Ciliary neurotrophic factor protects striatal output neurons in an animal model of Huntington disease. *Proceedings of the National Academy of Sciences of the United States of America*, 93, 7346–7351.

Anderson, R.M., Donnelly, C.A., Ferguson, N.M., Woolhouse, M.E.J., Watt, C.J., Udy, H.J. *et al.* (1996b). Transmission dynamics and epidemiology of BSE in British cattle. *Nature*, 382, 779–788.

Andrade, J. (1995). Learning during anaesthesia: A review. *British Journal of Psychology*, 86, 479–506.

Andrew, S.E., Goldberg, Y.P., Kremer, B., Telenius, H., Theilmann, J., Adam, S. *et al.* (1993). The relationship between trinucleotide (CAG) repeat length and clinical features of Huntington's disease. *Nature Genetics*, 4, 398–403.

Angelergues, R., Hécaen, H., and de Ajuriaguerra, J. (1955). Les troubles mentaux au cours des tumeurs du lobe frontal. *Annales Médico-Psychologiques*, 113, 577–642.

Ankarcrona, M., Dypbukt, J.M., Bonfoco, E., Zhivotovsky, B., Orrenius, S., Lipton, S.A., and Nicotera, P. (1995). Glutamate-induced neuronal death — a succession of necrosis or apoptosis depending on mitochondrial-function. *Neuron*, 15, 961–973.

Ansell, B.J. and Keenan, J.E. (1989). The Western Neuro Sensory Stimulation Profile: A tool for assessing slow-to-recover head-injured patients. *Archives of Physical Medicine and Rehabilitation*, 70, 104–108.

Anton, R., Kordower, J.H., Kane, D.J., Markham, C.H., and Bredesen, D.E. (1995). Neural transplantation of cells expressing the anti-apoptotic gene *bcl-2*. *Cell Transplantation*, 4, 49–54.

Antuono, P., Doody, R., Gilman, S., uff, J., heltens, P., Ueda, K., and Khachaturian, Z.S. (1997). Diagnostic criteria for dementia in clinical trials. Position paper from the international working group on harmonization of dementia drug guidelines. *Alzheimer Disease and Associated Disorders*, 11 (**Supplement 3**), 22–25.

Archer, D.R., Cuddon, P.A., Lipsitz, D., and Duncan, I.D. (1997). Myelination of the canine central nervous system by glial cell transplantation: a model for repair of human myelin disease. *Nature Medicine*, 3, 54–59.

Ariza, A., von Uexkull-Guldeband, C., Mate, J.L., Isamat, M., Aracil, C., Cruz-Sánchez, F.F. *et al.* (1996). Accumulation of wild-type p53 protein in progressive multifocal leukoencephalopathy: a flow cytometry and DNA sequencing study. *Journal of Neuropathology and Experimental Neurology*, 55, 144–149.

Ariza, A., Mate, J.L., Isamat, M., Calatrava, A., Fernandez-Vasalo, A., and Navas-Palacios, J.J. (1998). Overexpression of Ki-67 and cyclins A and B1 in JC virus-infected cells of progressive multifocal leukoencephalopathy. *Journal of Neuropathology and Experimental Neurology*, 57, 226–230.

Arkin, S.M. (1991). Memory training in early Alzheimer's disease: an optimistic look at the field. *The American Journal of Alzheimer's Care and Related Disorders and Research*, 17–25.

Arkin, S.M. (1992). Audio-assisted memory training with early Alzheimer's patients: two single subject experiments. *Clinical Gerontologist*, 12, 77–96.

Arnason, B.G.W. (1987). Pareneoplastic syndrome as an immunologic disease. In: Arnason, J.A., Behan, W.M.H., and Behan, P.O. eds. *Clinical Neuroimmunology*. London, Blackwell Scientific pp. 370–379.

Aruoma, O.I., Halliwell, B., Hoey, B.M., and Butler, J. (1989). The antioxidant action of N-acetylcysteine, its reaction with hydrogen peroxide, hydroxyl radical, superoxide and hypochlorous acid. *Free Radical Biology and Medicine*, 6, 593–597.

Asanuma, M., Hirata, H., and Cadet, J.L. (1998). Attenuation of 6-hydroxydopamine-induced dopaminergic nigrostriatal lesions in superoxide dismutase transgenic mice. *Neuroscience*, 85, 907–917.

Asher, R.A., idler, P.S., ogers, J.H., and awcett, J.W. (1998). TGF$\beta$ stimulates neurocan synthesis in cultured rat astrocytes. *Society for Neuroscience Abstracts*, 24, 56.

Assal, G. and Bindschaedler, C. (1990). Délire temporel systematisé et trouble auditif d'origine corticale. *Revue Neurologique*, 146, 249–255.

Aström, K.E., Mancall, E.L., and Richardson, E.P.J. (1958). Progessive multifocal leukoencephalopathy, a hitherto unrecognized complication of chronic lymphocytic leukaemia and Hodgkin's disease. *Brain*, 81, 93–111.

Åström, M., Olsson, T., and Asplund, K. (1993). Different linkage of depression to hypercortisolism early versus late after stroke — a 3-year longitudinal study. *Stroke*, 24, 52–57.

Avellana-Adalid, V., Nait-Oumesmar, B., Lachapelle, F., and Baron-Van Evercooren, A. (1996). Expansion of rat oligodendrocyte progenitors into proliferative oligospheres that retain differentiation potential. *Journal of Neuroscience Research*, 45, 558–570.

Aylward, E.H., Anderson, N.B., Bylsma, F.W., Wagster, M.V., Barta, P.E., Sherr, M. *et al.* (1998). Frontal lobe volume in patients with Huntington's disease. *Neurology*, 50, 252–258.

Azcoitia, I., Sierra, A., and Garcia-Segura, L.M. (1998). Estradiol prevents kainic acid-induced neuronal loss in the rat dentate gyrus. *NeuroReport*, 9, 3075–3079.

Baba, H., Doubell, T.P., and Woolf, C.J. (1999). Peripheral inflammation facilitates Aβ fiber-mediated synaptic input to the substantia gelatinosa of the adult rat spinal cord. *Journal of Neuroscience*, 19, 859–867.

Bach-y-Rita, P. (1980). *Recovery of Function: Theoretical Considerations for Brain Injury Rehabilitation*. Huber, Bern.

Backlund, E.O., Granberg, P.O., Hamberger, B., Knutsson, E., Mårtensson, A., Sedvall, G. *et al.* (1985). Transplantation of adrenal medullary tissue to striatum in parkinsonism. *Journal of Neurosurgery*, 62, 169–173.

Bäckman, L. and Dixon, R.A. (1992). Psychological compensation: a theoretical framework. *Psychological Bulletin*, 112, 259–283.

Baddeley, A.D. (1990). *Human Memory: Theory and Practice*. Lawrence Erlbaum Associates, London.

Baddeley, A.D. and Wilson, B.A. (1994). When implicit learning fails: amnesia and the problem of error elimination. *Neuropsychologia*, 32, 53–68.

Baethmann, A., Go, K.G., and Unterberg, A. (1984). *Mechanisms of Secondary Brain Damage*. Plenum Press, New York.

Bahr, M., Przyrembel, C., and Bastmeyer, M. (1995). Astrocytes from adult-rat optic nerves are nonpermissive for regenerating retinal ganglion cell axons. *Experimental Neurology*, 131, 211–220.

Baig, S., Olsson, T., Hojeberg, B., and Link, H. (1991). Cells secreting antibodies to myelin basic protein in cerebrospinal fluid of patients with Lyme neuroborreliosis. *Neurology*, 41, 581–587.

Bailey, S.J., Wood, N.I., Samson, N.A., Rothaul, A.L., Roberts, J.C., King, P.D. *et al.* (1995). Failure of isradipine to reduce infarct size in mouse, gerbil, and rat models of cerebral-ischemia. *Stroke*, 26, 2177–2183.

Bain, P. (1993). A combined clinical and neurophysiological approach to the study of patients with tremor. *Journal of Neurology, Neurosurgery and Psychiatry*, 56, 839–844.

Bain, P.G., Mally, J., Gresty, M., and Findley, L.J. (1993). Assessing the impact of essential tremor on upper limb function. *Journal of Neurology*, 241, 54–61.

Bain, P., Findley, L.J., Thompson, P.D., Gresty, M.A., Rothwell, J.C., Harding, A.E. *et al.* (1994). A study of hereditary essential tremor. *Brain*, 117, 805–824.

Baird, A. (1993). Fibroblast growth factors: what's in a name? *Endocrinology*, 132, 487–488.

Bakay, R.A.E., Allen, G.S., Apuzzo, M.L.J., Borges, L.F., Bullard, D.E., Ojemann, G.A. *et al.* (1990). Preliminary report on adrenal medullary grafting from the American Association of Neurological Surgeons graft project. *Progress in Brain Research*, 82, 603–610.

Baker, H.F., Ridley, R.M., and Crow, T.J. (1985). Experimental transmission of an autosomal dominant spongiform encephalopathy — does the infectious agent originate in the human genome. *British Medical Journal*, 291, 299–302.

Baker, H.F., Poulter, M., Crow, T.J., Frith, C.D., Lofthouse, R., Ridley, R.M. *et al.* (1991). Amino acid polymorphism in human prion protein and age at death in inherited prion disease. *Lancet*, 337, 1286.

Ball, M.J. (1976). Neurofibrillary tangles in the dementia of

'normal pressure' hydrocephalus. *Canadian Journal of Neurological Sciences*, 3, 227–235.

Bamford, K.A., Caine, E.D., Kido, D.K., Cox, C., and Shoulson, I. (1995). A prospective evaluation of cognitive decline in early Huntington's disease: functional and radiographic correlates. *Neurology*, 45, 1867–1873.

Bandtlow, C.E., Schmidt, M.F., Hassinger, T., Kater, S., and Schwab, M.E. (1993). Role of intracellular calcium in growth cone collapse evoked by myelin-associated neurite growth inhibitors. *Journal of Cellular Biochemistry*, 248.

Bankiewicz, K.S., Oldfield, E.H., Chiueh, C.C., Doppman, J.L., Jacobowitz, D.M., and Kopin, I.J. (1986). Hemiparkinsonism in monkeys after unilateral internal carotid artery infusion of 1-methyl-4-phenyl-1,2,3,6-tetrahydropyridine (MPTP). *Life Sciences*, 39, 7–16.

Barbeau, A., Roy, M., Bernier, G., Campanella, G., and Paris, S. (1987). Ecogenetics of Parkinson's disease: prevalence and environmental aspects in rural areas. *Canadian Journal of Neurological Sciences*, 14, 36–41.

Barkats, M., Bemelmans, A.P., Geoffroy, M.C., Robert, J.J., Loquet, I., Horellou, P. *et al.* (1996). An adenovirus encoding CuZnSOD protects cultured striatal neurones against gluatmate toxicity. *NeuroReport*, 7, 497–501.

Barker, R.A., Fricker, R.A., Abrous, D.N., Fawcett, J.W., and Dunnett, S.B. (1995). A comparative study of the preparation techniques for improving the viability of nigral grafts using vital stain, *in vitro* cultures and *in vivo* grafts. *Cell Transplantation*, 4, 173–200.

Barker, R.A. and Barasi, S. (1999). *Neuroscience at a Glance*. Blackwell Scientific, Oxford.

Barker, R.A., Scolding, N.J., and Compston, D.A.S. Control of movement and its clinical disorders. In *Neurosurgery: The Scientific Basis of Clinical Practice* (ed. A. Crockard, R. Hayward and J. Hoff). Blackwell Science, Oxford. (In press.)

Barnhill, L.J. and Gualtieri, C.T. (1989). Two cases of late-onset psychosis after closed head injury. *Neuropsychiatry, Neuropsychology and Behavioural Neurology*, 2, 211–217.

Barone, F.C., Lysko, P.G., Price, W.J., Feuerstein, G., Albaracanji, K.A., Benham, C.D. *et al.* (1995). Se 201823-a antagonizes calcium currents in central neurons and reduces the effects of focal ischemia in rats and mice. *Stroke*, 26, 1683–1689.

Baron-Van Evercooren, A., Avellana-Adalid, V., Ben Younes-Chennoufi, A., Gansmuller, A., Nait-Oumesmar, B., and Vignais, L. (1996). Cell-cell interactions during the migration of myelin-forming cells transplanted in the demyelinated spinal cord. *Glia*, 16, 147–164.

Barres, B.A., Hart, I.K., Coles, H.S.R., Burne, J.F., Voyyodic, J.T., Richardson, W.D., and Raff, M.C. (1992). Cell-death and control of cell-survival in the oligodendrocyte lineage. *Cell*, 70, 31–46.

Barrett-Connor, E. and Khaw, K.T. (1990). The epidemiology of DHEAS with particular reference to cardiovascular disease: the Rancho Bernardo study. In *The Biologic Role of Dehydroepiandrosterone (DHEA)* (ed. M. Kilimi and W. Regelson), pp. 281–298. de Gruyter, Berlin.

Barry, S. and Dinan, T.G. (1990). Alpha-2 adrenergic receptor function in post-stroke depression. *Psychological Medicine*, 20, 305–309.

Barry, S., Phillips, O.M., Williams, D.C., and Dinan, T.G.

(1990). Platelet 5-HT uptake in post-stroke depression. *Acta Psychiatrica Scandinavica*, **82**, 88–89.

Bartlett, P.F., Rosenfeld, J.V., Bailey, K.A., Cheesman, H., Harvey, A.R., and Kerr, R.S.C. (1990). Allograft rejection overcome by immunoselection of neuronal precursor cells. *Progress in Brain Research*, **82**, 153–160.

Baruk, H. (1926). *Les Troubles Mentaux dans les Tumeurs Cérébrales*. Octave Doin, Paris.

Baxter, J.D. and Tyrrell, J.B. (1987). The adrenal cortex. In *Endocrinology and Metabolism* (ed. P. Felig), pp. 511–650. McGraw Hill, New York.

Baxter, L.R., Mazziotta, J.C., Pahl, J.J., Grafton, S.T., St.George-Hislop, P., Haines, J.L. *et al.* (1992). Psychiatric, genetic, and positron emission tomographic evaluation of persons at risk for Huntington's disease. *Archives of General Psychiatry*, **49**, 148–154.

Bayer, S.A. (1982). Changes in total number of dentate granule cells in juvenile and adult rats: a correlated volumetric and $^3$H-thymidine autoradiographic study. *Experimental Brain Research*, **46**, 315–323.

Bayer, S.A. (1983). $^3$H-thymidine-radiographic studies of neurogenesis in the rat olfactory bulb. *Experimental Brain Research*, **50**, 329–340.

Bayer, S.A., Yackel, J.W., and Puri, P.S. (1982). Neurons in the rat dentate gyrus granular layer substantially increase during juvenile and adult life. *Science*, **216**, 890–892.

Beal, M.F. (1992). Does impairment of energy metabolism result in excitotoxic neuronal death in neurodegenerative illnesses? *Annals of Neurology*, **31**, 119–130.

Beal, M.F., Kowall, N.W., Ellison, D.W., Mazurek, M.F., Swartz, K.J., and Martin, J.B. (1986). Replication of the neurochemical characteristics of Huntington's disease by quinolinic acid. *Nature*, **321**, 168–171.

Beal, M.F., Swartz, K.J., Hyman, B.T., Storey, E., Finn, S.F., and Koroshetz, W. (1991). Aminooxyacetic acid results in excitotoxin lesions by a novel indirect mechanism. *Journal of Neurochemistry*, **57**, 1068–1073.

Beal, M.F., Hyman, B.T., and Koroshetz, W. (1993). Do defects in mitochondrial energy metabolism underlie the pathology of neurodegenerative diseases? *Trends in Neurosciences*, **16**, 125–131.

Beck, K.D., Valverde, J., Alexi, T., Poulsen, K., Moffat, B., Vandien, R.A. *et al.* (1995). Mesencephalic dopaminergic neurons protected by GDNF from axotomy-induced degeneration in the adult brain. *Nature*, **373**, 339–341.

Becker, J.B., Robinson, T.E., Barton, P., Sintov, A., Siden, R., and Levy, R.J. (1990). Sustained behavioral recovery from unilateral nigrostriatal damage produced by the controlled release of dopamine from a silicone polymer pellet placed into the denervated striatum. *Brain Research*, **508**, 60–64.

Bell, M.D., Taub, D.D., and Perry, V.H. (1996). Overriding the brain's intrinsic resistance to leukocyte recruitment with intraparenchymal injections of recombinant chemokines. *Neuroscience*, **74**, 283–292.

Ben-Shachar, D., Eshel, G., Riederer, P., and Youdim, M.B.H. (1992). Role of iron and iron chelation in dopaminergic-induced neurodegeneration: implication for Parkinson's disease. *Annals of Neurology*, **32**, S105–110.

Bencsics, C., Wachtel, S.R., Milstien, S., Hatakeyama, K., Becker, J.B., and Kang, U.J. (1996). Double transduction with GTP cyclohydrolase I and tyrosine hydroxylase is nec-

essary for spontaneous synthesis of L-DOPA by primary fibroblasts. *Journal of Neuroscience*, **16**, 4449–4456.

Benedict, R.H.B. (1989). The effectiveness of cognitive rehabilitation remediation strategies for victims of traumatic head injury: a review of the literature. *Clinical Psychology Review*, **9**, 605–626.

Benham, C.D., Brown, T.H., Cooper, D.G., Evans, M.L., Harries, M.H., Herdon, H.J. *et al.* (1993). Sb-201823-a, a neuronal ca2+ antagonist is neuroprotective in 2 models of cerebral-ischemia. *Neuropharmacology*, **32**, 1249–1257.

Bennett, H.L., Davis, H.S., and Giannini, J.A. (1985). Nonverbal response to intraoperative conversation. *British Journal of Anaesthesia*, **57**, 174–179.

Benowitz, L.I. and Routtenberg, A. (1997). GAP-43: an intrinsic determinant of neuronal development and plasticity. *Trends in Neurosciences*, **20**, 84–91.

Benton, A.L. (1968). Differential behavioural effects in frontal lobe disease. *Neuropsychologia*, **6**, 53–60.

Benveniste, H., Drejer, J., Schousboe, A., and Diemer, N.H. (1984). Elevation of the extracellular concentrations of glutamate and aspartate in rat hippocampus during transient cerebral ischemia monitored by intracerebral microdialysis. *Journal of Neurochemistry*, **43**, 1369–1374.

Berardelli, A., Rothwell, J.C., Hallett, M., Thompson, P.D., Manfredi, M., and Marsden, C.D. (1998). The pathophysiology of primary dystonia. *Brain*, **121**, 1195–1212.

Berg, I.J., Koning-Haanstra, M., and Deelman, B.G. (1991). Long term effects of memory rehabilitation: a controlled study. *Neuropsychological Rehabilitation*, **1**, 97–111.

Berger, J.R. (1997). Myelopathy and co-infection with HIV and HTLV-1. *Neurology*, **49**, 1190–1191.

Berger, J.R., Raffanti, S., Svenningsson, A., McCarthy, M., Snodgrass, S., and Resnick, L. (1991). The role of HTLV in HIV-I associated neurological disease. *Neurology*, **41**, 197–202.

Berger, J.R., Pall, L., Lanska, D., and Whiteman, M. (1998). Progressive multifocal leukoencephalopathy in patients with HIV infection. *Journal of Neurovirology*, **4**, 59–68.

Bernheimer, H., Birkmayer, W., Hornykiewicz, O., Jellinger, K., and Seitelberger, F. (1973). Brain dopamine and the syndromes of Parkinson and Huntington. Clinical, morphological and neurochemical correlations. *Journal of the Neurological Sciences*, **20**, 415–455.

Berrios, G.E. (1982). Disorientation states in psychiatry. *Comprehensive Psychiatry*, **23**, 479–491.

Berrios, G.E. (1987). Dementia during the seventeenth and eighteenth centuries: a conceptual history. *Psychological Medicine*, **17**, 829–837.

Berrios, G.E. and Dening, T. (1990). Biological and quantitative issue in neuropsychiatry. *Behavioual Neurology*, **3**, 247–259.

Berrios, G.E. and Luque, R. (1995). Cotard's delusion or syndrome? *Comprehensive Psychiatry*, **36**, 218–223.

Berrios, G.E. and Morley, S. (1984). Koro-like symptoms in non-chinese subjects. *British Journal of Psychiatry*, **145**, 331–334.

Berrios, G.E. and Quemada, J.I. (1990). Depressive illness in multiple sclerosis. *British Journal of Psychiatry*, **156**, 10–16.

Berrios, G.E. and Samuel, C. (1987). Affective symptoms in the neurological patient. *Journal of Nervous and Mental Disease*, **175**, 173–176.

Berrios, G.E., Marková, I.S., and Gimbert, R. (1995). The role of psychiatry in genetic prediction programmes for Huntington's disease. *Psychiatric Bulletin*, **19**, 203–206.

Berrios, G.E., Wagle, A.C., and Marková, I.S. Psychiatric symptoms and CAG repeats in neurologically asymptomatic Huntington's disease gene cariers: a comparison with gene negative at risk subjects. *Archives of General Psychiatry*. (In press.)

Berry, M., Hall, S., Rees, L., Carlile, J., and Wyse, J.P.H. (1992). Regeneration of axons in the optic nerve of the adult Browman-Wyse (bw) mutant rat. *Journal of Neurocytology*, **21**, 426–448.

Berry, M., Carlile, J., and Hunter, A. (1996). Peripheral nerve explants grafted into the vitreous body of the eye promote the regeneration of retinal ganglion cell axons severed in the optic nerve. *Journal of Neurocytology*, **25**, 147–170.

Bessen, R.A., Kocisko, D.A., Raymond, G.J., Nandan, S., Lansbury, P.T., and Caughey, B. (1995). Nongenetic propagation of strain-specific properties of scrapie prion protein. *Nature*, **375**, 698–700.

Betts, T.A., Alford, C.A., and Crowe, A. (1982). Psychotropic effects of sodium valproate. *British Journal of Clinical Practice*, (Supplement), S145.

Bever-CT, J. (1994). The current status of studies of aminopyridines in patients with multiple sclerosis. *Annals of Neurology*, **36** (Supplement), S118–S121.

Beyreuther, K., Pollwein, P., Multhaup, G., Mönning, U., König, G., Dyrks, T., Schubert, W., and Masters, C.L. (1993). Regulation and expression of the Alzheimer's β/A4 amyloid protein precursor in health, disease, and Down's syndrome. *Annals of the New York Academy of Sciences*, **695**, 91–102.

Bickford, J.A.R. and Ellison, R.M. (1953). The high incidence of Huntington's chorea in the Duchy of Cornwall. *Journal of Mental Science*, **99**, 291–294.

Bilang-Bleuel, A., Revah, F., Colin, P., Locquet, I., Robert, J.J., Mallet, J. *et al.* (1997). Intrastriatal injection of an adenoviral vector expressing glial cell line-derived neurotrophic factor prevents dopaminergic neuron degeneration and behavioral impairment in a rat model of Parkinson's disease. *Proceedings of the National Academy of Sciences of the United States of America*, **94**, 8818–8823.

Bing, G., Notter, M.F.D., Hansen, J.T., and Gash, D.M. (1988). Comparison of adrenal medullary, carotid body and PC12 cell grafts in 6-OHDA lesioned rats. *Brain Research Bulletin*, **20**, 399–406.

Birkmayer, W. and Hornykiewicz, O. (1961). Der l-Dioxyphenylalanin (l-Dopa)-Effekt bei der Parkinson-Akinese. *Wiener Klinische Wochenschrift*, **73**, 787–788.

Bixby, J.L., Lilien, J., and Reichardt, L.F. (1988). Identification of the major proteins that promote neuronal process outgrowth on Schwann cells *in vitro*. *Journal of Cell Biology*, **107**, 353–361.

Biziere, K. and Coyle, J.T. (1978). Influence of cortico-striatal afferents on striatal kainic acid neurotoxicity. *Neuroscience Letters*, **8**, 303–310.

Bjornson, C.R.R., Rietze, R.L., Reynolds, B.A., Magli, M.C., and Vescovi, A.L. (1999). Turning brain into blood: a hematopoietic fate adopted by adult neural stem cells *in vivo*. *Science*, **283**, 534–537.

Björklund, A. and Stenevi, U. (1979). Reconstruction of the nigrostriatal dopamine pathway by intracerebral transplants. *Brain Research*, **177**, 555–560.

Bjorklund, A. and Stenevi, U. (1977). Experimental reinnervation of the rat hippocampus by grafted sympathetic ganglia. I. Axonal regeneration along the hippocampal fimbria. *Brain Research*, **138**, 259–270.

Björklund, A., Stenevi, U., and Svendgaard, N.-A. (1976). Growth of transplanted monoaminergic neurones into the adult hippocampus along the perforant path. *Nature*, **262**, 787–790.

Björklund, A., Schmidt, R.H., and Stenevi, U. (1980a). Functional reinnervation of the neostriatum in the adult rat by use of intraparenchymal grafting of dissociated cell suspensions from the substantia nigra. *Cell and Tissue Research*, **212**, 39–45.

Björklund, A., Dunnett, S.B., Stenevi, U., Lewis, M.E., and Iversen, S.D. (1980b). Reinnervation of the denervated striatum by substantia nigra transplants: functional consequences as revealed by pharmacological and sensorimotor testing. *Brain Research*, **199**, 307–333.

Björklund, A., Stenevi, U., Dunnett, S.B., and Gage, F.H. (1982). Cross-species neural grafting in a rat model of Parkinson's disease. *Nature*, **298**, 652–654.

Björklund, A., Stenevi, U., Schmidt, R.H., Dunnett, S.B., and Gage, F.H. (1983a). Intracerebral grafting of neuronal cell-suspensions. I. Introduction and general methods of preparation. *Acta Physiologica Scandinavica, supplementum*, **522**, 1–7.

Björklund, A., Stenevi, U., Schmidt, R.H., Dunnett, S.B., and Gage, F.H. (1983b). Intracerebral grafting of neuronal cell suspensions. II. Survival and growth of nigral cell suspensions implanted in different brain sites. *Acta Physiological Scandinavica, supplementum*, **522**, 9–18.

Black, J.E., Sirevaag, A.M., and Greenough, W.T. (1987). Complex experience promotes capillary formation in young rat visual cortex. *Neuroscience Letters*, **83**, 351–355.

Blakemore, W.F. (1961). Ultrastructural study of remyelination in an experimental lesion in the adult cat spinal cord. *Journal of Biophysics, Biochemistry and Cytology*, **10**, 67–94.

Blakemore, W.F. (1974). Pattern of remyelination in the CNS. *Nature*, **249**, 577–578.

Blakemore, W.F. (1976). Invasion of Schwann cells into the spinal cord of the rat following local injections of lysolecithin. *Neuropathology and Applied Neurobiology*, **4**, 47–59.

Blakemore, W.F. (1977). Remyelination of CNS axons by Schwann cells transplanted from the sciatic nerve. *Nature*, **266**, 68–69.

Blakemore, W.F., Crang, A.J., and Franklin, R.J.M. (1995). Transplantation of glia. In *Neuroglia* (ed. H. Kettenmann and B.R. Ransom), pp. 869–882. Oxford University Press, New York.

Blakemore, W.F. and Franklin, R.J.M. (2000). Transplantation options for therapeutic central nervous system remyelination. *Cell Transplantation*, **9**, 289–294.

Blanc-Garin, J. (1994). Patterns of recovery from hemiplegia following stroke. *Neuropsychological Rehabilitation*, **4**, 359–385.

Blauer, K.L., Poth, M., Rogers, W.M., and Bernton, E.W. (1991). Dehydroepiandrosterone antagonizes the suppressive effects of dexamethasone on lymphocyte proliferation. *Endocrinology*, **129**, 3174–3179.

Bleuler, M. (1900). Psychiatry of cerebral diseases. *British Medical Journal*, 1233–1238.

Blomer, U., Naldini, L., Kafri, T., Trono, D., Verma, I.M., and Gage, F.H. (1997). Highly efficient and sustained gene transfer in adult neurons with a lentivirus vector. *Journal of Virology*, **71**, 6641–6649.

Blond, S., Caparros, L.D., Parker, F., Assaker, R., Petit, H., Guieu, J.D. *et al.* (1992). Control of tremor and involuntary movement disorders by chronic stereotactic stimulation of the ventral intermediate thalamic nucleus. *Journal of Neurosurgery*, **77**, 62–68.

Bluma, S., Shearer, M., Frohman, A., and Hilliard, J. (1976). *Portage Guide to Early Education.* Co-operative Educational Service Agency, Wisconsin, USA.

Boast, C.A., Gerhardt, S.C., Pastor, G., Lehmann, J., Etienne, P.E., and Liebman, J.M. (1988). The n-methyl-d-aspartate antagonists CGS-19755 and CPP reduce ischemic brain-damage in gerbils. *Brain Research*, **442**, 345–348.

Boer, G.J. (1994). Ethical guidelines for the use of human embryonic or fetal tissue for experimental and clinical neurotransplantation and research. *Journal of Neurology*, **242**, 1–13.

Bohn, M.C., Cupit, L., Marciano, F., and Gash, D.M. (1987). Adrenal grafts enhance recovery of striatal dopaminergic fibers. *Science*, **237**, 913–916.

Bohnen, N., Twijnstra, A., Kroeze, J., and Jolles, J. (1991). A psychophysiological method for assessing visual and acoustic hyperaesthesia in patients with mild head injury. *British Journal of Psychiatry*, **159**, 860–863.

Bohnen, N. and Jolles, J. (1992). Neurobehavioural aspects of postconcussive symptoms after mild head injury. *Journal of Nervous and Mental Disease*, **180**, 683–692.

Bolt, J.M.W. (1970). Huntington's chorea in West of Scotland. *British Journal of Psychiatry*, **116**, 259–270.

Bonhoeffer, K. (1910). *Die symptomatischen Psychosen.* Leipzig, Deuticke.

Bornstein, R.A., Miller, H.B., and Van Schoor, J.T. (1989). Neuropsychological deficit and emotional disturbance in head-injured patients. *Journal of Neurosurgery*, **70**, 509–513.

Borod, J.C., Koff, E., Lorch, M.P., and Nicholas, M. (1985). Channels of emotional expression in patients with unilateral brain damage. *Archives of Neurology*, **42**, 345–348.

Botez, M.I., Botez, M.T., Elie, R., Pedraza, O.L., Goyette, K., and Lalonde, R. (1996). Amantadine hydrochloride treatment in heredodegenerative ataxias: a double blind study. *Journal of Neurology, Neurosurgery and Psychiatry*, **61**, 259–264.

Boyle, M.E. and Greer, R.D. (1983). Operant procedures and the comatose patient. *Journal of Applied Behaviour Analysis*, **16**, 3–12.

Braak, H. and Braak, E. (1991). Neuropathological stageing of Alzheimer-related changes. *Acta Neuropathologica*, **82**, 239–259.

Bradbury, M.W. (1993). The blood-brain barrier. *Exp.Physiol.*, **78**, 453–472.

Bradbury, E.J., Kershaw, T.R., Marchbanks, R.M., and Sinden, J.D. (1995). Astrocyte transplants alleviate lesion induced memory deficits independently of cholinergic recovery. *Neuroscience*, **65**, 955–972.

Bradbury, E.J., Khemani, S., King, V.R., Priestley, J.V., and McMahon, S.B. (1998). NT-3 promotes growth of adult rat sensory axons ascending in the dorsal columns of the spinal cord. *European Journal of Neuroscience*, **11**, 3773–3883.

Bradley, J.R., Lockwood, C.M., and Thiru, S. (1994). Endothelial cell activation in patients with systemic vasculitis. *QJM.*, **87**, 741–745.

Bradbury, M. (1979). *The concept of the blood brain barrier.* John Wiley, New York.

Brain, L. and Wilkinson, M. (1965). Subacute cerebellar degeneration associated with neoplasms. *Brain*, **88**, 465–478.

Brandt, J. and Butters, N. (1996). Neuropsychological characteristics of Huntington's disease. In *Neuropsychological Assessment of Neuropsychiatric Disorders* (ed. I. Grant and K.M. Adams), pp. 321–341. Oxford University Press, Oxford.

Brandt, J., Folstein, S.E., and Folstein, M.F. (1988). Differential cognitive impairment in Alzheimer's disease and Huntington's disease. *Annals of Neurology*, **23**, 555–561.

Brandt, J., Bylsma, F.W., Gross, R., Stine, O.C., Ranen, N., and Ross, C.A. (1996). Trinucleotide repeat length and clinical progression in Huntington's disease. *Neurology*, **46**, 527–531.

Braughler, J.M., Hall, E.D., Jacobsen, E.J., McCall, E.M., and Means, E.D. (1989). The 21-aminosteroids: potent inhibitors of lipid peroxidation for the treatment of central nervous system trauma and ischemia. *Drug Future*, **14**, 143–152.

Bravin, M., Savio, T., Strata, P., and Rossi, F. (1997). Olivocerebellar axon regeneration and target reinnervation following dissociated Schwann cell grafts in surgically injured cerebella of adult rats. *European Journal of Neuroscience*, **9**, 2634–2649.

Brawn, K. and Fridovich, I. (1981). DNA strand scission by enzymatically generated oxygen free radicals. *Archives of Biochemistry and Biophysics*, **206**, 414–419.

Brecknell, J.E. and Fawcett, J.W. (1996). Axonal regeneration. *Biological Reviews of the Cambridge Philosophical Society*, **71**, 227–255.

Brecknell, J.E., Du, J.-S., Muir, E.M., Fidler, P.S., Hlavin, M.-L., Dunnett, S.B. *et al.* (1996). Bridge grafts of fibroblast growth factor-4-secreting Schwannoma cells promote functional axonal regeneration in the nigrostriatal pathway of the adult rat. *Neuroscience*, **74**, 775–784.

Bregman, B.S., Kunkel-Bagden, E., Reier, P.J., Dai, H.N., McAtee, M., and Gao, D. (1993). Recovery of function after spinal cord injury: mechanisms underlying transplant-mediated recovery of function differ after spinal cord injury in newborn and adult rats. *Experimental Neurology*, **123**, 3–16.

Bregman, B.S., Kunkel-Bagden, E., Schnell, L., Dai, H.N., Gao, D., and Schwab, M.E. (1995). Recovery from spinal cord injury mediated by antibodies to neurite growth inhibitors. *Nature*, **378**, 498–501.

Brenner, R., Hyman, N., Knobler, R., O'Brien, M., and Stephan, T. (1998). An approach to switching patients from baclofen to tizanidine. *Hosp.Med.*, **59**, 778–782.

Brick, J.E. and Brick, J.F. (1989). Neurologic manifestations of rheumatologic disease. *Neurologic Clinics*, **7**, 629–639.

Bricolo, A., Turazzi, S., and Feriotti, G. (1980). Prolonged traumatic unconsciousness: Therapeutic assets and liabilities. *Journal of Neurosurgery*, **52**, 625–634.

Brierly, J.B., Corsellis, J.A., Hierons, L., and Nevin, S. (1960). Subacute encephalitis of later adult life mainly affecting the limbic areas. *Brain*, 83, 357–368.

Brinkmann, R., von Cramon, D., and Schulz, H. (1976). The Munich Coma Scale (MCS). *Journal of Neurology, Neurosurgery and Psychiatry*, 39, 788–793.

Brooke, M.M., Questad, K.A., Patterson, D.R., and Bashak, K.J. (1992). Agitation and restlessness after closed head-injury: a prospective study of 100 consecutive admissions. *Archives of Physical Medicine and Rehabilitation*, 73, 320–323.

Brooks, N. (1984). *Closed Injury: Psychological, Social and Family Consequences*. Oxford University Press, Oxford.

Brothers, C.R.D. (1964). The history and incidence of Huntington's chorea in Tasmania. *Journal of Neurological Science*, 1, 405–420.

Brothers, C.R.D. and Meadows, AW. (1955). An investigation of Huntington's chorea in Victoria. *Journal of Mental Science*, 101, 548–563.

Brouillet, E., Henshaw, D.R., Schulz, J.B., and Beal, M.F. (1994). Aminooxyacetic acid striatal lesions attenuated by 1,3-butanediol and coenzyme Q(10). *Neuroscience Letters*, 177, 58–62.

Brouwer, E., Huitema, M.G., Mulder, A.H., Heeringa, P., van, G.H., Tervaert, J.W., Weening, J.J., and Kallenberg, C.G. (1994a). Neutrophil activation *in vitro* and *in vivo* in Wegener's granulomatosis. *Kidney Int.*, 45, 1120–1131.

Brouwer, E., Stegeman, C.A., Huitema, M.G., Limburg, P.C., and Kallenberg, C.G. (1994b). T cell reactivity to proteinase 3 and myeloperoxidase in patients with Wegener's granulomatosis (WG). *Clin.Exp.Immunol.*, 98, 448–453.

Brown, P. (1987). Causes of human spongiform encephalopathy. In *Prion Diseasess* (ed. H.F. Baker and R.M. Ridley), pp. 139–154. Humana Press, Totowa, NJ.

Brown, P. (1996). Myclonus. *Current Opinion In Neurology*, 9, 314–316.

Brown, J.D. and Larson, E.B. (1993). Drug induced cognitive impairment: defining the problem and finding solutions. *Drugs and Aging*, 3, 349.

Brown, R.G. and Marsden, C.D. (1988). Subcortical dementia: the neuropsychological evidence. *Neuroscience*, 25, 363–387.

Brown, P., Preece, M.A., and Will, R.G. (1992). Friendly fire in medicine — hormones, homografts, and Creutzfeldt–Jakob disease. *Lancet*, 340, 24–27.

Browne, S.E., Bowling, A.C., MacGarvey, U., Baik, M.J., Berger, S.C., Muqit, M.M. *et al.* (1997). Oxidative damage and metabolic dysfunction in Huntington's disease: Selective vulnerability of the basal ganglia. *Annals of Neurology*, 41, 646–653.

Browne, S.E., Ferrante, R.J., and Beal, M.F. (1999). Oxidative stress in Huntington's disease. *Brain Pathology*, 9, 147–163.

Bruce, M.E., Will, R.G., Ironside, J.W., McConnell, I., Drummond, D., Suttie, A. *et al.* (1997). Transmissions to mice indicate that 'new variant' CJD is caused by the BSE agent. *Nature*, 389, 498–501.

Bruce, M.E., Fraser, H., McBride, P.A., Scott, J.R., and Dickinson, A.G. (1999). The basis of strain variation in scrapie. In *Prion Diseases of Humans and Animals* (ed. S.B. Prusiner, J. Collinge, J. Powell and B.H. Anderton), pp. 497–508. Ellis Horwood, New York.

Brück, W., Schmied, M., Suchanek, G., Bruck, Y., Breitschopf, H., Poser, S. *et al.* (1994). Oligodendrocytes in the early course of multiple sclerosis. *Annals of Neurology*, 35, 65–73.

Brundin, P. (1992). Dissection, preparation, and implantation of human embryonic brain tissue. In *Neural Transplantation: a Practical Approach* (ed. S.B. Dunnett and A. Björklund), pp. 139–160. IRL Press, Oxford.

Brundin, P., Nilsson, O.G., Gage, F.H., and Björklund, A. (1985a). Cyclosporin-A increases survival of cross-species intrastriatal grafts of embryonic dopamine containing neurons. *Experimental Brain Research*, 60, 204–208.

Brundin, P., Barbin, G., Isacson, O., Mallat, M., Chamak, B., Prochiantz, A. *et al.* (1985b). Survival of intracerebrally grafted rat dopamine neurons previously cultured *in vitro*. *Neuroscience Letters*, 61, 79–84.

Brundin, P., Nilsson, O.G., Strecker, R.E., Lindvall, O., Åstedt, B., and Björklund, A. (1986). Behavioral effects of human fetal dopamine neurons grafted in a rat model of Parkinson's disease. *Experimental Brain Research*, 65, 235–240.

Brundin, P., Widner, H., Nilsson, O.G., Strecker, R.E., and Björklund, A. (1989). Intracerebral xenografts of dopamine neurons: the role of immunosuppression and the blood-brain barrier. *Experimental Brain Research*, 75, 195–207.

Bruno, J.P., Jackson, D., Zigmond, M.J., and Stricker, E.M. (1987). Effect of dopamine-depleting brain lesions in rat pups: role of striatal serotonergic neurons in behavior. *Behavioral Neuroscience*, 101, 806–811.

Brustle, O., Spiro, A.C., Karram, K., Choudhary, K., Okabe, S., and McKay, R.D.G. (1997). *In vitro*-generated neural precursors participate in mammalian brain development. *Proceedings of the National Academy of Sciences of the United States of America*, 94, 14809–14814.

Bruyn, G.W. and Lanser, J.B.K. (1990). The post concussional syndrome. In *Handbook of Clinical Neurology, Vol. 13, Head Injury* (ed. R. Braackman), pp. 421–427. Elsevier, New York.

Büeler, H., Fischer, M., Lang, Y., Bluethmann, H., Lipp, H.P., Dearmond, S.J. *et al.* (1992). Normal development and behavior of mice lacking the neuronal cell-surface prp protein. *Nature*, 356, 577–582.

Bumke, O. (1946). *Nuevo Tratado de Enfermedades Mentales (Spanish Translation)*. F. Seix, Barcelona.

Bunge, M.B., Bunge, R.P., and Ris, H. (1961). Ultrastructural study of remyelination in an experimental lesion in the adult cat spinal cord. *Journal of Biophysics, Biochemistry and Cytology*, 10, 67–94.

Burgess, P.W. (1998). Theory and methodology in executive function research. In *Methodology of Frontal and Executive Functions* (ed. P. Rabbitt), pp. 81–111. Psychology Press, Hove.

Burke, J.M., Imhoff, C.L., and Kerrigan, J.M. (1990). MMPI correlates among post-acute TBI patients. *Brain Injury*, 4, 223–231.

Burkle and Lipowski, Z. (1978). Colloid cyst of the third ventricle presenting as a psychiatric disorder. *American Journal of Psychiatry*, 135, 373–374.

Burns, R.S., Chiueh, C.C., Markey, S.P., Ebert, M.H., Jacobowitz, D.M., and Kopin, I.J. (1983). A primate model of parkinsoism: selective destruction of dopaminergic neurons in the pars compacta of the substantia nigra by n-methyl-4-phenyl-1,23,6-tetrahydropyridine. *Proceedings of the National Academy of Sciences of the United States of America*, **80**, 4546–4550.

Burns, A., Folstein, S.E., Brandt, J., and Folstein, M.F. (1990). Clinical assessment of irritability, aggression and apathy in Huntington's and Alzheimer's disease. *Journal of Nervous and Mental Disease*, **178**, 20–26.

Burns, J.C., Friedmann, T., Driever, W., Burrascano, M., and Yee, J.K. (1993). Vesicular stomatitis-virus g glycoprotein pseudotyped retroviral vectors — concentration to very high-titer and efficient gene-transfer into mammalian and nonmammalian cells. *Proceedings of the National Academy of Sciences of the United States of America*, **90**, 8033–8037.

Burright, E.N., Orr, H.T., and Clark, H.B. (1997). Mouse models of human CAG repeat disorders. *Brain Pathology*, **7**, 965–977.

Butterfield, P.G., Valanis, B.G., Spencer, P.S., Lindeman, C.A., and Nutt, J.G. (1993). Environmental antecedents of young-onset Parkinson's disease. *Neurology*, **43**, 1150–1158.

Bye, C., Clubley, M., and Peck, A.W. (1978). Drowsiness, impaired performance and tricyclic antidepressant drugs. *British Journal of Clinical Pharmacology*, **6**, 155.

Cabelli, R.J., Shelton, D.L., Segal, R.A., and Shatz, C.J. (1997). Blockade of endogenous ligands of trkB inhibits formation of ocular dominance columns. *Neuron*, **19**, 63–76.

Caceres, A. and Steward, O. (1983). Dendritic reorganization in the denervated dentate gyrus of the rat following entorhinal cortical lesions — a Golgi and electron microscopic analysis. *Journal of Comparative Neurology*, **214**, 387–403.

Cain, D.P. (1989). Long-term potentiation and kindling: how similar are the mechanisms? *Trends in Neurosciences*, **12**, 6–10.

Caine, E.D., Hunt, R.D., Weingartner, H., and Ebert, M.H. (1978). Huntington's dementia. *Archives of General Psychiatry*, **35**, 377–384.

Caine, E.D. and Shoulson, I. (1983). Psychiatric syndrome in Huntington's disease. *American Journal of Psychiatry*, **140**, 728–733.

Cairns, H., Oldfield, F., Pennybacker, J., and Whitteridge, D. (1941). Akinetic mutism an epidermoid cyst of the 3rd ventricle. *Brain*, **64**, 273–290.

Cairns, H. (1950). Mental Disorders with tumours of the pons. *Folia Psychiatrica, Neurologica et Neurochirurgica Nederlandica*, **53**, 193–203.

Cajal, S.R.y. (1928). *Degeneration and Regeneration of the Nervous System*. Oxford University Press, Oxford.

Calne, S., Schoenberg, B., Martin, W., Uitti, R.J., Spencer, P., and Calne, D.B. (1987). Familial Parkinson's disease: possible role of environmental factors. *Canadian Journal of Neurological Sciences*, **14**, 303–305.

Caltagirone, C., Gainotti, G., Masullo, C., and Villa, G. (1982). Neuropsychological study of normal pressure hydrocephalus. *Acta Psychiatrica Scandinavica*, **65**, 93–100.

Cameron, H.A. and Gould, E. (1994). Adult neurogenesis is regulated by adrenal steroids in the dentate gyrus. *Neuroscience*, **61**, 203–209.

Cameron, H.A., Tanapat, P., and Gould, E. (1998). Adrenal steroids and N-methyl-D-aspartate receptor activation regulate neurogenesis in the dentate gyrus of adult rats through a common pathway. *Neuroscience*, **82**, 349–354.

Campagna, J.A., Ruegg, M.A., and Bixby, J.L. (1995). Agrin is a differentiation-inducing "stop signal" for motoneurons *in vitro*. *Neuron*, **15**, 1365–1374.

Campenot, R.B. (1981). Regeneration of neurites in long-term cultures of sympathetic neurons deprived of nerve growth factor. *Science*, **214**, 579–581.

Campenot, R.B. (1982). Development of sympathetic neurons in compartmentalised cultures II. Local control of neurite survival by nerve growth factor. *Developmental Biology*, **93**, 13–21.

Campodonico, J.R., Codori, A.M., and Brandt, J. (1996). Neuropsychological stability over two disease mutation. *Journal of Neurology, Neurosurgery and Psychiatry*, **61**, 621–624.

Canning, D.R., Hoke, A., Malemud, C.J., and Silver, J. (1996). A potent inhibitor of neurite outgrowth that predominates in the extracellular matrix of reactive astrocytes. *International Journal of Developmental Neuroscience*, **14**, 153–175.

Capogna, M., Fankhauser, C., Gagliardini, V., Gahwiler, B.H., and Thompson, S.M. (1999). Excitatory synaptic transmission and its modulation by PKC is unchanged in the hippocampus of GAP-43-deficient mice. *European Journal of Neuroscience*, **11**, 433–440.

Carette, B. and Poulain, P. (1984). Excitatory effect of dehydroepiandrosterone, its sulfate ester and pregnenolone sulfate, applied by iontophoresis and pressure, on single neurons in the septo-preoptic area of the guinea pig. *Neuroscience Letters*, **45**, 205–210.

Carlsson, A. (1959). The occurrence, distribution and physiological role of catecholamines in the nervous system. *Pharmacological Review*, **11**, 490–493.

Carlsson, A. (1987). Perspectives on the discovery of central monoaminergic neurotransmission. *Annual Review of Neuroscience*, **10**, 19–40.

Carlson, L.E. and Sherwin, B.B. (1998). Steroid hormones, memory and mood in a healthy elderly population. *Psychoneuroendocrinology*, **23**, 583–603.

Carlstedt, T. (1985). Regenerating axons form nerve terminals at astrocytes. *Brain Research*, **347**, 188–191.

Carlstedt, T. (1997). Nerve fibre regeneration across the peripheral-central transitional zone. *Journal of Anatomy*, **190**, 51–60.

Carlstedt-Duke, J., Denis, M., Bonifer, C., Strömstedt, P.E., Dahlman, K., Wikström, A.C. *et al.* (1988). Structure and expression of the glucocorticoid receptor. In *Steroid Receptors and Disease* (ed. P.J. Sheridan, K. Blum and M.C. Trachtenberg), pp. 189–206. Marcel Dekker, New York.

Carlstedt, T., Cullheim, S., Risling, M., and Ulfhake, B. (1989). Nerve fibre regeneration across the PNS-CNS interface at the root-spinal cord junction. *Brain Research Bulletin*, **22**, 93–102.

Caroni, P. (1997). Intrinsic neuronal determinants that promote axonal sprouting and elongation. *BioEssays*, **19**, 767–775.

Carpenter, D.E. and Stevens, J.G. (1996). Long-term expression of a foreign gene from a unique position in the latent herpes simplex virus genome. *Human Gene Therapy*, **7**, 1447–1454.

Carpenter, M.K. (1999). *In vitro* expansion of a multipotent population of human neural progenitor cells. *Experimental Neurology*, **158**, 265–278.

Carroll, W.M., Jennings, A.R., and Ironside, L.J. (1998). Identification of the adult resting progenitor cell by autoradiographic tracking of oligodendrocyte precursors in experimental CNS demyelination. *Brain*, **121**, 293–302.

Carroll, S.L., Silossantiago, I., Frese, S.E., Ruit, K.G., Milbrandt, J., and Snider, W.D. (1992). Dorsal-root ganglion neurons expressing trk are selectively sensitive to ngf deprivation inutero. *Neuron*, **9**, 779–788.

Carter, D.A., Bray, G.M., and Aguayo, A.J. (1994). Long-term growth and remodeling of regenerated retino-collicular connections in adult hamsters. *Journal of Neuroscience*, **14**, 590–598.

Carter, R.J., Lione, L.A., Humby, T., Mangiarini, L., Mahal, A., Bates, G.P. *et al.* (1999). Characterisation of progressive motor deficits in mice transgenic for the human Huntington's disease mutation. *Journal of Neuroscience*, **19**, 3248–3257.

Carvalho, D., Savage, C.O., Black, C.M., and Pearson, J.D. (1996). IgG antiendothelial cell autoantibodies from scleroderma patients induce leukocyte adhesion to human vascular endothelial cells *in vitro*. Induction of adhesion molecule expression and involvement of endothelium-derived cytokines. *Journal of Clinical Investigation*, **97**, 111–119.

Casaccia-Bonnefil, P., Carter, B.D., Dobrowsky, R.T., and Chao, M.V. (1996). Death of oligodendrocytes mediated by the interaction of nerve growth factor with its receptor p75. *Nature*, **383**, 716–719.

Casmiro, M., D'Alessandro, R., Cacciatore, F.M., Daidone, R., Calbucci, F., and Lugaresi, E. (1989). Risk factors for the syndrome of ventricular enlargement with gait apraxia (idopathic normal pressure hydrocephalus): a case-control study. *Journal of Neurology, Neurosurgery and Psychiatry*, **52**, 847–857.

Catalano, S.M., Chang, C.K., and Shatz, C.J. (1997). Activity-dependent regulation of NMDAR1 immunoreactivity in the developing visual cortex. *Journal of Neuroscience*, **17**, 8376–8390.

Chalfie, M., Yu, Y., Euskirchen, G., Ward, W.W., and Prasher, D.C. (1994). Green fluorescent protein as a marker for gene expression. *Science*, **263**, 802–805.

Chamberlain, M.A., Neumann, V., and Tennant, A. (1995). *Traumatic Brain Injury Rehabilitation: Services, Treatments and Outcomes*. Chapman & Hall, London.

Chandler, J.H., Reed, T.E., and DeJong, R.N. (1960). Huntington's chorea in Michigan. III. Clinical observations. *Neurology*, **10**, 148–153.

Chao, H.M. and McEwen, B.S. (1994). Glucocorticoids and the expression of messenger RNAs for neurotrophins, their receptors and GAP-43 in the rat hippocampus. *Molecular Brain Research*, **26**, 271–276.

Chapelon, C., Ziza, J.M., Piette, J.C., Levy, Y., Raguin, G., Wechsler, B. *et al.* (1990). Neurosarcoidosis: signs, course and treatment in 35 confirmed cases. *Medicine Baltimore*, **69**, 261–276.

Chaturvedi, S., Ostbye, T., Stoessl, A.J., Merskey, H., and Hachinski, V. (1995). Environmental exposures in elderly Canadians with Parkinson's disease. *Canadian Journal of Neurological Sciences*, **22**, 232–234.

Chen, K.S. and Gage, F.H. (1995). Somatic gene transfer of NGF to the aged brain: behavioral and morphological amelioration. *Journal of Neuroscience*, **15**, 2819–2825.

Chen, R., Corwell, B., Yaseen, Z., Hallett, M., and Cohen, L.G. (1998). Mechanisms of cortical reorganization in lower limb amputees. *Journal of Neuroscience*, **18**, 3443–3450.

Cheng, H., Cao, Y.H., and Olson, L. (1996). Spinal cord repair in adult paraplegic rats — partial restoration of hind-limb function. *Science*, **273**, 510–513.

Choi, D.W. (1988). Glutamate neurotoxicity and diseases of the nervous system. *Neuron*, **1**, 623–634.

Choi, D.W. (1990). Cerebral hypoxia: some new approaches and unanswered questions. *Journal of Neuroscience*, **10**, 2493–2501.

Choi, D.W. (1992). Excitotoxic cell death. *Journal of Neurobiology*, **23**, 1261–1276.

Choi, D.W. (1999). Calcium-mediated neurotoxicity: relationship to specific channel types and role in ischemic damage. *Trends in Neurosciences*, **11**, 465–469.

Choi-Lundberg, D.L., Lin, Q., Chang, Y.N., Chiang, Y.L., Hay, C.M., Mohajeri, H. *et al.* (1997). Dopaminergic neurons protected from degeneration by GDNF gene therapy. *Science*, **275**, 838–841.

Chollet, F. and Weiller, C. (1994). Imaging recovery of function following brain injury. *Current Opinion in Neurobiology*, **4**, 226–230.

Chollet, F., Di Piero, V., Wise, R.J.S., Brooks, D.J., Dolan, R.J., and Frackowiak, R.S.J. (1991). The functional anatomy of motor recovery after stroke in humans: a study with positron emission tomography. *Annals of Neurology*, **29**, 63–71.

Chong, M.S., Reynolds, M.L., Irwin, N., Coggeshall, R.E., Emson, P.C., Benowitz, L.I. *et al.* (1994). GAP-43 expression in primary sensory neurons following central axotomy. *Journal of Neuroscience*, **14**, 4375–4384.

Chong, M.S., Woolf, C.J., Turmaine, M., Emson, P.C., and Anderson, P.N. (1996). Intrinsic versus extrinsic factors in determining the regeneration of the central processes of rat dorsal root ganglion neurons: The influence of a peripheral nerve graft. *Journal of Comparative Neurology*, **370**, 97–104.

Chou, Y.C., Lin, W.J., and Sapolsky, R.M. (1994). Glucocorticoids increase extracellular [$^3$H] D-aspartate overflow in hippocampal cultures during cyanide-induced ischemia. *Brain Research*, **654**, 8–14.

Chowdhury, M., Kundu, M., and Khalili, K. (1993). GA/GC-rich sequence confers Tat responsiveness to human neurotropic virus promoter, JCVL, in cells derived from central nervous system. *Oncogene*, **8**, 887–892.

Chretien, F., Belec, L., Hilton, D.A., Flament-Saillour, M., Guillon, F. *et al.* (1996). Herpes simplex virus type 1 encephalitis in acquired immunodeficiency syndrome. *Neuropathology and Applied Neurobiology*, **22**, 394–404.

Cid, M.C., Grau, J.M., Casademont, J., Campo, E., Coll, V.B., Lopez, S.A. *et al.* (1994). Immunohistochemical characterization of inflammatory cells and immunologic activation markers in muscle and nerve biopsy specimens from patients with systemic polyarteritis nodosa. *Arthritis Rheum.*, **37**, 1055–1061.

Cipolotti, L. and Warrington, E.K. (1995). Neuropsychological Assessment. *Journal of Neurology, Neurosurgery and Psychiatry*, **58**, 655–664.

Clark, K.R., Voulgaropoulou, F., and Johnson, P.R. (1996). A stable cell line carrying adenovirus-inducible rep and cap genes allows for infectivity titration of adeno-associated virus vectors. *Gene Therapy*, **3**, 1124–1132.

Clark, S.A., Allard, T., Jenkins, W.M., and Merzenich, M.M. (1988). Receptive field in the body surface map in adult cortex defined by temporally correlated inputs. *Nature*, **332**, 444–445.

Clarke, D.J. and Dunnett, S.B. (1993). Synaptic relationships between cortical and dopaminergic inputs and intrinsic GABAergic systems within intrastriatal striatal grafts. *Journal of Chemical Neuroanatomy*, **6**, 147–158.

Clinton, J., Ambler, M.W., and Roberts, G.W. (1991). Post-traumatic Alzheimer's disease: preponderance of a single plaque type. *Neuropathology and Applied Neurobiology*, **17**, 69–74.

Clothier, J. and Grotta, J. (1991). Recognition and management of post-stroke depression in the elderly. *Clinical and Geriatric Medicine*, **7**, 493–506.

Clough, C.G. (1987). A case of normal pressure hydrocephalus presenting as levodopa responsive Parkinsonism. *Journal of Neurology, Neurosurgery and Psychiatry*, **50**, 234.

Cockrell, J.R. and Folstein, M.F. (1988). Mini-Mental State Examination (MMSE). *Psychopharmacology Bulletin*, **24**, 689–692.

Coffey, C.E. and Figiel, G.S. (1991). Neuropsychiatric significance of subcortical encephalomalacia. In *Psychopathology and the Brain* (ed. B.J. Carroll and J.E. Barrett), pp. 243–264. Raven Press, New York.

Coffey, P.J., Lund, R.D., and Rawlins, J.N.P. (1989). Retinal transplant-mediated learning in a conditioned suppression task in rats. *Proceedings of the National Academy of Sciences of the United States of America*, **86**, 7248–7249.

Coffey, R.J., Cahill, D., Steers, W., Park, T.S., Ordia, J., Meythaler *et al.* (1993). Intrathecal baclofen for intractable spasticity of spinal origin: results a long-term multi-centre study. *Journal of Neurosurgery*, **78**, 226–232.

Cohadon, F., Richer, E., and Castel, J.P. (1991). Head injuries: incidence and outcome. *Journal of Neurological Sciences*, **103**, s27–s31.

Cohen, A., Bray, G.M., and Aguayo, A.J. (1994). Neurotrophin-4/5 (NT-4/5) Increases adult rat retinal ganglion cell survival and neurite outgrowth *in vitro*. *Journal of Neurobiology*, **25**, 953–959.

Cohen, J.A. and Lisak, R.P. (1987). Acute disseminated encephalomyelitis. In: Arnason, J.A., Behan, W.M.H., and Behan, P.O. eds. *Clinical Neuroimmunology*. London, Blackwell Scientific pp. 192–213.

Collinge, J. and Palmer, M.S. (1992). Molecular genetics of inherited, sporadic and iatrogenic prion disease. In *Prion Diseases of Humans and ANimals* (ed. S.B. Prusiner, J. Collinge, J.F. Powell and B.H. Anderton), pp. 95–119. Ellis Horwood, New York.

Collinge, J. and Palmer, M.S. (1997). *Prion Diseases*. Oxford University Press, Oxford.

Colton, C.A., Pagan, F., Snell, J., Colton, J.S., Cummins, A., and Gilbert, D.L. (1995). Protection form oxidation enhances the survival of cultured mesencephalic neurons. *Experimental Neurology*, **132**, 54–61.

Comella, C.L. and Tanner, C.M. (1995). Anticholinergic drugs in the treatment of Parkinson's disease. In *Therapy of Parkinson's Disease* (ed. W.C. Koller and G. Paulson), pp. 109–122. Marcel Dekker Inc, New York.

Compston, D.A.S. (1997). Genetic epidemiology of multiple sclerosis. *Journal of Neurology Neurosurgery and Psychiatry*, **62**, 553–561.

Conquet, F., Bashir, Z.I., Davies, C.H., Daniel, H., Ferraguti, F., Bordi, F. *et al.* (1994). Motor deficit and impairment of synaptic plasticity in mice lacking MGluR1. *Nature*, **372**, 237–243.

Conway, J.E., Zolotukhin, S., Muzyczka, N., Hayward, G.S., and Byrne, B.J. (1997). Recombinant adeno-associated virus type 2 replication and packaging is entirely supported by a herpes simplex virus type 1 amplicon expressing Rep and Cap. *Journal of Virology*, **71**, 8780–8789.

Cooper, J.E., Kendell, R.E., Gurland, B.J., Sharp, L., Copeland, J.R.M., and Simon, R. (1972). *Psychiatric Diagnoses in New York and London, Maudsley Monographs No. 20*. Oxford University Press, London.

Corder, E.H., Saunders, A.M., Strittmatter, W.J., Schmechel, D.E., Gaskell, P.C., Small, G.W. *et al.* (1993). Gene dose of apolipoprotein E type 4 allele and the risk of Alzheimer's disease in late onset families. *Science*, **261**, 921–923.

Corpechot, C., Synguelakis, M., Talha, S., Axelson, M., Sjovall, J., Vihko, R. *et al.* (1983). Pregnenolone and its sulfate ester in the rat brain. *Brain Research*, **270**, 119–125.

Corpechot, C., Young, J., Calvel, M., Wehrey, C., Veltz, J.N., Touyer, G., Mouren, M. *et al.* (1993). Neurosteroids — 3-α-hydroxy-5-α-pregnan-20-one and its precursors in the brain, plasma, and steroidogenic glands of male and female rats. *Endocrinology*, **133**, 1003–1009.

Corrigan, J.D. and Mysiw, W.J. (1988). Agitation following traumatic head injury: equivocal evidence for a discrete stage of cognitive recovery. *Archives of Physical Medicine and Rehabilitation*, **69**, 487–492.

Corrigan, J.D., Mysiw, W.J., Gribble, M.W., and Chock, S.K.L. (1992). Agitation, cognition and attention during post-traumatic amnesia. *Brain Injury*, **6**, 155–160.

Cosset, F.L. and Russell, S.J. (1996). Targeting retrovirus entry. *Gene Therapy*, **3**, 946–956.

Cotman, C.W., Matthews, D.A., Taylor, D., and Lynch, G. (1973). Synaptic rearrangement in the dentate gyrus: histochemical evidence of adjustments after lesions in immature and adult rats. *Proceedings of the National Academy of Sciences of the United States of America*, **70**, 3473–3477.

Cotzias, G.C., van Woert, M.H., and Schiffere, L.M. (1967). Aromatic amino acids and modification of Parkinsonism. *New England Journal of Medicine*, **282**, 31–33.

Coull, J.T., Sahakian, B.J., and Hodges, J.R. (1996). The alpha-2 antagonist idazoxan remediates certain attentional and executive dysfunction in patients with dementia of frontal type. *Psychopharmacology*, **123**, 239–249.

Covault, J. and Sanes, J.R. (1985). Neural cell-adhesion molecule (N-CAM) accumulates in denervated and paralyzed skeletal muscles. *Proceedings of the National Academy of Sciences of the United States of America*, **82**, 4544–4548.

Cowan, W.M., Fawcett, J.W., Oleary, D.D.M., and Stanfield, B.B. (1984). Regressive events in neurogenesis. *Science*, **225**, 1258–1265.

Coyle, J.T., Price, D.L., and DeLong, M.R. (1983). Alzheimer's disease: a disorder of cortical cholinergic innervation. *Science*, **219**, 1184–1190.

Coyle, P.K. (1995). Neurological Lyme disease: is there a true animal model? *Annals of Neurology*, 38, 560–562.

Coyle, J.T. and Puttfarcken, P. (1993). Oxidative stress, glutamate, and neurodegenerative disorders. *Science*, 262, 689–695.

Coyle, J.T. and Schwarcz, R. (1976). Lesions of striatal neurones with kainic acid provides a model for Huntington's chorea. *Nature*, 263, 244–246.

Coyle, J.T., McGeer, E.G., McGeer, P.L., and Schwarcz, R. (1978). Neostriatal injections: a model for Huntington's chorea. In *Kainic Acid as a Tool in Neurobiology* (ed. E.G. McGeer, J.W. Olney and P.L. McGeer), pp. 139–159. Raven Press, New York.

Creese, I., Burt, D.R., and Snyder, S.H. (1977). Dopamine receptor binding enhancement accompanies lesion-induced behavioral supersensitivity. *Science*, 197, 596–598.

Critchley, E.M.R. (1991). A comparison of human and animal botulism: a review. *Journal of the Royal Society of Medicine*, 84, 295–298.

Crowther, R.A. and Wischik, C.M. (1985). Image reconstruction of the Alzheimer paired helical filament. *EMBO Journal*, 4, 3661–3665.

Cruickshank, J.K., Rudge, P., Dalgleish, A.G., Newton, M., McLean, B.N., Barnard, R.O. *et al.* (1989). Tropical spastic paraparesis and human T-cell lymphotropic virus type 1 in the United Kingdom. *Brain*, 112, 1057–1090.

Crutcher, K.A. (1987). Sympathetic sprouting in the central nervous system: a model for studies of axonal growth in the mature mammalian brain. *Brain Research Reviews*, 12, 203–233.

Crutcher, K.A., Brothers, J., and Davis, J.N. (1981). Sympathetic noradrenergic sprouting in response to central cholinergic denervation — a histochemical study of neuronal sprouting in the rat hippocampal formation. *Brain Research*, 210, 115–128.

Csernok, E., Ernst, M., Schmitt, W., Bainton, D.F., and Gross, W.L. (1994). Activated neutrophils express proteinase 3 on their plasma membrane *in vitro* and *in vivo*. *Clin.Exp.Immunol.*, 95, 244–250.

Cui, Q. and Harvey, A.R. (1995). At least two mechanisms are involved in the death of retinal ganglion cells following target ablation in neonatal rats. *Journal of Neuroscience*, 15, 8143–8155.

Cummings, J.L. (1985). Organic delusions. *British Journal of Psychiatry*, 146, 184–197.

Cummings, J.L. and Benson, D.F. (1992). *Dementia: a Clinical Approach*. Butterworth, Boston.

Cummings, J.L. and Cunningham, K. (1992). Obsessive-compulsive disorder in Huntington's disease. *Biological Psychiatry*, 31, 263–270.

Curran, E.J., Albin, R.L., and Becker, J.B. (1993). Adrenal medulla grafts in the hemiparkinsonian rat: profile of behavioral recovery predicts restoration of the symmetry between the two striata in measures of pre- and postsynaptic dopamine function. *Journal of Neuroscience*, 13, 3864–3877.

Cutting, J. (1990). *The Right Cerebral Hemisphere and Psychiatric Disorders*. Oxford University Press, Oxford.

Dahlström, A. and Fuxe, K. (1964). Evidence for the existence of monoamine-containing neurons in the central nervous system. I. Demonstration of monoamines in the cell bodies of brain stem neurons. *Acta Physiological Scandinavica, supplementum*, 232, 1–55.

Dalby, J.T., Arboleda-Florez, J., and Seland, T.P. (1989). Somatic delusions following left parietal lobe-injury. *Neuropsychiatry, Neuropsychology, Behavioural Neurology*, 2, 306–311.

Dalmau, J., Furneaux, H.M., Rosenblum, M.K., Graus, F., and Posner, J.B. (1991). Detection of the anti-Hu antibody in specific regions of the nervous system and tumor from patients with paraneoplastic encephalomyelitis/sensory neuronopathy. *Neurology*, 41, 1757–1764.

Dam, H., Pedersen, H.E., Damkjaer, M., and Ahlgren, P. (1991). Dexamethasone suppression test in depressive stroke patients. *Acta Neurologica Scandinavica*, 84, 14–17.

Danel, T., Comayras, S., Goudemand, M., Leys, D., Destee, A., Lauth, B. *et al.* (1989). Troubles de l'humeur et infarctus de l'hemisphere droit [Mood disorders and right hemisphere infarction]. *L'Encéphale*, 15, 549–553.

Danel, T., Vaiva, G., Goudemand, M., and Parquet, P.J. (1992). Un cas de melancolie delirante: 'variante de perte de l'autoactivation psychique'? *Annales Médico-Psychologiques*, 150, 225–229.

Darian-Smith, C. and Gilbert, C.D. (1994). Axonal sprouting accompanies functional reorganization in adult cat striate cortex. *Nature*, 368, 737–740.

da Silva, R. (1987). Human spongiform encephalopathy. In *Prion Diseasess* (ed. H.F. Baker and R.M. Ridley), pp. 15–33. Humana Press, Totowa, NJ.

Datta, S.R., Dudek, H., Tao, X., Masters, S., Fu, H.A., Gotoh, Y. *et al.* (1997). Akt phosphorylation of BAD couples survival signals to the cell- intrinsic death machinery. *Cell*, 91, 231–241.

Davenport, C.B. (1916). Huntington's chorea in relation to heredity and eugenics. *American Journal of Insanity*, 73, 195–222.

David, Hécaen, H. and Fouquet. (1943). Démence, distension ventriculaire, disparition progressive des troubles mentaux après ouverture de la lame optique. *Annales Médico-Psychologiques*, 101, 435–438.

David, S. and Aguayo, A.J. (1981). Axonal elongation into peripheral nervous system 'bridges' after central nervous system injury in adult rats. *Science*, 214, 931–933.

Davies, A.M. (1994). Intrinsic programs of growth and survival developing vertebrate neurons. *Trends in Neurosciences*, 17, 195–199.

Davies, S.J.A., Field, P.M., and Raisman, G. (1996). Regeneration of cut adult axons fails even in the presence of continuous aligned glial pathways. *Experimental Neurology*, 142, 203–216.

Davies, S.W., Turmaine, M., Cozens, B.A., DiFiglia, M., Sharp, A.H., Ross, C.A. *et al.* (1997). Formation of neuronal intranuclear inclusions (NII) underlies the neurological dysfunction in mice transgenic for the HD mutation. *Cell*, 90, 537–548.

Davis, G.C., Williams, A.C., Markey, S.P., Ebert, M.H., Caine, E.D., Reichert, C.M. *et al.* (1979). Chronic parkinsonism secondary to intrevenous injection of meperidine analogues. *Psychiatry Research*, 1, 249–254.

Davison, K. and Bagley, C.R. (1969). Schizophrenia like psychoses associated with organic disorder of the central nervous system: a review of the literature. In *Current*

*Problems in Neuropsychiatry (Royal Medico-Psychological Association Publication)* (ed. R.N. Herrington), pp. 113–184. Headley Brothers, Kent.

de Bilbao, F. and Dubois-Dauphin, M. (1996). Acute application of an interleukin-1 beta-converting enzyme-specific inhibitor delays axotomy-induced motoneurone death. *NeuroReport*, 7, 3051–3054.

DeFilipe, J., Jenkins, R., O'Shea, R., Williams, T.S.C., and Hunt, S.P. (1993). The role of immediate early genes in the regeneration of the central nervous system. *Advances in Neurology*, 59, 263–271.

de la Torre, J.C., and Oldstone, M.B.A. (1992). Selective disruption of growth hormone transcription machinery by viral infection. *Proceedings of the National Academy of Sciences of the United States of America*, 89, 9939–9943.

de la Torre, J.C., Mallory, M., Brot, M., Gold, L., Koob, G., Oldstone, M.B.A. *et al.* (1996). Viral persistence in neurons alters synaptic plasticity and cognitive functions without destruction of brain cells. *Virology*, 220, 508–515.

de Kloet, E.R. (1991). Brain corticosteroid receptor balance and homeostatic control. *Frontiers in Neuroendocrinology*, 12, 95–164.

Deacon, T., Schumacher, J., Dinsmore, J., Thomas, C., Palmer, P., Kott, S., Edge, A., Penney, D., Kassissieh, S., Dempsey, P., and Isacson, O. (1997). Histological evidence of fetal pig neural cell survival after transplantation into a patient with Parkinson's disease. *Nature Medicine*, 3, 350–353.

Deller, T. and Frotscher, M. (1997). Lesion-induced plasticity of central neurons: Sprouting of single fibres in the rat hippocampus after unilateral entorhinal cortex lesion. *Progress in Neurobiology*, 53, 687–727.

Del Rio, J.A., Heimrich, B., Borrell, V., Forster, E., Drakew, A., Alcantara, S. *et al.* (1997). A role for Cajal-Retzius cells and *reelin* in the development of hippocampal connections. *Nature*, 385, 70–74.

De Luca, N.A., Mccarthy, A.M., and Schaffer, P.A. (1985). Isolation and characterization of deletion mutants of herpes-simplex virus type-1 in the gene encoding immediate-early regulatory protein- icp4. *Journal of Virology*, 56, 558–570.

De Marchi, N., Morris, M., Meneeella, R., La Pia, S., and Nestadt, G. (1998). Association of obsessive-compulsive disorder and pathological gambling with Huntington's disease in an Italian pedigree: possible association with Huntington's disease mutation. *Acta Psychiatrica Scandinavica*, 97, 62–65.

De Mol, J. (1981). Les troubles du caractere chez les traumatises craniens adultes. *Schweizer Archives Neurologie Neurochirurgie et Psychiatrie*, 129, 37–45.

De Mol, J., Violon, A., and Brihaye, J. (1982). Les decompensations schizophreniques post-traumatiques. A propos de 6 cas de schizophrenie traumatique. *L'Encéphale*, 8, 12–24.

Demonet, J.F., GelyNargeot, M.C., and Bakchine, S. (1997). Methodological aspects of cognitive assessments. *Therapie*, 52, 495–498.

de Morsier, G. (1972). Les hallucinations survenant après les traumatismes cranio-cérébraux. Les schizophrenie traumatique. *Annales Médico-Psychologiques*, 130, 183–194.

Deng, H.X., Hentati, A., Tainer, J.A., Iqbal, Z., Cayabyab, A., Hung, W.Y. *et al.* (1993). Amyotrophic-lateral-sclerosis and structural defects in cu,zn superoxide-dismutase. *Science*, 261, 1047–1051.

DePippo, K.L. (1994). Management of communication dysfunction. In *The Comprehensive Management of Parkinson's Disease* (ed. A.M. Cohen and W.J. Weiner), pp. 75–88. Demos, New York.

De Renzi, E. and Vignolo, L. (1962). The Token Test: a sensitive test to detect receptive disturbances in aphasics. *Brain*, 85, 665–678.

De Ryck, M. (1990). Animal models of cerebral stroke: pharmacological protection of function. *Experimental Neurology*, 30 (Supplement 2), 21–27.

Desimone, R. and Duncan, J. (1995). Neural mechanisms of selective visual attention. *Annual Review of Neuroscience*, 18, 193–222.

Dessi, F., Charriautmarlangue, C., and BenAri, Y. (1994). Glutamate-induced neuronal death in cerebellar culture is mediated by 2 distinct components — a sodium-chloride component and a calcium component. *Brain Research*, 650, 49–55.

Devor, M. and Wall, P.D. (1981). Effect of peripheral nerve injury on receptive fields of cells in the cat spinal cord. *Journal of Comparative Neurology*, 199, 277–291.

Dewhurst, K. (1970). Personality disorder in Huntington's disease. *Psychiatrica Clinica*, 3, 221–229.

Dewhurst, K., Oliver, J., Trick, K.L.K., and McKnight, A.L. (1969). Neuro-psychiatric aspects of Huntington's disease. *Confin.Neurol.*, 31, 268.

Dewhurst, K., Oliver, J.E., and McKnight, A.L. (1970). Sociopsychiatric consequences of Huntington's disease. *British Journal of Psychiatry*, 116, 255–258.

Diener, P.S. and Bregman, B.S. (1998). Fetal spinal cord transplants support growth of supraspinal and segmental projections after cervical spinal cord hemisection in the neonatal rat. *Journal of Neuroscience*, 18, 779–793.

DiFiglia, M., Sapp, E., Chase, K.O., Davies, S.W., Bates, G.P., Vonsattel, J.-P., and Aronin, N. (1997). Aggregation of huntingtin in neuronal intranuclear inclusions and dystrophic neurites in brain. *Science*, 277, 1990–1993.

Dimagl, U., Iadecola, C., and Moskowitz, M.A. (1999). Pathobiology and ischaemic stroke: an integrated view. *Trends in Neurosciences*, 22, 391–397.

Diringer, M.N. (1992). Early prediction of outcome from coma. *Current Opinion in Neurology and Neurosurgery*, 5, 826–830.

Ditter, S.M. and Mirra, S.S. (1987). Neuropathologic and clinical features of Parkinson's disease in Alzheimer's disease patients. *Neurology*, 37, 754–760.

Dlouhy, S.R., Hsiao, K., Farlow, M.R., Foroud, T., Conneally, P.M., Johnson, P. *et al.* (1992). Linkage of the indiana kindred of Gerstmann-Straussler-Scheinker disease to the prion protein gene. *Nature Genetics*, 1, 64–67.

Döbrössy, M.D. and Dunnett, S.B. (1998). Striatal grafts alleviate deficits in response execution in a lateralised reaction time task. *Brain Research Bulletin*, 47, 585–593.

Dobson, A.T., Margolis, T.P., Sedarati, F., Stevens, J.G., and Feldman, L.T. (1990). A latent, nonpathogenic hsv-1-derived vector stably expresses beta- galactosidase in mouse neurons. *Neuron*, 5, 353–360.

Dodwell, D. (1988). Comparison of self-ratings with informant-ratings of pre-morbid personality on two personality rating scales. *Psychological Medicine*, **18**, 495–501.

Doering, L.C. and Chang, P.L. (1991). Expression of a novel gene product by transplants of genetically modified primary fibroblasts in the central nervous system. *Journal of Neuroscience Research*, **29**, 292–298.

Doherty, P., Moolenaar, C.E.C.K., Ashton, S.V., Michalides, R.J.A.M., and Walsh, F.S. (1992). The vase exon down-regulates the neurite growth-promoting activity of NCAM-140. *Nature*, **356**, 791–793.

Dolan, R.J., Calloway, S.P., Fonagy, P., De Souza, F.V.A., and Wakeling, A. (1985). Life events, depression and hypothalamic pituitary-adrenal axis function. *British Journal of Psychiatry*, **147**, 429–433.

Dolman, K.M., Stegeman, C.A., van-de, W.B., Hack, C.E., von-dem, B.A., Kallenberg, C.G. *et al.* (1993) Relevance of classic anti-neutrophil cytoplasmic autoantibody (C-ANCA)-mediated inhibition of proteinase 3-alpha 1-antitrypsin complexation to disease activity in Wegener's granulomatosis. *Clin.Exp.Immunol.*, **93**, 405–410.

Donahue, R.E., Kessler, S.W., Bodine, D., Mcdonagh, K., Dunbar, C., Goodman, S. *et al.* (1992). Helper virus-induced t-cell lymphoma in nonhuman-primates after retroviral mediated gene-transfer. *Journal of Experimental Medicine*, **176**, 1125–1135.

Donoghue, J.P. and Sanes, J.N. (1988). Organization of adult motor cortex representation patterns following neonatal forelimb nerve injury in rats. *Journal of Neuroscience*, **8**, 3221–3232.

Doostzadeh, J., Cotillon, A.C., and Morfin, R. (1997). Dehydroepiandrosterone 7-α- and 7-β-hydroxylation in mouse brain microsomes. Effects of cytochrome P450 inhibitors and structure-specific inhibition by steroid hormones. *Journal of Neuroendocrinology*, **9**, 923–928.

Dore, S., Kar, S., and Quirion, R. (1997). Rediscovering an old friend, IGF-I: potential use in the treatment of neurodegenerative diseases. *Trends in Neurosciences*, **20**, 326–331.

Doster, S.K., Lozano, A.M., Aguayo, A.J., and Willard, M.B. (1991). Expression of the growth-associated protein GAP-43 in adult rat retinal ganglion cells following axon injury. *Neuron*, **6**, 635–647.

Dou, C.L. and Levine, J.M. (1997). Identification of a neuronal cell surface receptor for a growth inhibitory chondroitin sulfate proteoglycan (NG2). *Journal of Neurochemistry*, **68**, 1021–1030.

Drevets, W.C., Burton, H., Videen, T.O., Snyder, A.Z., Simpson, J.R., and Raichle, M.E. (1995). Blood flow changes in human somatosensory cortex during anticipated stimulation. *Nature*, **373**, 249–252.

Driscoll, M. and Chalfie, M. (1992). Developmental and abnormal-cell death in c-elegans. *Trends in Neurosciences*, **15**, 15–19.

Dropcho, E.J., Chen, Y.T., Posner, J.B., and Old, L.J. (1987). Cloning of a brain protein identified by autoantibodies from a patient with paraneoplastic cerebellar degeneration. *Proceedings of the National Academy of Sciences of the United States of America*, **84**, 4552–4556.

Drummond, L.M. (1988). Delayed emergence of obsessive-compulsive neurosis following heaad injury. *British Journal of Psychiatry*, **153**, 839–842.

Duff, J. and Sime, E. (1997). Surgical interventions in the treatment of Parkinson's disease (PD) and essential tremor (ET): medical pallidotomy in PD and chronic deep brain stimulation (DBS) in PD and ET. *Axone*, **18**, 85–89.

Duff, K., Eckman, C., Zehr, C., Yu, X., Prada, C.M., Perez-Tur, J. *et al.* (1996). Increased amyloid-beta-42(43) In brains of mice expressing mutant presenilin-1. *Nature*, **383**, 710–713.

Duncan, I.D. (1996). Glial cell transplantation and remyelination of the central nervous system. *Neuropathology and Applied Neurobiology*, **22**, 87–100.

Duncan, I.D., Grever, W.E., and Zhang, S.C. (1997). Repair of myelin disease: strategies and progress in animal models. *Molecular Medicine Today*, **3**, 554–561.

Duncan, I.D. (1999). Transplant strategies in myelin disorders. In *Cell Transplantation for Neurological Disorders: Towards Reconstruction of the Human Central Nervous System* (ed. T.B. Freeman and H. Widner), pp. 287–302. Humana Press Inc., Totowa, NJ — USA.

Dunlop, T.W., Udvarhelyi, G.B., Stedem, A.F.A., O'Connor, J.M., Isaacs, M.L., Puig, J.G. *et al.* (1991). Comparison of patients with and without emotional/behavioural deterioration during the first year after traumatic brain injury. *Journal of Neuropsychiatry and Clinical Neuroscience*, **3**, 150–156.

Dunn, E.H. (1917). Primary and secondary findings in a series of attempts to transplant cerebral cortex in the albino rat. *Journal of Comparative Neurology*, **27**, 565–582.

Dunnett, S.B. and Barth, T.M. (1991). Animal models of Alzheimer's disease and dementia (with an emphasis on cortical cholinergic systems). In *Behavioural Models in Psychopharmacology* (ed. P. Willner), pp. 359–418. Cambridge University Press, Cambridge.

Dunnett, S.B. and Björklund, A. (1994a). *Functional Neural Transplantation*. Raven Press, New York.

Dunnett, S.B. and Björklund, A. (1994b). Mechanisms of function of neural grafts in the injured brain. In *Functional Neural Transplantation* (ed. S.B. Dunnett and A. Björklund), pp. 531–567. Raven Press, New York.

Dunnett, S.B. and Björklund, A. (1999). Parkinson's disease: prospects for novel restorative and neuroprotective treatments. *Nature*, **399**, S32–S39.

Dunnett, S.B., Björklund, A., Stenevi, U., and Iversen, S.D. (1981a). Behavioral recovery following transplantation of substantia nigra in rats subjected to 6-OHDA lesions of the nigrostriatal pathway. 1. Unilateral lesions. *Brain Research*, **215**, 147–161.

Dunnett, S.B., Björklund, A., Stenevi, U., and Iversen, S.D. (1981b). Grafts of embryonic substantia nigra reinnervating the ventrolateral striatum ameliorate sensorimotor impairments and akinesia in rats with 6-OHDA lesions of the nigrostriatal pathway. *Brain Research*, **229**, 209–217.

Dunnett, S.B., Björklund, A., Schmidt, R.H., Stenevi, U., and Iversen, S.D. (1983). Intracerebral grafting of neuronal cell suspensions. IV. Behavioral recovery in rats with unilateral 6-OHDA lesions following implantation of nigral cell suspensions in different forebrain sites. *Acta Physiological Scandinavica, supplementum*, **522**, 29–37.

Dunnett, S.B., Hernandez, T.D., Summerfield, A., Jones, G.H., and Arbuthnott, G.W. (1988a). Graft-derived recovery from 6-OHDA lesions: specificity of ventral mesencephalic graft tissues. *Experimental Brain Research*, **71**, 411–424.

Dunnett, S.B., Isacson, O., Sirinathsinghji, D.J.S., Clarke, D.J., and Björklund, A. (1988b). Striatal grafts in rats with unilateral neostriatal lesions. III. Recovery from dopamine-dependent motor asymmetry and deficits in skilled paw reaching. *Neuroscience*, 24, 813–820.

Dunnett, S.B., Everitt, B.J., and Robbins, T.W. (1991). The basal forebrain cortical cholinergic system: interpreting the functional consequences of excitotoxic lesions. *Trends in Neurosciences*, 14, 494–501.

Dupré, E. (1903). Tumeurs de l'encéphale. In *Traité de Pathologie Mentale* (ed. G. Ballet and D. Anglade), pp. 1164–1191. Doin, Paris.

Duquette, P., Despault, L., Knobler, R.L., Lublin, F.D., Kelley, L., Francis, G.S. *et al.* (1995). Interferon beta-1b in the treatment of multiple sclerosis: Final outcome of the randomized controlled trial. *Neurology*, 45, 1277–1285.

Duret, H. (1905). *Les Tumeurs de l'Encéphale*. Alcan, Paris.

During, M.J., Naegele, J.R., O'Malley, K.L., and Geller, A.I. (1994). Long-term behavioral recovery in parkinsonian rats by an HSV vector expressing tyrosine hydroxylase. *Science*, 266, 1399–1402.

During, M.J. and Ashenden, L.-M.A. (1998). Towards gene therapy for the central nervous system. *Molecular Medicine Today*, 4, 485–493.

Durst, R. and Rosca, P.R. (1988). Koro secondary to a tumour of the corpus callosum. *British Journal of Psychiatry*, 153, 251–254.

Dyck, P.J., Benstead, T.J., and Conn, D.L. (1987). Nonsystemic vasculitic neuropathy. *Brain*, 110, 843–854.

Dyer, J.K., Bourque, J.A., and Steeves, J.D. (1999). Regeneration of brainstem–spinal axons after lesion and immunological disruption of myelin in adult rat. *Experimental Neurology*, 154, 12–22.

Easter, S.S. and Scherer, S.S. (1983). Growth related order of the retinal fiber layer in goldfish. *Journal of Neuroscience*, 4, 2173–2190.

Ecob-Prince, M.S., Hassan, K., Denheen, M.T., and Preston, C.M. (1995). Expression of beta-galactosidase in neurons of dorsal-root ganglia which are latently infected with herpes-simplex virus type-1. *Journal of General Virology*, 76, 1527–1532.

Edgren, E., Hedstrand, U., Nordin, M., Rydin, E., and Ronquist, G. (1987). Prediction of outcome after cardiac arrest. *Critical Care Medicine*, 15, 820–825.

Edwards, S.G.M., Gong, Q.Y., Liu, C., Zvartau, M.E., Jaspan, T., Roberts, N., and Blumhardt, L.D. (1999). Infratentorial atrophy on magnetic resonance imaging and disability in multiple sclerosis. *Brain*, 122, 291–301.

Egelko, S., Simon, D., Riley, E., Gordon, W., Ruckdeschel-Hibbard, M., and Diller, L. (1989). First year after stroke. *Archives of Physical Medicine and Rehabilitation*, 70, 297–302.

Ehringer, H. and Hornykiewicz, O. (1960). Verteilung von Noradrenalin und Dopamin (3-Hydroxytyramin) im Gehirn des Menschen und ihr Verhalten bei Erkrankungen des Extrapyramidalen Systems. *Klinische Wochenschrift*, 38, 1236–1239.

Elbert, T., Pantev, C., Wienbruch, C., Rockstroh, B., and Taub, E. (1995). Increased cortical representation of the fingers of the left hand in string players. *Science*, 270, 305–307.

Emerich, D.F., Winn, S.R., Harper, J.D., Hammang, J.P.,

Baetge, E.E., and Kordower, J.H. (1994). Implants of polymer-encapsulated human NGF-secreting cells in the non-human primate: rescue and sprouting of degenerating cholinergic basal forebrain neurons. *Journal of Comparative Neurology*, 349, 148–164.

Emerich, D.F., Lindner, M.D., Winn, S.R., Chen, E.Y., Frydel, B.R., and Kordower, J.H. (1996). Implants of encapsulated human CNTF-producing fibroblasts prevent behavioral deficits and striatal degeneration in a rodent model of Huntington's disease. *Journal of Neuroscience*, 16, 5168–5181.

Emerich, D.F., Winn, S.R., Hantraye, P., Peschanski, M., Chen, E.Y., Chu, Y.P. *et al.* (1997b). Protective effect of encapsulated cells producing neurotrophic factor CNTF in a monkey model of Huntington's disease. *Nature*, 386, 395–399.

Emerich, D.F., Cain, C.K., Greco, C., Saydoff, J.A., Hu, Z.Y., Liu, H.J., and Lindner, M.D. (1997). Cellular delivery of human CNTF prevents motor and cognitive dysfunction in a rodent model of Huntington's disease. *Cell Transplantation*, 6, 249–266.

Eng, L.F., Reier, P.J., and Houle, J.D. (1987). Astrocyte activation and fibrous gliosis: glial fibrillary acidic protein immunostaining of astrocytes following intraspinal cord grafting of fetal CNS tissue. *Progress in Brain Research*, 71, 439–455.

Engelhardt, J.F., Ye, X.H., Doranz, B., and Wilson, J.M. (1994). Ablation of e2a in recombinant adenoviruses improves transgene persistence and decreases inflammatory response in mouse-liver. *Proceedings of the National Academy of Sciences of the United States of America*, 91, 6196–6200.

England, J.D., Bohm, R.P., Roberts, E.D., and Philipp, M.T. (1997). Mononeuropathy multiplex in rhesus monkeys with chronic Lyme disease. *Annals of Neurology*, 41, 375–384.

Englund, E., Brun, A., and Gustafson, L. (1989). A white matter disease in dementia of Alzheimer's type — clinical and neuropathological changes. *International Journal of Geriatric Psychiatry*, 4, 87–102.

Epstein, C.J., Avraham, K.B., Lovett, M., Smith, S., Elroy-Stein, O., Rotman, G. *et al.* (1989). Transgenic mice with increased Cu/Zn-superoxide dismutase activity: an animal model of dosage effects in Down's syndrome. *Proceedings of the National Academy of Sciences of the United States of America*, 84, 8044–8048.

Eriksson, P.S., Perfilieva, E., Björk-Eriksson, T., Alborn, A.M., Nordborg, C., Peterson, D.A. *et al.* (1998). Neurogenesis in the adult human hippocampus. *Nature Medicine*, 4, 1313–1317.

Esiri, M.M. (1982). Herpes simplex encephalitis: an immuno-histochemical study of the distribution of viral antigen within the brain. *Journal of the Neurological Sciences*, 54, 209–226.

Esiri, M.M. and Kennedy, P.G.E. (1997). Viral disease. In *Greenfield's Neuropathology* (ed. D.I. Graham and P.L. Lantos), Arnold, New York.

Ettlin, T.M., Kischka, U., Reichmann, S., Radii, E.W., Heim, S., Wengen, D.A. *et al.* (1992). Cerebral symptoms after whiplash injury of the neck: a prospective clinical and neuropsychological study of whiplash injury. *Journal of Neurology, Neurosurgery and Psychiatry*, 55, 943–948.

Evans, C. (1987). Rehabilitation of head injury in a rural community. *Clinical Rehabilitation*, 1, 133–137.

Evans, J.J. and Wilson, B.A. (1992). A memory group for individuals with brain injury. *Clinical Rehabilitation*, 6, 75–81.

Everall, I., Luthert, P., and Lantos, P. (1993). A review of neuronal damage inhuman immunodeficiency virus infection: its assessment, possible mechanism and relationship to dementia. *Journal of Neuropathology and Experimental Neurology*, 52, 561–566.

Fabry, S., Raine, C.S., and Hart, M.N. (1994). Nervous tissue as an immune compartment: the dialect of the immune response in the CNS. *Immunology Today*, 15, 218–224.

Faden, A.I., Demediuk, P., Panter, S.S., and Vink, R. (1989). The role of excitatory amino acids and NMDA receptors in traumatic brain injury. *Science*, 244, 798–800.

Fahn, S., Elton, R.L., and UPDRS Development Committee. (1987). Unified Parkinson's Disease Rating Scale. In *Recent Developments in Parkinson's DiawAW* (ed. S. Fahn, C.D. Marsden, M. Goldstein and D.B. Calne), pp. 153–163. New York, MacMillan Haalth Care Information.

Falk, R.J., Terrell, R.S., Charles, L.A., and Jennette, J.C. (1990). Anti-neutrophil cytoplasmic autoantibodies induce neutrophils to degranulate and produce oxygen radicals *in vitro*. *Proceedings of the National Academy of Sciences of the United States of America*, 87, 4115–4119.

Farah, M.J. (1994). Neuropsychological inference with an interactive brain: a critique of the 'locality' assumption. *Behavioral and Brain Sciences*, 17, 43–104.

Fathallah, S.H., Wolf, S., Wong, E., Posner, J.B., and Furneaux, H.M. (1991). Cloning of a leucine-zipper protein recognized by the sera of patients with antibody-associated paraneoplastic cerebellar degeneration. *Proceedings of the National Academy of Sciences of the United States of America*, 88, 3451–3454.

Faulds, D., Goa, K.L., and Benfield, P. (1993). Cyclosporin: a review of its pharmacodynamic and pharmacokinetic properties, and therapeutic use in immunoregulatory disorders. *Drugs*, 45, 953–1040.

Fawcett, J.W. and Asher, R.A. (1999). The glial scar and central nervous system repair. *Brain Research Bulletin*, 49, 377–391.

Fawcett, J.W. and Keynes, R.J. (1990). Peripheral nerve regeneration. *Annual Review of Neuroscience*, 13, 43–60.

Fawcett, J.W., Housden, E., Smith-Thomas, L., and Meyer, R.L. (1989a). The growth of axons in three dimensional astrocyte cultures. *Developmental Biology*, 133, 140–147.

Fawcett, J.W., Rokos, J., and Bakst, I. (1989b). Oligodendrocytes repel axons and cause axonal growth cone collapse. *Journal of Cell Science*, 9, 93–100.

Fawcett, J.W., Fersht, N., Housden, E., Schachner, M., and Pesheva, P. (1992). Axonal growth on astrocytes is not inhibited by oligodendrocytes. *Journal of Cell Science*, 103, 571–579.

Fawcett, J.W., Mathews, G., Housden, E., Goedert, M., and Matus, A. (1994). Regenerating sciatic nerve axons contain the adult rather than the embryonic pattern of microtubule associated proteins. *Neuroscience*, 61, 789–804.

Fedoroff, J.P., Starkstein, S.E., Forrester, A.W., Geisler, F.H., Jorge, R.E., Arndt, S.V. *et al.* (1992). Depression in patients with acute traumatic brain injury. *American Journal of Psychiatry*, 149, 918–923.

Fedoroff, J.P., Jorge, R.E., and Robinson, R.G. (1993). Depression in traumatic brain injury. In *Depression in Neurologic Disease* (ed. S.E. Starkstein and R.G. Robinson), pp. 139–151. John Hopkins University Press, Baltimore.

Fedoroff, J.P., Peyser, C., Franz, M.L., and Folstein, S.E. (1994). Sexual disorders in Huntington's disease. *Journal of Neuropsychiatry and Clinical Neuroscience*, 6, 147–153.

Feher, E.P., Inbody, S.B., Nolan, B., and Pirozzolo, F.J. (1988). Other neurological diseases with dementia as a sequelae. *Clinical and Geriatric Medicine*, 4, 799–814.

Feighner, J.P., Boyer, W.F., Tyler, D.L., and Nebrosky, R.J. (1990). Adverse consequences of fluoxetine-MAOI combination therapy. *Journal of Clinical Psychiatry*, 512, 222–225.

Feigin, A., Kieburtz, K., Como, P., Hickey, C., Claude, K., Abwender, D. *et al.* (1996). Assessment of coenzyme Q10 tolerability in Huntington's disease. *Movement Disorders*, 11, 321–323.

Feldman, R.S., Meyer, J.S., and Quenzer, L.F. (1997). *Principles of Neuropsychopharmacology*. Sinauer, Sunderland, Mass.

Feneley, M.R., Fawcett, J.W., and Keynes, R.J. (1991). The role of Schwann cells in the regeneration of peripheral nerve axons through muscle basal lamina grafts. *Experimental Neurology*, 114, 275–285.

Fenton, G., McClelland, R., Montgomery, A., MacFlynn, G., and Rutherford, W. (1993). The post-concussional syndrome: social antecedents and psychological sequelae. *British Journal of Psychiatry*, 162, 493–497.

Fenwick, P., Galliano, S., Coate, M.A., Rippere, V., and Brown, D. (1985). 'Psychic sensitivity', mystical experience, head injury and brain pathology. *British Journal of Medical Psychology*, 58, 35–44.

Fernandes, K.J., Kobayashi, N.R., Jasmin, B.J., and Tetzlaff, W. (1998). Acetylcholinesterase gene expression in axotomized rat facial motoneurons is diffentially regulated by neurotrophins: correlation with trkB and trkC mRNA levels and isoforms. *Journal of Neuroscience*, 18, 9936–9947.

Ferrari, G., Yan, C.Y.I., and Greene, L.A. (1995). N-acetylcysteine (D- and L-stereoisomers) prevents apoptotic death of neuronal cells. *Journal of Neuroscience*, 15, 2857–2866.

Ferrey, G. and Gagey, P.M. (1987). Le syndrome subjectif et les troubles psychiques des traumatisés du crâne. *Encyclopédie Médico-Chirurgicale (Paris-France)*.

Ferris, S.H. (1992). Diagnosis by specialists: psychological testing. *Acta Neurologica Scandinavica supplementum*, 139, 32–35.

Ferris, S.H., Lucca, U., Mohs, R., Dubois, B., Wesnes, K., Erzigkeit, H. *et al.* (1997). Objective psychometric tests in clinical trials of dementia drugs. *Alzheimer Disease and Associated Disorders*, 11 (**Supplement 3**), 34–38.

ffrench-Constant, C. and Raff, M.C. (1986). Proliferating bipotential glial progenitor cells in adult rat optic nerve. *Nature*, 319, 499–502.

Fidler, P.S., Schuette, K., Asher, R.A., Dobbertin, A., Thornton, S.R., Calle-Patino, Y. *et al.* (1999). Comparing astrocytic cell lines that are inhibitory or permissive for axon growth: the major axon inhibitory proteoglycan is NG2. *Journal of Neuroscience*, 19, 8778–8788.

Finsen, B., Oteruelo, F., and Zimmer, J. (1988). Immunocytochemical characterization of the cellular immune response to intracerebral xenografts of brain tissue. *Progress in Brain Research*, 78, 261–270.

Finset, A., Goffeng, L., Landro, N.I., and Haakonsen, M.

(1989). Depressed mood and intrahemispheric location of lesion in right hemisphere stroke patients. *Scandinavian Journal of Rehabilitation Medicine*, 21, 1–6.

Fisher, L.J. (1995). Engineered cells: a promising therapeutic approach for neural disease. *Restorative Neurology and Neuroscience*, 8, 49–57.

Fisher, L.J. (1997). Neural precursor cells: applications for the study and repair of the central nervous system. *Neurobiology of Disease*, 4, 1–22.

Fisher, L.J., Jinnah, H.A., Kale, L.C., Higgins, G.A., and Gage, F.H. (1991). Survival and function of intrastriatally grafted primary fibroblasts genetically modified to produce l-DOPA. *Neuron*, 6, 371–380.

Fisher, K.J., Choi, H., Burda, J., Chen, S.J., and Wilson, J.M. (1996). Recombinant adenovirus deleted of all viral genes for gene therapy of cystic fibrosis. *Virology*, 217, 11–22.

Fitzgerald, M. (1985). The sprouting of saphenous nerve terminals in the spinal cord following early postnatal sciatic nerve section in the rat.
cgrid0 *Journal of Comparative Neurology*, 240, 407–413.

Fleet, W.S., Valenstein, E., Watson, R.T., and Heilman, K.M. (1987). Dopamine agonist therapy for neglect in humans. *Neurology*, 37, 1765–1770.

Florence, S.L. and Kaas, J.H. (1995). Large-scale reorganization at multiple levels of the somatosensory pathway follows therapeutic amputation of the hand in monkeys. *Journal of Neuroscience*, 15, 8083–8095.

Florence, S.L., Jain, N., Pospichal, M.W., Beck, P.D., Sly, D.L., and Kaas, J.H. (1996). Central reorganization of sensory pathways following peripheral nerve regeneration in fetal monkeys. *Nature*, 381, 69–71.

Florence, S.L., Taub, H.B., and Kaas, J.H. (1998). Large-scale sprouting of cortical connections after peripheral injury in adult macaque monkeys. *Science*, 282, 1117–1121.

Florian, V., Katz, S., and Lahav, V. (1991). Impact of traumatic brain damage on family dynamics and functioning: a review. *International Disability Studies*, 13, 150–157.

Foa, L.C., Balazovich, K.J., and Tosney, K.W. (1997). A role for FGF receptor in contact-mediated signalling during axon guidance. *Developmental Biology*, 186, A226.

Fok-Seang, J., Mathews, G.A., ffrench-Constant, C., Trotter, J., and Fawcett, J.W. (1995). Migration of oligodendrocyte precursors on astrocytes and meningeal cells. *Developmental Biology*, 171, 1–15.

Fok-Seang, J., DiProspero, N.A., Meiners, S., Muir, E., and Fawcett, J.W. (1998). Cytokine-induced changes in the ability of astrocytes to support migration of oligodendrocyte precursors and axon growth. *European Journal of Neuroscience*, 10, 2400–2415.

Folstein, S.E. (1989). *Huntington's disease. A disorder of families*. John Hopkins University Press, Baltimore.

Folstein, S.E. and McHugh, P.R. (1983). The neuropsychiatry of some specific brain disorders. In *Handbook of Psychiatry, vol 2, Mental Disorders and Somatic Illness* (ed. M.H. Lader), pp. 107–118. Cambridge University Press, Cambridge.

Folstein, S.E., Folstein, M.F., and McHugh, P.R. (1979). Psychiatric syndromes in Huntington's disease. *Advances in Neurology*, 23, 281–289.

Folstein, S.E., Franz, M.L., Jensen, B.A., Chase, G.A., and Folstein, M.F. (1983a). Conduct disorder and affective dis-

order among the offspring of patients with Huntington's disease. *Psychological Medicine*, 13, 45–52.

Folstein, S.E., Abbott, M.H., Chase, G.A., Jensen, B.A., and Folstein, M.F. (1983b). The association of affective disorder with Huntington's disease in a case series and in families. *Psychological Medicine*, 13, 537–542.

Folstein, S.E., Chase, G.A., Wahl, W.E., McDonnell, A.M., and Folstein, M.F. (1987). Huntington's disease in Maryland: Clinical aspects and racial variation. *American Journal of Human Genetics*, 41, 168–179.

Forno, L.S. (1996). Neuropathology of Parkinson's disease. *Journal of Neuropathology and Experimental Neurology*, 55, 259–272.

Foster, A.C., Gill, R., and Woodruff, G.N. (1988). Neuroprotective effects of MK-801 *in vivo*: selectivity and evidence for delayed degeneration mediated by NMDA receptor activation. *Journal of Neuroscience*, 8, 4745–4754.

Foster, N.L., Wilhelmsen, K., Sima, A.A.F., Jones, M.Z., D'Amato, C., Gilman, S. *et al.* (1997). Frontotemporal dementia and parkinsonism linked to chromosome 17: a consensus statement. *Annals of Neurology*, 41, 706–715.

Fotaki, M.E., Pink, J.R., and Mous, J. (1997). Tetracycline-responsive gene expression in mouse brain after amplicon-mediated gene transfer. *Gene Therapy*, 4, 901–908.

Fournier, A.E., Beer, J., Arregui, C.O., Essagian, C., Aguayo, A.J., and McKerracher, L. (1997). Brain-derived neurotrophic factor modulates GAP-43 but not T alpha1 expression in injured retinal ganglion cells of adult rats. *Journal of Neuroscience Research*, 47, 561–572.

Fowler, C.J. (1997). The cause and management of bladder, sexual and bowel symptoms in multiple sclerosis. *Baillieres.Clin.Neurol.*, 6, 447–466.

Foy, A., O'Connell, D., and Henry, D. (1995). Benzodiazepine use as a cause of cognitive impairment in elderly hospital inpatients. *Journal of Gerontology*, 50, 99.

Frade, J.M. and Barde, Y.A. (1998). Microglia-derived nerve growth factor causes cell death in the developing retina. *Neuron*, 20, 35–41.

Fraefel, C., Song, S., Lim, F., Lang, P., Yu, L., Wang, Y.M. *et al.* (1996). Helper virus-free transfer of herpes simplex virus type 1 plasmid vectors into neural cells. *Journal of Virology*, 70, 7190–7197.

Frank, E. and Tew, J.M. (1982). Normal-pressure hydrocephalus: clinical symptoms, diagnosis, pathophysiology and treatment. *Heart and Lung*, 11, 321–326.

Franklin, R.J.M. and Blakemore, W.F. (1995). Glial cell transplantation and plasticity in the O-2A lineage: implications for CNS repair. *Trends in Neurosciences*, 18, 151–156.

Franklin, R.J.M., Gilson, J.M., and Blakemore, W.F. (1997). Local recruitment of remyelinating cells in the repair of demyelination in the central nervous system. *Journal of Neuroscience Research*, 50, 337–344.

Franklin, R.J.M. and ffrench-Constant, C. (1996). Transplantation and repair in multiple sclerosis. In *Molecular Biology of Multiple Sclerosis* (ed. W.C. Russell), pp. 231–242. John Wiley & Sons, London.

Franklin, R.J.M., Gilson, J.M., Fransceshini, I.A., and Barnett, S.A. (1996a). Schwann cell-like myelination following transplantation of an olfactory bulb ensheathing cell line into areas of demyelination in the adult CNS. *Glia*, 17, 217–224.

Franklin, R.J.M., Bayley, S.A., and Blakemore, W.F. (1996b). Transplanted CG4 cells (an oligodendrocyte progenitor cell line) survive, migrate and contribute to repair of areas of demyelination in X-irradiated and damaged spinal cord, but not in normal spinal cord. *Experimental Neurology*, 137, 263–276.

Fraser, N.W., Spivack, J.G., Wroblewska, Z., Block, T., Deshmane, S.L., Valyinagy, T. *et al.* (1991). A review of the molecular mechanism of hsv-1 latency. *Current Eye Research*, 10, 1–13.

Fray, P.J. and Robbins, T.W. (1996). CANTAB battery: proposed utility in neurotoxicology. *Neurotoxicology and Teratology*, 18, 499–504.

Fray, P.J., Robbins, T.W., and Sahakian, B.J. (1996). Neuropsychiatric applications of CANTAB. *International Journal of Geriatric Psychiatry*, 11, 329–336.

Frederiksen, K. and McKay, R.D.G. (1988). Proliferation and differentiation of rat neuroepithelial precursor cells *in vivo*. *Journal of Neuroscience*, 8, 1144–1151.

Frederiksen, K., Jat, P.S., Valtz, N., Levy, D., and McKay, R. (1988). Immortalization of precursor cells from the mammalian CNS. *Neuron*, 1, 439–448.

Freed, W.J., Morihisa, J.M., Spoor, E., Hoffer, B.J., Olson, L., Seiger, Å. *et al.* (1981). Transplanted adrenal chromaffin cells in rat brain reduce lesion-induced rotational behavior. *Nature*, 292, 351–352.

Freeman, T.B., Olanow, C.W., Hauser, R.A., Nauert, G.M., Smith, D.A., Borlongan, C.V. *et al.* (1995). Bilateral fetal nigral transplantation into the postcommissural putamen in Parkinson's disease. *Annals of Neurology*, 38, 379–388.

Frim, D.M., Uhler, T.A., Short, M.P., Ezzedine, Z.D., Klagsbrun, M., Breakefield, X.O. *et al.* (1993). Effects of biologically delivered NGF, BDNF and bFGF on striatal excitotoxic lesions. *NeuroReport*, 4, 367–370.

Frim, D.M., Uhler, T.A., Galpern, W.R., Beal, M.F., Breakefield, X.O., and Isacson, O. (1994). Implanted fibroblasts genetically engineered to produce brain derived neurotrophic factor prevent 1-methyl-4-phenylpyridinium toxicity to dopaminergic neurons in the rat. *Proceedings of the National Academy of Sciences of the United States of America*, 91, 5104–5108.

Frodl, E.M., Nakao, N., and Brundin, P. (1994). Lazaroids improve the survival of cultured rat embryonic mesencephalic neurones. *NeuroReport*, 5, 2393–2396.

Frohman, E.M., Van Den Noort, S., and Gupta, S. (1989). Astrocytes and intracerebral immune responses. *J. Clin. Immunol.*, 9, 1–9.

Fuchs, E. and Flugge, G. (1998). Stress, glucocorticoids and structural plasticity of the hippocampus. *Neuroscience and Biobehavioral Reviews*, 23, 295–300.

Funder, J.W. (1992). Glucocorticoid receptors. *Journal of Steroid Biochemistry and Molecular Biology*, 43, 389–394.

Furneaux, H.F., Reich, L., and Posner, J.B. (1990). Autoantibody synthesis in the central nervous system of patients with paraneoplastic syndromes. *Neurology*, 40, 1085–1091.

Gage, F.H., Björklund, A., and Stenevi, U. (1983). Reinnervation of the partially deafferented hippocampus by compensatory collateral sprouting from spared cholinergic and noradrenergic afferents. *Brain Research*, 268, 27–37.

Gage, F.H., Wolff, J.A., Rosenberg, M.B., Xu, L., Yee, J.K., Shults, C., and Friedmann, T. (1987). Grafting genetically modified cells to the brain: possibilities for the future. *Neuroscience*, 23, 795–807.

Gage, F.H., Ray, J., and Fisher, L.J. (1995a). Isolation, characterization, and use of stem cells from the CNS. *Annual Review of Neuroscience*, 18, 159–192.

Gage, F.H., Coates, P.W., Palmer, T.D., Kuhn, H.G., Fisher, L.J., Suhonen, J.O. *et al.* (1995b). Survival and differentiation of adult neuronal progenitor cells transplanted to the adult brain. *Proceedings of the National Academy of Sciences of the United States of America*, 92, 11879–11883.

Gajdusek, D.C. (1994). Nucleation of amyloidogenesis in infections and noninfectious amyloidoses of brain. *Annals of the New York Academy of Sciences*, 724, 173–190.

Gallia, G.L., Houff, S.A., Major, E.O., and Khalili, K. (1997). Review: JC virus infection of lymphocytes — revisited. *Journal of Infectious Disease*, 176, 1603–1609.

Games, D., Adams, D., Alessandrini, R., Barbour, R., Berthelette, P., Blackwell, C. *et al.* (1995). Alzheimer-type neuropathology in transgenic mice overexpressing V71F β-amyloid precursor protein. *Nature*, 373, 523–527.

Garcia-Monco, J.C. and Benach, J.L. (1995). Lyme neuroborreliosis. *Annals of Neurology*, 37, 691–702.

Garcia-Monco, J.C., Coleman, J.L., and Benach, J.L. (1988). Antibodies to myelin basic protein in Lyme disease patients. *Journal of Infectious Disease*, 158, 667–669.

Garcia-Monco, J.C., Fernandez-Villar, B., and Benach, J.L. (1989). Adherence of the Lyme disease spirochete to glial cells and cells of glial origin. *Journal of Infectious Disease*, 160, 497–506.

Gardner, M.B. (1991). Retroviral leukemia and lower motor neuron disease in wild mice: natural history, pathogenesis, and genetic resistance. *Advances in Neurology*, 56, 473–479.

Garin, C. and Bujadoux, C. (1922). Paralysie par les tiques. *Journal of Medicine (Lyon)*, 71, 765–767.

Garraghty, P.E. and Muja, N. (1996). NMDA receptors and plasticity in adult primate somatosensory cortex. *Journal of Comparative Neurology*, 367, 319–326.

Garwood, J., Schnadelbach, O., Clement, A., Schutte, K., Bach, A., and Faissner, A. (1999). DSD-1-proteoglycan is the mouse homolog of phosphacan and displays opposing effects on neurite outgrowth dependent on neuronal lineage. *Journal of Neuroscience*, 19, 3888–3899.

Gash, D.M., Zhang, Z., Ovadia, A., Cass, W.A., Yi, A., Simmerman, L., Russell, D. *et al.* (1996). Functional recovery in parkinsonian monkeys treated with GDNF. *Nature*, 380, 252–255.

Gash, D.M., Zhang, Z.M., and Gerhardt, G. (1998). Neuroprotective and neurorestorative properties of GDNF. *Annals of Neurology*, 44, S121–S125.

Gensemer, I.B., Smith, J.L., Walker, J.C., McMurray, F., Indeck, M., and Brotman, S. (1989). Psychological consequences of blunt head trauma and relation to other indices of severity of injury. *Annales of Emergency Medicine*, 18, 9–12.

Gensert, J.M. and Goldman, J.E. (1997). Endogenous progenitors remyelinate demyelinated axons in the adult CNS. *Neuron*, 19, 197–203.

Gentile, A.M., Green, S., Neiburgs, A., Schmelzer, W., and Stein, D.G. (1978). Disruption and recovery of locomotor and manipulative behaviour following cortical lesions in rats. *Behavioural Biology*, 22, 417–455.

George, C.P., Goldberg, M.P., Choi, D.W., and Steinberg, G.K. (1988). Dextromorphan reduces neocortical ischemic neuronal damage *in vivo*. *Brain Research*, **440**, 375–379.

George, E.B., Glass, J.D., and Griffin, J.W. (1995). Axotomy-induced axonal degeneration is mediated by calcium influx through ion-specific channels. *Journal of Neuroscience*, **15**, 6445–6452.

Gessain, A., Vernant, J.C., Barin, A., Gout, O., and De Thé, G. (1985). Antibodies to human lymphotropic virus type 1 in patients with tropical spastic paraparesis. *Lancet*, **ii**, 407–410.

Ghetti, B., Tagliavini, F., Masters, C.L., Beyreuther, K., Giaccone, G., Verga, L. *et al.* (1989). Gerstmann–Straussler–Scheinker disease.2. Neurofibrillary tangles and plaques with prp-amyloid coexist in an affected family. *Neurology*, **39**, 1453–1461.

Ghetti, B., Dlouhy, S.R., Giaccone, G., Bugiani, O., Frangione, B., Farlow, M.R. *et al.* (1995). Gerstmann–Straussler–Scheinker disease and the indiana kindred. *Brain Pathology*, **5**, 61–75.

Ghika, J., Villemure, J.G., Fankhauser, H., Favre, J., Assal, G., and Ghika-Schmid, F. (1998). Efficiency and safety of bilateral contemporaneous pallidal stimulation (deep brain stimulation) in levodopa-responsive patients with Parkinson's disease with severe motor fluctuations: a 2-year follow-up review. *Journal of Neurosurgery*, **89**, 713–718.

Giang, D.W. (1991). Systemic lupus erythematosus and depression. *Neuropsychiatry, Neuropsychology, Behavioural Neurology*, **4**, 78–82.

Giftochristos, N. and David, S. (1988). Immature optic nerve glia of rat do not promote axonal regeneration when transplanted into a peripheral nerve. *Developmental Brain Research*, **39**, 149–153.

Gilson, J. and Blakemore, W.F. (1993). Failure of remyelination in areas of demyelination produced in the spinal cord of old rats. *Neuropathology and Applied Neurobiology*, **19**, 173–181.

Glass, J.D., Brushart, T.M., George, E.B., and Griffin, J.W. (1993). Prolonged survival of transected nerve fibers in C57BL/Ola mice is an intrinsic characteristic of the axon. *Journal of Neurocytology*, **22**, 311–321.

Glenner, G.G. and Wong, C.W. (1984). Alzheimer's disease: initial report of the purification and characterization of a novel cerebrovascular amyloid protein. *Biochemistry and Biophsyics Research Communications*, **120**, 885–890.

Glicksman, M.A. and Sanes, J.R. (1983). Differentiation of motor nerve terminals formed in the absence of muscle fibers. *Journal of Neurocytology*, **12**, 661–671.

Glisky, E.L. (1995). Computers in memory rehabilitation. In *Handbook of memory disorders* (ed. A.D. Baddeley, B.A. Wilson and F.N. Watts), pp. 557–575. John Wiley, Chichester.

Goate, A., Chartier-Harlin, M.-C., Mullan, M., Brown, J., Crawford, F., Fidani, L. *et al.* (1991). Segregation of a missense mutation in the amyloid precursor protein gene with familial Alzheimer's disease. *Nature*, **349**, 704–706.

Goedert, M. (1993). Tau protein and the neurofibrillary pathology of Alzheimer's disease. *Trends in Neurosciences*, **16**, 460–465.

Goedert, M., Wischik, C.M., Crowther, R.A., Walker, J.E., and Klug, A. (1988). Cloning and sequencing of the cDNA-encoding a core protein of the paired helical filament of Alzheimer's disease — identification as the microtubule-associated protein tau. *Proceedings of the National Academy of Sciences of the United States of America*, **85**, 4051–4055.

Goedert, M., Jakes, R., Spillantini, M.G., Hasegawa, M., Smith, M.J., and Crowther, R.A. (1996). Assembly of microtubule-associated protein tau into Alzheimer-like filaments induced by sulphated glycosaminoglycans. *Nature*, **383**, 550–553.

Goetz, C.G. and Cohen, M.M. (1994). Neurotoxic agents. *Clinical Neurology*, **20**, 1.

Goetz, C.G., Stebbins, G.T., Klawans, H.L., Koller, W.C., Grossman, R.G., Bakay, R.A.E. *et al.* (1991). United Parkinson Foundation neural transplantation registry multicenter data base: 2-year follow-up. *Annals of Neurology*, **30**, 296–296.

Goldberg, M.P. and Choi, D.W. (1993). Combined oxygen and glucose deprivation in cortical cell-culture — calcium-dependent and calcium-independent mechanisms of neuronal injury. *Journal of Neuroscience*, **13**, 3510–3524.

Golden, J.P., Baloh, R.H., Kotzbauer, P.T., Lampe, P.A., Osborne, P.A., Milbrandt, J. *et al.* (1998). Expression of neurturin, GDNF, and their receptors in the adult mouse CNS. *Journal of Comparative Neurology*, **398**, 139–150.

Goldfarb, L.G., Brown, P., Haltia, M., Cathala, F., Mccombie, W.R., Kovanen, J. *et al.* (1992a). Creutzfeldt-Jakob disease cosegregates with the codon-178Asn PrnP mutation in families of European origin. *Annals of Neurology*, **31**, 274–281.

Goldfarb, L.G., Petersen, R.B., Tabaton, M., Brown, P., Leblanc, A.C., Montagna, P. *et al.* (1992b). Fatal familial insomnia and familial Creutzfeldt-Jakob disease — disease phenotype determined by a DNA polymorphism. *Science*, **258**, 806–808.

Goldman, M.S. and Kelly, P.J. (1992). Symptomatic and functional outcome of stereotactic ventralis lateralis thalamotomy for intention tremor [see comments]. *Journal of Neurosurgery*, **77**, 223–229.

Goldman, S.A. and Nottebohm, F. (1983). Neuronal production, migration, and differentiation in a vocal control nucleus of the adult female canary brain. *Proceedings of the National Academy of Sciences of the United States of America*, **80**, 2390–2394.

Goodale, M.A. (1973). Cortico-tectal and intertectal modulation of visual responses in the rat's superior colliculus. *Experimental Neurology*, **17**, 75–86.

Goodkin, D.E., Hertsgaard, D., and Seminary, J. (1988). Upper extremity function in multiple sclerosis: improving assessment sensitivity with box-and-block and nine-hole peg tests. *Archives of Physical Medicine and Rehabilitation*, **69**, 850–854.

Goodyer, I.M., Herbert, J., Altham, P.M.E., Pearson, J., Secher, S.M., and Shiers, H.M. (1996). Adrenal secretion during major depression in 8-year-olds to 16-year-olds. 1. Altered diurnal rhythms in salivary cortisol and dehydroepiandrosterone (DHEA) at presentation. *Psychological Medicine*, **26**, 245–256.

Goodyer, I.M., Herbert, J., and Altham, P.M.E. (1998). Adrenal steroid secretion and major depression in 8- to 16-year-olds, III. Influence of cortisol/DHEA ratio at presentation on subsequent rates of disappointing life events and persistent major depression. *Psychological Medicine*, **28**, 265–273.

Gordon, W.A., Hibbard, M.R., Egelko, S. *et al.* (1991). Issues in the diagnosis of post-stroke depression. *Rehabilitation and Psychology*, **36**, 71–87.

Gorman, D.G. and Cummings, J.L. (1992). Hypersexuality following septal injury. *Archives of Neurology*, **49**, 308–310.

Gossen, M. and Bujard, H. (1992). Tight control of gene expression in mammalian cells by tetracycline-responsive promoters. *Proceedings of the National Academy of Sciences of the United States of America*, **89**, 5547–5551.

Gould, E., Woolley, C.S., and McEwen, B.S. (1991a). Adrenal steroids regulate postnatal development of the rat dentate gyrus. 1. Effects of glucocorticoids on cell-death. *Journal of Comparative Neurology*, **313**, 479–485.

Gould, E., Woolley, C.S., Cameron, H.A., Daniels, D.C., and McEwen, B.S. (1991b). Adrenal steroids regulate postnatal development of the rat dentate gyrus. 2. Effects of glucocorticoids and mineralocorticoids on cell birth. *Journal of Comparative Neurology*, **313**, 486–493.

Gouvier, W.D., Cubic, B., Jones, G. *et al.* (1992). Post-concussional syndrome and daily stress in normal and head-injured college populations. *Archives of Clinical Neuropsychology*, **7**, 192–211.

Grace, A.A. and Bunney, B.S. (1984a). The control of firing pattern in nigral dopamine neurons: single spike firing. *Journal of Neuroscience*, **4**, 2866–2876.

Grace, A.A. and Bunney, B.S. (1984b). The control of firing pattern in nigral dopamine neurons: burst firing. *Journal of Neuroscience*, **4**, 2877–2890.

Gracies, J.M., Elovic, E., McGuire, J., and Simpson, D.M. (1997a). Traditional pharmacological treatments for spasticity. Part I: Local treatments. *Muscle Nerve*, **6 (Supplement)**, S61–S91.

Gracies, J.M., Nance, P., Elovic, E., McGuire, J., and Simpson, D.M. (1997b). Traditional pharmacological treatments for spasticity. Part II: General and regional treatments. *Muscle Nerve*, **6 (Supplement)**, S92–S120.

Grafft-Radford, N.R. and Godersky, J.C. (1986). Normal-pressure hydrocephalus. *Archives of Neurology*, **43**, 940–942.

Graham, F.L., Smiley, J., Russell, W.C., and Nairn, R. (1977). Characteristics of a human cell line transformed by DNA from human adenovirus type 5. *Journal of General Virology*, **36**, 59–74.

Grasbon-Frodl, E.M., Nakao, N., and Brundin, P. (1996). The lazaroid U-83836E improves the survival of rat embryonic mesencephalic tissue stored at 4°C and subsequently used for cultures or intracerebral transplantation. *Brain Research Bulletin*, **39**, 341–347.

Graus, F., Cordon, C.C., and Posner, J.B. (1985). Neuronal antinuclear antibody in sensory neuronopathy from lung cancer. *Neurology*, **35**, 538–543.

Graus, F., Ribalta, T., Campo, E., Monforte, R., Urbano, A., and Rozman, C. (1990). Immunohistochemical analysis of the immune reaction in the nervous system in paraneoplastic encephalomyelitis [see comments]. *Neurology*, **40**, 219–222.

Graus, F., Illa, I., Agusti, M., Ribalta, T., Cruz, S.F., and Juarez, C. (1991). Effect of intraventricular injection of an anti-Purkinje cell antibody (anti-Yo) in a guinea pig model. *Journal of the Neurological Sciences*, **106**, 82–87.

Gray, J.M., Robertson, I.H., Pentland, B., and Anderson, S.I. (1992). Microcomputer based cognitive rehabilitation for brain damage: a randomised group controlled trial. *Neuropsychological Rehabilitation*, **2**, 97–116.

Graybiel, A.M. (1984). Neurochemically specified subsystems in the basal ganglia. In *Functions of the Basal Ganglia* (ed. Ciba Foundation Symposium 107), pp. 114–149. Pitman, London.

Graybiel, A.M. (1995). The basal ganglia. *Trends in Neurosciences*, **18**, 60–62.

Green, H. (1993). Human genetic diseases due to codon reiteration: relationship to an evolutionary mechanism. *Cell*, **74**, 955–956.

Green, A.R. and Cross, A.J. (1997). *Neuroprotective Agents and Cerebral Ischaemia*. Academic Press, San Diego.

Greenamyre, J.T., and Young, A.B. (1989). Excitatory amino-acids and Alzheimers disease. *Neurobiology of Aging*, **10**, 593–602.

Greenlee, J.E. (1998). Progressive multifocal leukoencephalopathy — progress made and lessons relearned. *New England Journal of Medicine*, **338**, 1378–1380.

Greenlee, J.E. and Brashear, H.R. (1983). Antibodies to cerebellar Purkinje cells in patients with paraneoplastic cerebellar degeneration and ovarian carcinoma. *Annals of Neurology*, **14**, 609–613.

Greenough, W.T., Larson, J.R., and Withers, G.S. (1985). Effects of unilateral and bilateral training in a reaching task on dendritic branching of neurons in the rat motor-sensory forelimb cortex. *Behavioral and Neural Biology*, **44**, 301–304.

Greenwood, J. (1991). Mechanisms of blood-brain barrier breakdown. *Neuroradiology*, **33**, 95–100.

Griffin, D.E., Levine, B.E., Tyor, W.R., Tucker, P.C., and Hardwick, J.M. (1994). Age-dependent susceptibility to fatal encephalitis: alpha virus infection of neurons. *Archives of Virologyt*, **9 (Supplement)**, 31–39.

Griffith, M.E., Coulthart, A., and Pusey, C.D. (1996). T cell responses to myeloperoxidase (MPO) and proteinase 3 (PR3) in patients with systemic vasculitis. *Clin.Exp.Immunol.*, **103**, 253–258.

Grill, R., Murai, K., Blesch, A., Gage, F.H., and Tuszynski, M.H. (1997). Cellular delivery of neurotrophin-3 promotes corticospinal axonal growth and partial functional recovery after spinal cord injury. *Journal of Neuroscience*, **17**, 5560–5572.

Grober, S.E., Gordon, W.A., Sliwinski, M.J., Hibbard, M.R., Aletta, E.G., and Paddison, P.L. (1991). Utility of the dexamethasone suppression test in the diagnosis of post-stroke depression. *Archives of Physical Medicine and Rehabilitation*, **72**, 1076–1079.

Gronwall, D. and Wrightson, P. (1980). Duration of post-traumatic amnesia after mild head injury. *Journal of Clinical Neuropsychology*, **2**, 51–60.

Groves, A.K., Barnett, S.C., Franklin, R.J.M., Crang, A.J., Mayer, M., Blakemore, W.F. *et al.* (1993). Repair of demyelinated lesions by transplantation of purified O-2A progenitor cells. *Nature*, **362**, 453–455.

Gualtieri, T. and Cox, D.R. (1991). The delayed neurobehavioural sequelae of traumatic head injury. *Brain Injury*, **5**, 219–232.

Guazzo, E.P., Kirkpatrick, P.J., Goodyer, I.M., Shiers, H.M., and Herbert, J. (1996). Cortisol, dehydroepiandrosterone

(DHEA), and DHEA sulfate in the cerebrospinal fluid of man: relation to blood levels and the effects of age. *Journal of Clinical Endocrinology and Metabolism,* **81,** 3951–3960.

Gumpel, M., Baumann, N., Raoul, M., and Jacque, C. (1993). Survival and differentiation of oligodendrocytes from neural tissue transplanted into new-born mouse brain. *Neuroscience Letters,* **37,** 307–311.

Haas, A. (1998). Lyme neuroborreliosis. *Current Opinion In Neurology,* **11,** 253–258.

Haas, B.M., Bergström, E., Jamous, A., and Bennie, A. (1996). The inter-rater reliability of the original and of the modified Ashworth scale for the assessment of spasticity in patients with spinal cord injury. *Spinal Cord,* **34,** 560–564.

Hagg, T. (1998). Neurotrophins prevent death and differentially affect tyrosine hydroxylase of adult rat nigrostriatal neurons *in vivo. Experimental Neurology,* **149,** 183–192.

Hakim, S. and Adams, R.D. (1965). The special clinical problems of symptomatic hydrocephalus with normal cerebrospinal fluid pressure. *Journal of Neurological Science,* **2,** 307–327.

Halberstam, J.L., Zaretsky, H.H., Brucker, B.S., and Guttman, A. (1971). Avoidance conditioning of motor responses in elderly brain damaged patients. *Archives of Physical Medicine and Rehabilitation,* **52,** 318–328.

Haley, E.C., Kassell, N.F., Apperson-Hansen, C., Maile, M.H., and Alves, W.M. (1997). A randomized, double-blind, vehicle-controlled trial of tirilazad mesylate in patients with aneurysmal subarachnoid hemorrhage: a cooperative study in North America. *Journal of Neurosurgery,* **86,** 467–474.

Hall, S.M. (1986). The effect of inhibiting Schwann cell mitosis on the re-innervation of acellular autografts in the peripheral nervous system of the mouse. *Neuropathology and Applied Neurobiology,* **12,** 401–414.

Hall, Z.W. and Sanes, J.R. (1993). Synaptic structure and development: the neuromuscular junction. *Cell,* **72,** 99–121.

Hall, E.D. (1997). Lazaroids: mechanisms of action and implications for disorders of the CNS. *The Neuroscientist,* **3,** 42–51.

Halliwell, B. and Gutteridge, J.M.C. (1985). Oxygen radicals and the nervous system. *Trends in Neurosciences,* **8,** 22–26.

Halliwell, B. and Gutteridge, J.M.C. (1989). *Free Radicals in Biology and Medicine.* Clarendon Press, Oxford.

Hamilton, A.S. (1908). A report of 27 cases of chronic progressive chorea. *American Journal of Insanity,* **64,** 403–475.

Hammer, R.E., Palmiter, R.D., and Brinster, R.L. (1984). Partial correction of murine hereditary growth hormone disorder by germ-line incorporation of a new gene. *Nature,* **311,** 65–76.

Hanes, K.R., Andrews, D.G., and Pantelis, C. (1995). Cognitive flexibility and complex integration in Parkinson's disease, Huntington's disease and schizophrenia. *Journal of the International Neuropsychological Society,* **1,** 545–553.

Hans, M.B. and Gilmore, T.H. (1968). Social aspects of Huntington's chorea. *British Journal of Psychiatry,* **114,** 93–98.

Hansotia, P., Wall, R., and erendes, J. (1985). Sleep disturbance and severity of Huntington's disease. *Neurology,* **35,** 1672–1674.

Hantraye, P., Brouillet, E., Ferrante, R., Palfi, S., Dolan, R., Matthews, R.T. *et al.* (1996). Inhibition of neuronal nitric oxide synthase prevents MPTP-induced parkinsonism in baboons. *Nature Medicine,* **2,** 1017–1021.

Hara, H., Morita, M., Iwaka, T., Hatae, T., Itoyama, Y.,

Kitamoto, T. *et al.* (1994). Detection of human T lymphotropic virus type I (HTLV-I) proviral DNA and analysis of T cell receptor Vβ CDR3 sequences in spinal cord lesions of HTLV-I associated myelopathy/tropical spastic paraparesis. *Journal of Experimental Medicine,* **180,** 831–839.

Hardwicke, M.A. and Sandri-Goldin, R.M. (1994). The herpes simplex virus regulatory protein ICP-27 contributes to the decrease in cellular in RNA levels during infection. *Journal of Virology,* **68,** 4797–4810.

Hardy, J. (1992). Framing β-amyloid. *Nature Genetics,* **1,** 233–234.

Hardy, S., Kitamura, M., Harris-Stansil, T., Dai, Y., and Phipps, M.L. (1997). Construction of adenovirus vectors through Cre-lox recombination. *Journal of Virology,* **71,** 1842–1849.

Hargraves, R.W. and Freed, W.J. (1987). Chronic intrastriatal dopamine infusions in rats with unilateral lesions of the substantia nigra. *Life Sciences,* **40,** 959–966.

Harper, P.S. (1992). *Huntington's Disease.* W.B. Saunders, London.

Harrington, C.R., Wischik, C.M., McArthur, F.K., Taylor, G.A., Edwardson, J.A., and Candy, J.M. (1994). Alzheimer's disease-like changes in tau protein processing: association with aluminium accumulation in brains of renal dialysis patients. *Lancet,* **343,** 993–997.

Harris, J.E. (1992). Ways of improving memory. In *Clinical Management of Memory Problems* (ed. B.A. Wilson and N. Moffat), pp. 56–82. Chapman and Hall, London.

Harrison, N.L., Majewska, M.D., Harrington, J.W., and Barker, J.L. (1987). Structure-activity relationships for steroid interaction with the gamma aminobutyric acid α receptor complex. *Journal of Pharmacology and Experimental Therapeutics,* **241,** 346–353.

Hartlage, L.C. (1990). *Neuropsychological Evaluation of Head Injury.* Professional Resource Exchange, Saratosa.

Hastings, T.G., Lewis, D.A., and Zigmond, M.J. (1996). Role of oxidation in the neurotoxic effects of intrastriatal dopamine injections. *Proceedings of the National Academy of Sciences of the United States of America,* **93,** 1956–1961.

Hauser, R.A., Freeman, T.B., Snow, B.J., Nauert, M., Gauger, L., Kordower, J.H *et al.* (1999). Long-term evaluation of bilateral fetal nigral transplantation in Parkinson's disease. *Archives of Neurology,* **56,** 179–187.

Hayes, G.M., Woodroofe, M.N., and Cuzner, M.L. (1987). Microglia are the major cell type expressing MHC class II in human white matter. *Journal of the Neurological Sciences,* **80,** 25–37.

Hebb, D.O. (1949). *The organization of behaviour: a neuropsychological theory.* Wiley, New York.

Heck, A.W. and Phillips, L.H. (1989). Sarcidosis and the nervous system. *Neurol. Clin.,* **7,** 641–654.

Hefti, F. (1983). Is Alzheimer's disease caused by a lack of nerve growth factor? *Annals of Neurology,* **13,** 109–110.

Hefti, F. (1986). Nerve growth factor promotes survival of septal cholinergic neurons after fimbrial transections. *Journal of Neuroscience,* **6,** 2155–2162.

Hefti, F., Melamed, E., Sahakian, B.J., and Wurtman, R.J. (1980). Circling behavior in rats with partial, unilateral nigro-striatal lesions: effects of amphetamine, apomorphine, and DOPA. *Pharmacology, Biochemistry and Behavior,* **12,** 185–188.

Heinel, L., Rubin, S., Rosenwasser, R.H., Vashare, U.S., and

Tuma, R.F. (1994). Leukocyte involvemenkocyte invot in cerebral infarct generation after ischemia and reperfusion. *Brain Research Bulletin*, **34**, 137–141.

Held, J.M., Gordon, J., and entile, A.M. (1985). Environmental influences on locomotor recovery following cortical lesions in rats. *Behavioral Neuroscience*, **4**, 678–690.

Hely, M.A. and Morris, J.G. (1996). Controversies in the treatment of Parkinson's disease. *Current Opinion In Neurology*, **9**, 308–313.

Hemachudha, T. (1994). Human rabies: clinical aspects, pathogenesis and potential therapy. In *Lyssa Viruses* (ed. C.E. Rupprecht, B. Dietzschold and H. Koprowski), pp. 121–143. Springer-Verlag, Berlin.

Hemachudha, T. and Phuapradit, P. (1997). Rabies. *Current Opinion In Neurology*, **10**, 260–267.

Hemmingsen, R. and Rafaelsen, O.J. (1980). Hypnagogic and hypnopompic hallucinations during amitriptyline treatment. *Acta Psychiatrica Scandinavica*, **62**, 364–368.

Henderson, C.E. (1996). Programmed cell death in the developing nervous system. *Neuron*, **17**, 579–585.

Henson, R.A. and Urich, H. (1982). *Cancer and the Nervous System* Anonymous, Blackwell Scientific, London.

Henson, R.A., Hoffman, H.L., and Urich, H. (1965). Encephalomyelitis with carcinoma. *Brain*, **88**, 449–464.

Herbert, J. (1987). Neuroendocrine responses to social stress. *Clin.Endocrinol.Metab.*, **2**, 467–490.

Herbert, J. (1989). Partitioning of neuroendocrine steroids and peptides between vascular and cerebral compartments. In *Psychoendocrinology* (ed. F.R. Brush and S. Levine), pp. 1–40. Academic Press, New York.

Herbert, J. and Martinesz, N.D. (1982). Distribution of prolactin and cortisol between serum and CSF in rhesus monkeys. *Front.Horm.Res.*, **9**, 159–172.

Herman, J.P., Patel, P.D., Akil, H., and Watson, S.J. (1989). Localization and regulation of glucocorticoid and mineralocorticoid receptor messenger RNAs in the hippocampal formation of the rat. *Molecular Endocrinology*, **3**, 1886–1894.

Herzog, R.W., Yang, E.Y., Couto, L.B., Hagstrom, J.N., Elwell, D., Fields, P.A., Burton, M., Bellinger, D.A., Read, M.S., Brinkhous, K.M., Podsakoff, G.M., Nichols, T.C., Kurtzman, G.J. and High, K.A. (1999). Long-term correction of canine hemophilia B by gene transfer of blood coagulation factor IX mediated by adeno-associated viral vector. *Nature Medicine*, **5**, 56–63.

Hess, C.W., Mills, K.R., Murray, N.M., and Schriefer, T.N. (1987). Magnetic brain stimulation: central motor conduction studies in multiple sclerosis. *Annals of Neurology*, **22**, 744–752.

Hess, G. and Donoghue, J.P. (1994). Long-term potentiation of horizontal connections provides a mechanism to reorganize cortical motor maps. *Journal of Neurophysiology*, **71**, 2543–2547.

Heuyer, G. and Lamache, A. (1929a). Le mentisme, part 1. *L'Encéphale*, **24**, 325–336.

Heuyer, G. and Lamache, A. (1929b). Le mentisme, part 2. *L'Encéphale*, **24**, 444–465.

Heyes, M.P., Brew, B.J., Martin, A., Price, R.W., Salazar, A.M., Sidtis, J.J. *et al.* (1991). Quinolinic acid in cerebrospinal-fluid and serum in hiv-1 infection — relationship to clinical and neurological status. *Annals of Neurology*, **29**, 202–209.

Hickey, W.F. and Kumura, H. (1987). Graft versus host disease elicits expression of Class I and Class II histocompatibility antigens and the presence of scattered T-lymphocytes in rat central nervous system. *Proc. Nat. Acad. Sci.*, **84**, 2802–2806.

Hickey, W.F., Hsu, B.L., and Kimura, H. (1991). T-lymphocyte entry into the central nervous system. *Journal of Neuroscience Research*, **28**, 254–260.

Hillbom, M. and Holm, L. (1986). Contribution of traumatic head injury to neuropsychological deficits in alcoholics. *Journal of Neurology, Neurosurgery and Psychiatry*, **49**, 1348–1353.

Himi, T., Ishizaki, Y., and Murota, S.I. (1998). A caspase inhibitor blocks ischaemia-induced delayed neuronal death in the gerbil. *European Journal of Neuroscience*, **10**, 777–781.

Ho, D.Y. (1994). Amplicon-based herpes simplex virus vectors. *Methods In Cell Biology*, **43**, 191–210.

Ho, D.Y., Fink, S.L., Lawrence, M.S., Meier, T.J., Saydam, T.C., Dash, R. *et al.* (1995). Herpes simplex virus vector system: analysis of its *in vivo* and *in vitro* cytopathic effects. *Journal of Neuroscience Methods*, **57**, 205–215.

Ho, D.Y., McLaughlin, J.R., and Sapolsky, R.M. (1996). Inducible gene expression from defective herpes-simplex virus vectors using the tetracycline-responsive promoter system. *Molecular Brain Research*, **41**, 200–209.

Hoche, A.E. (1912). Die Bedeutung der Symptomenkomplexe in der Psychiatrie. *Zeitschrift für die gesamte Neurologie und Psychiatrie*, **12**, 540–551.

Hodges, J.R., Salmon, D.P., and Butters, N. (1990). Differential impairment of semantic and episodic memory in Alzheimer's and Huntington's disease: a controlled prospective study. *Journal of Neurology, Neurosurgery and Psychiatry*, **53**, 1089–1095.

Hoffer, B.J., Hoffman, A., Bowenkamp, K., Huettl, P., Hudson, J., Martin, D. *et al.* (1994). Glial cell line-derived neurotrophic factor reverses toxin-induced injury to midbrain dopaminergic neurons *in vivo*. *Neuroscience Letters*, **182**, 107–111.

Hofmann, A., Nolan, G.P., and Blau, H.M. (1996). Rapid retroviral delivery of tetracycline-inducible genes in a single autoregulatory cassette. *Proceedings of the National Academy of Sciences of the United States of America*, **93**, 5186–5190.

Hohlfeld, R. (1997). Biotechnological agents for the immunotherapy of multiple sclerosis — principles, problems and perspectives. *Brain*, **120**, 865–916.

Holcomb, L., Gordon, M.N., McGowan, E., Yu, X., Benkovic, S., Jantzen, P. *et al.* (1998). Accelerated Alzheimer-type phenotype in transgenic mice carrying both mutant amyloid precursor protein and presenilin 1 transgenes. *Nature Medicine*, **4**, 97–100.

Hollerman, J.R. and Grace, A.A. (1990). The effects of dopamine-depleting brain lesions on the electrophysiological activity of rat substantia nigra dopamine neurons. *Brain Research*, **533**, 203–212.

Hollman, M., O'Shea-Greenfield, A., Rogers, S.W., and Heinemann, S. (1989). Cloning by functional expression of a member of the glutamate receptor family. *Nature*, **342**, 643–648.

Hollmann, M. and Heinemann, S. (1994). Cloned glutamate receptors. *Annual Review of Neuroscience*, **17**, 31–108.

Höllsberg, P., and Hafler, D.A. (1993). Pathogenesis of diseases induced by human lymphotropic virus type I infection. *New England Journal of Medicine*, **328**, 1173–1182.

Höllsberg, P. and Hafler, D.A. (1995). What is the pathogenesis of human T-cell lymphotropic virus type — associated myelopathy/tropical spastic paraparesis. *Annals of Neurology*, **37**, 143–145.

Holmin, S., Almqvist, P., Lendahl, U., and Mathiesen, T. (1997). Adult nestin-expressing subependymal cells differentiate to astrocytes in response to brain injury. *European Journal of Neuroscience*, **9**, 65–75.

Holt, C.E., Bertsch, T.W., Ellis, H.M., and Harris, W.A. (1988). Cellular determination in the Xenopus retina is independent of lineage and birth date. *Neuron*, **1**, 15–26.

Honey, C.R., Clarke, D.J., Dallman, M.J., and Charlton, H.M. (1990). Human neural graft function in rats treated with anti-interleukin II receptor antibody. *NeuroReport*, **1**, 247–249.

Honmou, O., Felts, P.A., Waxman, S.G., and Kocsis, J.D. (1996). Restoration of normal conduction properties in demyelinated spinal cord axons in the adult rat by transplantation of exogenous Schwann cells. *Journal of Neuroscience*, **16**, 3199–3208.

Horellou, P., Marlier, P., Privat, A., and Mallet, J. (1990). Behavioural effects of engineered cells that synthesize L-DOPA or dopamine after grafting into the rat striatum. *European Journal of Neuroscience*, **2**, 116–119.

Horellou, P., Lundberg, C., Lebourdelles, B., Wictorin, K., Brundin, P., Kalén, P. *et al.* (1991). Behavioural effects of genetically engineered cells releasing DOPA and dopamine after intracerebral grafting in a rat model of Parkinson's disease. *Journal de Physiologie*, **85**, 158–170.

Horellou, P., Vigne, E., Castel, M.-N., Barnéoud, P., Colin, P., Perricaudet, M., Delaere, P., and Mallet, J. (1994). Direct intracerebral gene transfer of an adenoviral vector expressing tyrosine hydroxylase in a rat model of Parkinson's disease. *NeuroReport*, **6**, 49–53.

Horger, B.A., Nishimura, M.C., Armanini, M.P., Wang, L.C., Poulsen, K.T., Rosenblad, C. *et al.* (1998). Neurturin exerts potent actions on survival and function of midbrain dopaminergic neurons. *Journal of Neuroscience*, **18**, 4929–4937.

Hori, Y., Kageyama, H., Kihara, T., Ikeda, M., Nakano, A., and Kurosawa, A. (1993). Transient improvement of amphetamine-induced rotational behavior by PC12 cell grafts: Studies with microdialysis. *Restorative Neurology and Neuroscience*, **6**, 49–55.

Horn, S., Shiel, A., McLellan, L., Campbell, M., Watson, M., and Wilson, B.A. (1993). A review of behavioural assessment scales for monitoring recovery in and after coma with pilot data on a new scale of visual awareness. *Neuropsychological Rehabilitation*, **3**, 121–138.

Hortnagl, H., Berger, M.L., Havelec, L., and Hornykiewicz, O. (1993). Role of glucocorticoids in the cholinergic degeneration in rat hippocampus induced by ethylcholine aziridinium (AF64A). *Journal of Neuroscience*, **13**, 2939–2945.

House, A., Dennis, M., Hawton, K., and Warlow, C. (1989). Methods of identifying mood disorders in stroke patients: experiences in the Oxfordshire Community Stroke Project. *Age and Ageing*, **18**, 371–379.

House, A., Dennis, M., Warlow, C., Hawton, K., and Molyneux, A. (1990). Mood disorders after atroke and their relationship to lesion location: a CT scan study. *Brain*, **113**, 1113–1129.

House, A., Dennis, M., Mogridge, L., Warlow, C., Hawton, K., and Jones, L. (1991). Mood disorders in the year after first stroke. *British Journal of Psychiatry*, **158**, 83–92.

Hoverd, P.A. and Fowler, C.J. (1998). Desmopressin in the treatment of daytime urinary frequency in patients with multiple sclerosis. *J.Neurol.Neurosurg.Psychiatry*, **65**, 778–780.

Hoyt, K.R., Reynolds, I.J., and Hastings, T.G. (1997). Mechanisms of dopamine-induced cell death in cultured rat forebrain neurons: interactions with and differences from glutamate-induced cell death. *Experimental Neurology*, **143**, 269–281.

Hsiao, K., Baker, H.F., Crow, T.J., Poulter, M., Owen, F., Terwilliger, J.D. *et al.* (1989). Linkage of a prion protein missense variant to Gerstmann-Straussler syndrome. *Nature*, **338**, 342–345.

Hsiao, K., Groth, D.F., Scott, M., Yang, S.L., Serban, A., and Rapp, D. (1992). Genetic and transgenic studies of prion protein in Gerstman-Straussler-Scheinker disease. In *Prion Diseases of Humans and ANimals* (ed. S.B. Prusiner, J. Collinge, J.F. Powell and B.H. Anderton), pp. 120–128. Ellis Horwood, New York.

Hu, H., Tomasiewicz, H., Magnuson, T., and Rutishauser, U. (1996). The role of polysialic acid in migration of olfactory bulb interneuron precursors in the subventricular zone. *Neuron*, **16**, 735–743.

Hubel, D.H., Wiesel, T.N., and LeVay, S. (1977). Plasticity of ocular dominance columns in monkey striate cortex. *Philosophical Transactions of the Royal Society of London.B:Biological Sciences*, **277**, 377–409.

Huber, G. (1981). *Psychiatrie*. Schattauer, Stuttgart.

Huber, S.J. and Paulson, G.W. (1985). The concept of subcortical dementia. *American Journal of Psychiatry*, **142**, 1312–1317.

Huffaker, T.K., Boss, B.D., Morgan, A.S., Neff, N.T., Strecker, R.E., Spence, M.S., and Miao, R. (1989). Xenografting of fetal pig ventral mesencephalon corrects motor asymmetry in the rat model of Parkinson's disease. *Experimental Brain Research*, **77**, 329–336.

Hughes, E.M. (1925). Social significance of Huntington's chorea. *American Journal of Psychiatry*, **81**, 537–573.

Hunter, A.J. (1997). Calcium antagonists: their role in neuroprotection. In *Neuroprotective Agents and Cerebral Ischaemia* (ed. A.R. Green and A.J. Cross), pp. 95–108. Academic Press, San Diego.

Huntington, G. (1872). On chorea. *Advances in Neurology*, **1**, 33–35.

Huntington's Disease Collaborative Research Group. (1993). A novel gene containing a trinucleotide repeat that is expanded and unstable on Huntington's disease chromosomes. *Cell*, **72**, 971–983.

Hutchison, W.D., Lozano, A.M., Davis, K.D., St.Cyr, J.A., Lang, A.E., and Dostrovsky, J.O. (1994). Differential neuronal activity in segments of globus pallidus in Parkinson's disease patients. *NeuroReport*, **5**, 1533–1537.

Hutchison, W.D., Allan, R.J., Opitz, H., Levy, R., Dostrovsky, J.O., Lang, A.E. *et al.* (1998). Neurophysiological identification of the subthalamic nucleus in surgery for Parkinson's disease. *Annals of Neurology*, **44**, 622–628.

Hyatt-Sachs, H., Schreiber, R.C., Bennett, T.A., and Zigmond,

R.E. (1993). Phenotypic plasticity in adult sympathetic ganglia *in vivo*: effects of deafferentation and axotomy on the expression of vasoactive intestinal peptide. *Journal of Neuroscience*, 13, 1642–1653.

Hynes, M., Porter, J.A., Chiang, C., Chang, D., Tessier-Lavigne, M., Beachy, P.A. *et al.* (1995). Induction of midbrain dopaminergic neurons by Sonic hedgehog. *Neuron*, 15, 35–44.

Ichinose, H., Ohye, T., Takahashi, E., Seki, N., Hori, T., Segawa, M. *et al.* (1994). Hereditary progressive dystonia with marked diurnal fluctuation caused by mutations in the GTP cyclohydrolase I gene [see comments]. *Nat.Genet.*, 8, 236–242.

Illarioshkin, S.N., Igarashi, S., Onodera, O., Markova, E.D., Nikolskaya, N.N., Tanaka, H. *et al.* (1994). Trinucleotide repeat length and rate of progression of Huntington's disease. *Annals of Neurology*, 36, 630–635.

Imaizumi, T., Lankford, K.L., Waxman, S.G., Greer, C.A., and Kocsis, J.D. (1998). Transplanted olfactory ensheathing cells remyelinate and enhance axonal conduction in the demyelinated dorsal columns of the rat spinal cord. *Journal of Neuroscience*, 18, 6176–6185.

Ince, L.P. (1969). Escape and avoidance conditioning of response in the plegic arm of stroke patients: a preliminary study. *Psychonomic Science*, 16, 49–50.

Ip, N.Y. and Yancopoulos, G.D. (1996). The neurotrophins and CNTF — 2 families of collaborative neurotrophic factors. *Annual Review of Neuroscience*, 19, 491–515.

Irwin, R.P., Maragakis, N.J., Rogawski, M.A., Purdy, R.H., Farb, D.H., and Paul, S.M. (1992). Pregnenolone sulfate augments NMDA receptor mediated increases in intracellular $Ca^{2+}$ in cultured rat hippocampal neurons. *Neuroscience Letters*, 141, 30–34.

Isacson, O., Dunnett, S.B., and Björklund, A. (1986). Graft-induced behavioral recovery in an animal model of Huntington disease. *Proceedings of the National Academy of Sciences of the United States of America*, 83, 2728–2732.

Itoyama, Y., Ohnishi, A., Tateishi, J., Kuroiwa, Y., and Webster, H.D. (1985). Spinal cord multiple sclerosis lesions in Japanese patients — Schwann cell remyelination occurs in areas that lack glial fibrillary acidic protein (GFAP). *Acta Neuropathologica*, 65, 217–223.

Izumo, S., Usuku, K., Osame, M. *et al.* (1989). The neuropathology of HTLV-I associated myelopathy in Japan: report of an autopsy case and review of the literature. In *HTLV-I and the Nervous System* (ed. G.C. Roman, J.C. Vernant and M. Osame), pp. 261–267. Alan R Liss, New York.

Jablonska, B., Gierdalski, M., Siucinska, E., Skangiel-Kramska, J., and Kossut, M. (1995). Partial blocking of NMDA receptors restricts plastic changes in adult-mouse barrel cortex. *Behavioural Brain Research*, 66, 207–216.

Jackson, A.C. and Park, H. (1998). Apoptotic cell death in experimental rabies in suckling mice. *Acta Neuropathologica*, 95, 159–164.

Jacobs, L. and Kinkel, W. (1976). Computerized axial transverse tomography in normal pressure hydrocephalus. *Neurology*, 26, 501–507.

Jacobs, K.M. and Donoghue, J.P. (1991). Reshaping the cortical motor map by unmasking latent intracortical connections. *Science*, 251, 944–947.

Jacobsen, E.J., McCall, J.M., Ayer, D.E., VanDoornik, F.J., Palmer, J.R., Belonga, K.L. *et al.* (1990). Novel 21-aminosteroids that inhibit iron-dependent lipid peroxidation and protect against central nervous system trauma. *Journal of Medicinal Chemistry*, 33, 1145–1151.

Jacobson, P.L. and Farmer, T.W. (1979). The 'hypernormal' CT scan and dementia: bilateral isodense subdural haematomas. *Neurology*, 29, 1522–1524.

Jaeckle, K.A., Graus, F., Houghton, A., Cardon, C.C., Nielsen, S.L., and Posner, J.B. (1985). Autoimmune response of patients with paraneoplastic cerebellar degeneration to a Purkinje cell cytoplasmic protein antigen. *Annals of Neurology*, 18, 592–600.

Jain, A.K., Kewala, S., and Gershon, S. (1988). Antipsychotic drugs in schizophrenia: current issues. *International Journal of Clinical Psychopharmacology*, 3, 1–30.

Jankovic, J. (1994). Botulinum toxin in movement disorders. *Current Opinion In Neurology*, 7, 358–366.

Jankovic, J. (1998). Re-emergence of surgery for dystonia [editorial; comment]. *J.Neurol.Neurosurg.Psychiatry*, 65, 434.

Janota, I. (1981). Dementia, deep white matter damage and hypertension 'Binswanger disease'. *Psychological Medicine*, 11, 39–48.

Janzer, R.C. and Raff, M.C. (1987). Astrocytes induce blood–brain barrier properties in endothelial cells. *Nature*, 325, 253–257.

Jason, G.W., Suchowersky, O., Pajurkova, E.M., Graham, L., Klimek, M.L., Garber, A.T. *et al.* (1997). Cognitive manifestations of Huntington disease in relation to genetic structure and clinical onset. *Archives of Neurology*, 54, 1081–1088.

Jaszai, J., Farkas, L., Galter, D., Reuss, B., Strelau, J., Unsicker, K., and Krieglstein, K. (1998). GDNF-related factor persephin is widely distributed throughout the nervous system. *Journal of Neuroscience Research*, 53, 494–501.

Jeffcoate, W.J., Silverstone, J.T., Edwards, C.R.W., and Besser, G.M. (1979). Psychiatric manifestations of Cushing's syndrome: response to lowering of plasma cortisol. *Quarterly Journal of Medicine*, 48, 465–472.

Jeffery, N.D. and Blakemore, W.F. (1997). Locomotor deficits induced by experimental spinal cord demyelination are abolished by spontaneous remyelination. *Brain*, 120, 27–37.

Jenkins, W.M., Merzenich, M.M., Ochs, M.T., Allard, T., and Guic-Robles, E. (1990). Functional reorganization of primary somatosensory cortex in adult owl monkeys after behaviorally controlled tactile stimulation. *Journal of Neurophysiology*, 63, 82–104.

Jenkins, I.H., Fernandez, W., Playford, E.D., Lees, A.J., Frackowiak, R.S., Passingham, R.E. *et al.* (1992). Impaired activation of the supplementary motor area in Parkinson's disease is reversed when akinesia is treated with apomorphine. *Annals of Neurology*, 32, 749–757.

Jenner, P. (1998). Oxidative mechanisms in nigral cell death in Parkinson's disease. *Movement Disorders*, 13, 24–34.

Jennett, B. and Teasdale, G. (1977). Aspects of coma after severe head injury. *Lancet*, 1, 878–881.

Jennett, B. and Teasdale, G. (1981). *Management of Head Injuries*. Davis, Philadelphia.

Jennette, J.C., Falk, R.J., Andrassy, K., Bacon, P.A., Churg, J., Gross, W.L. *et al.* (1994a). Nomenclature of systemic vasculitides: proposal of an international consensus conference. *Arthritis and Rheumatism*, 37, 187–192.

Jennette, J.C., Falk, R.J., and Milling, D.M. (1994b). Pathogenesis of vasculitis. *Semin. Neurol.*, **14**, 291–299.

Jensen, P., Sorensen, S.A., Fenger, F., and Bowling, T.G. (1993). A study of psychiatric morbidity in patients with Huntington's disease, their relatives and controls. *British Journal of Psychiatry*, **163**, 790–797.

Jessen, K.R. and Mirsky, R. (1999). Schwann cells and their precursors emerge as major regulators of nerve development. *Trends in Neurosciences*, **22**, 402–410.

Jiao, S.S., Schultz, E., and Wolff, J.A. (1992). Intracerebral transplants of primary muscle cels: a potential 'platform' for transgene expression in the brain. *Brain Research*, **575**, 143–147.

Jiao, S.S., Gurevich, V., and Wolff, J.A. (1993). Long-term correction of rat model of Parkinson's disease by gene therapy. *Nature*, **362**, 450–453.

Johansson, C.B., Momma, S., Clarke, D.L., Risling, M., Lendahl, U., and Frisen, J. (1999). Identification of a neural stem cell in the adult mammalian central nervous system. *Cell*, **96**, 25–34.

John, J. (1984). Grading of muscle power: comparison of MRC and analogue scales by physiotherapists. *International Journal of Rehabilitation Research*, **7**, 173–181.

Johnson, R.T., Glass, J.D., McArthur, J.C., and Chesebro, B.W. (1996). Quantitation of human immunodeficiency virus in brains of demented and non-demented patients with acquired immunodeficiency syndrome. *Annals of Neurology*, **39**, 392–395.

Johnson, K.P., Brooks, B.R., Cohen, J.A., Ford, C.C., Goldstein, J., Lisak, R.P. *et al.* (1998). Extended use of glatiramer acetate (Copaxone) is well tolerated and maintains its clinical effect on multiple sclerosis relapse rate and degree of disability. *Neurology*, **50**, 701–708.

Joly, E. and Oldstone, M.B.A. (1992). Neuronal cells are deficient in loading peptides onto MHC class 1 molecules. *Neuron*, **8**, 1185–1190.

Joly, E., Mucke, L., and Oldstone, M.B.A. (1991). Viral persistence in neurons explained by lack of major histocompatibility class 1 expression. *Science*, **253**, 1283–1285.

Jones, E.G. and Pons, T.P. (1998). Thalamic and brainstem contributions to large-scale plasticity of primate somatosensory cortex. *Science*, **282**, 1121–1125.

Jones, T.A. and Schallert, T. (1992). Overgrowth and pruning of dendrites in adult rats recovering from neocortical damage. *Brain Research*, **581**, 156–160.

Jonhagen, M.E., Nordberg, A., Amberla, K., Backman, L., Ebendal, T., Meyerson, B. *et al.* (1998). Intracerebroventricular infusion of nerve growth factor in three patients with Alzheimer's disease. *Dementia and Geriatric Cognitive Disorders*, **9**, 246–257.

Jorge, R.E., Robinson, R.G., and Arndt, S. (1993a). Are there symptoms that are specific for depressed mood in patients with traumatic brain injury? *Journal of Nervous and Mental Diseases*, **181**, 91–99.

Jorge, R.E., Robinson, R.G., Arndt, S.V., Forrester, A.W., Geisler, F., and Starkstein, S.E. (1993b). Comparison between acute- and delayed-onset depression following traumatic brain injury. *J. Neuropsychiatry Clin. Neurosci.*, **5**, 43–49.

Juhler, M. and Neuwelt, E.A. (1989). The blood brain barrier and the immune system. In: Neuwelt, E.A. ed. *Implications of the blood brain barrier and its manipulation*. Plenum Press.

Kaas, J.H. (1991). Plasticity of sensory and motor maps in adult mammals. *Annual Review of Neuroscience*, **14**, 137–167.

Kaas, J.H. (1995). The reorganisation of sensory and motor maps in adult mammals. In *The Cognitive Neurosciences* (ed. M.S. Gazzaniga), pp. 51–71. MIT Press, Cambridge, MA.

Kallenberg, C.G.M., Brouwer, E., Weening, J.J., and Cohen Tervaert, J.W. (1994). Anti-neutrophil cytoplasmic antibodies: current diagnostic and pathophysiological potential. *Kidney International*, **46**, 1–15.

Kandel, E.R., Schwartz, J.H., and Jessell, T.M. (1991). *Principles of Neural Science*. Appleton & Lange, Stamford, CT.

Kandel, E.R., Schwartz, J.H., and Jessell, T.M. (1995). *Essentials of Neural Science and Behavior*. Appleton & Lange, Stamford, CT.

Kandel, E.R., Schwarz, J.H., and Jessell, T.M. (2000). *Principles of Neural Science*, 4th edn. McGraw-Hill Comparies Inc.

Kang, J., Lemaire, H.-G., Unterbeck, A., Salbaum, J.M., Masters, C.L., Grzeschik, K.-H., Multhaup, G., Beyreuther, K., and Müller-Hill, B. (1987). The precursor of Alzheimer's disease amyloid A4 protein resembles a cell-surface receptor. *Nature*, **325**, 733–736.

Kaplan, M.S. (1981). Neurogenesis in the 3 month old rat visual cortex. *Journal of Comparative Neurology*, **195**, 323–338.

Kaplitt, M.G., Leone, P., Samulski, R.J., Xiao, X., Pfaff, D.W., O'Malley, K.L. *et al.* (1994a). Long-term gene expression and phenotypic correction using adeno-associated virus vectors in the mammalian brain. *Nature Genetics*, **8**, 148–154.

Kaplitt, M.G., Kwong, A.D., Kleopoulos, S.P., Mobbs, C.V., Rabkin, S.D., and Pfaff, D.W. (1994b). Preproenkephalin promoter yields region-specific and long-term expression in adult brain after direct *in vivo* gene-transfer via a defective herpes-simplex viral vector. *Proceedings of the National Academy of Sciences of the United States of America*, **91**, 8979–8983.

Kass, I.S. and Lipton, P. (1982). Mechanisms involved in irreversible anoxic damage to the *in vitro* rat hippocampal stlice. *Journal of Physiology (London)*, **332**, 459–472.

Kassell, N.F., Haley, C., Apperson-Hansen, C., Stat, M., and Alves, W.M. (1996). Randomized, double-blind, vehicle-controlled trial of tirilazad mesyulate in patients with aneurysmal subarachnoid haemorrhage: a cooperative study in Europe, Australia, and New Zealand. *Journal of Neurosurgery*, **84**, 221–228.

Kawaja, M.D. and Gage, F.H. (1991). Reactive astrocytes are substrates for the growth of adult CNS axons in the presence of elevated levels of nerve growth factor. *Neuron*, **7**, 1019–1030.

Kazumata, K., Antonini, A., Dhawan, V., Moeller, J.R., Alterman, R.L., Kelly, P. *et al.* (1997). Preoperative indicators of clinical outcome following stereotaxic pallidotomy. *Neurology*, **49**, 1083–1090.

Kehrer, F. (1928). *Erblichkeit und Nervenleiden. I. Ursachen und erblichkeitskreis von Chorea, Myoklonie und Athetose.* Springer, Berlin.

Keirstead, H.S., Dyer, J.K., Sholomenko, G.N., McGraw, J.,

Delaney, K.R., and Steeves, J.D. (1995). Axonal regeneration and physiological activity following transection and immunological disruption of myelin within the hatchling chick spinal cord. *Journal of Neuroscience*, 15, 6963–6974.

Keirstead, H.S. and Blakemore, W.F. (1997). Identification of post-mitotic oligodendrocytes incapable of remyelination within the demyelinated adult spinal cord. *Journal of Neuropathology and Experimental Neurology*, 56, 1191–1201.

Keirstead, H.S., Levine, J.M., and Blakemore, W.F. (1998). Response of the oligodendrocyte progenitor cell population (as defined by NG2 labelling) to demyelination in the adult spinal cord. *Glia*, 22, 161–170.

Keirstead, H.S., Hughes, H.C., and Blakemore, W.F. (1998). A quantifiable model of axonal regeneration in the demyelinated adult rat spinal cord. *Experimental Neurology*, 151, 303–313.

Kellner, M.B. and Strian, F. (1991). Bizarre delusion and post-hemiplegic hemidystonia [letter]. *Br.J.Psychiatry*, 159, 448.

Kempermann, G., Kuhn, H.G., and Gage, F.H. (1998). Experience-induced neurogenesis in the senescent dentate gyrus. *Journal of Neuroscience*, 18, 3206–3212.

Kempermann, G., Brandon, E.P., and Gage, F.H. (1998). Environmental stimulation of 129/SvJ mice causes increased cell proliferation and neurogenesis in the adult dentate gyrus. *Current Biology*, 8, 939–942.

Kempermann, G. and Gage, F.H. (1999). New nerve cells for the adult brain. *Scientific American*, 280, 48–53.

Kendall, A.L., Rayment, F.D., Torres, E.M., Baker, H.F., Ridley, R.M., and Dunnett, S.B. (1998). Functional integration of striatal allografts in a primate model of Huntington's disease. *Nature Medicine*, 4, 727–729.

Kennard, M.A. (1936). Age and other factors in motor recovery from precentral lesions in monkeys. *American Journal of Physiology*, 115, 138–146.

Kennard, M.A. (1942). Cortical reorganisation of motor function: studies on a series of monkeys of various ages from infancy to maturity. *Archives of Neurology and Psychiatry*, 48, 227–240.

Kerr, J.F.R. and Harmon, B.V. (1991) Definition and incidence of apoptosis: A historical perspective. In Tomei, LD, Cope, FO (eds) *Apoptosis, the molecular basis of cell death*. Cold Spring Harbor, NY, Cold Spring Harbor Laboratory Press.

Kertesz, A. (1979). *Aphasia and Associated Disorders*. Grune and Stratton, New York.

Keschner, M., Bender, M.B., and Strauss, I. (1936). Mental symptoms in cases of tumour of the temporal lobe. *Archives of Neurology and Psychiatry*, 35, 572–596.

Kieburtz, K., Feigin, A., McDermott, M., Como, P., Abwender, D., Zimmerman, C. *et al.* (1996a). A controlled trial of remacemide hydrochloride in Huntington's disease. *Movement Disorders*, 11, 273–277.

Kieburtz, K., Penney, J.B., Como, P., Ranen, N., Shoulson, I., Feigin, A. *et al.* (1996b). Unified Huntington's disease rating scale: reliability and consistency. *Movement Disorders*, 11, 136–142.

Kieburtz, K. (1999). Antiglutamate therapies in Huntington's disease. *Journal of Neural Transmission, supplement*, 55, 97–102.

Kimonides, V.G., Khatibi, N.H., Svendsen, C.N., Sofroniew, M.V., and Herbert, J. (1998). Dehydroepiandrosterone (DHEA) and DHEA-sulfate (DHEAS) protect hippocampal neurons against excitatory amino acid-induced neurotoxicity. *Proceedings of the National Academy of Sciences of the United States of America*, 95, 1852–1857.

Kimonides, V.G., Spillantini, M.G., Sofroniew, M.V., Fawcett, J.W., and Herbert, J. (1999). Dehydroepiandrosterone antagonizes the neurotoxic effects of corticosterone and translocation of stress-activated protein kinase 3 in hippocampal primary cultures. *Neuroscience*, 89, 429–436.

King, M. (1985). Alcohol abuse in Huntington's disease. *Psychological Medicine*, 15, 815–819.

Kinsella, G., and Ford, B. (1980). Acute recovery patterns in stroke patients. *Medical Journal of Australia*, 2, 663–666.

Kirsch, N.L., Levine, S.P., Fallon-Krueger, M., and Jaros, L.A. (1987). The microcomputer as an 'orthotic' device for patients with cognitive deficits. *Journal of Head Trauma Rehabilitation*, 2, 77–86.

Kissel, J.T. (1989). Neurologic manifestations of vasculitis. *Neurologic Clinics*, 7, 655–673.

Kizer, S., Nemeroff, C.R., and Youngblood, W.W. (1978). Neurotoxic amino acids and structurally related analogs. *Pharmacological Review*, 29, 301–318.

Klassen, H., and Lund, R.D. (1987). Retinal transplants can drive a pupillary reflex in host rat brains. *Proceedings of the National Academy of Sciences of the United States of America*, 84, 6958–6960.

Klein, R.L., Meyer, E.M., Peel, A.L., Zolotukhin, S., Meyers, C., Muzyczka, N. *et al.* (1998). Neuron-specific transduction in the rat septohippocampal or nigrostriatal pathway by recombinant adeno-associated virus vectors. *Experimental Neurology*, 150, 183–194.

Klocker, N., Cellerino, A., and Bahr, M. (1998). Free radical scavenging and inhibition of nitric oxide synthase potentiates the neurotrophic effects of brain-derived neurotrophic factor on axotomized retinal ganglion cells *in vivo*. *Journal of Neuroscience*, 18, 1038–1046.

Knüsel, B., Beck, K.D., Winslow, J.W., Rosenthal, A., Burton, L.E., Widmer, H.R. *et al.* (1992). Brain-derived neurotrophic factor administration protects basal forebrain cholinergic but not nigral dopaminergic neurons from degenerative changes after axotomy in the adult brain. *Journal of Neuroscience*, 12, 4391–4402.

Kobayashi, N.R., Bedard, A.M., Hincke, M.T., and Tetzlaff, W. (1996). Increased expression of BDNF and trkB mRNA in rat facial motoneurons after axotomy. *European Journal of Neuroscience*, 8, 1018–1029.

Kobayashi, N.R., Fan, D.P., Giehl, K.M., Bedard, A.M., Wiegand, S.J., and Tetzlaff, W. (1997). BDNF and NT-4/5 prevent atrophy of rat rubrospinal neurons after cervical axotomy, stimulate GAP-43 and T1-tubulin mRNA expression, and promote axonal regeneration. *Journal of Neuroscience*, 15, 9583–9595.

Kochler, R., Linder, M., and Stula, D. (1984). Primäre Hirntumoren in der Psychiatrie. *Schweizer Archives für Neurologie, Neurochirurgie und Psychiatrie*, 135, 217–227.

Kocisko, D.A., Come, J.H., Priola, S.A., Chesebro, B., Raymond, G.J., Lansbury, P.T. *et al.* (1994). Cell-free formation of protease-resistant prion protein. *Nature*, 370, 471–474.

Koike, T., Martin, D.P., and Johnson, E.M. (1989). Role of $Ca^{2+}$ channels in the ability of membrane depolarization to prevent neuronal death induced by trophic-factor deprivation: evidence that levels of internal $Ca^{2+}$ determine nerve growth factor dependence of sympathetic ganglion cells. *Proceedings of the National Academy of Sciences of the United States of America*, 86, 6421–6425.

Koike, C., Hayashi, R., Yokoyama, I., Yamakawa, H., Negita, M., and Takagi, H. (1996). Converting alpha-GAL epitope of pig into H antigen. *Transplantation Proceedings*, 28, 553.

Kokkanen, L. and Launes, J. (1997). Cognitive recovery instead of decline after acute encephalitis: a prospective follow up study. *Journal of Neurology, Neurosurgery and Psychiatry*, 63, 222–227.

Kolb, B. (1992). Mechanisms underlying recovery from cortical injury: reflections on progress and directions for the future. In *Recovery from brain damage: Reflections and directions* (ed. F.D. Rose and D.A. Johnson), pp. 169–186. Plenum, New York.

Kolb, B. (1996). *Brain Plasticity and Behaviour*. Lawrence Erlbaum, Hillsdale, NJ.

Kolb, B. and Whishaw, I.Q. (1989). Plasticity in the neocortex: mechanisms underlying recovery from early brain damage. *Progress in Neurobiology*, 32, 235–276.

Koller, W., Vetere-Overfeld, B., Gray, C., Alexander, C., Chin, T., Dolezal, J. *et al.* (1990). Environmental risk factors in Parkinson's disease. *Neurology*, 40, 1218–1221.

Komoly, S., Hudson, L.D., Webster, H.D., and Bondy, C.A. (1992). Insulin-like growth factor-1 gene expression is induced in astrocytes during experimental demyelination. *Proceedings of the National Academy of Sciences of the United States of America*, 89, 1894–1898.

Kondziolka, D., Bonaroti, E., Baser, S., Brandt, F., Kim, Y.S., and Lunsford, L.D. (1999). Outcomes after stereotactically guided pallidotomy for advanced Parkinson's disease. *Journal of Neurosurgery*, 90, 197–202.

Kopyov, O.V., Jacques, D., Lieberman, A., Duma, C.M., and Rogers, R.L. (1996). Clinical study of fetal mesencephalic intracerebral transplants for the treatment of Parkinson's disease. *Cell Transplantation*, 5, 327–337.

Kopyov, O.V., Jacques, S., Kurth, M., Philpott, L.M., Lee, A., Patterson, M., Duma, C., Lieberman, A., and Eagle, K.S. (1998). Fetal transplantation for Huntington's disease: clinical studies. In *Cell Transplantation for Neurological Disorders* (ed. T.B. Freeman and J.H. Kordower), pp. 95–134. Humana Press, Totowa, NJ.

Kordower, J.H., Palfi, S., Chen, E.Y., Ma, S.Y., Sendera, T., Cochran, E.J., Mufson, E.J., Penn, R., Goetz, C.G., and Comella, C.D. (1999). Clinicopathological findings following intraventricular glial-derived neurotrophic factor treatment in a patient with Parkinson's disease. *Annals of Neurology*, 46, 419–424.

Kordower, J.H., Freeman, T.B., Snow, B.J., Vingerhoets, F.J.G., Mufson, E.J., Sanberg, P.R., Hauser, R.A., Smith, D.A., Nauert, G.M., Perl, D.P., and Olanow, C.W. (1995). Neuropathological evidence of graft survival and striatal reinnervation after the transplantation of fetal mesencephalic tissue in a patient with Parkinson's disease. *New England Journal of Medicine*, 332, 1118–1124.

Kornack, D.R. and Rakic, P. (1999). Continuation of neurogenesis in the hippocampus of the adult macaque monkey. *Proceedings of the National Academy of Sciences of the United States of America*, 96, 5768–5773.

Kornstein, M.J., Asher, O., and Fuchs, S. (1995). Acetylcholine

receptor alpha-subunit and myogenin mRNAs in thymus and thymomas. *Am. J. Pathol.*, 146, 1320–1324.

Kornguth, S.E. (1989). Neuronal proteins and paraneoplastic syndromes. *New Eng. J. Med.*, 321, 1607–1608.

Kosaka, K., Matsushita, M., Oyanagi, S., Hato, K., and Mehraein, P. (1980). [Pick's disease with concomitant traumatic brain damage–five autopsied cases and a critical review of literatures (author's transl)]. *Seishin.Shinkeigaku.Zasshi.*, 82, 33–47.

Kosaka, K., Yoshimura, M., Ikeda, K., and Budka, H. (1984). Diffuse type of Lewy body disease — progressive dementia with abundant cortical lewy bodies and senile changes of varying degree — a new disease. *Clinical Neuropathology*, 3, 185–192.

Koshel, K. and Munzel, P. (1984). Inhabitation of opiate receptor mediated signal transmission by rabies virus in persistently infected NG-108-15 mouse neuroblastoma — rat glioma hybrid cells. *Proceedings of the National Academy of Sciences of the United States of America*, 81, 950–954.

Kosslyn, S.M. (1996). Neural systems and psychiatric disorders. *Cognitive Neuropsychiatry*, 1, 89–93.

Kou, S.Y., Chiu, A.Y., and Patterson, P.H. (1995). Differential regulation of motor neuron survival and choline acetyltransferase expression following axotomy. *Journal of Neurobiology*, 27, 561–572.

Kowall, N.W., Beal, M.F., Busciglio, J., Duffy, L.K., and Yankner, B.A. (1991). An *in vivo* model for the neurodegenerative effects of $\beta$ amyloid and protection by substance P. *Proceedings of the National Academy of Sciences of the United States of America*, 88, 7247–7251.

Krack, P., Benazzouz, A., Pollak, P., Limousin, P., Piallat, B., Hoffmann, D. *et al.* (1998). Treatment of tremor in Parkinson's disease by subthalamic nucleus stimulation. *Movement Disorders*, 13, 907–914.

Kreutzberg, G.W. (1996). Microglia: a sensor for pathological events in the CNS. *Trends in Neurosciences*, 19, 312–318.

Krieger, D.T., Allen, W., Rizzo, F., and Krieger, H.P. (1971). Characterisation of the temporal pattern of plasma corticosterone levels. *Journal of Clinical Endocrinology and Metabolism*, 32, 266–285.

Krieger, D.T., Perlow, M.J., Gibson, M.J., Davies, T.F., Zimmerman, E.A., Ferin, M. *et al.* (1982). Brain grafts reverse hypogonadism of gonadotropin releasing hormone deficiency. *Nature*, 298, 468–471.

Kromer, L.F. (1987). Nerve growth factor treatment after brain injury prevents neuronal death. *Science*, 235, 214–216.

Kromer, L.F., Björklund, A., and Stenevi, U. (1981). Regeneration of the septohippocampal pathway in adult rats is promoted by utilizing embryonic hippocampal implants as bridges. *Brain Research*, 210, 173–200.

Kuang, R.Z. and Kalil, K. (1990). Specificity of corticospinal axon arbors sprouting into denervated contralateral spinal cord. *Journal of Comparative Neurology*, 302, 461–472.

Kuffler, D.P. (1986). Accurate reinnervation of motor end plates after disruption of sheath cells and muscle fibers. *Journal of Comparative Neurology*, 250, 228–235.

Kuhn, T. (1970). *The Structure of Scientific Revolutions*. University of Chicago Press, Chicago.

Kuhn, H.G., Dickinson-Anson, H., and Gage, F.H. (1997). Neurogenesis in the dentate gyrus of the adult rat: age-related decrease of neuronal progenitor proliferation. *Journal of Neuroscience*, 16, 2027–2033.

Kurtzke, J.F. (1955). A new scale for evaluating disability in multiple sclerosis. *Neurology*, 5, 580–585.

Kurtzke, J.F. (1961). On the evaluation of disability in multiple sclerosis. *Neurology*, 11, 686–694.

Kwentus, J.A. and Hart, R.P. (1987). Normal pressure hydrocephalus presenting as mania. *Journal of Nervous and Mental Diseases*, 175, 500–502.

La Gamma, E.F., Strecker, R.E., Lenn, N.J., DeChristofano, J.D., and Weisinger, G. (1994). Dopaminergic regulation of a transfected preproenkephalin promoter in primary rat astrocytes *in vitro* and *in vivo*. *Experimental Neurology*, 130, 304–310.

Labrie, Y., Couet, J., Simard, J., and Labrie, F. (1994). Multihormonal regulation of dehydroepiandrosterone sulfotransferase messenger ribonucleic acid levels in adult rat liver. *Endocrinology*, 134, 1693–1699.

Lachmann, R.H. and Efstathiou, S. (1997). Utilization of the herpes simplex virus type 1 latency-associated regulatory region to drive stable reporter gene expression in the nervous system. *Journal of Virology*, 71, 3197–3207.

Lader, M. (1995). *Handbook of Clinical Neurology, Vol. 65.* Elsevier.

Lafon-Cazal, M., Pietri, S., Culcasi, M., and Bockaert, J. (1997). NMDA-dependent superoxide production and neurotoxicity. *Nature*, 364, 535–537.

Lam, T.T., Abler, A.S., and Tso, M.O.M. (1999). Apoptosis and caspases after ischemia-reperfusion injury in rat retina. *Investigative Ophthalmology and Visual Science*, ISUAL, 967–975.

Lan, N.C., Gee, K.W., Bolger, M.B., and Chen, J.S. (1991). Differential responses of expressed recombinant human $\gamma$-aminobutyric acid $\alpha$ receptors to neurosteroids. *Journal of Neurochemistry*, 57, 1818–1821.

Landis, S.C. and Keefe, D. (1983). Evidence for neurotransmitter plasticity *in vivo*: developmental changes in properties of cholinergic sympathetic neurons. *Developmental Biology*, 98, 349–372.

Lang, A.E. (1996). Teaching tape for the motor section of the Unified Parkinson's Disease Rating Scale. *Movement Disorders*, 11, 344–345.

Lang, A.E. and Lozano, A.M. (1998a). Parkinson's disease. First of two parts. *New England Journal of Medicine*, 339, 1044–1053.

Lang, A.E. and Lozano, A.M. (1998b). Parkinson's disease. Second of two parts. *New England Journal of Medicine*, 339, 1130–1143.

Lange, K.W., Sahakian, B.J., Quinn, N.P., Marsden, C.D., and Robbins, T.W. (1995). Comparison of executive and visuospatial memory function in Huntington's disease and dementia of Alzheimer-type matched for degree of dementia. *Journal of Neurology, Neurosurgery and Psychiatry*, 58, 598–606.

Lange, K.W., Robbins, T.W., Marsden, C.D., James, M., Owen, A.M., and Paul, G.M. (1992). L-Dopa withdrawal in Parkinson's disease selectively impairs cognitive performance in tests of frontal lobe function. *Psychopharmacology*, 107, 394–404.

Langston, J.W. and Ballard, P.A. (1983). Parkinson's disease in a chemist working with 1-methyl-4-phenyl-1,2,5,6-tetrahydropyridine. *New England Journal of Medicine*, 309, 310.

Langston, J.W., Ballard, P., Tetrud, J.W., and Irwin, I. (1983).

Chronic parkinsonism in humans due to a product of meperidine-analog synthesis. *Science*, 219, 979–980.

Langston, J.W., Forno, L.S., Rebert, C.S., and Irwin, I. (1984). Selective nigral toxicity after systemic administration of 1-methyl-4-phenyl-1,2,5,6-tetrahydropyrine (MPTP) in the squirrel monkey. *Brain Research*, 292, 390–394.

Langston, J.W., Widner, H., and Goetz, C.G. (1992). Core assessment program for intracerebral transplantation (CAPIT). *Movement Disorders*, 7, 2–13.

Langton-Hewer, R. (1995). The management of motor neuron disease. In *Motor Neuron Disease: Biology and Management* (ed. P.N. Leigh and M. Swash), pp. 375–403. Springer-Verlag, London.

Lansbury, P.T. (1998). Structural neurology: are seeds at the root of neuronal degeneration? *Neuron*, 19, 1151–1154.

Lapchak, P.A., Miller, P.J., Jiao, S.S., Araujo, D.M., Hilt, D., and Collins, F. (1996). Biology of glial cell line-derived neurotrophic factor (GDNF): Implications for the use of GDNF to treat Parkinson's disease. *Neurodegeneration*, 5, 197–205.

Lapchak, P.A., Araujo, D.M., Hilt, D.C., Sheng, J., and Jiao, S.S. (1997a). Adenoviral vector-mediated GDNF gene therapy in a rodent lesion model of late stage Parkinson's disease. *Brain Research*, 777, 153–160.

Lapchak, P.A., Gash, D.M., Jiao, S.S., Miller, P.J., and Hilt, D. (1997b). Glial cell line-derived neurotrophic factor: a novel therapeutic approach to treat motor dysfunction in Parkinson's disease. *Experimental Neurology*, 144, 29–34.

Laplanche, J.L., Delasnerielaupretre, N., Brandel, J.P., Chatelain, J., Beaudry, P., Alperovitch, A. *et al.* (1994). Molecular-genetics of prion diseases in france. *Neurology*, 44, 2347–2351.

Lawrence, A.D. (1997). Executive Functions and Memory in Huntington's Disease. *Unpublished thesis, University of Cambridge.*

Lawrence, A.D. and Sahakian, B.J. (1996). The neuropsychology of fronto-striatal dementias. In *Handbook of the Clinical Psychology of Ageing* (ed. R.T. Woods), pp. 243–265. Wiley, Chichester.

Lawrence, A.D., Sahakian, B.J., and Robbins, T.W. (1998a). Cognitive functions and corticostriatal circuits: insights from Huntington's disease. *Trends in Cognitive Sciences*, 2, 379–388.

Lawrence, A.D., Hodges, J.R., Rosser, A.E., Kershaw, A., ffrench-Constant, C., Rubinsztein, D.C. *et al.* (1998b). Evidence for specific cognitive deficits in preclinical Huntington's disease. *Brain*, 121, 1329–1343.

Lee, S.T., Lui, T.N., Chang, C.N., Wang, D.J., Heimburger, R.F., and Fai, H.D. (1990). Features of head injury in a developing country–Taiwan (1977–1987). *J.Trauma*, 30, 194–199.

Lees, A.J. (1995). Comparison of therapeutic effects and mortality data of levodopa and levodopa combined with selegiline in patients with early, mild Parkinson's disease. *British Medical Journal*, 311, 1602–1607.

Leff, S.E., Rendahl, K.G., Spratt, S.K., Kang, U.J., and Mandel, R.J. (1998). *In vivo* L-DOPA production by genetically modified primary rat fibroblast or 9L gliosarcoma cell grafts via coexpression of GTP cyclohydrolase I with tyrosine hydroxylase. *Experimental Neurology*, 151, 249–264.

Leftoff, S. (1983). Psychopathology in the light of brain injury: a case study. *J.Clin.Neuropsychol.*, 5, 51–63.

Le Gal La Salle, G., Robert, J.J., Berrard, S., Ridoux, V.,

Stratford-Perricaudet, L.D., Perricaudet, M. *et al.* (1993). An adenovirus vector for gene transfer into neurons and glia in the brain. *Science*, **259**, 988–990.

Le Gros Clark, W.E. (1940). Neuronal differentiation in implanted foetal cortical tissue. *Journal of Neurology and Psychiatry*, **3**, 263–284.

Lehky, T.J., Fox, C.H., Koenig, S., Levin, M.C., Flerlage, N., Izumo, S. *et al.* (1995). Detection of human T-lymphotropic virus type I (HTLV-I) tax RNA in the central nervous system of HTLV-I associated myelopathy/tropical spastic paraparesis patients by in situ hybridization. *Annals of Neurology*, **37**, 167–175.

Lehrmann, E., Christensen, T., Zimmer, J., Diemer, N.H., and Finsen, B. (1997). Microglial and macrophage reactions mark progressive changes and define the penumbra in the rat neocortex and striatum after transient middle cerebral artery occlusion. *Journal of Comparative Neurology*, **386**, 461–476.

Lemke, E. and Wiersma, W. (1976). *Principles of Psychological Assessment*. Rand McNally, Chicago.

Lennon, V.A., Kryzer, T.J., Griesmann, G.E., O'Suilleabhain, P.E., Windebank, A.J., Woppmann, A. *et al.* (1995). Calcium-channel antibodies in the Lambert-Eaton syndrome and other paraneoplastic syndromes. *N.Engl.J.Med.*, **332**, 1467–1474.

LeVay, S., Wiesel, T.N., and Hubel, D.H. (1980). The development of ocular dominance columns in normal and visually deprived monkeys. *Journal of Comparative Neurology*, **191**, 1–51.

Levi-Montalcini, R. (1972). The morphological effects of immunosympathectomy. In *Immunosympathectomy* (ed. G. Steiner and E. Schönbaum), pp. 55–78. Elsevier, Amsterdam.

Levi-Montalcini, R. (1982). Developmental neurobiology and the natural-history of nerve growth- factor. *Annual Review of Neuroscience*, **5**, 341–362.

Levi-Montalcini, R. (1987). The nerve growth factor: thirty five years later. *EMBO Journal*, **6**, 1145–1154.

Levin, B.E. and Dunn-Meynell, A. (1993). Regulation of growth-associated protein-43 (GAP-43) messenger-RNA associated with plastic change in the adult rat barrel receptor complex. *Molecular Brain Research*, **18**, 59–70.

Levin, B.E., Craik, R.L., and Hand, P.J. (1988). The role of norepinephrine in adult rat somatosensory (SmI) cortical metabolism and plasticity. *Brain Research*, **443**, 261–271.

Levin, H.S., Benton, A.L., and Grossman, R.G. (1982). *Neurobehavioral Consequences of Closed Head Injury*. Oxford University Press, New York.

Levine, J.M. (1994). Increased expression of the NG2 chondroitin sulfate proteoglycan after brain injury. *Journal of Neuroscience*, **14**, 4716–4730.

Levine, D.N. and Finklestein, S. (1982). Delayed psychosis after right temporoparietal stroke or trauma: relation to epilepsy. *Neurology*, **32**, 267–273.

Lewis, D.A. and Smith, R.E. (1983). Steroid-induced psychiatric syndromes — a report of 14 cases and a review of the literature. *Journal of Affective Disorders*, **5**, 319–332.

Le Winn, E.B. and Dimancescu, M.D. (1978). Environmental deprivation and enrichment in coma. *Lancet*, **15**, 156–157.

Lewis, S.W., Harvey, I., Ron, M., Murray, R., and Reveley, A. (1990). Can brain damage protect against schizophrenia? A case report of twins. *Br.J.Psychiatry*, **157**, 600–603.

LeWitt, P.A. (1994). Clinical trials of neuroprotection in Parkinson's disease: Long-term selegiline and $\alpha$-tocopherol treatment. *Journal of Neural Transmission*, **98 (Supplement 43)**, 171–181.

Lewy, F.H. (1914). Zur pathologische anatomie der Paralysis agitans. *Dt.Z.NervHeilk.*, **50**, 50–55.

Leys, K., Lang, B., Johnston, I., and Newsom, D.J. (1991). Calcium channel autoantibodies in the Lambert-Eaton myasthenic syndrome. *Annals of Neurology*, **29**, 307–314.

Lezak, M.D. (1989). *Assessment of the Behavioural Consequences of Head Trauma*. Alan R. Liss, New York.

Li, L., Oppenheim, R.W., Lei, M., and Houenou, L.J. (1994). Neurotrophic agents prevent motoneuron death following sciatic nerve section in neonatal mouse. *Journal of Neurobiology*, **25**, 759–766.

Li, L.X., Wu, W.T., Lin, L.F.H., Lei, M., Oppenheim, R.W., and Houenou, L.J. (1995). Rescue of adult mouse motoneurons from injury-induced cell death by glial cell line-derived neurotrophic factor. *Proceedings of the National Academy of Sciences of the United States of America*, **92**, 9771–9775.

Li, M., Shibata, A., Li, C.M., Braun, P.E., McKerracher, L., Roder, J., Kater, S.B. *et al.* (1996). Myelin-associated glycoprotein inhibits neurite/axon growth and causes growth cone collapse. *Journal of Neuroscience Research*, **46**, 404–414.

Li, Y., Field, P.M., and Raisman, G. (1997). Repair of adult rat corticospinal tract by transplants of olfactory ensheathing cells. *Science*, **277**, 2000–2002.

Lieberman, A.R. (1971). The axon reaction: a review of the principal features of perikaryal responses to axon injury. *International Review of Neurobiology*, **14**, 49–124.

Lieberman, A.R., Campbell, G., and Zhang, Y. (1998). Cellular and molecular correlates of the regeneration of adult mammalian CNS axons into peripheral nerve grafts. *Progress in Brain Research*, **117**, 211–232.

Linazasoro, G., Grandas, F., Martin, P.M., and Bravo, J.L. (1999). Controlled release levodopa in Parkinson's disease: influence of selection criteria and conversion recommendations in the clinical outcome of 450 patients. STAR Study Group. *Clinical Neuropharmacology*, **22**, 74–79.

Lindholm, D., Heumann, R., Meyer, M., and Thoenen, H. (1987). Interleukin-1 regulates synthesis of nerve growth factor in non-neuronal cells of rat sciatic nerve. *Nature*, **330**, 658–659.

Lindmark, B. (1988). Evaluation of functional capacity after stroke, with special emphasis on motor function and activities of daily living. *Scandinavian Journal of Rehabilitation Medicine*, **21 (Supplement)**, 1–40.

Lindsay, R.M., Wiegand, S.J., Altar, C.A., and DiStefano, P.S. (1994). Neurotrophic factors: from molecule to man. *Trends in Neurosciences*, **17**, 182–188.

Lindsay, R.M. (1994). Neurotrophic growth factors and neurodegenerative diseases: therapeutic potential of the neurotrophins and ciliary neurotrophic factor. *Neurobiology of Aging*, **15**, 249–251.

Lindsay, R.M. (1996). Role of neurotrophins and trk receptors in the development and maintenance of sensory neurons: An overview. *Philosophical Transactions of the Royal Society of London. B: Biological Sciences*, **351**, 365–373.

Lindvall, O. (1994). Neural transplants in Parkinson's disease.

In *Functional Neural Transplantation* (ed. S.B. Dunnett and A. Björklund), pp. 103–137. Raven Press, New York.

Lindvall, O. (1997). Neural transplantation: a hope for patients with Parkinson's disease? *NeuroReport*, 8(14), iii-x.

Lindvall, O., Brundin, P., Widner, H., Rehncrona, S., Gustavii, B., Frackowiak, R. *et al.* (1990). Grafts of fetal dopamine neurons survive and improve motor function in Parkinson's disease. *Science*, 247, 574–577.

Lindvall, O., Widner, H., Rehncrona, S., Brundin, P., Odin, P., Gustavii, B. *et al.* (1992). Transplantation of fetal dopamine neurons in Parkinson's disease: one year clinical and neuro-physiological observations in 2 patients with putaminal implants. *Annals of Neurology*, 31, 155–165.

Lindvall, O., Sawle, G., Widner, H., Rothwell, J.C., Björklund, A., Brooks, D.J. *et al.* (1994). Evidence for long-term survival and function of dopaminergic grafts in progressive Parkinson's disease. *Annals of Neurology*, 35, 172–180.

Ling, Z.D., Potter, E.D., Lipton, J.W., and Carvey, P.M. (1998). Differentiation of mesencephalic progenitor cells into dopaminergic neurons by cytokines. *Experimental Neurology*, 149, 411–423.

Lipe, H., Schultz, A., and Bird, T.D. (1993). Risk factors for suicide in Huntington's disease: a retrospective case controlled study. *American Journal of Medical Genetics*, 48, 231–233.

Lipsey, J.R., Robinson, R.G., Pearlson, G.D., Rao, K., and Price, T.R. (1983). Mood change following bilateral hemisphere brain injury. *Br.J.Psychiatry*, 143, 266–273.

Lipton, S.A. (1997). Neuropathogenesis of acquired immunodeficiency syndrome dementia. *Current Opinion In Neurology*, 10, 247–253.

Lipton, S.A. and Gendelman, H.E. (1995). The dementia associated with the acquired immunodeficiency syndrome. *New England Journal of Medicine*, 332, 934–940.

Lisak, R.P. (1994). Immune-mediated para-infectious encephalomyelitis. In *Handbook of Neurovirology* (ed. R.R. McKendall and W.G. Stroop), pp. 173–186. Marcel Dekker, New York.

Lishman, W.A. (1973). The psychiatric sequelae of head injury: a review. *Psychological Medicine*, 3, 304–318.

Lisovski, F., Wahrmann, J.P., Pages, J.C., Cadusseau, J., Rieu, M., Weber, A. *et al.* (1997). Long-term histological follow-up of genetically modified myoblasts grafted into the brain. *Molecular Brain Research*, 44, 125–133.

Liu, D., Yang, R., Yan, X., and McAdoo, D. (1994). Hydroxy radicals generated *in vivo* kill neurons in the rat spinal cord: electrophysiological, histological and neurochemical results. *Journal of Neurochemistry*, 62, 37–44.

Liu, C.K., Wel, G., and Atwood, W.J. (1998). Infection of glial cells by the human polyoma virus JC is mediated by an N-linked glycoprotein containing terminal alpha(2–6) linked sialic acids. *Journal of Virology*, 72, 4643–4649.

Liu, Y., Kim, D.H., Himes, B.T., Chow, S.Y., Schallert, T., Murray, M. *et al.* (1999). Transplants of fibroblasts genetically modified to express BDNF promote regeneration of adult rat rubrospinal axons and recovery of forelimb function. *Journal of Neuroscience*, 19, 4370–4387.

Liuzzi, F.J. and Lasek, R.J. (1987). Astrocytes block axonal regeneration in mammals by activating the physiological stop pathway. *Science*, 237, 642–645.

Livingston, M.G. (1988). The burden on families of the brain injured: a review. *Journal of Head Trauma Rehabilitation*, 3, 6–15.

Ljungberg, T. and Ungerstedt, U. (1976). Reinstatement of eating by dopamine agonists in aphagic dopamine denervated rats. *Physiology and Behavior*, 16, 277–283.

Lobosky, J.M., Vangilder, J.C., and Damasio, A.R. (1984). Behavioural manifestations of third ventricular colloid cysts. *J.Neurol.Neurosurg.Psychiatry*, 47, 1075–1080.

Lois, C. and Alvarez-Buylla, A. (1993). Proliferating subventricular zone cells in the adult mammalian forebrain can differentiate into neurons and glia. *Proceedings of the National Academy of Sciences of the United States of America*, 90, 2074–2077.

Lois, C. and Alvarez-Buylla, A. (1994). Long-distance neuronal migration in the adult mammalian brain. *Science*, 264, 1145–1148.

Lokensgard, J.R., Bloom, D.C., Dobson, A.T., and Feldman, L.T. (1994). Long-term promoter activity during herpes simplex virus latency. *Journal of Virology*, 68, 7148–7158.

Long, C.J. and Ross, L.K. (1992). *Handbook of Head Trauma*. Plenum Press, New York.

Losseff, N.A., Webb, S.L., O'Riordan, J.I., Page, R., Wang, L., Barker, G.J. *et al.* (1996). Spinal cord atrophy and disability in multiple sclerosis. A new reproducible and sensitive MRI method with potential to monitor disease progression. *Brain*, 119, 701–708.

Lotz, B., Brooks, B., Sanjak, M., Weasler, C., Roelke, K., Parnell, J. *et al.* (1996). A double-blind placebo-controlled clinical-trial of subcutaneous recombinant human ciliary neurotrophic factor (rhCNTF) in amyotrophic-lateral-sclerosis. *Neurology*, 46, 1244–1249.

Louis, E.D., Lynch, T., arder, K., and Fahn, S. (1996). Reliability of patient completion of the historical section of the Unified Parkinson's Disease Rating Scale. *Movement Disorders*, 11, 185–192.

Lowry, O.H., Passonneau, J.V., Hasselberger, F.X., and Schultz, D.W. (1964). Effect of ischemia on known substrates and cofactors of the glycolytic pathway in brain. *Journal of Biological Chemistry*, 239, 18–30.

Loy, R. and Moore, R.Y. (1977). Anomalous innervation of the hippocampal formation by peripheral sympathetic axons following mechanical injury. *Experiment Neurology*, 57, 645–650.

Lu, X. and Richardson, P.M. (1995). Changes in neuronal messenger-rnas induced by a local inflammatory reaction. *Journal of Neuroscience Research*, 41, 8–14.

Lubbers, K., Wolff, J.R., and Frotscher, M. (1985). Neurogenesis of GABAergic neurons in the rat dentate gyrus: a combined autoradiographic and immunocytochemical study. *Neuroscience Letters*, 62, 317–322.

Lublin, F.D. and Reingold, S.C. (1996). Defining the clinical course of multiple sclerosis: results of an international survey. National Multiple Sclerosis Society (USA) Advisory Committee on Clinical Trials of New Agents in Multiple Sclerosis. *Neurology*, 46, 907–911.

Lucas, D.R. and Newhouse, J.P. (1957). The toxic effect of sodium-L-glutamate on the inner layers of the retina. *Archives of Ophthalmology*, 58, 193–201.

Lucius, R. and Sievers, J. (1997). YVAD protect post-natal retinal ganglion cells against axotomy- induced but not free radical-induced axonal degeneration *in vitro*. *Molecular Brain Research*, **48**, 181–184.

Ludolph, A.C., He, F., Spencer, P.S., Hammerstad, J.P., and Sabri, M. (1991). 3-nitropropionic acid — exogenous animal neurotoxin and possible human striatal toxin. *Canadian Journal of Neurological Sciences*, **18**, 492–498.

Ludwin, S.K. and Bakker, D.A. (1988). Can oligodendrocytes attached to myelin proliferate? *Journal of Neuroscience*, **8**, 1239–1244.

Luiten, P.G.M., Douma, B.R.K., Vanderzee, E.A., and Nyakas, C. (1995). Neuroprotection against NMDA induced cell death in rat nucleus basalis by Ca$^{2+}$ antagonist nimodipine, influence of aging and developmental drug treatment. *Neurodegeneration*, **4**, 307–314.

Lund, R.D. and Bannerjee, R. (1992). Immunological considerations in neural transplantation. In *Neural Transplantation: A Practical Approach* (ed. S.B. Dunnett and A. Björklund), pp. 161–176. IRL Press, Oxford.

Lundberg, C., Winkler, C., Whittemore, S.R., and Björklund, A. (1996a). Conditionally immortalised neural progenitor cells grafted to the striatum exhibit site-specific neuronal differentiation and establish connections with the host globus pallidus. *Neurobiology of Disease*, **3**, 33–50.

Lundberg, C., Field, P.M., Ajayi, Y.O., Raisman, G., and Björklund, A. (1996b). Conditionally immortalized neural progenitor cell lines integrate and differentiate after grafting to the adult rat striatum. A combined autoradiographic and electron microscopic study. *Brain Research*, **737**, 295–300.

Lunn, E.R., Perry, V.H., Brown, M.C., Rosen, H., and Gordon, S. (1989). Absence of wallerian degeneration does not hinder regeneration in peripheral-nerve. *European Journal of Neuroscience*, **1**, 27–33.

Lupien, S., Lecours, A.R., Lussier, I., Schwartz, G., Nair, N.P.V., and Meaney, M.J. (1994). Basal cortisol levels and cognitive deficits in human aging. *Journal of Neuroscience*, **14**, 2893–2903.

Lupien, S.J., de Leon, M., de Santi, S., Convit, A., Tarshish, C., Thakur, M. *et al.* (1998). Cortisol levels during human aging predict hippocampal atrophy and memory deficits. *Nature Neuroscience*, **1**, 69–73.

Luria, A.R. (1963). *Restoration of Function After Brain Injury*. Pergamon, Oxford.

Luria, A.R., Naydin, V.L., Tsvetkvova, L.S., and Vinarskaya, E.N. (1975). Restoration of higher cortical functions following local brain damage. In *Handbook of Clinical Neurology* (ed. P.J. Vinken and G.W. Bruyn), pp. 368–433. Elsevier, New York.

Luskin, M.B. (1993). Restricted proliferation and migration of postnatally generated neurons derived from the forebrain subventricular zone. *Neuron*, **11**, 173–189.

Lying, T.U. (1979). Psychotic symptoms in normal-pressure hydrocephalus. *Acta Psychiatr.Scand.*, **59**, 415–419.

Lynch, J.C. and McLaren, J.W. (1989). Deficits of visual attention and saccadic eye movements after lesions of parietooccipital cortex in monkeys. *Journal of Neurophysiology*, **61**, 74–90.

Lysko, P.G., Cox, J.A., Vigano, M.A., and Henneberry, R.C. (1989). Excitatory amino acid neurotoxicity at the N-methyl_D-aspartate receptor in cultured neurons: pharmacological characterization. *Brain Research*, **499**, 258–266.

Mack, W.J., Freed, D.M., Williams, B.W., and Henderson, V.W. (1992). Boston Naming Test: shortened versions for use with Alzheimer's disease. *Journal of Gerontology*, **47**, 154–158.

MacLeod, C.M. (1991). Half a century of research on the Stroop effect — an integrative review. *Psychological Bulletin*, **109**, 163–203.

MacMillan, J.C., Snell, R.G., Tyler, A., Houlihan, G.D., Fenton, I., Cheadle, J.P. *et al.* (1993). Molecular analysis and clinical correlations of the Huntington's disease mutation. *Lancet*, **342**, 954–958.

Madden, K.P., Clark, W.M., Marcoux, F.W., Probert, A.W., Weber, M.L., Rivier, J. *et al.* (1990). Treatment with conotoxin, an n-type calcium-channel blocker, in neuronal hypoxic-ischemic injury. *Brain Research*, **537**, 256–262.

Madison, R.D., Archibald, S.J., and Brushart, T.M. (1996). Reinnervation accuracy of the rat femoral nerve by motor and sensory neurons. *Journal of Neuroscience*, **16**, 5698–5703.

Madrazo, I., Drucker-Colín, R., Díaz, V., Martínez-Mata, J., Torres, C., and Becerril, J.J. (1987). Open microsurgical autograft of adrenal medulla to the right caudate nucleus in two patients with intractable Parkinson's disease. *New England Journal of Medicine*, **316**, 831–834.

Madrazo, I., Franco-Bourland, R., Ostrosky-Solis, F., Aguilera, M.C., Cuevas, C., Alvarez, F. *et al.* (1990). Neural transplantation (auto-adrenal, fetal nigral and fetal adrenal) in Parkinson's disease: the Mexican experience. *Progress in Brain Research*, **82**, 593–602.

Magarinos, A.M. and McEwen, B.S. (1995). Stress-induced atrophy of apical dendrites of hippocampal CA3c neurons — involvement of glucocorticoid secretion and excitatory amino acid receptors. *Neuroscience*, **69**, 89–98.

Maidment, N.T., Tan, A.M., Bloom, D.C., Anton, B., Feldman, L.T., and Stevens, J.G. (1996). Expression of the lacZ reporter gene in the rat basal forebrain, hippocampus,and nigrostriatal pathway using a nonreplicating herpes simplex vector. *Experimental Neurology*, **139**, 107–114.

Majewska, M.D. (1992). Neurosteroids — endogenous bimodal modulators of the GABA-A receptor — mechanism of action and physiological significance. *Progress in Neurobiology*, **38**, 379–395.

Majewska, M.D., Mienville, J.M., and Vicini, S. (1988). Neurosteroid pregnenolone sulfate antagonizes electrophysiological responses to GABA in neurons. *Neuroscience Letters*, **90**, 279–284.

Malkmus, D., Booth, B.J., and Kodimer, C. (1980). *Rehabilitation of the Head Injured Adult: Comprehensive Cognitive Management*. Professional Staff Association of Rancho Los Amigos Hospital, Downey, California.

Mandel, R.J., Spratt, S.K., Snyder, R.O., and Leff, S.E. (1997). Midbrain injection of recombinant adeno-associated virus encoding rat glial cell line-derived neurotrophic factor protects nigral neurons in a progressive 6-hydroxydopamine-induced degeneration model of Parkinson's disease in rats. *Proceedings of the National Academy of Sciences of the United States of America*, **94**, 14083–14088.

Mangiarini, L., Sathasivam, K., Seller, M., Cozens, B., Harper, A., Hetherington, C. *et al.* (1996). Exon 1 of the *HD* gene with an expanded CAG repeat is sufficient to cause a progressive neurological phenotype in transgenic mice. *Cell*, **87**, 493–506.

Mangiarini, L., Sathasivam, K., Mahal, A., Mott, R., Seller, M., and Bates, G.P. (1997). Instability of highly expanded CAG repeats in mice transgenic for the Huntington's disease mutation. *Nature Genetics*, **15**, 197–200.

Mann, R., Mulligan, R.C., and Baltimore, D. (1983). Construction of a retrovirus packaging mutant and its use to produce helper-free defective retrovirus. *Cell*, **33**, 153–159.

Mann, D.M.A., Younis, N., Jones, D., and Stoddart, R.W. (1992). The time course of pathological events in Down's syndrome with particular reference to the involvement of microglial cells and deposits of β/A4. *Neurodegeneration*, **1**, 201–215.

Mannion, R.J., Doubell, T.P., Coggeshall, R.E., and Woolf, C.J. (1996). Collateral sprouting of uninjured primary afferent A fibers into the superficial dorsal horn of the adult rat spinal cord after topical capsaicin treatment to the sciatic nerve. *Journal of Neuroscience*, **16**, 5189–5195.

Manson, J.C., Clarke, A.R., Hooper, M.L., Aitchison, L., McConnell, I., and Hope, J. (1994). 129/Ola mice carrying a null mutation in prp that abolishes messenger-rna production are developmentally normal. *Molecular Neurobiology*, **8**, 121–127.

Mao, X.R. and Barger, S.W. (1998). Neuroprotection by dehydroepiandrosterone sulfate: role of an NF kappa B-like factor. *NeuroReport*, **9**, 759–763.

Maragos, W.F., Greenamyre, J.T., Penney, J.B., and Young, A.B. (1987). Glutamate dysfunction in alzheimers-disease — an hypothesis. *Trends in Neurosciences*, **10**, 65–68.

Margolin, D.I. (1992). *Cognitive Neuropsychology in Clinical Practice*. Oxford University Press, New York.

Margolis, T.P., Bloom, D.C., Dobson, A.T., Feldman, L.T., and Stevens, J.G. (1993). Decreased reporter gene-expression during latent infection with hsv lat promoter constructs. *Virology*, **197**, 585–592.

Mark, M.H. (1997). Other choreatic disorders. In *Movement Disorders. Neurologic Principles and Practice* (ed. R.L. Watts and W.C. Koller), pp. 527–539. McGraw-Hill, New York.

Maroteaux, L. and Scheller, R.H. (1991). The rat brain synucleins — family of proteins transiently associated with neuronal membrane. *Molecular Brain Research*, **11**, 335–343.

Marsden, C.D. (1982). Basal ganglia disease. *Lancet*, **ii**, 1141–1146.

Marsden, C.D. and Parkes, J.D. (1977). Success and problems of long-term levodopa therapy in Parkinson's disease. *Lancet*, **1**, 345–349.

Marsden, C.D. and Quinn, N.P. (1990). The dystonias [see comments]. *BMJ.*, **300**, 139–144.

Marshall, F.J. and Shoulson, I. (1997). Clinical features and treatment of Huntington's disease. In *Movement Disorders. Neurologic Principles and Practice* (ed. R.L. Watts and W.C. Koller), pp. 491–502. McGraw-Hill, New York.

Marshall, J.F., Richardson, J.S., and Teitelbaum, P. (1974). Nigrostriatal bundle damage and the lateral hypothalamic syndrome. *Journal of Comparative and Physiological Psychology*, **87**, 808–830.

Martin, D.P., Schmidt, R.E., DiStefano, P.S., Lowry, O.H., Carter, J.G., and Johnson, E.M. (1988a). Inhibitors of protein-synthesis and rna-synthesis prevent neuronal death caused by nerve growth-factor deprivation. *Journal of Cell Biology*, **106**, 829–844.

Martin, R., Ortlauf, J., Sticht-Groh, V., Bogdahn, U., Gold-mann, S.F., and Mertens, H.G. (1988b). Borrelia burgdorferi-specific and autoreactive T cell lines from cerebrospinal fluid in Lyme radiculomyelitis. *Annals of Neurology*, **24**, 509–516.

Martin, A., Pigott, T.A., Lalonde, F.M., Dalton, I., Dubbert, B., and Murphy, D.L. (1993). Lack of evidence for Huntington's disease-like cognitive dysfunction in obsessive-compulsive disorder. *Biological Psychiatry*, **33**, 345–353.

Martinez-Martin, P., Gil-Nagel, A., Gracia, L.M., Gomez, J.B., Martinez-Sarries, J., and Bermejo, F. (1994). Unified Parkinson's Disease Rating Scale characteristics and structure. The Cooperative Multicentric Group. *Movement Disorders*, **9**, 76–83.

Martinez-Serrano, A., Fischer, W., Söderström, S., Ebendal, T., and Björklund, A. (1996). Long-term functional recovery from age-induced spatial memory impairments by nerve growth factor gene transfer to the rat basal forebrain. *Proceedings of the National Academy of Sciences of the United States of America*, **93**, 6355–6360.

Martinez-Serrano, A., Fischer, W., and Björklund, A. (1995). Reversal of age-dependent cognitive impairments and cholinergic neuron atrophy by NGF-secreting neural progenitors grafted to the basal forebrain. *Neuron*, **15**, 473–484.

Martinez-Serrano, A., Lundberg, C., Horellou, P., Fischer, W., Bentlage, C., Campbell, K., McKay, R.D.G., Mallet, J., and Björklund, A. (1995). CNS-derived neural progenitor cells for gene transfer of nerve growth factor to the adult rat brain: Complete rescue of axotomized cholinergic neurons after transplantation into the septum. *Journal of Neuroscience*, **15**, 5668–5680.

Martinez-Serrano, A. and Björklund, A. (1997). Immortalized neural progenitor cells for CNS gene transfer and repair. *Trends in Neurosciences*, **20**, 530–538.

Martini, R., Schachner, M., and Brushart, T.M. (1994). The L2/HNK-1 carbohydrate is preferentially expressed by previously motor axon-associated Schwann cells in reinnervated peripheral nerves. *Journal of Neuroscience*, **14**, 7180–7191.

Maruff, P., Tyler, P., Burt, T., Currie, B., Burns, C., and Currie, J. (1996). Cognitive deficits in Machado-Joseph disease. *Annals of Neurology*, **40**, 421–427.

Maruyama, W., and Naoi, M. (1999). Neuroprotection by(-)-deprenyl and related compounds. *Mechanisms of Ageing and Development*, **111**, 189–200.

Masliah, E. (1999). *Neuroscience News*, **1**, 14.

Mason, D.W., Charlton, H.M., Jones, A.J., Lavy, C.B.D., Puklavec, M., and Simmonds, S.J. (1986). The fate of allogeneic and xenogeneic neuronal tissue transplanted into the third ventricle of rodents. *Neuroscience*, **19**, 685–694.

Masters, C.L., Simms, G., Weinmann, N.A., Multhaup, G., McDonald, B.L., and Beyreuther, K. (1985). Amyloid plaque core protein in Alzheimer's disease and Down's syndrome. *Proceedings of the National Academy of Sciences of the United States of America*, **82**, 4245–4249.

Mathias, C.J. and Kimber, J.R. (1999). Postural hypotension: causes, clinical features, investigation, and management. *Annu.Rev.Med.*, **50**, 317–336.

Matsuo, Y., Onodera, H., Shiga, Y., Shozuhara, H., Ninomiya, M., Kihara, T. *et al.* (1994). Role of cell-adhesion molecules in brain injury after transient middle cerebral-artery occlusion in the rat. *Brain Research*, **656**, 344–352.

Mattis, S. (1976). Mental status examination for organic mental syndrome in the elderly patient. In *Geriatric Psychi-*

*atry* (ed. R. Bellack and B. Karasu), pp. 77–121. Grune and Stratton, New York.

Mattson, B. (1974). Huntington's chorea in Sweden: social and clinical data. *Acta Psychiatrica Scandinavica, supplementum*, **255**, 221–235.

May, M., Holmes, E., Rogers, W., and Poth, M. (1990). Protection from glucocorticoid induced thymic involution by dehydroepiandrosterone. *Life Sciences*, **46**, 1627–1631.

Mayberg, H.S., Robinson, R.G., Wong, D.F., Parikh, R., Bolduc, P., Starkstein, S.E. *et al.* (1988). PET imaging of cortical S2 serotonin receptors after stroke: lateralized changes and relationship to depression. *Am.J.Psychiatry*, **145**, 937–943.

Mayberg, H.S., Parikh, R.M., Morris, P.L., and Robinson, R.G. (1991). Spontaneous remission of post-stroke depression and temporal changes in cortical S2-serotonin receptors. *J.Neuropsychiatry Clin.Neurosci.*, **3**, 80–83.

Mayer-Proschel, M., Kalyani, A.J., Mujtaba, T., and Rao, M.S. (1997). Isolation of lineage-restricted neuronal precursors from multipotent neuroepithelial stem cells. *Neuron*, **19**, 773–785.

Mayer, E., Brown, V.J., Dunnett, S.B., and Robbins, T.W. (1992). Striatal graft-associated recovery of a lesion-induced performance deficit in the rat requires learning to use the transplant. *European Journal of Neuroscience*, **4**, 119–126.

Mayet, W.J., Csernok, E., Szymkowiak, C., Gross, W.L., and Meyer-zum, B.K. (1993). Human endothelial cells express proteinase 3, the target antigen of anticytoplasmic antibodies in Wegener's granulomatosis. *Blood*, **82**, 1221–1229.

Mazaux, J.M., Barat, M., Giroire, J.M. *et al.* (1982). Place de la reeducation des troubles des fonctions symboliques dans la prise en charge des traumatises craniens graves. *Annales de Medicine Physique*, **25**, 177–188.

Mazzucchi, A., Cattelani, E., Missale, G., Gugliotta, M., Brianti, R., and Parma, M. (1992). Head-injured subjects aged over 50 years: correlations between variables of trauma and neuropsychological follow-up. *Journal of Neurology*, **239**, 256–260.

McAllister, A.K., Katz, L.C., and Lo, D.C. (1996). Neurotrophin regulation of cortical dendritic growth requires activity. *Neuron*, **17**, 1057–1064.

McCarthy, R.A. and Warrington, E.K. (1990). *Cognitive Neuropsychology — a Clinical Introduction*. Academic Press, San Diego.

McCullers, D.L. and Herman, J.P. (1998). Mineralocorticoid receptors regulate bcl-2 and p53 mRNA expression in hippocampus. *NeuroReport*, **9**, 3085–3089.

McDonald, W.I. and Kocen, R.S. (1991). Diptheric neuropathy. In Anonymous.

McDonald, W.I. and Kocen, R.S. (1993). Diptheric neuropathy. In *Peripheral Neuropathy* (ed. P.J. Dyck, P.K. Thomas and J.W. Griffin), W.B. Saunders, London.

McEwen, B.S. (1994). The plasticity of the hippocampus is the reason for its vulnerability. *Seminars in the Neurosciences*, **6**, 239–246.

McGeer, E.G. and McGeer, P.L. (1976). Duplication of the biochemical changes of Huntington's choreas by intrastriatal injection of glutamic and kainic acids. *Nature*, **263**, 517–519.

McGeer, E.G., Olney, J.W., and McGeer, P.L. (1978). *Kainic Acid as a Tool in Neurobiology*. Raven Press, New York.

McGlynn, S.M. (1990). Behavioural approaches to neuropsychological rehabilitation. *Psychological Bulletin*, **108**, 420–421.

McHugh, P.R. and Folstein, M.F. (1975). Psychiatric syndromes of Huntington's chorea: a clinical and phenomenological study. In *Psychiatric Aspects of Neurological Diseases* (ed. D.F. Benson and D. Blummer), pp. 267–286. Grune & Stratton, New York.

McIntosh, L.J. and Sapolsky, R.M. (1996). Glucocorticoids increase the accumulation of reactive oxygen species and enhance adriamycin-induced toxicity in neuronal culture. *Experimental Neurology*, **141**, 201–206.

McIntyre, A.W. and Emsley, R.A. (1990). Shoplifting associated with normal-pressure hydrocephalus: report of a case. *J.Geriatr.Psychiatry Neurol.*, **3**, 229–230.

McKay, R. (1998). Stem cells in the central nervous system. *Science*, **276**, 66–71.

McKay, R., Renfranz, P., and Cunningham, M. (1993). Immortalized stem cells from the central nervous system. *Comptes Rendus de l'Academie des Sciences*, **316**, 1452–1457.

McKay, J.S., Blakemore, W.F., and Franklin, R.J.M. (1997). The effects of the growth factor-antagonist rapidil on remyelination in the CNS. *Neuropathology and Applied Neurobiology*, **23**, 50–58.

McKeon, J., McGuffin, P., and Robinson, P. (1984). Obsessive-compulsive neurosis following head injury. A report of four cases. *Br.J.Psychiatry*, **144**, 190–192.

McKerracher, L., David, S., Jackson, D.L., Kottis, V., Dunn, R.J., and Braun, P.E. (1994). Identification of myelin-associated glycoprotein as a major myelin-derived inhibitor of neurite growth. *Neuron*, **13**, 805–811.

McKinlay, W.W., Brooks, D.N., Bond, M.R., Martinage, D.P., and Marshall, M.M. (1981). The short-term outcome of severe blunt head injury as reported by relatives of the injured persons. *Journal of Neurology, Neurosurgery and Psychiatry*, **44**, 527–533.

Mclean, C.A., Storey, E., Gardner, R.J.M., Tannenberg, A.E.G., Cervenakova, L., and Brown, P. (1997). The D178N (cis-129M) "fatal familial insomnia" mutation associated with diverse clinicopathologic phenotypes in an Australian kindred. *Neurology*, **49**, 552–558.

McMahon, S.B. and Kett-White, R. (1991). Sprouting of peripherally regenerating primary sensory neurons in the adult central nervous system. *Journal of Comparative Neurology*, **304**, 307–315.

McMillan, T.M. and Wilson, S.L. (1993). Coma and the persistent vegetative stage. *Neuropsychological Rehabilitation*, **3**, 97–98.

Meaney, M.J., Aitken, D.H., van Berkel, C., Bhatnagar, S., and Sapolsky, R.M. (1988). Effect of neonatal handling on age-related impairments associated with the hippocampus. *Science*, **239**, 766–768.

Mears, S.C. and Frank, E. (1996). A critical period for the influence of peripheral targets on the central projections of developing sensory neurons. *International Journal of Developmental Neuroscience*, **14**, 731–737.

Medawar, P.B. (1948). Immunity to homologous grafted skin. II. The fate of skin homografts transplanted to the brain, to subcutaneous tissue, and to the anterior chamber of the eye. *British Journal of Experimental Pathology*, **29**, 58–69.

Medical Disability Society. (1988). *The managment of Trau-*

*matic Brain Injury*. Development Trust for the Young Disabled, London.

Medori, R., Tritschler, H.J., Leblanc, A., Villare, F., Manetto, V., Chen, H.Y. *et al.* (1992). Fatal familial insomnia, a prion disease with a mutation at codon 178 of the prion protein gene. *New England Journal of Medicine*, **326**, 444–449.

Meichenbaum, D. (1977). *Cognitive-behaviour Modification: an Integrative Approach*. Plenum Press, New York.

Meiri, K.F., Saffell, J.L., Walsh, F.S., and Doherty, P. (1998). Neurite outgrowth stimulated by neural cell adhesion molecules requires growth-associated protein-43 (GAP-43) function and is associated with GAP-43 phosphorylation in growth cones. *Journal of Neuroscience*, **18**, 10429–10437.

Meister, A. (1988). Glutathione metabolism and its selective modification. *Journal of Biological Chemistry*, **263**, 17205–17208.

Meister, M., Wong, R.O.L., Baylor, D.A., and Shatz, C.J. (1991). Synchronous bursts of action potentials in ganglion cells of the developing mammalian retina. *Science*, **252**, 939–943.

Meldrum, B. and Garthwaite, J. (1990). Excitatory amino acid neurotoxicity and neurodegenerative disease. *Trends in Pharmacological Sciences*, **11**, 379–387.

Mellon, S.H. and Deschepper, C.F. (1993). Neurosteroid biosynthesis — genes for adrenal steroidogenic enzymes are expressed in the brain. *Brain Research*, **629**, 283–292.

Merzenich, M.M., Kaas, J.H., Wall, J.T., Nelson, R.J., Sur, M., and Felleman, D.J. (1983). Topographic reorganization of somoatosensory cortical areas 3B and 1 in adult monkeys following restricted deafferentation. *Neuroscience*, **8**, 33–55.

Merzenich, M.M., Jenkins, W.M., Johnston, P., Schreiner, C., Miller, S.L., and Tallal, P. (1996). Temporal processing deficits of language learning impaired children ameliorated by training. *Science*, **271**, 77–81.

Messert, B. and Wannamaker, B.B. (1974). Reappraisal of the adult occult hydrocephalus syndrome. *Neurology*, **24**, 224–231.

Meyendorf, R. (1976). Hirnembolie und Psychose. *Journal of Neurology*, **213**, 163–177.

Meyer, M., Matusoka, I., Wetmore, C., Olson, L., and Thoenen, H. (1992). Enhanced synthesis of brain-derived neurotrophic factor in the lesioned peripheral nerve: different mechanisms are responsible for the regulation of BDNF and NGF mRNA. *Journal of Cell Biology*, **119**, 45–54.

Meyer, R.L., Miotke, J., and Fawcett, J.W. (1989). Deficient neurite outgrowth of retinal explant from adult mouse on astrocytes. *Society for Neuroscience Abstracts*, **15**, 1027.

Middel, B., Kuipers, U.H., Bouma, J., Staal, M., Oenema, D., Postma, T. *et al.* (1997). Effect of intrathecal baclofen delivered by an implanted programmable pump on health related quality of life in patients with severe spasticity. *Journal of Neurology, Neurosurgery and Psychiatry*, **63**, 204–209.

Middelboe, T., Andersen, H.S., Birket-Smith, M., and Friis, M.L. (1992). Psychiatric sequelae of minor head injury. A Prospective follow-up study. *European Psychiatry*, **7**, 183–189.

Mifka, P. (1976). Post-traumatic psychiatric disturbances. In *Handbook of Clinical Neurology* (ed. P.J. Vinken and G.W. Bruyn), pp. 517–574. Amsterdam, North Holland.

Miko, T.L., Le Maitre, C., and Kinfu, Y. (1993). Damage and regeneration of peripheral nerves in advanced treated leprosy. *Lancet*, **342**, 521–525.

Milberg, W. (1996). Issues in the assessment of cognitive function in dementia. *Brain and Cognition*, **31**, 114–132.

Milbrandt, J., De Sauvage, F.J., Fahrner, T.J., aloh, R.H., eitner, M.L., ansey, M.G. *et al.* (1998). Persephin, a novel neurotrophic factor related to GDNF and neurturin. *Neuron*, **20**, 245–253.

Miles, C., Green, R., Sanders, G., and Hines, M. (1998). Estrogen and memory in a transsexual population. *Hormones and Behavior*, **34**, 199–208.

Millar, K. and Watkinson, N. (1983). Recognition of words presented during general anaesthesia. *Ergonomics*, **26**, 585–594.

Miller, E. (1984). *Recovery and Management of Neuropsychological Impairments*. Wiley, Chichester.

Miller, A.D. (1990). Retrovirus packaging cells. *Human Gene Therapy*, **1**, 5–14.

Miller, J.D. (1991). Changing patterns in acute management of head injury. *Journal of the Neurological Sciences*, **103 Suppl**, S33-S37.

Miller, A.D. and Buttimore, C. (1986). Redesign of retrovirus packaging cell-lines to avoid recombination leading to helper virus production. *Molecular And Cellular Biology*, **6**, 2895–2902.

Miller, N. and Whelan, J. (1997). Progress in transcriptionally targeted and regulatable vectors for genetic therapy. *Human Gene Therapy*, **8**, 803–815.

Miller, D.H., Newton, M.R., van der Poel, J.C., du Boulay, E.P., Halliday, A.M., Kendall, B.E. *et al.* (1988). Magnetic resonance imaging of the optic nerve in optic neuritis. *Neurology*, **38**, 175–179.

Miller, D.G., Adam, M.A., and Miller, A.D. (1990). Genetransfer by retrovirus vectors occurs only in cells that are actively replicating at the time of infection. *Molecular And Cellular Biology*, **10**, 4239–4242.

Milligan, N.M., Newcombe, R., and Compston, D.A.S. (1987). A double blind controlled trial of high dose methylprednisolone in patients with multiple sclerosis: 1 clinical effects. *Journal of Neurology, Neurosurgery and Psychiatry*, **50**, 511–516.

Milner, B. (1963). Effects of different brain lesions on card sorting. *Archives of Neurology*, **9**, 90–100.

Milner, B. (1972). Interhemispheric differences in the localization of psychological processes in man. *British Medical Bulletin*, **27**, 272–277.

Milner, B. (1975). Psychological aspects of focal epilepsy and its neurosurgical management. *Advances in Neurology*, **8**, 299–321.

Milner, B., Squire, L.R., and Kandel, E.R. (1998). Cognitive neuroscience and the study of memory. *Neuron*, **20**, 445–468.

Mindham, R.H.S., Steele, C., Folstein, M.F., and Lucas, J. (1985). A comparison of frequency of major affective disorder in Huntington's disease and Alzheimer's disease. *Journal of Neurology, Neurosurgery and Psychiatry*, **48**, 1172–1174.

Mitchell, S., Bradley, V.A., Welch, J.L., and Britton, P.G. (1990). Coma arousal procedure: a therapeutic intervention in the treatment of head injury. *Brain Injury*, **4**, 273–279.

Mitrushina, M.N., Boone, K.B., and D'Elia, L.F. (1998). *Handbook of Normative Data for Neuropsychological Assessment*. Oxford University Press, New York.

Mobayef, M. and Dinan, T.G. (1990). Buspirone/prolactin response in post-head injury depression. *Journal of Affective Disorders*, **19**, 237–241.

Mocchetti, I., Spiga, G., Hayes, V.Y., Isackson, P.J., and Colangelo, A. (1996). Glucocorticoids differentially increase nerve growth factor and basic fibroblast growth factor expression in the rat brain. *Journal of Neuroscience*, **16**, 2141–2148.

Moehle, K.A. and Fitzhugh-Bell, K.B. (1988). Laterality of brain damage and emotional disturbance in adults. *Archives of Clinical Neuropsychology*, **3**, 137–144.

Moghaddam, B. (1993). Stress preferentially increases extraneuronal levels of excitatory amino acids in the prefrontal cortex — comparison to hippocampus and basal ganglia. *Journal of Neurochemistry*, **60**, 1650–1657.

Mogilner, A., Grossman, J.A.L., Ribary, U., Joliot, M., Volkmann, J., Rapaport, D. *et al.* (1993). Somatosensory cortical plasticity in adult humans revealed by magnetoencephalography. *Proceedings of the National Academy of Sciences of the United States of America*, **90**, 3593–3597.

Mohajeri, M.H., Bartsch, U., Schachner, M., Sansig, G., and Mucke, L. (1996). Neurite outgrowth on non-permissive substrates *in vitro* is enhanced by ectopic expression of the neural adhesion molecule L1 by mouse astrocytes. *European Journal of Neuroscience*, **8**, 1085–1097.

Mohs, R.C. (1995). Neuropsychological assessment of patients with Alzheimer's disease. In *Psychopharmacology: the Fourth Generation of Progress* (ed. F.E. Bloom and D.J. Kupfer), pp. 1377–1388. Raven Press, New York.

Monaghan, D.T., Bridges, R.J., and Cotman, C.W. (1989). The excitatory amino acid receptors: their classes, pharmacology and distinct properties in the function of the central nervous system. *Annual Review of Pharmacology and Toxicology*, **29**, 365–402.

Mondrup, K. and Norskov, O. (1980). Cerebral tumours: material of undiagnosed cerebral tumours admitted to a psychiatric hospital during an 18-year period. *Ugeskr.Laeger.*, **142**, 2546–2549.

Montaron, M.F., Petry, K.G., Rodriguez, J.J., Marinelli, M., Aurousseau, C., Rougon, G. *et al.* (1999). Adrenalectomy increases neurogenesis but not PSA-NCAM expression in aged dentate gyrus. *European Journal of Neuroscience*, **11**, 1479–1485.

Montero, C.N. and Hefti, F. (1988). Rescue of lesioned septal cholinerigic neurons by nerve growth factor: specificity and requirement for chronic treatment. *Journal of Neuroscience*, **8**, 2986–2999.

Montgomery, R.D., Cruickshank, K., Robertson, W.B., and McMenemy, W.H. (1964). Clinical and pathological observations on Jamaican neuropathy. *Brain*, **87**, 425–462.

Moon, L.D.F., Brecknell, J.E., Franklin, R.J.M., Dunnett, S.B., and Fawcett, J.W. (1999). Robust regeneration of CNS axons through a track depleted of CNS glia. *Experimental Neurology*, **141**, 49–61.

Moore, P.M. (1994). Vasculitis of the central nervous system. *Seminars in Neurology*, **14**, 307–312.

Moore, P.M. Calabrese, L.H. (1994). Neurologic manifestations of systemic vasculitides. *Seminars in Neurology*, **14**, 300–306.

Moore, S. and Thanos, S. (1996). The concept of microglia in relation to central nervous system disease and regeneration. *Progress in Neurobiology*, **48**, 441–449.

Moore, R.Y., Björklund, A., and Stenevi, U. (1974). Growth and plasticity of adrenergic neurons. In *The Neurosciences. Third Study Progrram* (ed. F.O. Schmitt and F.G. Worden), pp. 961–977. The MIT Press, Cambridge, MA.

Mora, W., Traugott, U., Scheinberg, L., and Raine, C. (1989). Tropical spastic paraparesis: a model of virus induced, cytotoxic T-cell mediated demyelination. *Annals of Neurology*, **26**, 523–530.

Moran, J. and Desimone, R. (1985). Selective attention gates visual processing in the extrastriate cortex. *Science*, **s24229**, 782–784.

Moreau, T., Thorpe, J., Miller, D.H., Moseley, I., Hale, G., Waldmann, H. *et al.* (1994). Preliminary evidence from magnetic resonance imaging for reduction in disease activity after lymphocyte depletion in multiple sclerosis. *Lancet*, **344**, 298–301.

Morley, S. and Snaith, P. (1992). Principles of psychological assessment. In *Research Methods in Psychiatry* (ed. C. Freeman and P. Tyrer), pp. 135–152. Gakell, London.

Morley, P., Hogan, M.J., and Hakim, A.M. (1994). Calcium-mediated mechanisms of ischemic-injury and protection. *Brain Pathology*, **4**, 37–47.

Morris, P.L.P., Robinson, R.G., and Raphael, B. (1992). Lesion location and depression in hospitalized stroke patients. *Neuropsychiatry, Neuropsychology, Behavioural Neurology*, **5**, 75–82.

Morris, P.L.P., Robinson, R.G., and Raphael, B. (1992). Lesion location and depression in hospitalized stroke patients. *Neuropsychiatry, Neuropsychology and Behavioural Neurology*, **5**, 75–82.

Morrow, A.L., Suzdak, P.D., and Paul, S.M. (1987). Steroid hormone metabolites potentiate GABA receptor-mediated chloride ion flux with nanomolar potency. *European Journal of Pharmacology*, **142**, 483–485.

Morrow, D.R., Campbell, G., Lieberman, A.R., and Anderson, P.N. (1993). Differential regenerative growth of CNS axons into tibial and peroneal nerve grafts in the thalamus of adult rats. *Experimental Neurology*, **120**, 60–69.

Motomura, M., Lang, B., Johnston, I., Palace, J., Vincent, A., and Newsom, D.J. (1997). Incidence of serum anti-P/O-type and anti-N-type calcium channel autoantibodies in the Lambert-Eaton myasthenic syndrome. *Journal of the Neurological Sciences*, **147**, 35–42.

Mueller-Jensen, A., Neunzig, H.P., and Emskotter, T. (1987). Outcome prediction in comatose patients: Significance of reflex eye movement analysis. *Journal of Neurology, Neurosurgery and Psychiatry*, **50**, 389–392.

Muhlnickel, W., Elbert, T., Taub, E., and Flor, H. (1998). Reorganization of auditory cortex in tinnitus. *Proceedings of the National Academy of Sciences of the United States of America*, **95**, 10340–10343.

Mukhopadhyay, G., Doherty, P., Walsh, F.S., Crocker, P.R., and Filbin, M.T. (1994). A novel role for myelin-associated glycoprotein as an inhibitor of axonal regeneration. *Neuron*, **13**, 757–767.

Mulder, D.W. and Swenson, W.M. (1974). Psychologic and psychiatric aspects of brain tumours. In *Handbook of Clinical Neurology — Tumours of the Brain and Skull* (ed. P.J.

Vinken and G.W. Bruyn), pp. 727–740. Amsterdam, North Holland.

Muller, G.E. (1974). Les syndromes post-traumatiques précoces atypiques. *Acta Neurologica Belga*, **74**, 163–181.

Müller, C.M. (1993). Glial cell functions and activity dependent plasticity of the mammalian visual cortex. *Perspectives in Developmental Neurobiology*, **1**, 169–177.

Mumford, C.J. and Compston, A. (1993). Problems with rating scales for multiple sclerosis: a novel approach — the CAMBS score. *Journal of Neurology*, **240**, 209–215.

Mummidi, S., Ahuja, S.S., Gonzalez, E., Anderson, S.A., Santiago, E.N., Stephan, K.T. *et al.* (1998). Genealogy of the CCR5 locus and chemokine system gene variants associated with altered rates of HIV-1 disease progression. *Nature Medicine*, **4**, 786–793.

Munck, A., Guyre, P.M., and Holbrook, N.J. (1984). Physiological functions of glucocorticoids in stress and their relation to pharmacological actions. *Endocrine Reviews*, **5**, 25–44.

Murros, K., Fogelholm, R., Kettunen, S., and Vuorela, A.L. (1993). Serum cortisol and outcome of ischemic brain infarction. *Journal of the Neurological Sciences*, **116**, 12–17.

Muzyczka, N. (1992). Use of adenoassociated virus as a general transduction vector for mammalian-cells. *Current Topics In Microbiology and Immunology*, **158**, 97–129.

Nait-Oumesmar, B., Vignais, L., Duhamel-Clerin, E., Avellana-Adalid, V., Rougon, G., and Baron-Van Evercooren, A. (1995). Expression of the highly polysialylated neural cell-adhesion molecule during postnatal myelination and following chemically-induced demyelination of the adult-mouse spinal-cord. *European Journal of Neuroscience*, **7**, 480–491.

Nakamura, R., Kamakura, K., Tadano, Y., Hosoda, Y., Nagata, N., Tsuchiya, K. *et al.* (1993). MR imaging findings of tremors associated with lesions in cerebellar outflow tracts: report of two cases. *Movement Disorders*, **8**, 209–212.

Nakao, N., Frodl, E.M., Duan, W.-M., Widner, H., and Brundin, P. (1994). Lazaroids improve the survival of grafted rat embryonic dopamine neurons. *Proceedings of the National Academy of Sciences of the United States of America*, **91**, 12408–12412.

Nakao, N., Frodl, E.M., Widner, H., Carlson, E., Eggerding, F.A., Epstein, C.J. *et al.* (1995). Overexpressing Cu/Zn superoxide dismutase enhances survival of transplanted neurons in a rat model of Parkinson's disease. *Nature Medicine*, **1**, 226–231.

Naldini, L., Blömer, U., Gage, F.H., Trono, D., and Verma, I.M. (1996). Efficient transfer, integration, and sustained long-term expression of the transgene in adult rat brains injected with a lentiviral vector. *Proceedings of the National Academy of Sciences of the United States of America*, **93**, 11382–11388.

Naparstek, Y., Cohen, I.R., Fuks, Z., and Vlodavsky, I. (1984). Activated T lymphocytes produce a matrix-degrading heparan sulphate endoglycosidase. *Nature*, **310**, 241–244.

Nasrallah, H.A. and Wilcox, J.A. (1989). Gender differences in the aetiology and symptoms of schizophrenia: genetic versus brain injury factors. *Annales of Clinical Psychiatry*, **1**, 51–52.

Nasrallah, H.A., Fowler, R.C., and Judd, L.L. (1981). Schizo-phrenia-like illness following head injury. *Psychosomatics.*, **22**, 359–361.

Neering, S.J., Hardy, S.F., Minamoto, D., Spratt, S.K., and Jordan, C.T. (1996). Transduction of primitive human hematopoietic cells with recombinant adenovirus vectors. *Blood*, **88**, 1147–1155.

Nelson, H.E. (1991). *The National Adult Reading Test.* NFER-Nelson, Windsor.

Ness, R. and David, S. (1997). Leptomeningeal cells modulate the neurite growth promoting properties of astrocytes *in vitro*. *Glia*, **19**, 47–57.

Neumann, H. and Wekerle, H. (1998). Neuronal control of the immune response in the central nervous system: linking brain immunity to neurodegeneration. *Journal of Neuropathology and Experimental Neurology*, **57**, 1–9.

Newsom, D.J. and Murray, N.M. (1984). Plasma exchange and immunosuppressive drug treatment in the Lambert-Eaton myasthenic syndrome. *Neurology*, **34**, 480–485.

Newsom, D.J. Pinching, A.J., Vincent, A., and Wilson, S.G. (1978). Function of circulating antibody to acetylcholine receptor in myasthenia gravis: investigation by plasma exchange. *Neurology*, **28**, 266–272.

Newton, A. and Johnson, D.A. (1985). Social adjustment and interaction after severe head injury. *Br.J.Clin.Psychol.*, **24**, 225–234.

Nicolelis, M.A.L., Lin, R.C.S., Woodward, D.J., and Chapin, J.K. (1993). Induction of immediate spatiotemporal changes in thalamic networks by peripheral block of ascending cutaneous information. *Nature*, **361**, 533–536.

Njiokiktjien, C., Valk, J., and Ramaekers, G. (1988). Malformation or damage of the corpus callosum? A clinical and MRI study. *Brain Dev.*, **10**, 92–99.

Nobes, C.D. and Tolkovsky, A.M. (1995). Neutralizing anti-p21(Ras) Fabs suppress rat sympathetic neuron survival induced by ngf, lif, cntf and camp. *European Journal of Neuroscience*, **7**, 344–350.

Norman, D.A. (1988). *The Psychology of Everyday Things.* Basic Books, New York.

Nottebohm, F. (1991). Reassessing the mechanisms and origins of vocal learning in birds. *Trends in Neurosciences*, **14**, 206–211.

Nottebohm, F., Nottebohm, M.E., and Crane, L. (1986). Developmental and seasonal-changes in canary song and their relation to changes in the anatomy of song control nuclei. *Behavioral and Neural Biology*, **46**, 445–471.

Novelli, G.P., Angiolini, P., Tani, R., Consale, G., and Bordi, L. (1997). Phenyl-*tert*-butyl-α-phenylnitrone is active against traumatic shock in rat. *Free Radicals Research Communications*, **1**, 321–327.

Nudo, R. and Grenda, R. (1992). Reorganisation of distal forelimb representations in primary motor cortex adult squirrel monkeys following focal ischemic infarct. *Society for Neuroscience Abstracts*, **18**, 216.

Nunally, J.C. (1978). *Psychometric Theory.* McGraw-Hill, New York.

O'Brien, M.D. (1990). Management of major status epilepticus in adults. *British Medical Journal*, **301**, 918.

Obeso, J.A. (1997). Classification, clinical features and treatment of myclonus. In *Movement Disorders. Neurologic principles and practice* (ed. R.L. Watts and W.C. Koller), pp. 541–550. McGraw-Hill, New York.

O'Callaghan, E., Larkin, C., Redmond, O., Stack, J., Ennis,

J.T., and Waddington, J.L. (1988). 'Early-onset schizophrenia' after teenage head injury. A case report with magnetic resonance imaging. *British Journal of Psychiatry*, **153**, 394–396.

O'Carroll, R.E., Woodrow, J., and Maroun, F. (1991). Psychosexual and psychosocial sequelae of closed head injury. *Brain Injury*, **5**, 303–313.

Oestreicher, A.B., Degraan, P.N.E., Gispen, W.H., Verhaagen, J., and Schrama, L.H. (1997). B-50, the growth associated protein-43: Modulation of cell morphology and communication in the nervous system. *Progress in Neurobiology*, **53**, 627–686.

Ogata, A., Nagashima, K., Hall, W.W., Ichikawa, M., Kimura-Kimoda, J., and Yasui, K. (1991). Japanese encephalitis virus neurotropism is dependent on the degree of neuronal maturity. *Journal of Virology*, **65**, 880–886.

Oksi, J., Kalimo, H., Marttila, R.J., Marjamäki, M., Sonninen, P., Nikoskelainen, J. *et al.* (1996). Inflammatory brain changes in Lyme borreliosis. A report on three patients and review of the literature. *Brain*, **119**, 2143–2154.

Okuda, O., Bressler, J., Chang, L., and Brightman, M. (1991). Viral Kirsten ras infection differentiates PC12 cells and enhances their survival upon implantation into brain. *Experimental Neurology*, **113**, 330–337.

Olanow, C.W. (1997). Attempts to obtain neuroprotection in Parkinson's disease. *Neurology*, **49**, S26–S33.

Olanow, C.W. and Arendash, G.W. (1994). Metals and free radicals in neurodegeneration. *Current Opinion In Neurology*, **7**, 548–558.

Olanow, C.W., Kordower, J.H., and Freeman, T.B. (1996). Fetal nigral transplantation as a therapy for Parkinson's disease. *Trends in Neurosciences*, **19**, 102–109.

Oldstone, M.B.A., Holnstein, J., and Welsh, R.M. (1977). Alterations in acetyl choline enzymes in neuroblastoma cells persistently infected with lymphocytic choriomeningitis virus. *Journal of Cell Physiology*, **91**, 459–472.

Oldstone, M.B.A., Rodriguez, M., Daughaday, W.H., and Lampert, P.W. (1984). Viral perturbation of endocrine function: disordered cell function leads to disturbed haemostasis and disease. *Nature*, **307**, 278–281.

Oliver, J.E. (1970). Huntington's chorea in Northamptonshire. *British Journal of Psychiatry*, **116**, 241–253.

Oliver, K.R. and Fazakerley, J.K. (1998). Transneuronal spread of Semliki forest virus in the developing mouse olfactory system is determined by neuronal maturity. *Neuroscience*, **82**, 867–877.

Oliver, K.R., Scallan, M.F., Dyson, H., and Fazakerley, J.K. (1997). Susceptibility to a neurotropic virus and its changing distribution in the developing brain is a function of CNS maturity. *Journal of Neurovirology*, **3**, 38–48.

Olney, J.W. (1969). Brain lesions, obesity, and other disturbances in mice treated with monosodium glutamate. *Science*, **164**, 719–721.

Olney, J.W. (1971). Glutamate induced neuronal necrosis in the infant mouse hippocampus. *Journal of Neuropathology and Experimental Neurology*, **30**, 75–90.

Olney, J.W. (1978). Neurotoxicity of excitatory amino acids. In *Kainic Acid as a Tool in Neurobiology* (ed. E.G. McGeer, J.W. Olney and P.L. McGeer), pp. 95–122. Raven Press, New York.

Olney, J.W. (1989). Excitatory amino acids and neuropsychiatric disorders. *Biological Psychiatry*, **26**, 505–525.

Olney, J.W., Ho, O.L., and Rhee, V. (1971). Cytotoxic effects of acidic and sulphur containing amino acids on the infant mouse central nervous system. *Experimental Brain Research*, **14**, 61–76.

Olney, J.W., Rhee, V., and Ho, O.L. (1974). Kainic acid: a powerful neurotoxic analogue of glutamate. *Brain Research*, **77**, 507–512.

Olney, J.W., Misra, C.H., and de Gubareff, T. (1975). Cysteine-S-sulphate brain damaging metabolite in sulfite oxidase deficiency. *Journal of Neuropathology and Experimental Neurology*, **34**, 167–177.

Olney, J.W., Price, M.T., Samson, L., and Labruyere, J. (1986). The role of specific ions in glutamate toxicity. *Neuroscience Letters*, **65**, 65–71.

Olson, L. and Malmfors, T. (1970). Growth characteristics of adrenergic nerves in the adult rat. Fluorescence histochemical and 3H-noradrenaline uptake studies using tissue transplantation to the anterior chamber of the eye. *Acta Physiological Scandinavica, supplementum*, **348**, 1–112.

Olson, L. and Seiger, Å. (1972). Brain tissue transplanted to the anterior chamber of the eye. I. Fluorescence histochemistry of immature catecholamine and 5-hydroxytryptamine neurons innervating the iris. *Zeitung Zellforschung*, **195**, 175–194.

Olson, L., Seiger, Å., and Strömberg, I. (1983). Intraocular transplantation in rodents: a detailed account of the procedure and examples of its use in neurobiology with special reference to brain tissue grafting. *Advances in Cellular Neurobiology*, **4**, 407–442.

Olson, L., Björklund, H., and Hoffer, B.J. (1984). Camera bulbi anterior: new vistas on a classical locus for neural tissue transplantation. In *Neural Transplants: Development and Function* (ed. J.R. Sladek and D.M. Gash), pp. 125–165. Plenum Press, New York.

Olsson, T., Astrom, M., Eriksson, S., and Forssell, A. (1989). Hypercortisolism revealed by the dexamethasone suppression test in patients [corrected] with acute ischemic stroke [published erratum appears in Stroke 1990 Apr;21(4):681]. *Stroke*, **20**, 1685–1690.

Olsson, T., Marklund, N., Gustafson, Y., and Nasman, B. (1992). Abnormalities at different levels of the hypothalamic-pituitary-adrenocortical axis early after stroke. *Stroke*, **23**, 1573–1576.

Ona, V.O., Li, M., Vonsattel, J.P.G., Andrews, L.J., Khan, S.Q., Chung, W.M. *et al.* (1999). Inhibition of caspase-1 slows disease progression in a mouse model of Huntington's disease. *Nature*, **399**, 263–267.

O'Neill, J.H., Murray, N.M., and Newsom, D.J. (1988). The Lambert-Eaton myasthenic syndrome. A review of 50 cases. *Brain*, **111**, 577–596.

O'Neill, P.A., Davies, I., Fullerton, K.J., and Bennett, D. (1991). Stress hormone and blood glucose response following acute stroke in the elderly. *Stroke*, **22**, 842–847.

Onifer, S.M., Whittemore, S.R., and Holets, V.R. (1993). Variable morphological differentiation of a Raphé-derived neuronal cell line following transplantation into the adult rat CNS. *Experimental Neurology*, **122**, 130–142.

Onodera, H., Sato, G., and Kogure, K. (1986). Lesions to Schaffer collaterals prevent ischemic death of ca1 pyramidal cells. *Neuroscience Letters*, **68**, 169–174.

Onodera, H., Sato, G., and Kogure, K. (1997). Lesions to

Schaffer collaterals prevent ischemic death of CA1 pyramidal cells. *Neuroscience Letters*, **68**, 169–174.

Orentreich, N., Brind, J.L., Vogelman, J.H., Andres, R., and Baldwin, H. (1992). Long-term longitudinal measurements of plasma dehydroepiandrosterone sulfate in normal men. *Journal of Clinical Endocrinology and Metabolism*, **75**, 1002–1004.

Öttenbacher, K.J. and Jannel, M.S. (1993). The results of clinical trials in stroke rehabilitation research. *Archives of Neurology*, **50**, 37–44.

Ottenhoff, J.H.M. (1994). Immunology of leprosy: Lessons from and for leprosy. *International Journal of Leprosy*, **42**, 108–121.

Oumesmar, B.N., Vignais, L., Duhamel-Clerin, E., Avellana-Adalid, V., Rougon, G., and Baron-Van-Evercooren, A. (1995). Expression of the highly polysialylated neural cell adhesion molecule during postnatal myelination and following chemically induced demyelination of the adult mouse spinal cord. *European Journal of Neuroscience*, **7**, 480–491.

Owen, A.M., Sahakian, B.J., and Robbins, T.W. (1998). The role of executive deficits in memory disorders in neurodegenerative disease. In *Memory in Neurodegenerative Disease: Biological, Cognitive and Clinical Perspectives* (ed. A.I. Trosyter), pp. 157–171. Cambridge University Press, Cambridge.

Oyesiku, N.M., Wilcox, J.N., and Wigston, D.J. (1997). Changes in expression of ciliary neurotrophic factor (CNTF) and CNTF-receptor ? after spinal cord injury. *Journal of Neurobiology*, **32**, 251–261.

Paal, G. (1981). Zur Psychopathologie des Hirntumorkranken. *Forschritte der Neurologie und Psychiatrie*, **49**, 265–274.

Pachner, A.R. and Itano, A. (1990). Borrelia burgdorferi infection of the brain: characterization of the organism and response to antibodies and immune sera in the mouse model. *Neurology*, **40**, 1535–1540.

Paganini-Hill, A. and Henderson, V.W. (1996). Estrogen replacement therapy and risk of Alzheimer disease. *Archives of Internal Medicine*, **156**, 2213–2217.

Page, K.J., Potter, L., Aronni, S., Everitt, B.J., and Dunnett, S.B. (1998). The expression of huntingtin-associated protein (HAP1) mRNA in developing, adult and aging rat CNS: implications for Huntington's disease neuropathology. *European Journal of Neuroscience*, **10**, 1835–1845.

Page, K.J., Meldrum, A., and Dunnett, S.B. (1999). The 3-nitroproprionic acid (3NPA) model of Huntington's disease: do alterations in the expression of metabolic mRNAs predict the development of striatal pathology. In *Mitochondrial Inhibitors as Tools for Neurobiology* (ed. P.R. Sanberg, H. Nishino and C.V. Borlongan), pp. 141–156. Humana, Totowa, NJ.

Palfi, S., Condé, F., Riche, D., Brouillet, E., Dautry, C., Mittoux, V. *et al.* (1998). Fetal striatal allografts reverse cognitive deficits in a primate model of Huntington's disease. *Nature Medicine*, **4**, 963–966.

Pall, A.A. and Savage, C.O. (1994). Mechanisms of endothelial cell injury in vasculitis. *Springer Semin.Immunopathol.*, **16**, 23–37.

Pallis, C. (1999). ABC of brain stem death. The arguments about the EEG. *British Medical Journal*, **286**, 284–287.

Palmer, M.S., Dryden, A.J., Hughes, J.T., and Collinge, J. (1991). Homozygous prion protein genotype predisposes to sporadic Creutzfeldt-Jakob disease. *Nature*, **352**, 340–342.

Panse, F. (1942). *Die Erbchorea. Eine klinisch-genetische Studie*. Thieme, Leipzig.

Parikh, R.M., Lipsey, J.R., Robinson, R.G., and Price, T.R. (1988). A two year longitudinal study of poststroke mood disorders: prognostic factors related to one and two year outcome. *Int.J.Psychiatry Med.*, **18**, 45–56.

Parisi, J.E. Moore, P.M. (1994). The role of biopsy in vasculitis of the central nervous system. *Semin. Neurol.*, **14**, 341–348.

Park, D.S., Morris, E.J., Stefanis, L., Troy, C.M., Shelanski, M.L., Geller, H.M. *et al.* (1998). Multiple pathways of neuronal death induced by DNA-damaging agents, NGF deprivation, and oxidative stress. *Journal of Neuroscience*, **18**, 830–840.

Parkinson's Disease Consensus Working Party (1998). Guidelines for the management of Parkinson's disease. *Hosp.Med.*, **59**, 469–480.

Parkinson's Study Group (1993). Effect of tocopherol and deprenyl on the progression of disability in early Parkinson's disease. *New England Journal of Medicine*, **328**, 176–183.

Parks, R.J., Chen, L., Anton, M., Sankar, U., Rudnicki, M.A., and Graham, F.L. (1996). A helper-dependent adenovirus vector system: removal of helper virus by Cre-mediated excision of the viral packaging signal. *Proceedings of the National Academy of Sciences of the United States of America*, **93**, 13565–13570.

Parmelee, D.X., Kowatch, R.A., Sellman, J., and Davidow, D. (1989). Ten cases of head-injured, suicide-surviving adolescents: challenges for rehabilitation. *Brain Injury*, **3**, 295–300.

Parry, C.J. and Hodges, J.R. (1996). Spectrum of memory dysfunction in degenerative disease. *Current Opinion In Neurology*, **9**, 281–285.

Pascual-Leone, A., Grafman, J., and Hallett, M. (1984). Modulation of cortical motor output maps during development of implicit and explicit knowledge. *Science*, **265**, 1600–1601.

Pascual-Leone, A., Cammarota, A., Wassermann, E.M., Brasil-neto, J.P., Cohen, L.G., and Hallett, M. (1993). Modulation of motor cortical outputs to the reading hand of braille readers. *Annals of Neurology*, **34**, 33–37.

Pascual-Leone, A. and Torres, F. (1993). Plasticity of the sensorimotor cortex representation of the reading finger in braille readers. *Brain*, **116**, 39–52.

Patrick, D. and Gates, P.C. (1984). Chronic subdural haematoma in the elderly. *Age Ageing*, **13**, 367–369.

Patten, S.B. and Lauderdale, W.M. (1992). Delayed sleep phase disorder after traumatic brain injury. *J.Am.Acad.Child Adolesc.Psychiatry*, **31**, 100–102.

Patterson, P.H. and Nawa, H. (1993). Neuronal differentiation factors, cytokines and synaptic plasticity. *Cell*, **72**, 123–137.

Paty, D.W., McFarlin, D.E., and McDonald, W.I. (1991). Magnetic resonance imaging and laboratory aids in the diagnosis of multiple sclerosis [editorial]. *Annals of Neurology*, **29**, 3–5.

Paty, D.W. and Li, D.K.B. (1993). The IFBN Multiple Sclerosis Study Group. Interferon-beta 1b is effective in relapsing-remitting multiple sclerosis: MRI results of a multicenter, randomised, double-blind placebo-controlled trial. *Neurology*, **43**, 662–667.

Paul, G. and Davies, A.M. (1995). Trigeminal sensory neurons require extrinsic signals to switch neurotrophin dependence during the early stages of target field innervation. *Developmental Biology*, **171**, 590–605.

Paulson, H.L. and Fischbeck, K.H. (1996). Trinucleotide repeats in neurogenetic disorders. *Annual Review of Neuroscience*, **19**, 79–107.

Paykel, E.S. (1978). Contribution of life events to causation of psychiatric illness. *Psychological Medicine*, **8**, 245–253.

Pearson, J., Johnson, E.M., and Brandeis, L. (1983). Effects of antibodies to nerve growth factor on intrauterine development of derivatives of cranial neural crest and placode in the guinea pig. *Developmental Biology*, **96**, 32–36.

Pearson, R.C.A., Esiri, M.M., Hiorns, R.W., Wilcock, G.K., and Powell, T.P.S. (1985). Anatomical correlates of the distribution of the pathological changes in the neocortex in Alzheimer disease. *Proceedings of the National Academy of Sciences of the United States of America*, **82**, 4531–4534.

Pendlebury, S.C., Moses, D.K., and Eadie, M.J. (1989). Hyponatremia during oxcarbazepine therapy. *Human Toxicology*, **8**, 337–344.

Penney, J.B., Vonsattel, J.P., MacDonald, M.E., Gusella, J.F., and Myers, R.H. (1997). CAG repeat number governs the development rate of pathology in Huntington's disease. *Annals of Neurology*, **41**, 689–692.

Penney, J.B., Maragos, W.F., Greenamyre, J.T., Debowey, D.L., Hollingsworth, Z., and Young, A.B. (1990). Excitatory amino-acid binding-sites in the hippocampal region of alzheimers-disease and other dementias. *Journal of Neurology, Neurosurgery and Psychiatry*, **53**, 314–320.

Perez-Navarro, E., Arenas, E., Reiriz, J., Calvo, N., and Alberch, J. (1996). Glial cell line-derived neurotrophic factor protects striatal calbindin-immunoreactive neurons from excitotoxic damage. *Neuroscience*, **75**, 345–352.

Perlow, M.J., Freed, W.J., Hoffer, B.J., Seiger, Å., Olson, L., and Wyatt, R.J. (1979). Brain grafts reduce motor abnormalities produced by destruction of nigrostriatal dopamine system. *Science*, **204**, 643–647.

Peroutka, S.J., Sohmer, B.H., Kumar, A.J., Folstein, M., and Robinson, R.G. (1982). Hallucinations and delusions following a right temporoparietooccipital infarction. *Johns. Hopkins.Med.J.*, **151**, 181–185.

Perry, V.H. and Brown, M.C. (1992). Role of macrophages in peripheral nerve degeneration and repair. *BioEssays*, **14**, 401–406.

Perutz, M. (1994). Polar zippers — their role in human disease. *Protein Science*, **3**, 1629–1637.

Perutz, M.F., Johnson, T., Suzuki, M., and Finch, J.T. (1994). Glutamine repeats as polar zippers: their possible role in inherited neurodegenerative disease. *Proceedings of the National Academy of Sciences of the United States of America*, **91**, 5355–5358.

Peschanski, M., Defer, G., N'Guyen, J.P., Ricolfi, F., Montfort, J.C., Rémy, P. *et al.* (1994). Bilateral motor improvement and alteration of l-dopa effect in two patients with Parkinson's disease following intrastriatal transplantation of foetal ventral mesencephalon. *Brain*, **117**, 487–499.

Pesheva, P., Spiess, E., and Schachner, M. (1989). J1–160 and J1–180 are oligodendrocyte-secreted nonpermissive substrates for cell adhesion. *Journal of Cell Biology*, **109**, 1765–1778.

Peters, G.R., Hwang, L.J., Musch, B., Brosse, D.M., and Orgogozo, J.M. (1996). Safety and efficacy of 6 mg/kg/day tirilazad mesylate in patients with acute ischemic stroke (TESS study). *Stroke*, **27**, 161.

Peterson, K., Rosenblum, M.K., Kotanides, H., and Posner, J.B. (1992). Paraneoplastic cerebellar degeneration. I. A clinical analysis of 55 anti-Yo antibody-positive patients. *Neurology*, **42**, 1931–1937.

Pettmann, B. and Henderson, C.E. (1998). Neuronal cell death. *Neuron*, **20**, 633–647.

Peyser, C.E. and Folstein, S.E. (1990). Huntington's disease as a model for mood disorders. Clues from neuropathology and neurochemistry. *Molecular and Chemical Neuropathology*, **12**, 99–119.

Pérez-Navarro, E., Arenas, E., Reiriz, J., Calvo, N., and Alberch, J. (1996). Glial cell line-derived neurotrophic factor protects striatal calbindin-immunoreactive neurons from excitotoxic damage. *Neuroscience*, **75**, 345–352.

Pfister, H.W. and Scheld, W.M. (1997). Brain injury in bacterial meningitis: therapeutic implications. *Current Opinion In Neurology*, **10**, 254–259.

Pfister, H.W., Wilske, B., and Weber, K. (1994). Lyme borreliosis: basic science and clinical aspects. *Lancet*, **343**, 1013–1016.

Pflanz, S., Besson, J.A.O., Ebmeier, K.P., and Simpson, S. (1991). The clinical manifestation of mental disorder in Huntington's disease: a retrospective case record study of disease progression. *Acta Psychiatrica Scandinavica*, **83**, 53–60.

Piccardo, P., Maysinger, D., and Cuello, A.C. (1992). Recovery of nucleus basalis cholinergic neurons by grafting NGF secreting fibroblasts. *NeuroReport*, **3**, 353–356.

Pickard, J. (1982). Adult communicating hydrocephalus. *British Journal of Hospital Medicine*, **27**, 35–44.

Pinter, M.M., Pogarell, O., and Oertel, W.H. (1999). Efficacy, safety, and tolerance of the non-ergoline dopamine agonist pramipexole in the treatment of advanced Parkinson's disease: a double-blind, placebo controlled, randomised, multicentre study. *Journal of Neurology, Neurosurgery and Psychiatry*, **66**, 436–441.

Plaisted, K.C. and Sahakian, B.J. (1997). Dementia of frontal lobe type — living in the here and now. *Aging and Mental Health*, **1**, 293–295.

Plum, F. and Posner, J.B. (1980). *Stupor and Coma*. Davis, Philadelphia.

Podlisny, M.B., Stephenson, D.T., Frosch, M.P., Lieberberg, I., Clemens, J.A., and Selkoe, D.J. (1992). Synthetic β-amyloid fails to produce specific neurotoxicity in monkey cerebral cortex. *Neurobiology of Aging*, **13**, 561–567.

Poewe, W. and Granata, R. (1997). Pharmacological treatment of Parkinson's disease. In *Movement Disorders. Neurological Principles and Practice* (ed. R.L. Watts and W.C. Koller), pp. 201–219. McGraw-Hill, New York.

Poiesz, C.M., Ruscetti, F.W., Gazdar, A.F., Bunn, P.A., Minno, J.D., and Gallo, R.C. (1980). Detection and isolation of type C retroviruses particles from fresh and cultured lymphocytes of a patient with cutaneous T-cell lymphoma. *Proceedings of the National Academy of Sciences of the United States of America*, **77**, 7415–7419.

Polymeropoulos, M.H., Lavedan, C., Leroy, E., Ide, S.E., Dehejia, A., Dutra, A. *et al.* (1997). Mutation in the alpha-synuclein gene identified in families with Parkinson's disease. *Science*, **276**, 2045–2047.

Pope-HG, J., McElroy, S.L., Satlin, A., Hudson, J.I., Keck-PE, J., and Kalish, R. (1988). Head injury, bipolar disorder, and response to valproate. *Comprehensive Psychiatry*, **29**, 34–38.

Posner, M.I. (1993). Interaction of arousal and selection in the posterior attention network. In *Attention, Selection, Awareness and Control* (ed. A. Baddeley and L. Weiskrantz), pp. 390–405. Clarendon Press, Oxford.

Poulter, M., Baker, H.F., Frith, C.D., Leach, M., Lofthouse, R., Ridley, R.M. *et al.* (1992). Inherited prion disease with 144 base pair gene insertion. 1. Genealogical and molecular studies. *Brain*, **115**, 675–685.

Powell, G.E. (1981). *Brain Function Therapy*. Gower, London.

Preston, C.M. and Nicholl, M.J. (1997). Repression of gene expression upon infection of cells with herpes simplex virus type 1 mutants impaired for immediate-early protein synthesis. *Journal of Virology*, **71**, 7807–7813.

Price, B.H. and Mesulam, M. (1985). Psychiatric manifestations of right hemisphere infarctions. *Journal of Nervous and Mental Diseases*, **173**, 610–614.

Price, T.R. and Tucker, G.J. (1977). Psychiatric and behavioral manifestations of normal pressure hydrocephalus. A case report and brief review. *Journal of Nervous and Mental Diseases*, **164**, 51–55.

Prigatano, G.P., O'Brien, K.P., and Klonoff, P.S. (1988). The Clinical management of paranoid delusions in post-acute traumatic brain-injured patients. *Journal of Head Trauma and Rehabilitation*, **3**, 23–32.

Primeau, F. (1988). Post-stroke depression: a critical review of the literature. *Can.J.Psychiatry*, **33**, 757–765.

Prineas, J.W., Barnard, R.O., Kwon, E.E., Sharer, L.R., and Cho, E.S. (1993a). Multiple-sclerosis — remyelination of nascent lesions. *Annals of Neurology*, **33**, 137–151.

Prineas, J.W., Barnard, R.O., Revesz, T., Kwon, E.E., Sharer, L., and Cho, E.S. (1993b). Multiple-sclerosis — pathology of recurrent lesions. *Brain*, **116**, 681–693.

Prusiner, S.B. (1982). Novel proteinaceous infectious particles cause scrapie. *Science*, **216**, 136–144.

Prusiner, S.B. (1991). Molecular biology of prion diseases. *Science*, **252**, 1515–1522.

Prusiner, S.B. (1996a). Molecular biology and genetics of prion diseases. *Cold Spring Harbor Symposia on Quantitative Biology*, **61**, 473–493.

Prusiner, S.B. (1996b). Molecular biology and pathogenesis of prion diseases. *Trends In Biochemical Sciences*, **21**, 482–487.

Prusiner, S.B. (1997a). Cell biology and transgenic models of prion disease. In *Prion Diseases* (ed. J. Collinge and S.B. Prusiner), pp. 130–162. Oxford University Press, New York.

Prusiner, S.B. (1997b). Prion diseases and the BSE crisis. *Science*, **278**, 245–251.

Prusiner, S.B., McKinley, M.P., Bowman, K.A., Bolton, D.C., Bendheim, P.E., Groth, D.F. *et al.* (1983). Scrapie prions aggregate to form amyloid-like birefringent rods. *Cell*, **35**, 349–358.

Przedborski, S., Kostic, V., Jackson-Lewis, V., Naini, A.B., Simonetti, S., Fahn, S. *et al.* (1992). Transgenic mice with increased Cu/Zn superoxide dismutase actvity are resistant to MPTP-induced neurotoxicity. *Journal of Neuroscience*, **12**, 1658–1667.

Przedborski, S., Jackson-Lewis, V., Yokoyama, R., Shibata, R., Dawson, V.L., and Dawson, T.M. (1996). Role of neuronal nitric oxide in 1-methyl-4-phenyl-1,2,3,6-tetrahydropyridine (MPTP)-induced toxicity. *Proceedings of the National Academy of Sciences of the United States of America*, **93**, 4565–4571.

Ptak, L.R., Hart, K.R., Lin, D., and Carvey, P.M. (1995). Isolation and manipulation of rostral mesencephalic tegmental progenitor cells from rat. *Cell Transplantation*, **4**, 335–342.

Pulsinelli, W.A., Brierley, M.D., and Plum, F. (1982). Temporal profile of neuronal damage in a model of transient forebrain ischaemia. *Annals of Neurology*, **11**, 491–498.

Purves, D. and Lichtman, J.W. (1985). *Principles of Neural Development*. Sinauer Associates, Sunderland, MA.

Quinn, N.P. (1990). The clinical application of cell grafting techniques in patients with Parkinson's disease. *Progress in Brain Research*, **82**, 619–625.

Quinn, N.P. (1997). Parkinsonism. *Baillieres.Clin.Neurol.*, **6**, 1–218.

Quinn, N.P., Brown, R., Craufurd, D., Goldman, S., Hodges, J.R., Kieburtz, K. *et al.* (1996). Core assessment programme for intracerebral transplantation in Huntington's disease (CAPIT-HD). *Movement Disorders*, **11**, 143–150.

Rabchevsky, A.G. and Streit, W.J. (1997). Grafting of cultured microglial cells into the lesioned spinal cord of adult rats enhances neurite outgrowth. *Journal of Neuroscience Research*, **47**, 34–48.

Rabins, P.V., Starkstein, S.E., and Robinson, R.G. (1991). Risk factors for developing atypical (schizophreniform) psychosis following stroke. *J.Neuropsychiatry Clin.Neurosci.*, **3**, 6–9.

Raff, M.C., Miller, R.H., and Noble, M. (1983). A glial progenitor cell that develops *in vitro* into an astrocyte or an oligodendrocyte depending on the culture medium. *Nature*, **303**, 390–396.

Raisman, G. (1969). Neuronal plasticity in the septal nuclei of the adult brain. *Brain Research*, **14**, 25–48.

Raisman, G. and Field, P.M. (1973). A quantitative investigation of the development of collateral reinnervation after partial deafferentation of the septal nuclei. *Brain Research*, **50**, 241–264.

Raivich, G., Bohatschek, M., Kloss, C.U.A., Werner, A., Jones, L.L., and Kreutzberg, G.W. (1999). Neuroglial activation repertoire in the injured brain: graded response, molecular mechanisms and cues to physiological function. *Brain Research Reviews*, **30**, 77–105.

Rajan, R., Irvine, D.R.F., Wise, L.Z., and Heil, P. (1993). Effect of unilateral partial cochlear lesions in adult cats on the representation of lesioned and unlesioned cochleas in primary auditory cortex. *Journal of Comparative Neurology*, **338**, 17–49.

Rakic, P. (1985). Limits of neurogenesis in primates. *Science*, **227**, 1054–1056.

Rall, G.F., Mucke, L., and Oldstone, M.B.A. (1995). Consequences of cytotoxic T lymphocyte interaction with major histocompatibility complex class 1 expressing neurons *in vivo*. *Journal of Experimental Medicine*, **182**, 1201–1212.

Ramachandran, V.S., Rogers-Ramachandran, D., and Stewart, M. (1992a). Perceptual correlates of massive cortical reorganisation. *Science*, **258**, 1159–1160.

Ramachandran, V.S., Stewart, M., and Rogers-Ramachandran, D.C. (1992b). Perceptual correlates of massive cortical reorganisation. *NeuroReport*, **3**, 583–586.

Ramon-Cueto, A. and Nieto-Sampedro, M. (1994). Regeneration into the spinal cord of transected dorsal root axons is promoted by ensheathing glia transplants. *Experimental Neurology*, **127**, 232–244.

Ramon-Cueto, A., Plant, G.W., Avila, J., and Bunge, M.B. (1998). Long-distance axonal regeneration in the transected adult rat spinal cord is promoted by olfactory ensheathing glia transplants. *Journal of Neuroscience*, **18**, 3803–3816.

Randolph, C., Mohr, E., and Chase, T.N. (1993). Assessment of intellectual function in dementing disorders — validity of WAIS-R short forms for patients with Alzheimers, Huntington's, and Parkinson's disease. *Journal of Clinical and Experimental Neuropsychology*, **15**, 743–753.

Rao, M.S., Landis, S.C., Escary, J.L., Perreau, J., Tresser, S., Patterson, P.H. *et al.* (1993). Leukemia inhibitory factor mediates an injury response but not a target-directed developmental transmitter switch in sympathetic neurons. *Neuron*, **11**, 1175–1185.

Rasmussen, D.X., Bylsma, F.W., and Brandt, J. (1995). Stability of performance on the Hopkins Verbal-Learning Test. *Archives of Clinical Neuropsychology*, **10**, 21–26.

Ray, J., Peterson, D.A., Schinstine, M., and Gage, F.H. (1993). Proliferation, differentiation, and long-term culture of primary hippocampal neurons. *Proceedings of the National Academy of Sciences of the United States of America*, **90**, 3602–3606.

Read, G.S. and Frenkel, N. (1983). Herpes simplex virus mutants defective in the viron associated shut-off of hart polypeptide synthesis and exhibiting abnormal synthesis of $\alpha$ (immediate-early) viral polypeptide. *Journal of Virology*, **46**, 498–512.

Recanzone, G.H., Schreiner, C.E., and Merzenich, M.M. (1993). Plasticity in the frequency representation of primary auditory cortex following discrimination training in adult owl monkeys. *Journal of Neuroscience*, **13**, 87–103.

Reddy, R.V. and Vakili, S.T. (1981). Midbrain encephalitis as a remote effect of a malignant neoplasm. *Archives of Neurology*, **38**, 781–782.

Reddy, P.H., Williams, M., and Tagle, D.A. (1999). Recent advances in understanding the pathogenesis of Huntington's disease. *Trends in Neurosciences*, **22**, 248–255.

Reding, M., Orto, L., Willensky, P., Fortuna, I., Day, N., Steiner, S.F. *et al.* (1985). The dexamethasone suppression test. An indicator of depression in stroke but not a predictor of rehabilitation outcome. *Archives of Neurology*, **42**, 209–212.

Redlich, E. (1912). *Die Psychosen bei Gehirnerkrankungen.* Deuticke, Leipzig.

Redmond, D.E., Naftolin, F., Collier, T.J., Leranth, C., Robbins, R.J., Sladek, C.D. *et al.* (1988). Cryopreservation, culture, and transplantation of human fetal mesencephalic tissue into monkeys. *Science*, **242**, 768–771.

Reed, A.P. (1993). Huntington's disease: testing the test. *Nature Genetics*, **4**, 329–330.

Reed, T.E. and Chandler, J.H. (1958). Huntington's chorea in Michigan. I. Demography and genetics. *American Journal of Human Genetics*, **10**, 201–225.

Reier, P.J., Stensaas, L.J., and Guth, L. (1982). The astrocytic scar as an impediment to regeneration in the central nervous system. In *Spinal Cord Reconstruction* (ed. C.C. Kao, R.P. Bunge and P.J. Reier), pp. 163–195. Raven Press, New York.

Reeves, S.A. (1998). Retrovirus vectors and regulatable promoters. In *Gene Therapy for Neurological Disorders and Brain Tumors* (ed. E.A. Chiocca and X.O. Breakefield), pp. 7–38. Humana, Totowa, N.J.

Reier, P.J. and Houle, J.D. (1988). The glial scar: its bearing on axonal elongation and transplantation approaches to CNS repair. *Advances in Neurology*, **47**, 87–138.

Reisberg, B., Schneider, L., Doody, R., Anand, R., Feldman, H., Haraguchi, H. *et al.* (1997). Clinical global measures of dementia. Position paper from the International Working Group on Harmonization of Dementia Drug Guidelines. *Alzheimer Disease and Associated Disorders*, **11**, 8–18.

Reitan, R.M. (1958). Validity of the Trial Making Test as an indicator of organic brain damage. *Perceptual and Motor Skills*, **8**, 271–276.

Renfranz, P.J., Cunningham, M.G., and McKay, R.D.G. (1998). Region-specific differentiation of the hippocampal stem cell line HiB5 upon implantation into the developing mammalian brain. *Cell*, **66**, 713–729.

Reynolds, B.A. and Weiss, S. (1992). Generation of neurons and astrocytes from isolated cells of the adult mammalian central nervous system. *Science*, **255**, 1707–1710.

Reynolds, B.A. and Weiss, S. (1996). Clonal and population analyses demonstrate that an egf-responsive mammalian embryonic cns precursor is a stem cell. *Developmental Biology*, **175**, 1–13.

Reynolds, B.A., Tetzlaff, W., and Weiss, S. (1992). A multipotent EGF-responsive striatal embryonic progenitor cell produces neurons and astrocytes. *Journal of Neuroscience*, **12**, 4565–4574.

Richards, L.J., Kilpatrick, T.J., and Bartlett, P.F. (1992). De novo generation of neuronal cells from the adult mouse brain. *Proceedings of the National Academy of Sciences of the United States of America*, **89**, 8591–8595.

Richards, M., Marder, K., Cote, L., and Mayeux, R. (1994). Interrater reliability of the Unified Parkinson's Disease Rating Scale motor examination. *Movement Disorders*, **9**, 89–91.

Richardson, J.T.E. (1990). *Clinical and Neuropsychological Aspects of Closed Head Injury.* Taylor and Francis, London.

Richardson, P.M., McGuinness, U.M., and Aguayo, A.J. (1982). Peripheral nerve autografts to the rat spianl cord: studies with axonal tracing methods. *Brain Research*, **257**, 147–162.

Ridley, R.M. and Baker, H.F. (1995). The myth of maternal transmission of spongiform encephalopathy. *British Medical Journal*, **311**, 1071–1075.

Ridley, R.M. and Baker, H.F. (1996). To what extent is strain variation evidence for an independent genome in the agent of the transmissible spongiform encephalopathies? *Neurodegeneration*, **5**, 219–231.

Ridley, R.M. and Baker, H.F. (1997). The nature of transmission in prion diseases [Full text delivery]. *Neuropathology and Applied Neurobiology*, **23**, 273–280.

Ridley, R.M. and Baker, H.F. (1998). *Fatal Protein, the Story of CJD, BSE and Other Prion Diseases.* Oxford University Press, Oxford.

Ridoux, V., Robert, J.J., Zhang, X., Perricaudet, M., Mallet, J., and Le Gal La Salle, G. (1994). The use of adenovirus vectors for intracerebral grafting of transfected nervous cells. *NeuroReport*, 5, 801–804.

Robbins, T.W. (1996). Dissociating executive functions of the prefrontal cortex. *Philosophical Transactions of the Royal Society of London.B:Biological Sciences*, 351, 1463–1471.

Robbins, T.W., Semple, J., Kumar, R., Truman, M.I., Shorter, J., Ferraro, A. *et al*. (1997). Effects of scopolamine on delayed-matching-to-sample and paired associates tests of visual memory and learning in human subjects: comparison with diazepam and implicationd for dementia. *Psychopharmacology*, 134, 95–106.

Robbins, T.W., James, M., Owen, A.M., Sahakian, B.J., Lawrence, A.D., McInnes, L. *et al*. (1998). A study of performance on tests from the CANTAB battery sensitive to frontal lobe dysfunction in a large sample of normal volunteers: implications for theories of executive functioning and cognitive aging. *Journal of the International Neuropsychological Society*, 4, 474–490.

Roberts, A.H. (1979). *Severe Accidental Injury: an Assessment of Long-term Prognosis*. Macmillan, London.

Roberts, A.C. and Sahakian, B.J. (1993). Comparable tests of cognitive function in monkey and man. In *Behavioural Neuroscience: a Practical Approach,*, Vol. I (ed. A. Sahgal), pp. 165–184. IRL Press, Oxford.

Roberts, A., Perera, S., Lang, B., Vincent, A., and Newsom, D.J. (1985). Paraneoplastic myasthenic syndrome IgG inhibits 45Ca2+ flux in a human small cell carcinoma line. *Nature*, 317, 737–739.

Robertson, I.H. and Murre, J.M.J. (1999). Rehabilitation of brain damage: brain plasticity and principles of guided recovery. *Psychological Bulletin*, 125, 544–575.

Robertson, I.H. and North, N. (1992). Spatio-motor cueing in unilateral neglect: the role of hemispace, hand and motor activation. *Neuropsychologia*, 30, 553–563.

Robertson, I.H. and North, N. (1993). Active and passive activation of left limbs: influence on visual and sensory neglect. *Neuropsychologia*, 31, 293–300.

Robertson, I.H. and North, N. (1994). One hand is better than two: motor extinction of left hand advantage in unilateral neglect. *Neuropsychologia*, 32, 1–11.

Robertson, I.H., North, N., and Geggie, C. (1992). Spatio-motor cueing in unilateral neglect: three single case studies of its therapeutic effectiveness. *Journal of Neurology, Neurosurgery and Psychiatry*, 55, 799–805.

Robertson, I.H., Tegnér, R., Tham, K., Lo, A., and Nimmo-Smith, I. (1995). Sustained attention training for unilateral neglect: theoretical and rehabilitation implications. *Journal of Clinical and Experimental Neuropsychology*, 17, 416–430.

Robertson, I.H., Manly, T., Beschin, N., Daini, R., Haeske-Dewick, H., Hömberg, V. *et al*. (1997a). Auditory sustained attention is a marker of unilateral spatial neglect. *Neuropsychologia*, 35, 1527–1532.

Robertson, I.H., Ridgeway, V., Greenfield, E., and Parr, A. (1997b). Motor recovery after stroke depends on intact sustained attention: a two-year follow up study. *Neuropsychology*, 11, 290–295.

Robertson, I.H., Mattingley, J.B., Rorden, C., and Driver, J. (1998). Phasic alerting of neglect patients overcomes their spatial deficit in visual awareness. *Nature*, 395, 169–172.

Robinson, R.G. and Szetela, B. (1981). Mood change following left hemispheric brain injury. *Annals of Neurology*, 9, 447–453.

Robinson, R.G., Boston, J.D., Starkstein, S.E., and Price, T.R. (1988). Comparison of mania and depression after brain injury: causal factors. *Am.J.Psychiatry*, 145, 172–178.

Robinson, R.G., Parikh, R.M., Lipsey, J.R., Starkstein, S.E., and Price, T.R. (1993). Pathological laughing and crying following stroke: validation of a measurement scale and a double-blind treatment study [see comments]. *Am.J.Psychiatry*, 150, 286–293.

Rodriguez, M., Miller, D.J., and Lennon, V.A. (1996). Immunoglobulins reactive with myelin basic protein promote CNS remyelination. *Neurology*, 46, 538–545.

Rogers, D.C. and Dunnett, S.B. (1989). Hypersensitivity to α-methyl-p-tyrosine suggests that behavioural recovery of rats receiving neonatal 6-OHDA lesions is mediated by residual catecholamine neurons. *Neuroscience Letters*, 102, 108–113.

Rogers, M.J. and Franzen, M.D. (1992). Delusional reduplication following closed-head injury. *Brain Injury*, 6, 469–476.

Rogers, S.L. and Friedhoff, L.T. (1998). Long-term efficacy and safety of donepezil in the treatment of Alzheimer's disease: an interim analysis of the results of a US multicentre open label extension study. *Eur.Neuropsychopharmacol.*, 8, 67–75.

Rogers, R.D., Andrews, T.C., Grasby, P.M., Brooks, D.J., and Robbins, T.W. (1997). Contrasting cortical and subcortical PET activations produced by reversal learning and attentional set-shifting in humans. *Society for Neuroscience Abstracts*, 23, 87.1.

Rogers, S.L., Farlow, M.R., Doody, R.S., Mohs, R., and Friedhoff, L.T. (1998). A 24-week, double-blind, placebo-controlled trial of donepezil in patients with Alzheimer's disease. Donepezil Study Group. *Neurology*, 50, 136–145.

Roizman, B. and Sears, A.E. (1996). Herpes simplex viruses and their replication. In *Field's Virology* (ed. B.M. Filed, D.M. Knipe and P.M. Howley), pp. 2231–2295. Lippincott-Raven, Philadelphia.

Roizman, B. and Sears, A. (1999). Herpes simplex viruses and the replication. In *Virology* (ed. D.M. Knife, B.N. Fields and.), pp. 1795–1842.

Rose, F.D., Al-Khamees, K., Davey, M.J., and Attree, E.A. (1993). Environmental enrichment following brain damage: an aid to recovery of compensation? *Behavioural Brain Research*, 56, 93–100.

Rose, K.A., Stapleton, G., Dott, K., Kieny, M.P., Best, R., Schwarz, M. *et al*. (1997). Cyp7b, a novel brain cytochrome P450, catalyzes the synthesis of neurosteroids 7 α-hydroxy dehydroepiandrosterone and 7 α-hydroxy pregnenolone. *Proceedings of the National Academy of Sciences of the United States of America*, 94, 4925–4930.

Rosen, H. and Swigar, M.E. (1976). Depression and normal pressure hydrocephalus. A dilemma in neuropsychiatric differential diagnosis. *Journal of Nervous and Mental Diseases*, 163, 35–40.

Rosen, D.R., Siddique, T., Patterson, D., Figlewicz, D.A., Sapp, P., Hentati, A. *et al*. (1993). Mutations in cu/zn superoxide-dismutase gene are associated with familial amyotrophic-lateral-sclerosis. *Nature*, 362, 59–62.

Rosen, D.R., Siddique, T., and Patterson, D. (1999). Mutations in Cu/Zn superoxide dismutase gene are associated with familial amyotrophic lateral sclerosis. *Nature*, **362**, 59–62.

Rosenbaum, D. (1941). Psychosis with Huntington's chorea. *Psychiatric Quarterly*, **15**, 93–99.

Rosenberg, M.B., Friedmann, T., Robertson, R.C., Tuszynski, M., Wolff, J.A., Breakefield, X.O. *et al.* (1988). Grafting genetically modified cells to the damaged brain: restorative effects of NGF expression. *Science*, **242**, 1575–1578.

Rosenblad, C., Martinez-Serrano, A., and Björklund, A. (1996). Glial cell line-derived neurotrophic factor increases survival, growth and function of intrastriatal fetal nigral dopaminergic grafts. *Neuroscience*, **75**, 979–985.

Rosenblad, C., Martinez-Serrano, A., and Björklund, A. (1997). Intrastriatal glial cell line-derived neurotrophic factor promotes sprouting of spared nigrostriatal dopaminergic afferents and induces recovery of function in a rat model of Parkinson's disease. *Neuroscience*, **82**, 129–137.

Rosenberg, W.S., Breakefield, X.O., Deantonio, C., and Isacson, O. (1992). Authentic and artifactual detection of the E coli lac Z gene product in the rat brain by histochemical methods. *Molecular Brain Research*, **16**, 311–315.

Roses, A.D. (1996). Apolipoprotein-E alleles as risk factors in Alzheimer's disease. *Annual Review of Medicine*, **47**, 387–400.

Rosler, A., Pohl, M., Braune, H.J., Oertel, W.H., Gemsa, D., and Sprenger, H. (1998). Time course of chemokines in the cerebrospinal fluid and serum during herpes simplex type 1 encephalitis. *Journal of the Neurological Sciences*, **157**, 82–89.

Ross, E.D. and Rush, A.J. (1981). Diagnosis and neuroanatomical correlates of depression in brain-damaged patients. Implications for a neurology of depression. *Arch.Gen.Psychiatry*, **38**, 1344–1354.

Ross, E.D. and Stewart, R.S. (1987). Pathological display of affect in patients with depression and right frontal brain damage. An alternative mechanism. *Journal of Nervous and Mental Diseases*, **175**, 165–172.

Rosse, R.B. and Ciolino, C.P. (1985). Effects of cortical lesion location on psychiatric consultation referral for depressed stroke inpatients. *Int.J.Psychiatry Med.*, **15**, 311–320.

Rossi, F., Jankovski, A., and Sotelo, C. (1995). Differential regenerative response of Purkinje cell and inferior olivary axons confronted with embryonic grafts: Environmental cues versus intrinsic neuronal determinants. *Journal of Comparative Neurology*, **359**, 663–677.

Roth, M., Tomlinson, B.E., and Blessed, G. (1967). The relationship between measures of dementia and of degenerative changes in the cerebral grey matter of elderly subjects. *Proceedings of the Royal Society of London, series B: Biological Sciences*, **60**, 254–259.

Rothman, S.M. and Olney, J.W. (1987). Excitotoxicity and the NMDA receptor. *Trends in Neurosciences*, **10**, 299–302.

Rubin, L.L. (1999). Neuronal cell death: an updated view. *Progress in Brain Research*, **117**, 3–8.

Rudelli, R., Strom, J.O., Welch, P.T., and Ambler, M.W. (1982). Post-traumatic premature Alzheimer's disease. Neuropathologic findings and pathogenetic considerations. *Archives of Neurology*, **39**, 570–575.

Ruff, R.M., Young, D., Gautille, T. *et al.* (1989). Verbal learning deficits following severe head injury: heterogeneity in

recovery over 1 year. *Journal of Neurosurgery*, **75** (**Supplement**), S50–S58.

Rupprecht, R. (1997). The neuropsychopharmacological potential of neuroactive steroids. *Journal of Psychiatric Research*, **31**, 297–314.

Rushton, D.N. (1996). Sexual and sphincter dysfunction. In *Neurology in Clinical Practice* (ed. W.G. Bradley, R.B. Daroff, G.M. Fenichel and C.D. Marsden), pp. 407–420. Butterworth-Heinemann, Oxford.

Russell, T.R., Brotman, M., and Norris, F. (1984). Percutaneous gastrostomy. A new simplified and cost-effective technique. *Am.J.Surg.*, **148**, 132–137.

Ruthazer, E.S., Gillespie, D.C., Dawson, T.M., Snyder, S.H., and Stryker, M.P. (1996). Inhibition of nitric oxide synthase does not prevent ocular dominance plasticity in kitten visual cortex. *Journal of Physiology (London)*, **494**, 519–527.

Ryan, T.V., Sautter, S.W., Capps, C.F., Meneese, W., and Barth, J.T. (1992). Utilizing neuropsychological measures to predict vocational outcome in a head trauma population. *Brain Injury*, **6**, 175–182.

Sacks, O.W. (1973). *Awakenings*. Duckworth, London.

Sadato, N., Pascualleone, A., Grafman, J., Ibanez, V., Deiber, M.P., Dold, G. *et al.* (1996). Activation of the primary visual cortex by Braille reading in blind subjects. *Nature*, **380**, 526–528.

Saffran, B.N., Woo, J.E., Mobley, W.C., and Crutcher, K.A. (1989). Intraventricular ngf infusion in the mature rat brain enhances sympathetic innervation of cerebrovascular targets but fails to elicit sympathetic ingrowth. *Brain Research*, **492**, 245–254.

Sagot, Y., Tan, S.A., Baetge, E., Schmalbruch, H., Kato, A.C., and Aebischer, P. (1995). Polymer encapsulated cell lines genetically engineered to release ciliary neurotrophic factor can slow down progressive motor neuronopathy in the mouse. *European Journal of Neuroscience*, **7**, 1313–1322.

Sagot, Y., Tan, S.A., Hammang, J.P., Aebischer, P., and Kato, A.C. (1996). GDNF slows loss of motoneurons but not axonal degeneration or premature death of *pmn/pmn* mice. *Journal of Neuroscience*, **16**, 2335–2341.

Sahakian, B.J. (1990). Computerised assessment of neuropsychological function in Alzheimer's disease and Parkinson's disease. *International Journal of Geriatric Psychiatry*, **5**, 211–213.

Sahakian, B.J., Owen, A.M., Morant, N.J., Eagger, S.A., Boddington, S., Crayton, L. *et al.* (1993). Further analysis of the cognitive effects of tetrahydroaminoacridine (THA) in Alzheimer's disease: assessment of attentional and mnemonic function using CANTAB. *Psychopharmacology*, **110**, 395–401.

Sahakian, B.J., Elliott, R., Low, N., Mehta, M., Clark, R.T., and Pozniak, A.L. (1995). Neuropsychological deficits in tests of executive function in asymptomatic and symptomatic HIV-1 seropositive men. *Psychological Medicine*, **25**, 1233–1246.

Saint-Cyr, J.A., Taylor, A.E., and Nicholson, K. (1996). Behaviour and basal ganglia. *Advances in Neurology*, **65**, 1–28.

Sakai, K., Mitchell, D.J., Tsukamoto, T., and Steinman, L. (1990). Isolation of a complementary DNA clone encoding an autoantigen recognized by an anti-neuronal cell antibody from a patient with paraneoplastic cerebellar degeneration [published erratum appears in *Annals of Neurology* (1991), 30(5), 738]. *Annals of Neurology*, 28, 692–698.

Salloum, I.M., Jenkins, E.J., Thompson, B., Levi, D., and Burnett, Y. (1990). Treatment compliance and hostility levels of head-injured psychiatric outpatients. *J.Natl.Med.Assoc.*, 82, 557–564.

Salojin, K.V., Le, T.M., Nassovov, E.L., Blouch, M.T., Baranov, A.A., Saraux, A. et al. (1996). Anti-endothelial cell antibodies in patients with various forms of vasculitis. *Clin.Exp.Rheumatol.*, 14, 163–169.

Salthouse, T.A. (1984). Effects of age and skill in typing. *Journal of Experimental Psychology: General*, 113, 345–371.

Samii, A., Turnbull, I.M., Kishore, A., Schulzer, M., Mak, E., Yardley, S. et al. (1999). Reassessment of unilateral pallidotomy in Parkinson's disease. A 2-year follow-up study. *Brain*, 122, 417–425.

Samulski, R.J., Srivastava, A., Berns, K.I., and Muzyczka, N. (1983). Rescue of adeno-associated virus from recombinant plasmids: gene correction within the terminal repeats of AAV. *Cell*, 33, 135–143.

Samulski, R.J., Chang, L.S., and Shenk, T. (1989). Helper-free stocks of recombinant adeno-associated viruses: normal integration does not require viral gene expression. *Journal of Virology*, 63, 3822–3828.

Samulski, R.J., Zhu, X., Xiao, X., Brook, J.D., Housman, D.E., Epstein, N. et al. (1991). Targeted integration of adenoassociated virus (Aav) Into human chromosome-19. *EMBO Journal*, 10, 3941–3950.

Sandel, M.E., Olive, D.A., and Rader, M.A. (1993). Chlorpromazine-induced psychosis after brain injury. *Brain Injury*, 7, 77–83.

Sandrock, A.W. and Matthew, W.D. (1987). Identification of a peripheral nerve neurite growth-promoting activity by development and use of an *in vitro* bioassay. *Proceedings of the National Academy of Sciences of the United States of America*, 84, 6934–6938.

Sanes, J.R., Gautum, M., Martin, P.T., Noakes, P.G., Porter, B.E., and Merlie, J.P. (1995). Basal limina components that influence synaptogenesis. *Journal of Neurochemistry*, 65, S1.

Santa-Olalla, J. and Covarrubias, L. (1998). Random catecholaminergic differentiation of mesencephalic neural precursors. *NeuroReport*, 27, 2394–2398.

Sapolsky, R.M., Krey, L.C., and McEwen, B.S. (1985). Prolonged glucocorticoid exposure reduces hippocampal neuron number: implications for aging. *Journal of Neuroscience*, 5, 1222–1227.

Sapolsky, R.M. (1992). *Stress, the Aging Brain, and the Mechanisms of Neuron Death*. MIT Press, Cambridge MA.

Sapolsky, R.M. (1996). Why stress is bad for your brain. *Science*, 273, 749–750.

Sato, S., Inuzuka, T., Nakano, R., Fujita, N., Matsubara, N., Sakimura, K. et al. (1991). Antibody to a zinc finger protein in a patient with paraneoplastic cerebellar degeneration. *Biochemistry and Biophsyics Research Communications*, 178, 198–206.

Sauer, H. and Brundin, P. (1991). Effects of cool storage on survival and function of intrastriatal ventral mesencephalic grafts. *Restorative Neurology and Neuroscience*, 2, 123–135.

Sauer, H., Rosenblad, C., and Björklund, A. (1995). Glial cell line-derived neurotrophic factor but not transforming growth factor β3 prevents delayed degeneration of nigral dopaminergic neurons following striatal 6-hydroxydopamine lesion. *Proceedings of the National Academy of Sciences of the United States of America*, 92, 8935–8939.

Saugstad, L. and Odegard, O. (1986). Huntington's chorea in Norway. *Psychological Medicine*, 16, 39–48.

Saunders, A.M., Strittmatter, W.J., Schmechel, D.E., St.George-Hislop, P., Pericak-Vance, M.A., Joo, S.H. et al. (1993). Association of apolipoprotein-E allele epsilon-4 with late onset familial and sporadic Alzheimer's disease. *Neurology*, 43, 1467–1472.

Sautter, J., Strecker, S., Kupsch, A., and Oertel, W.H. (1996). Methylcellulose during cryopreservation of ventral mesencephalic tissue fragments fails to improve survival and function of cell suspension grafts. *Journal of Neuroscience Methods*, 64, 173–179.

Sawai, H., Clarke, D.B., Kittlerova, P., Bray, G.M., and Aguayo, A.J. (1996). Brain-derived neurotrophic factor and neurotrophin-4/5 stimulate growth of axonal branches from regenerating retinal ganglion cells. *Journal of Neuroscience*, 16, 3887–3894.

Scalapino, K., Conner, J.M., and Varon, S. (1996). The role of NGF and afferent denervation in the process of sympathetic fiber ingrowth into the hippocampal formation. *Experimental Neurology*, 141, 310–317.

Scaravilli, F. and Harrison, M.J.G. (1997). Infectious diseases causing dementia. In *The Neuropathology of Dementia* (ed. M.M. Esiri and J.H. Morris), pp. 372–378. Cambridge University Press, Cambridge.

Scatton, B. (1993). The NMDA receptor complex. *Fundamentals in Clinical Pharmacology*, 7, 389–400.

Schacter, D.L. (1987). Memory, amnesia and frontal lobe dysfunction. *Psychobiology*, 15, 21–36.

Schaden, H., Stuermer, C.A.O., and Bähr, M. (1994). Gap-43 immunoreactivity and axon regeneration in retinal ganglion cells of the rat. *Journal of Neurobiology*, 25, 1570–1578.

Schafer, M., Fruttiger, M., Montag, D., Schachner, M., and Martini, R. (1996). Disruption of the gene for the myelin-associated glycoprotein improves axonal regrowth along myelin in c57bl/wld(S) Mice. *Neuron*, 16, 1107–1113.

Schapira, A.H.V. (1999). Parkinson's Disease. *BMJ.*, 318, 311–314.

Scherer, S.S. and Easter, S.S. (1984). Degenerative and regenerative changes in the trochlear nerve of goldfish. *Journal of Neurocytology*, 13, 519–565.

Schierle, G.S., Hansson, O., Leist, M., Nicotera, P., Widner, H., and Brundin, P. (1999). Caspase inhibition reduces apoptosis and increases survival of nigral transplants. *Nature Medicine*, 5, 97–100.

Schiff, D. and Rosenblum, M.K. (1998). Herpes simplex encephalitis (HSE) and the immunocompromised: a clinical and autopsy study of HSE in the settings of cancer and human immunodeficiency virus type 1 infection. *Human Pathology*, 29, 215–222.

Schinstine, M., Rosenberg, M.B., Routledge-Ward, C., Friedmann, T., and Gage, F.H. (1992). Effects of choline and quiescence on *Drosophila* choline acetyltransferase expression and acetylcholine production by transduced fibroblasts. *Journal of Neurochemistry*, 58, 2019–2029.

Schlaepfer, W.W. and Bunge, R.P. (1973). The effects of calcium ion concentration on the degradation of amputated axons in tissue culture. *Journal of Cell Biology*, 59, 456–470.

Schneider, L.S., Hinsey, M., and Lyness, S. (1992). Plasma dehydroepiandrosterone sulfate in Alzheimer's disease. *Biological Psychiatry*, 31, 205–208.

Schnell, L. and Schwab, M.E. (1990). Axonal regeneration in the rat spinal cord produced by an antibody against myelin-associated neurite growth inhibitors. *Nature*, 343, 269–272.

Schoenfeld, M., Mayers, R.H., Cupples, L.A., Berkman, B., Sax, D., and Clark, E. (1984). Increased rate of suicide among patients with Huntington's disease. *Journal of Neurology, Neurosurgery and Psychiatry*, 47, 1283–1287.

Schoenhuber, M. and Gentilini, M. (1988). Anxiety and depression after mild head injury. *Journal of Neurology, Neurosurgery and Psychiatry*, 51, 722–724.

Schubert, D.S.P., Taylor, C., Lee, S., Mentari, A., and Tamaklo, W. (1992). Detection of depression in the stroke patient. *Psychosomatics.*, 33, 290–294.

Schulterbrandt, J.G., Raskin, A., and Reatig, N. (1974). Further replication of factors of psychopathology in the interview, ward behaviour and self-reported ratings of hospitalized depressed patients. Psycholgical Rep 34: 23–32. *Psychological Reports*, 34, 23–32.

Schulz, J.B., Henshaw, D.R., Siwek, D., Jenkins, B.G., Ferrante, R.J., Cipolloni, P.B. *et al.* (1995). Involvement of free radicals in excitotoxicity *in vivo*. *Journal of Neurochemistry*, 64, 2239–2247.

Schulz, J.B., Matthews, R.T., Henshaw, D.R., and Beal, M.F. (1996). Neuroprotective strategies for treatment of lesions produced by mitochondrial toxins: Implications for neurodegenerative diseases. *Neuroscience*, 71, 1043–1048.

Schulz, J.B., Weller, M., Matthews, R.T., Heneka, M.T., Groscurth, P., Martinou, J.C. *et al.* (1998). Extended therapeutic window for caspase inhibition and synergy with MK-801 in the treatment of cerebral histotoxic hypoxia. *Cell Death and Differentiation*, 5, 847–857.

Schumacher, J.M., Short, M.P., Hyman, B.T., Breakefield, X.O., and Isacson, O. (1991). Intracerebral implantation of nerve growth factor-producing fibroblasts protects striatum against neurotoxic levels of excitatory amino acids. *Neuroscience*, 45, 561–570.

Schumacher, J.M. and Isacson, O. (1997). Neuronal xenotransplantation in Parkinson's disease. *Nature Medicine*, 3, 474–475.

Schuster, T. (1902). *Psychischen Störungen bei Hirntumoren*. Enke, Stuttgart.

Schwab, M.E. (1990). Myelin-associated inhibitors of neurite growth and regeneration in the CNS. *Trends in Neurosciences*, 13, 452–456.

Schwab, M.E. and Bartholdi, D. (1996). Degeneration and regeneration of axons in the lesioned spinal cord. *Physiological Reviews*, 78, 319–370.

Schwab, M.E., Kapfhammer, J.P., and Bandtlow, C.E. (1993). Inhibitors of neurite growth. *Annual Review of Neuroscience*, 16, 565–595.

Schwartz, J.P. (1992). Neurotransmitters as neurotrophic factors: a new set of functions. *International Review of Neurobiology*, 34, 1–23.

Schwarcz, R., Hökfelt, T., Fuxe, K., Jonsson, G., Goldstein, M., and Terenius, L. (1979). Ibotenic acid-induced neuronal degeneration: a morphological and neurochemical study. *Experimental Brain Research*, 37, 199–216.

Schwarcz, R., Whetsell, W.O., and Mangano, R.M. (1983). Quinolinic acid: an endogenous metabolite that produces axon-sparing lesions in rat brain. *Science*, 219, 316–318.

Schwarzschild, M.A., Cole, R.L., and Hyman, S.E. (1997). Glutamate, but not dopamine, stimulates stress-activated protein kinase and AP-1-mediated transcription in striatal neurons. *Journal of Neuroscience*, 17, 3455–3466.

Schwid, S.R., Goodman, A.D., Mattson, D.H., Mihai, C., Donohoe, K.M., Petrie, M.D. *et al.* (1997). The measurement of ambulatory impairment in multiple sclerosis. *Neurology*, 49, 1419–1424.

Schwob, J.E., Fuller, T., Price, J.L., and Olney, J.W. (1980). Widespread patterns of neuronal damage following systemic or intracerebral injections of kainic acid: a histological study. *Neuroscience*, 5, 991–1014.

Scolding, N.J. (1999). *Immunological and Inflammatory Disorders of the Central Nervous System*. Heinemann Butterworths, London.

Scolding, N.J., Morgan, B.P., Houston, W.A.J., Linington, C., Campbell, A.K., and Compston, D.A.S. (1989). Vesicular removal by oligodendrocytes of membrane attack complexes formed by activated complement. *Nature*, 339, 620–622.

Scolding, N.J., Zajicek, J.P., Wood, N., and Compston, D.A.S. (1994). The pathogenesis of demyelinating disease. *Progress in Neurobiology*, 43, 143–173.

Scolding, N.J., Rayner, P.J., Sussman, J., Shaw, C.E., and Compston, D.A.S. (1995). A proliferative adult human oligodendrocyte progenitor. *NeuroReport*, 6, 441–445.

Scolding, N.J., Jayne, D.R., Zajicek, J.P., Meyer, P.A.R., Wraight, E.P., and Lockwood, C.M. (1997). The syndrome of cerebral vasculitis: recognition, diagnosis and management. *Q.J.Med.*, 90, 61–73.

Scott, M. (1970). Transitory psychotic behavior following operation for tumors of the cerebello-pontine angle. *Psychiatr.Neurol.Neurochir.*, 73, 37–48.

Scott, P., Barsan, W., Frederiksen, S., Kronick, S., Zink, B.J., Domeier, R.M. *et al.* (1996). A randomized trial of tirilazad mesylate in patients with acute stroke (RANTTAS). *Stroke*, 27, 1453–1458.

Seiger, Å., Nordberg, A., Von Holst, H., Bäckman, L., Ebendal, T., Alafuzoff, I. *et al.* (1993). Intracranial infusion of purified nerve growth factor to an Alzheimer patient: the first attempt of a possible future treatment strategy. *Behavioural Brain Research*, 57, 255–261.

Selmaj, K. (1996). Pathophysiology of the blood-brain barrier. *Springer Semin.Immunopathol.*, 18, 57–73.

Sen, S. and Phillis, J.W. (1993). Alpha-phenyl-*tert*-butylnitrone (PBN) attenuates hydroxyl radical production during ischemia-reperfusion injury of rat brain — and EPR study. *Free Radicals Research Communications*, 19, 255–265.

Sendtner, M., Kreutzberg, G.W., and Thoenen, H. (1990). Cilary neurotrophic factor prevents the degeneration of motoneurons after axotomy. *Nature*, 345, 440–441.

Sendtner, M., Stöckli, K.A., and Thoenen, H. (1992). Synthesis and localization of ciliary neurotrophic factor in the sciatic nerve of the adult rat after lesion and during regeneration. *Journal of Cell Biology*, 118, 139–148.

Sendtner, M., Gotz, R., Holtmann, B., and Thoenen, H. (1997). Endogenous ciliary neurotrophic factor is a lesion factor for axotomized motoneurons in adult mice. *Journal of Neuroscience*, 17, 6999–7006.

Sengstock, G.J., Johnson, K.B., Jantzen, P.T., Meyer, E.M., Dunn, A.J., and Arendash, G.W. (1992). Nucleus basalis lesions in neonate rats induce a selective cortical cholinergic hypofunction and cognitive deficits during adulthood. *Experimental Brain Research*, 90, 163–174.

Senut, M.C., Aubert, I., Horner, P.J., and Gage, F.H. (1998). Gene transfer for adult CNS regeneration and aging. In *Gene Therapy for Neurological Disorders and Brain Tumors* (ed. E.A. Chiocca and X.O. Breakefield), pp. 345–375. Humana, Totowa, N.J.

Serdaroglu, P. (1998). Behcet's disease and the nervous system. *Journal of Neurology*, 245, 197–205.

Serdaroglu, P., Yazici, H., Ozdemir, C., Yurdakul, S., Bahar, S., and Aktin, E. (1989). Neurologic involvement in Behcet's syndrome. A prospective study. *Archives of Neurology*, 46, 265–269.

Seta, K.A., Crumrine, R.C., Whittingham, T.S., Lust, W.D., and McCandless, D.W. (1992). Experimental models of human stroke. In *Neuromethods 22. Animal Models of Neurological Disease II* (ed. A.A. Boulton, G.B. Baker and R.F. Butterworth), pp. 1–50. Humana Press, Totowa, NJ.

Shaker, R.A., Newman, P.K., and Poser, C.M. (1996). *Tropical Neurology*. W.B. Saunders, London.

Shannon, K.M., Penn, R.D., Kroin, J.S., Adler, C.H., Janko, K.A., York, M. *et al.* (1998). Stereotactic pallidotomy for the treatment of Parkinson's disease: efficacy and adverse effects at 6 months in 26 patients. *Neurology*, 50, 434–438.

Sharlip, I.D. (1998). Evaluation and nonsurgical management of erectile dysfunction. *Urol.Clin.North Am.*, 25, 647–659, ix.

Sharpe, M., Hawton, K., House, A., Molyneux, A., Sandercock, P., Bamford, J. *et al.* (1990). Mood disorders in long-term survivors of stroke: associations with brain lesion location and volume. *Psychological Medicine*, 20, 815–828.

Sharrack, B. and Hughes, R.A.C. (1999). The Guy's Neurological Disability Scale (GNDS): a new disability measure for multiple sclerosis. *Multiple Sclerosis*, 5, 223–233.

Shaw, P.J. (1999). Stiff-man syndrome and its variants. *Lancet*, 353, 86–87.

Shenk, T. (1996). Adenoviridae: the viruses and their replication. In *Field's Virology* (ed. B.M. Filed, D.M. Knipe and P.M. Howley), pp. 2111–2148. Lippincott-Raven, Philadelphia.

Shepherd, M. and Sartorius, N. (1974). Personaility disorder and the International Classification of Diseases. *Psychological Medicine*, 4, 141–146.

Shiel, A., Wilson, B.A., Horn, S., Watson, M., and McLellan, L. (1993). Can patients in coma following traumatic head injury learn simple tasks? *Neuropsychological Rehabilitation*, 3, 161–176.

Shihabuddin, L.S., Hertz, J.A., Holets, V.R., and Whittemore, S.R. (1995). The adult CNS retains the potential to direct region-specific differentiation of a transplanted neuronal precursor cell line. *Journal of Neuroscience*, 15, 6666–6678.

Shihabuddin, L.S., Brunschwig, J.P., Holets, V.R., Bunge, M.B., and Whittemore, S.R. (1996a). Induction of mature neuronal properties in immortalized neuronal precursor cells following grafting into the neonatal CNS. *Journal of Neurocytology*, 25, 101–111.

Shihabuddin, L.S., Holets, V.R., and Whittemore, S.R. (1996b). Selective hippocampal lesions differentially affect the phenotypic fate of transplanted neuronal precursor cells. *Experimental Neurology*, 139, 61–72.

Shimohama, S., Rosenberg, M.B., Fagan, A.M., Wolff, J.A., Short, M.P., Breakefield, X.O., Friedmann, T., and Gage, F.H. (1989). Grafting genetically modified cells into the rat brain: characteristics of Escherichia-coli β-galactosidase as a reporter gene. *Molecular Brain Research*, 5, 271–278.

Shiwach, R. (1994). Psychopathology in Huntington's disease. *Acta Psychiatrica Scandinavica*, 90, 241–246.

Shiwach, R.S. and Patel, V. (1993). Aggressive behaviour in Huntington's disease: a cross-sectional study in a nursing home population. *Behavioural Neurology*, 6, 43–47.

Shiwach, R. and Norbury, G. (1994). A controlled psychiatric study of individuals at risk for Huntington's disease. *British Journal of Psychiatry*, 165, 500–505.

Shockett, P.E. and Schatz, D.G. (1996). Diverse strategies for tetracycline-regulated inducible gene expression. *Proceedings of the National Academy of Sciences of the United States of America*, 93, 5173–5176.

Shoulson, I., Penney, J.B., Kieburtz, K., Oakes, D., Chase, T., Choi, D. *et al.* (1998). Safety and tolerability of the free-radical scavenger OPC-14117 in Huntington's disease. *Neurology*, 50, 1366–1373.

Shults, C.W., Kimber, T., and Martin, D. (1996). Intrastriatal injection of GDNF attenuates the effects of 6- hydroxydopamine. *NeuroReport*, 7, 627–631.

Sieling, P.A., Abrams, J.S., Yamamura, M., Salgame, P., Bloom, B.R., Rea, T.H. *et al.* (1993). Immunosuppressive roles for IL-10 and IL-4 inhuman infection: *in vitro* modulation of T-cell responses in leprosy. *Journal of Immunology*, 150, 5501–5510.

Siesjo, B.K. and Bengtsson, F. (1989). Calcium fluxes, calcium-antagonists, and calcium-related pathology in brain ischemia, hypoglycemia, and spreading depression — a unifying hypothesis. *Journal of Cerebral Blood Flow and Metabolism*, 9, 127–140.

Siesling, S., Zwinderman, A.H., Van Vugt, J.P., Kieburtz, K., and Roos, R.A. (1997). A shortened version of the motor section of the Unified Huntington's Disease Rating Scale. *Movement Disorders*, 12, 229–234.

Siesling, S., Van Vugt, J.P.P., Zwinderman, K.A.H., Kieburtz, K., and Roos, R.A.C. (1998). Unified Huntington's disease rating scale: a follow up. *Movement Disorders*, 13, 915–919.

Sigal, L.H. (1987). The neurologic presentation of vasculitic and rheumatologic syndromes. A review. *Medicine Baltimore.*, 66, 157–180.

Silver, J.M., Yudofsky, S.C., and Hales, R.E. (1991). Depression in traumatic head injury. *Neuropsychiatry, Neuropsychology, Behavioural Neurology*, 4, 12–23.

Silvestri, R., Raffaele, M., De Domenico, P., Tisano, A., Mento, G., Casella, C. *et al.* (1995). Sleep features in Tourette's syndrome, neuroacanthocytosis and Huntington's chorea. *Neurophysiological Clinics*, 25, 66–77.

Simmons, R.D., Buzbee, T.M., Linthicum, D.S., Mandy, W.J., Chen, G., and Wang, C. (1987). Simultaneous visualization of vascular permeability change and leukocyte egress in the central nervous system during autoimmune encephalomyelitis. *Acta Neuropathol.Berl.*, **74**, 191–193.

Simon, R.P., Swan, J.H., Griffiths, T., and Meldrum, B.S. (1984). Blockade of N-methyl-D-aspartate receptors may protect against ischemic damage in the brain. *Science*, **226**, 850–852.

Simonian, N.A. and Coyle, J.T. (1996). Oxidative stress in neurodegenerative diseases. *Annual Review of Pharmacology and Toxicology*, **36**, 83–106.

Sims, T.J. and Gilmore, S.A. (1994). Regeneration of dorsal root axons into experimentally altered glial environments in the rat spinal cord. *Experimental Brain Research*, **99**, 25–33.

Simson, E.L., Gold, R.M., Standish, L.J., and Pellett, P.L. (1977). Axon-sparing brain lesioning technique: the use of monosodium-L-glutamate and other amino acids. *Science*, **198**, 515–517.

Sinclair, S.R., Svendsen, C.N., Torres, E.M., Martin, D., Fawcett, J.W., and Dunnett, S.B. (1996). GDNF enhances dopaminergic cell survival and fibre outgrowth in embryonic nigral grafts. *NeuroReport*, **7**, 2547–2552.

Sinden, J.D., Rashid-Doubell, F., Kershaw, T.R., Nelson, A., Chadwick, A., Jat, P.S. *et al.* (1997). Recovery of spatial learning by grafts of a conditionally immortalized hippocampal neuroepithelial cell line into the ischaemia-lesioned hippocampus. *Neuroscience*, **81**, 599–608.

Singh, M., Meyer, E.M., and Simpkins, J.W. (1995). The effect of ovariectomy and estradiol replacement on brain-derived neurotrophic factor messenger ribonucleic acid expression in cortical and hippocampal brain regions of female Sprague-Dawley rats. *Endocrinology*, **136**, 2320–2324.

Sinyor, D., Jacques, P., Kaloupek, D.G., Becker, R., Goldenberg, M., and Coopersmith, H. (1986). Poststroke depression and lesion location. An attempted replication. *Brain*, **109**, 537–546.

Sirinathsinghji, D.J.S., Dunnett, S.B., Isacson, O., Clarke, D.J., Kendrick, K., and Björklund, A. (1988). Striatal grafts in rats with unilateral neostriatal lesions. II. *In vivo* monitoring of GABA release in globus pallidus and substantia nigra. *Neuroscience*, **24**, 803–811.

Small, G.W., Rabins, P.V., Barry, P.P., Buckholtz, N.S., DeKosky, S.T., Ferris, S.H. *et al.* (1997). Diagnosis and treatment of Alzheimer's disease and related disorders. Consensus statement of the American Association for Geriatric Psychiatry, the Alzheimer's Association, and the American Geriatrics Society. *Journal of the American Medical Association*, **278**, 1363–1371.

Smith, K.J., Blakemore, W.F., and McDonald, W.I. (1979). Central remyelination secures secure conduction. *Nature*, **280**, 395–396.

Smith, J.L., Finley, J.C., and Lennon, V.A. (1988). Autoantibodies in paraneoplastic cerebellar degeneration bind to cytoplasmic antigens of Purkinje cells in humans, rats and mice and are of multiple immunoglobulin classes. *Journal of Neuroimmunology*, **18**, 37–48.

Smith, M.A., Makino, S., Kvetnansky, R., and Post, R.M. (1995a). Stress and glucocorticoids affect the expression of brain-derived neurotrophic factor and neurotrophin-3 messenger-RNAs in the hippocampus. *Journal of Neuroscience*, **15**, 1768–1777.

Smith, R.L., Geller, A.I., Escudero, K.W., and Wilcox, C.L. (1995b). Long-term expression in sensory neurons in tissue culture from herpes simplex virus type-1 (HSV-1) promoters in an HSV-1-derived vector. *Journal of Virology*, **69**, 4593–4599.

Smith-Thomas, L.C., Fok-Seang, J., Stevens, J., Du, J.-S., Muir, E.M., Faissner, A. *et al.* (1994). An inhibitor of neurite outgrowth produced by astrocytes. *Journal of Cell Science*, **107**, 1687–1695.

Smith-Thomas, L.C., Stevens, J., Fok-Seang, J., Faissner, A., Rogers, J.H., and Fawcett, J.W. (1995). Increased axon regeneration in astrocytes grown in the presence of proteoglycan synthesis inhibitors. *Journal of Cell Science*, **108**, 1307–1315.

Snaith, R.P., Constantopoulos, A.A., Jardine, M.Y., and McGuffin, P. (1978). A clinical scale for the self-assessment of Irritability. *British Journal of Psychiatry*, **132**, 164–171.

Snell, R.G., MacMillan, J.C., Cheadle, J.P., Fenton, I., Lazarou, L.P., Davies, P. *et al.* (1993). Relationship between trinucleotide repeat expansion and phenotypic variation in Huntington's disease. *Nature Genetics*, **4**, 393–397.

Snyder, E.Y., Yoon, C., Flax, J.D., and Macklis, J.D. (1997). Multipotent neural precursors can differentiate toward replacement of neurons undergoing targeted apoptotic degeneration in adult mouse neocortex. *Proceedings of the National Academy of Sciences of the United States of America*, **94**, 11663–11668.

Snyder, R.O., Miao, C., Meuse, L., Tubb, J., Donahue, B.A., Lin, H.F. *et al.* (1999). Correction of hemophilia B in canine and murine models using recombinant adeno-associated viral vectors. *Nature Medicine*, **5**, 64–70.

Sohlberg, M. and Mateer, C. (1987). Effectiveness of an attention-training programme. *Journal of Clinical and Experimental Neuropsychology*, **9**, 117–130.

Son, Y.J., Trachtenberg, J.T., and Thompson, W.J. (1996). Schwann cells induce and guide sprouting and reinnervation of neuromuscular junctions. *Trends in Neurosciences*, **19**, 280–285.

Song, S., Wang, Y.M., Bak, S.Y., Lang, P., Ullrey, D., Neve, R.L. *et al.* (1997). An HSV-1 vector containing the rat tyrosine hydroxylase promoter enhances both long-term and cell type-specific expression in the midbrain. *Journal of Neurochemistry*, **68**, 1792–1803.

Sonsalla, P.K. and Heikkila, R.E. (1990). Modulation of methamphetamine-induced neurotoxicity by various pharmacological agents including glutamate receptor antagonists. *European Journal of Pharmacology*, **183**, 211–212.

Sonsalla, P.K., Nicklas, W.J., and Heikkila, R.E. (1989). Role for excitatory amino acids in methamphetamine-induced nigrostriatal dopaminergic toxicity. *Science*, **243**, 398–400.

Spear, P.G. (1998). A welcome mat for leprosy and lassa fever. *Science*, **282**, 1999–2000.

Speelman, J.D. and Bosch, D.A. (1998). Resurgence of functional neurosurgery for Parkinson's disease: a historical perspective. *Mov.Disord.*, **13**, 582–588.

Spenger, C., Haque, N.S.K., Studer, L., Evtouchenko, L., Wagner, B., Bühler, B., Lendahl, U., Dunnett, S.B., and Seiler, R.W. (1996). Fetal ventral mesencephalon of human and rat origin maintained in vitro and transplanted to 6-hydroxy-dopamine-lesioned rats gives rise to grafts rich in dopaminergic neurons. *Experimental Brain Research*, **112**, 47–57.

Spillane, J. and Phillips, R. (1937). Huntington's chorea in South Wales. *Quarterly Journal of Medicine*, **6**, 403–423.

Spillantini, M.G., Schmidt, M.L., Lee, V.M.Y., Trojanowski, J.Q., Jakes, R., and Goedert, M. (1997). α-Synuclein in Lewy bodies. *Nature*, 388, 839–890.

Spillantini, M.G., Bird, T.D., and Ghetti, B. (1998). Frontotemporal Dementia and Parkinsonism linked to chromosome 17: a new group of tauopathies. *Brain Pathology*, 8, 387–402.

Spokes, E.G.S. (1980). Neurochemical alterations in Huntington's chorea: a study of postmortem brain tissue. *Brain*, 103, 179–210.

Sprague, J.M. (1966). Interaction of cortex and superior colliculus in mediation of visually guided behaviour in the cat. *Science*, 153, 1544–1547.

Spreen, O. and Strauss, E. (1998). *A Compendium of Neuropsychological Tests — Administration, Norms, and Commentary*. Oxford University Press, New York.

Springer, T.A. (1994). Traffic signals for lymphocyte recirculation and leukocyte emigration: the multistep paradigm. *Cell*, 76, 301–314.

Springer, J.E. and Loy, R. (1985). Intrahippocampal injections of antiserum to nerve growth factor inhibit sympathohippocampal sprouting. *Brain Research Bulletin*, 15, 629–634.

Squire, L.R., Zola, M.S., Stocchi, F., Nordera, G., and Marsden, C.D. (1991). The medial temporal lobe memory systemStrategies for treating patients with advanced Parkinson's disease with disastrous fluctuations and dyskinesias. *Science*, 253, 1380–1386.

Stadtman, E. (1986). Oxidation of proteins by mixed-function oxidation systems. *Trends in Biological Sciences*, 11, 11–12.

Stambrook, M., Cardoso, E., Hawryluk, G.A. *et al.* (1988). Neuropsychological changes following the neurosurgical treatment of normal pressure hydrocephalus. *Archives of Clinical Neuropsychology*, 3, 323–330.

Starkman, M.N., Schteingart, D.E., and Schork, M.A. (1981). Depressed mood and other psychiatric manifestations of Cushing syndrome — relationship to hormone levels. *Psychosomatic Medicine*, 43, 3–18.

Starkstein, S.E. and Robinson, R.G. (1993). Depression in cerebro-vascular disease. In *Depression in Neurological Disease* (ed. S.E. Starkstein and R.G. Robinson), pp. 28–49. John Hopkins Press, Baltimore.

Steadman, J.H. and Graham, J.G. (1970). Head injuries: an analysis and follow-up study. *Proc.R.Soc.Med.*, 63, 23–28.

Stebbins, G.T. and Goetz, C.G. (1998). Factor structure of the Unified Parkinson's Disease Rating Scale: Motor Examination section. *Movement Disorders*, 13, 633–636.

Steere, A.C., Malawista, S.E., Snysman, D.R., Shope, R.E., Andiman, W.A., Ross, M.R. *et al.* (1977). Lyme arthritis: an epidemic of oligoarticular arthritis in children and adults in three Connecticut communities. *Arthritis and Rheumatology*, 20, 7–17.

Stegeman, C.A., Tervaert, J.W., Huitema, M.G., de, J.P., and Kallenberg, C.G. (1994). Serum levels of soluble adhesion molecules intercellular adhesion molecule 1, vascular cell adhesion molecule 1, and E-selectin in patients with Wegener's granulomatosis. Relationship to disease activity and relevance during followup. *Arthritis Rheum.*, 37, 1228–1235.

Stein, D.G. and Glasier, M.M. (1992). An overview of developments in research on recovery from brain injury. In *Recovery from Brain Damage: Reflections and Directions*

(ed. F.D. Rose and D.A. Johnson ), pp. 1–22. Plenum, New York.

Steinhoff, B.J., Stroll, K.D., Stodieck, S.R., and Palulus, W. (1992). Hyponatremic coma under oxcarbazepine therapy. *Epilepsy Research*, 11, 67–70.

Stenevi, U., Björklund, A., and Svendgaard, N.-A. (1976). Transplantation of central and peripheral monoamine neurons to the adult rat brain: techniques and conditions for survival. *Brain Research*, 114, 1–20.

Stenevi, U., Björklund, A., and Dunnett, S.B. (1980). Functional reinnervation of the denervated neostriatum by nigral transplants. *Peptides*, 1, 111–116.

Stenevi, U., Kromer, L.F., Gage, F.H., and Björklund, A. (1985). Solid neural grafts in intracerebral transplantation cavities. In *Neural Grafting in the Mammalian CNS* (ed. A. Björklund and U. Stenevi), pp. 41–49. Elsevier, Amsterdam.

Sterzi, R., Bottini, G., Celani, M., Righetti, E., Lamassa, M., Ricci, M., and Vallar, G. (1993). Hemianopia, hemianaesthesia and hemiplegia after right and left hemisphere damage. A hemispheric difference. *Journal of Neurology, Neurosurgery and Psychiatry*, 56, 308–310.

Stevens, J.G., Wagner, E.K., Devi-Rao, G.B., Cook, M.L., and Feldman, L.T. (1987). RNA complementary to a herpes virus alpha gene mRNA in prominent in latently infected neurons. *Science*, 235, 1056–1059.

St.George-Hislop, P., Fraser, P.E., Westaway, D., Levesque, G., Yu, G., Ikeda, M., Nishimura, M., Rogaeva, E., Song, Y., Kawarai, T., and Orlacchio, A. (1998). Genetic and molecular biological studies in Alzheimer's disease. *Naunyn-Schmiedebergs Archives Of Pharmacology*, 358, SF123.

Stidworthy-Johnson, E., and Ludwin, S.K. (1981). The demonstration of recurrent demyelination and remyelination of axons in the central nervous system. *Acta Neuropathologica*, 53, 93–98.

Stiernstedt, G., Gustafsson, R., Karlsson, M., Svenungsson, B., and Skoldenberg, B. (1988). Clinical manifestations and diagnosis of neuroborreliosis. *Annals of the New York Academy of Sciences*, 539, 46–55.

Stocchi, F., Nordera, G., and Marsden, C.D. (1997). Strategies for treating patients with advanced Parkinson's disease with disastrous fluctuations and dyskinesias. *Clinical Neuropharmacology*, 20, 95–115.

Stoddard, S.L., Tyce, G.M., Ahlskog, J.E., Zinsmeister, A.R., and Carmichael, S.W. (1989). Decreased catecholamine content in parkinsonian adrenal medullae. *Experimental Neurology*, 104, 22–27.

Stokes, B.T. and Reier, P.J. (1992). Fetal grafts alter behavioral outcome after contusion damage to the adult rat spinal cord. *Experimental Neurology*, 116, 1–12.

Stone, S.P., Wilson, B.A., Wroot, A., Halligan, P.W., ange, L.S., Marshall, J.C. *et al.* (1991). The assessment of visuo-spatial neglect after acute stroke. *Journal of Neurology, Neurosurgery and Psychiatry*, 54, 345–350.

Stone, S.P., Patel, P., Greenwood, R.J., and Halligan, P.W. (1992). Measuring visual neglect in acute stroke and predicting its recovery: the visual neglect recovery index. *Journal of Neurology, Neurosurgery and Psychiatry*, 55, 431–436.

Stone, D.J., Rozovsky, I., Morgan, T.E., Anderson, C.P., and Finch, C.E. (1998). Increased synaptic sprouting in response to estrogen via an apolipoprotein E-dependent mechanism:

Implications for Alzheimer's disease. *Journal of Neuroscience*, 18, 3180–3185.

Stott, K., Blackburn, J.M., Butler, P.J.G., and Perutz, M. (1995). Incorporation of glutamine repeats makes protein oligomerize — implications for neurodegenerative diseases. *Proceedings of the National Academy of Sciences of the United States of America*, 92, 6509–6513.

Strahan, A., Rosenthal, J., Kaswan, M., and Winston, A. (1985). Three case reports of acute paroxysmal excitement associated with alprazolam treatment. *American Journal of Psychiatry*, 142, 859–861.

Stricker, E.M. and Zigmond, M.J. (1976). Recovery of function following damage to central catecholamine-containing neurons: a neurochemical model for the lateral hypothalamic syndrome. In *Progress in Psychobiology and Physiological Psychology* (ed. J.M. Sprague and A.N. Epstein), pp. 121–189. Academic Press, New York.

Strijbos, P.J.L.M., Leach, M.J., and Garthwaite, J. (1996). Vicious cycle involving $Na^+$ channels, glutamate release, and NMDA receptors mediates delayed neurodegeneration through nitric oxide formation. *Journal of Neuroscience*, 16, 5004–5013.

Stryker, M.P. and Strickland, S.L. (1983). Physiological segretation of ocular dominance columns depends on the pattern of afferent electrical activity. *Investigative Ophthalmology and Visual Science*, 25, 278.

Stryker, M.P. and Harris, W.A. (1986). Binocular impulse blockade prevents the formation of ocular dominance columns in cat visual cortex. *Journal of Neuroscience*, 6, 2117–2133.

Studer, L., Tabar, V., and McKay, R.D.G. (1998). Transplantation of expanded mesencephalic precursors leads to recovery in parkinsonian rats. *Nature Neuroscience*, 1, 290–295.

Sturm, W., Dahmen, W., Harjte, W., and Willmes, K. (1983). Ergebnisse eines Trainingsprogramms zur Verbesserung der visuellen Auffassungsshnelligkeit und Konzentrationsfahigkeit bei Hirngeschaditgten. *Archive fur Psychiatrie und Nervenkrankenheiten*, 233, 9–22.

Stuss, D.T. and Gow, C.A. (1992). 'Frontal dysfunction' after traumatic brain injury. *Neuropsychiatry, Neuropsychology, Behavioural Neurology*, 5, 272–282.

Stuss, D.T. and Levine, B. (1996). The dementias: nosological and clinical factors related to diagnosis. *Brain and Cognition*, 31, 99–113.

Suhonen, J.O., Peterson, D.A., Ray, J., and Gage, F.H. (1996). Differentiation of adult hippocampus-derived progenitors into olfactory neurons *in vivo*. *Nature*, 383, 624–627.

Sun, Y. and Zigmond, R.E. (1996). Leukaemia inhibitory factor induced in the sciatic nerve after axotomy is involved in the induction of galanin in sensory neurons. *European Journal of Neuroscience*, 8, 2213–2230.

Sunderland, S. (1972). *Nerves and Nerve Injuries*. Churchill Livingstone, Edinburgh.

Sutton, G., Shah, S., and Hill, V. (1991). Clean intermittent self-catheterisation for quadriplegic patients–a five year follow-up. *Paraplegia.*, 29, 542–549.

Svendsen, C.N. (1997). Neural stem cells for brain repair. *Alzheimer's Research*, 3, 131–135.

Svendsen, C.N., Fawcett, J.W., Bentlage, C., and Dunnett, S.B. (1995). Increased survival of rat EGF-generated CNS progenitor cells using B27 supplemented medium. *Experimental Brain Research*, 102, 407–414.

Svendsen, C.N., Clarke, D.J., Rosser, A.E., and Dunnett, S.B. (1996). Survival and differentiation of rat and human EGF responsive precursor cells following grafting into the lesioned adult CNS. *Experimental Neurology*, 137, 376–388.

Svendsen, C.N., Caldwell, M.A., Shen, J., ter Borg, M., Rosser, A.E., Tyers, P. *et al.* (1997a). Long term survival of human central nervous system progenitor cells transplanted into a rat model of Parkinson's disease. *Experimental Neurology*, 148, 135–146.

Svendsen, C.N., Rosser, A.E., ter Borg, M., Tyers, P., Skepper, J., and Rykin, T. (1997b). Restricted growth potential of rat striatal precursors as compared to mouse. *Developmental Brain Research*, 99, 253–259.

Swaab, D.F., Raadsheer, F.C., Endert, E., Hofman, M.A., Kamphorst, W., and Ravid, R. (1994). Increased cortisol levels in aging and Alzheimer's disease in postmortem cerebrospinal fluid. *Journal of Neuroendocrinology*, 6, 681–687.

Swanson, P.D. (1994). Drug treatment of Parkinson's disease: is 'polypharmacy' best? *Journal of Neurology, Neurosurgery and Psychiatry*, 57, 401–403.

Swartz, M.N. (1984). Bacterial meningitis: more involved than just the meninges. *New England Journal of Medicine*, 311, 912–914.

Swift, T.R. and Sabin, T.D. (1996). Leprosy. In *Tropical Neurology* (ed. R.A. Shaker, P.K. Neuman and C.M. Poser), pp. 151–166. WB Sanders, London.

Szabo, A., Dalmau, J., Manley, G., Rosenfeld, M., Wong, E., Henson, J. *et al.* (1991). HuD, a paraneoplastic encephalomyelitis antigen, contains RNA-binding domains and is homologous to Elav and Sex-lethal. *Cell*, 67, 325–333.

Szatkowski, M. and Atwell, D. (1994). Triggering and execution of neuronal death in brain ischaemia: two phases of glutamate release by different mechanisms. *Trends in Neuro-sciences*, 17, 359–365.

Szymanski, H.V. and Linn, R. (1992). A review of the postconcussion syndrome. *Int.J.Psychiatry Med.*, 22, 357–375.

Tadir, M., and Stern, J.M. (1985). The mourning process with brain injured patients. *Scand.J.Rehabil.Med.Suppl.*, 12, 50–52.

Takahashi, K., Wesselingh, S.L., Griffin, D.E., McArthur, J.C., Johnson, R.T., and Glass, J.D. (1996). Localization of HIV-1 in human brain using polymerase chain reaction in situ hybridization and immunocytochemistry. *Annals of Neurology*, 39, 705–711.

Tallal, P., Miller, S.L., Bedi, G., Byma, G., Wang, X.Q., Nagarajan, S.S. *et al.* (1996). Language comprehension in language learning impaired children improved with acoustically modified speech. *Science*, 271, 81–84.

Tamayose, K., Hirai, T., and Shimada, T. (1996). A new strategy for large scale preparation of high titer recombinant adeno-associated virus vectors by using packaging cell lines and sulfonated cellulose column chromatography. *Human Gene Therapy*, 7, 507–513.

Tamir, A., Whittier, J., and Koorenyi, C. (1969). Huntington's chorea: a sex difference in psychopathological symptoms. *Diseases of the Nervous System*, 30, 103.

Tan, S.A. and Aebischer, P. (1996). The problems of delivering neuroactive molecules to the CNS. *Ciba Foundation Symposia*, 196, 211–236.

Tanaghow, A., Lewis, J., and Jones, G.H. (1989). Anterior tumour of the corpus callosum with atypical depression. *Br.J.Psychiatry*, **155**, 854–856.

Tanaka, K., Tanaka, M., Igarashi, S., Onodera, O., Miyatake, T., and Tsuji, S. (1995). Trial to establish an animal model of paraneoplastic cerebellar degeneration with anti-Yo antibody. 2. Passive transfer of murine mononuclear cells activated with recombinant Yo protein to paraneoplastic cerebellar degeneration lymphocytes in severe combined immunodeficiency mice. *Clin.Neurol.Neurosurg.*, **97**, 101–105.

Tang, M.X., Jacobs, D., Stern, Y., Marder, K., Schofield, P., Gurland, B. *et al.* (1996). Effect of oestrogen during menopause on risk and age at onset of Alzheimer's disease. *Lancet*, **348**, 429–432.

Tans, J.T.J. and Poortvliet, D.C.J. (1988). Reduction in ventricular size after shunting for normal pressure hydrocephalus. *Journal of Neurology, Neurosurgery and Psychiatry*, **51**, 521–525.

Tate, R.L., Fenelon, B., Manning, M.L., and Hunter, M. (1991). Patterns of neuropsychological impairment after severe blunt head injury. *Journal of Nervous and Mental Diseases*, **179**, 117–126.

Taub, E., Miller, N.E., Novack, T.A., ook, E.W., eming, W.C., epomuceno, C.S., Connell, J.S., and Crago, J.E. (1993). Technique to improve chronic motor deficit after stroke. *Archives of Physical Medicine and Rehabilitation*, **74**, 347–354.

Taylor, D.C. (1975). Factors influencing the occurrence of schizophrenia-like psychosis in patients with temporal lobe epilepsy. *Psychological Medicine*, **5**, 249–254.

Taylor, N. and Bramble, D. (1997). Sleep disturbance and Huntington's disease. *British Journal of Psychiatry*, **171**, 393.

Taylor, D. and Lewis, S. (1993). Delirium. *Journal of Neurology, Neurosurgery and Psychiatry*, **56**, 742–751.

Teasdale, G. and Jennett, B. (1974). Assessment of coma and impaired consciousness: a practical scale. *Lancet*, **2**, 81–84.

Teasdale, G. and Jennett, B. (1976). Assessment and prognosis of coma after head injury. *Acta Neurochirurgica*, **34**, 45–55.

Teitelbaum, P. and Epstein, A.N. (1972). The lateral hypothalamic syndrome: recovery from lateral hypothalamic damage. *Psychological Review*, **69**, 74–90.

Telling, G.C., Scott, M., Mastrianni, J., Gabizon, R., Torchia, M., Cohen, F.E. *et al.* (1995). Prion propagation in mice expressing human and chimeric prp transgenes implicates the interaction of cellular prp with another protein. *Cell*, **83**, 79–90.

Temey, G. (1976). Psychométrie et hydrocéphalie normotensive. *Bulletin de Psychologie*, **30**, 468–476.

Tenser, R.B. (1998). Trigeminal neuralgia: mechanisms of treatment. *Neurology*, **51**, 17–19.

Terrace, H.S. (1963). Discrimination learning with and without 'errors'. *Journal of the Experimental Analysis of Behavior*, **6**, 1–27.

Terrace, H.S. (1966). Stimulus control. In *Operant Behaviour: Areas of Research and Application* (ed. W.K. Honig), pp. 271–344. Appleton-Century-Crofts, New York.

Tetzlaff, W., Kobayashi, N.R., Giehl, K.M., Tsui, B.J., Cassar, S.L., and Bedard, A.M. (1994). Response of rubrospinal and corticospinal neurons to injury and neurotrophins. *Progress in Brain Research*, **103**, 271–286.

Thoenen, H. (1995). Neurotrophins and neuronal plasticity. *Science*, **270**, 593–598.

Thomas, D.G.T. (1983). Brain Tumours. *British Journal of Hospital Medicine*, **28**, 148–158.

Thomas, D.D., Cadavid, D., and Barbour, A.G. (1994). Differential association of Borrelia species with cultured neural cells. *Journal of Infectious Disease*, **169**, 445–448.

Thompson, A.J., Polman, C.H., Miller, D.H., McDonald, W.I., Brochet, B. *et al.* (1997). Primary progressive multiple sclerosis. *Brain*, **120**, 1085–1096.

Thomsen, I.V. (1984). Late outcome of very severe blunt head trauma: a 10–15 year second follow-up. *Journal of Neurology, Neurosurgery and Psychiatry*, **47**, 260–268.

Tiller, J.W.G. (1992). Post-stroke depression. *Psychopharmacology*, **106** (**Supplement**), S130–S133.

Tomac, A., Lindqvist, E., Lin, L.-F.H., Ögren, S.O., Young, D., Hoffer, B.J. *et al.* (1995). Protection and repair of the nigrostriatal dopaminergic system by GDNF *in vivo*. *Nature*, **373**, 335–339.

Tombaugh, G.C., Yang, S.H., Swanson, R.A., and Sapolsky, R.M. (1992). Glucocorticoids exacerbate hypoxic and hypoglycemic hippocampal injury *in vitro* — biochemical correlates and a role for astrocytes. *Journal of Neurochemistry*, **59**, 137–146.

Tomlinson, B.E., Blessed, G., and Roth, M. (1970). Observations on the brains of demented old people. *Journal of the Neurological Sciences*, **11**, 205–242.

Tonkongy, J. and Barreira, P. (1989). Obsessive-compulsive disorder and caudate frontal lesion. *Neuropsychiatry, Neuropsychology and Behavioural Neurology*, **2**, 203–209.

Toyka, K.V., Brachman, D.B., Pestronk, A., and Kao, I. (1975). Myasthenia gravis: passive transfer from man to mouse. *Science*, **190**, 397–399.

Tretiakoff, C. (1919). Contribution à l'étude de l'anatomie pathologique du Locus niger de Soemmering avec quelques deduction relatives à la pathogenie des troubles du tonus musculaires dt de la maladie de Parkinson. *Unpublished thesis, University of Paris*,

Trojanowski, J.Q. and Lee, V.M. (1998). Aggregation of neurofilament and α-synuclein proteins in Lewy bodies — Implications for the pathogenesis of Parkinson disease and Lewy body dementia. *Archives of Neurology*, **55**, 151–152.

Trojanowski, J.Q., Kleppner, S.R., Hartley, R.S., Miyazono, M., Fraser, N.W., Kesari, S. *et al.* (1997). Transfectable and transplantable postmitotic human neurons: a potential 'platform' for gene therapy of nervous system diseases. *Experimental Neurology*, **144**, 92–97.

Trucksis, M. (1995). Tetanus. In *Tropical neurology* (ed. R.A. Shaker, P.K. Neuman and C.M. Poser), pp. 19–35. WB Sanders, London.

Tseng, J.L., Bruhn, S.L., Zurn, A.D., and Aebischer, P. (1998). Neurturin protects dopaminergic neurons following medical forebrain bundle axotomy. *NeuroReport*, **9**, 1817–1822.

Tsiang, H. (1993). Pathophysiology of rabies virus infection of the nervous system. *Advances in Virus Research*, **42**, 375–412.

Tsiang, H., Ermine, A., and Marcovistz, R. (1982). Aspects moleculaires et cellulaires de la pathogenie dans la rage.

*Comparative Immunology, Microbiology and Infectious Disease*, 5, 61–65.

Tsirka, S.E., Gualandris, A., Amaral, D.G., and Strickland, S. (1995). Excitotoxin-induced neuronal degeneration and seizure are mediated by tissue-plasminogen activator. *Nature*, 377, 340–344.

Tsuang, D., Di Giacomo, L., Lipe, H., and Bird, E.D. (1998). Familial aggregation of schizophrenia like symptoms in Huntington's disease. *American Journal of Medical Genetics*, 81, 323–327.

Tsubokawa, T., Katayama, Y., Yamamoto, T., Hirayama, T., and Koyama, S. (1991). Treatment of thalamic pain by chronic motor cortex stimulation. *Pacing Clin.Electrophysiol.*, 14, 131–134.

Tsuda, M., Yuasa, S., Sekikawa, M., Ono, K., Tsuchiya, T., and Kawamura, K. (1990). Retrovirus-mediated gene transfer into mouse cerebellar primary culture and its application to the neural transplantation. *Brain Research Bulletin*, 24, 787–792.

Tulving, E. and Schacter, D.L. (1990). Priming and human memory systems. *Science*, 247, 301–306.

Tuokko, H., Vernon, W.R., and Robinson, E. (1991). The use of the MCMI in the personality assessment of head-injured adults. *Brain Injury*, 5, 287–293.

Turner, D.L. and Cepko, C.L. (1987). A common progenitor for neurons and glia persists in rat retina late in development. *Nature*, 328, 131–136.

Tuszynski, M.H. and Kordower, J.H. (1999). *CNS Regeneration*. Academic Press, New York.

Uchida, K., Ishii, A., Kaneda, N., Toya, S., Nagatsu, T., and Kohsaka, S. (1990). Tetrahydrobiopterin-dependent production of l-DOPA in NRK fibroblasts transfected with tyrosine hydroxylase cDNA: future use for intracerebral grafting. *Neuroscience Letters*, 109, 282–286.

Ungerstedt, U. (1971a). Striatal dopamine release after amphetamine or nerve degeneration revealed by rotational behaviour. *Acta Physiological Scandinavica, supplementum*, 367, 49–68.

Ungerstedt, U. (1971b). Postsynaptic supersensitivity after 6-hydroxydopamine-induced degeneration of the nigro-striatal dopamine system. *Acta Physiological Scandinavica, supplementum*, 367, 69–93.

Ungerstedt, U. and Arbuthnott, G.W. (1970). Quantitative recording of rotational behaviour in rats after 6-hydroxydopamine lesions of the nigrostriatal dopamine system. *Brain Research*, 24, 485–493.

Urbach, J.R. and Culbert, J.P. (1991). Head-injured parents and their children. Psychosocial consequences of a traumatic syndrome. *Psychosomatics.*, 32, 24–33.

Valenzuela, D.M., Maisonpierre, P.C., Glass, D.J., Rojas, E., Nuñez, L., Kong, Y. *et al.* (1993). Alternative forms of rat TrkC with different functional capabilities. *Neuron*, 10, 963–974.

Van Broeckhoven, C., Genthe, M., Van den Berghe, A., Horst-Hemke, B., Backhoevens, H., Raeymaekers, P. *et al.* (1987). failure of familial Alzheimer's disease to segregate with theA4-amyloid gene in several European families. *Nature*, 329, 153–155.

Van Dam, A.P. (1991). Diagnosis and pathogenesis of CNS lupus. *Rheumatology and Internal Medicine*, 11, 1–11.

Van den Bogaerde, J. and White, D.J. (1997). Xenogeneic transplantation. *British Medical Bulletin*, 53, 904–920.

Vanek, P., Thallmair, M., Schwab, M.E., and Kapfhammer, J.P. (1998). Increased lesion-induced sprouting of corticospinal fibres in the myelin-free rat spinal cord. *European Journal of Neuroscience*, 10, 45–56.

Van Esseveldt, K.E., Hermens, W.T., Verhaagen, J., and Boer, G.J. (1998). Transgene expression in rat fetal brain grafts is maintained for 7 months after *ex vivo* adenoviral vector-mediated gene transfer. *Neuroscience Letters*, 240, 116–120.

van Hilten, J.J., van der Zwan, A.D., Zwinderman, A.H., and Roos, R.A. (1994). Rating impairment and disability in Parkinson's disease: evaluation of the Unified Parkinson's Disease Rating Scale. *Movement Disorders*, 9, 84–88.

van Oosten, B.W., Lai, M., Hodgkinson, S., Barkhof, F., Miller, D.H., Moseley, I.F. *et al.* (1997). Treatment of multiple sclerosis with the monoclonal anti-CD4 antibody cM-T412: Results of a randomized, double-blind, placebo-controlled, MR-monitored phase II trial. *Neurology*, 49, 351–357.

Van Putten, T., May, P.R.A., and Marder, S.R. (1984). Akathisia with haloperidol and thiothixane. Archives of General Psychiatry 41: 1036. *Archives of General Psychiatry*, 41, 1036–1039.

Vanneste, J. and Hyman, R. (1986). Non-tumoural aqueduct stenosis and normal pressure hydrocephalus in the elderly. *Journal of Neurology, Neurosurgery and Psychiatry*, 49, 529–535.

Vanneste, J. and van-Acker, R. (1990). Normal pressure hydrocephalus: did publications alter management? *Journal of Neurology, Neurosurgery and Psychiatry*, 53, 564–568.

Van Vugt, J.P., Siesling, S., Vergeer, M., Van der Velde, E.A., and Roos, R.A. (1997). Clozapine versus placebo in Huntington's disease: a double blind randomised comparative study. *Journal of Neurology, Neurosurgery and Psychiatry*, 63, 35–39.

van Zomeren, A.H. and Saan, R.J. (1990). Psychological and social sequelae of severe head injury. In *Handbook of Clinical Neurology — Head Injury* (ed. R. Braackman), pp. 397–420. Elsevier, New York.

van Zomeren, A.H. and van der Burg, W. (1985). Residual complaints of patients two years after severe head injury. *Journal of Neurology, Neurosurgery and Psychiatry*, 48, 21–28.

Varney, N.R., Hines, M.E., Bailey, C., and Roberts, R.J. (1992). Neuropsychiatric correlates of theta bursts in patients with closed head injury [see comments]. *Brain Injury*, 6, 499–508.

Vaudano, E., Campbell, G., Anderson, P.N., Schreyer, D.J., Woolhead, C., and Lieberman, A.R. (1995). The effects of a lesion or peripheral nerve graft on GAP-43 upregulation in the adult rat brain: an *in situ* hybridization and immunocytochemical study. *Journal of Neuroscience*, 15, 3594–3611.

Vaudano, E., Campbell, G., and Hunt, S.P. (1996). Change in the molecular phenotype of Schwann cells upon transplantation into the central nervous system: down-regulation of c-jun. *Neuroscience*, 74, 553–565.

Verge, V.M.K., Gratto, K.A., Karchewski, L.A., and Richardson, P.M. (1996). Neurotrophins and nerve injury in the adult. *Philosophical Transactions of the Royal Society of London.B:Biological Sciences*, 351, 423–430.

Verma, I.M. and Somia, N. (1997). Gene therapy — promises, problems and prospects. *Nature*, 389, 239–242.

Vernant, J.C. (1995). HTLV-1. In *Tropical Neurology* (ed. R.A. Shaker, P.K. Neuman and C.M. Poser), pp. 19–35. WB Sanders, London.

Vicario-Abejón, C., Cunningham, M.G., and McKay, R.D.G. (1995). Cerebellar precursors transplanted to the neonatal dentate gyrus express features characteristic of hippocampal neurons. *Journal of Neuroscience*, **15**, 6351–6363.

Vieregge, P., Gerhard, L., and Reinhardt, V. (1988). Intrakranielle raumfordernde Prozesse in der Psychiatrie. *Forschritte der Neurologie und Psychiatrie*, **56**, 373–379.

Vile, R.G. and Russell, S.J. (1995). Retroviruses as vectors. *British Medical Bulletin*, **51**, 12–30.

Vilkki, J., Ahola, K., Holst, P., Öhman, J., Servo, A., and Heiskanen, O. (1994). Prediction of psychosocial recovery after head injury with cognitive tests and neurobehavioural ratings. *Journal of Clinical and Experimental Neuropsychology*, **16**, 325–338.

Vincent, K.A., Piraino, S.T., and Wadsworth, S.C. (1997). Analysis of recombinant adeno-associated virus packaging and requirements for *rep* and *cap* gene products. *Journal of Virology*, **71**, 1897–1905.

von Cramon, D., Matthes von Cramon, G., and Mai, N. (1991). Problem solving deficits in brain injured patients: a therapeutic approach. *Neuropsychological Rehabilitation*, **1**, 45–64.

Wade, D.T., Legh, S.J., and Hewer, R.A. (1987). Depressed mood after stroke. A community study of its frequency. *Br.J.Psychiatry*, **151**, 200–205.

Wagner, E.K. and Bloom, D.C. (1997). Experimental investigation of herpes simplex virus latency. *Clinical Microbiology Reviews*, **10**, 419.

Wahlgren, N.G. (1997). A rejiew of earlier clinical studies on neuroprotective agents and current approaches. In *Neuroprotective Agents and Cerebral Ischaemia* (ed. A.R. Green and A.J. Cross), pp. 337–363. Academic Press, San Diego.

Walker, G.C., Cardenas, D.D., Guthrie, M.R., McLean, A., and Brooke, M.M. (1991). Fatigue and depression in brain-injured patients correlated with quadriceps strength and endurance. *Arch.Phys.Med.Rehabil.*, **72**, 469–472.

Wall, J.T., Kaas, J.H., Sur, M., Nelson, R.J., Felleman, D.J., and Merzenich, M.M. (1986). Functional reorganization in somatosensory cortical areas 3b and 1 of adult monkeys after median nerve repair: possible relationships to sensory recovery in humans. *Journal of Neuroscience*, **6**, 218–233.

Wallace, D.C. and Hall, A.C. (1972). Evidence of genetic heterogeneity in Huntington's chorea. *Journal of Neurology, Neurosurgery and Psychiatry*, **35**, 789–800.

Wallace, S.F., Rosenquist, A.C., and Sprague, J.M. (1990). Ibotenic acid lesions of the lateral substantia nigra restore visual orientation behaviour in the hemianopic cat. *Journal of Comparative Neurology*, **296**, 222–252.

Wallace, C.S., Kilman, V.L., Withers, G.S., and Greenough, W.T. (1992). Increases in dendritic length in occipital cortex after 4 days of differential housing in weanling rats. *Behavioral and Neural Biology*, **58**, 279–284.

Wang, C.R., Liu, M.F., Tsai, R.T., Chuang, C.Y., and Chen, C.Y. (1993). Circulating intercellular adhesion molecules-1 and autoantibodies including anti-endothelial cell, anti-cardiolipin, and anti-neutrophil cytoplasma antibodies in patients with vasculitis. *Clin.Rheumatol.*, **12**, 375–380.

Wang, X.Q., Merzenich, M.M., Sameshima, K., and Jenkins, W.M. (1995). Remodeling of hand representation in adult cortex determined by timing of tactile stimulation. *Nature*, **378**, 71–75.

Wang, Y.M.F., Tsirka, S.E., Strickland, S., Stieg, P.E., Soriano, S.G., and Lipton, S.A. (1998). Tissue plasminogen activator (tPA) increases neuronal damage after focal cerebral ischemia in wild-type and tPA-deficient mice. *Nature Medicine*, **4**, 228–231.

Warrington, E.K. and James, M. (1991). *The Visual Object and Space Perception Battery*. Thames Valley Test Company, Bury St Edmunds.

Warrington, E.K., James, M., and Maciejewski, C. (1986). The WAIS as a lateralising and localising diagnostic instrument: a study of 656 patients with unilateral cerebral lesions. *Neuropsychologia*, **24**, 223–239.

Warrington, A.E., Barbarese, E., and Pfeiffer, S.E. (1993). Differential myelinogenic capacity of specific developmental stages of the oligodendrocyte lineage upon transplantation into hypomyelinating hosts. *Journal of Neuroscience Research*, **34**, 1–13.

Watson, M.J., Horn, S., and Curl, J. (1992). Searching for signs of revival: Uses and abuses of the Glasgow Coma Scale. *Professional Nurse*, **7**, 670–674.

Watt, D.C. and Seller, A. (1993). A clinico-genetic study of psychiatric disorder in Huntington's chorea. *Psychological Medicine*, **23** (Supplement 23), 1–46.

Waxman, S.G. (1998). Demyelinating diseases–new pathological insights, new therapeutic targets [editorial; comment]. *N.Engl.J.Med.*, **338**, 323–325.

Wearing, D. (1992). Self help groups. In *Clinical Management of Memory Problems* (ed. B.A. Wilson and N. Moffat), pp. 271–301. Chapman and Hall, London.

Weaver, C.E., Wu, F.S., Gibbs, T.T., and Farb, D.H. (1998). Pregnenolone sulfate exacerbates NMDA-induced death of hippocampal neurons. *Brain Research*, **803**, 129–136.

Webb, M. and Trzepacz, P.T. (1987). Huntington's disease: Correlations of mental status with chorea. *Biological Psychiatry*, **22**, 751–761.

Weber, T. and Major, E.O. (1997). Progressive multifocal leukoencephalopathy: molecular biology,pathogenesis and clinical impact. *Intervirology*, **40**, 98–111.

Wechsler, D.A. (1981). *Wechsler Adult Intelligence Scale — Revised*. Harcourt Brace Jovanovich, New York.

Weeks, B.S., Lieberman, D.M., Johnson, B., Roque, E., Green, M., Lowenstein, P. *et al.* (1995). Neurotoxicity of the human immunodeficiency virus type 1 Tat transactivator to PC12 cells requires the Tat amino acid 49–58 basic domain. *Journal of Neuroscience Research*, **42**, 32–40.

Weibel, D., Kreutzberg, G.W., and Schwab, M.E. (1995). Brain-derived neurotrophic factor (BDNF) prevents lesion-induced axonal die-back in young rat optic nerve. *Brain Research*, **679**, 249–254.

Weigell-Weber, M., Schmid, W., and Spiegal, R. (1996). Psychiatric symptoms and CAG expansion in Huntington's disease. *American Journal of Medical Genetics*, **67**, 53–57.

Weinberg, J., Diller, L., Gordon, W., Gerstman, L., Leiberman, A., Lakin, P. *et al.* (1979). Training sensory awareness and spatial organization in people with right brain damage. *Archives of Physical Medicine and Rehabilitation*, **60**, 491–496.

Weintraub, S., Baratz, R., and Mesulam, M.M. (1982). Daily living activities in the assessment of dementia. In *Alzheimer's*

*Disease: a Report of Progress* (ed. S. Corkin), pp. 189–192. Raven Press, New York.

Weiss, J.H., Hartley, D.M., Koh, J., and Choi, D.W. (1990). The calcium-channel blocker nifedipine attenuates slow excitatory amino-acid neurotoxicity. *Science*, **247**, 1474–1477.

Welker, E., Rao, S.B., Dorfl, J., Melzer, P., and Van der Loos, H. (1992). Plasticity in the barrel cortex of the adult-mouse — effects of chronic stimulation upon deoxyglucose uptake in the behaving animal. *Journal of Neuroscience*, **12**, 153–170.

Wenning, G.K., Odin, P., Morrish, P., Rehncrona, S., Widner, H., Brundin, P. *et al.* (1997). Short- and long-term survival and function of unilateral intrastriatal dopaminergic grafts in Parkinson's disease. *Annals of Neurology*, **42**, 95–107.

Wermuth, L. (1998). A double-blind, placebo-controlled, randomized, multi-center study of pramipexole in advanced Parkinson's disease. *European Journal of Neurology*, **5**, 235–242.

Westaway, D. (1987). Transgenic approaches to prion 'species barrier' effects. In *Prion Diseasess* (ed. H.F. Baker and R.M. Ridley), pp. 251–263. Humana Press, Totowa, NJ.

Westaway, D., Dearmond, S.J., Cayetanocanlas, J., Groth, D., Foster, D., Yang, S.L. *et al.* (1994). Degeneration of skeletal-muscle, peripheral-nerves, and the central- nervous-system in transgenic mice overexpressing wild-type prion proteins. *Cell*, **76**, 117–129.

Westphal, U. (1970). Binding of hormones to serum proteins. In *Biochemical Actions of Hormones* (ed. G. Litwack), pp. 209–265.

White, J.G., Southgate, E., Thomson, J.N., and Brenner, S. (1986). The structure of the nervous system of the nematode caenorhabditis elegans. *Philosophical Transactions of the Royal Society of London.B:Biological Sciences*, **314**, 1–340.

Whitley, R.J. (1990). Viral encephalitis. *New England Journal of Medicine*, **323**, 242–250.

Whitley, R., Lakeman, A.D., Nahmias, A., and Roizman, B. (1982). DNA restriction enzyme analysis of herpes simplex virus isolates obtained from patients with encephalitis. *New England Journal of Medicine*, **307**, 1060–1062.

Whitley, R.J., Alford, C.A., Hirsch, M.S., Schooley, R.T., Luby, J.P., Aoki, F.Y. *et al.* (1986). Vidarabine versus acyclovir therapy in herpes simplex encephalitis. *New England Journal of Medicine*, **314**, 144–149.

Wictorin, K. (1992). Anatomy and connectivity of intrastriatal striatal transplants. *Progress in Neurobiology*, **38**, 611–639.

Wictorin, K., Brundin, P., Sauer, H., Lindvall, O., and Björklund, A. (1992). Long distance directed axonal growth from human dopaminergic mesencephalic neuroblasts implanted along the nigrostriatal pathway in 6-hydroxydopamine lesioned adult rats. *Journal of Comparative Neurology*, **323**, 475–494.

Wieloch, T. (1985). Endogenous excitotoxins as possible mediators of ischemic and hypoglycemic brain damage. *Epilepsia*, **26**, 501.

Wieloch, T. (1995). Hypoglycemia-induced neuronal damage prevented by an n-methyl-d-aspartate antagonist. *Science*, **230**, 681–683.

Wiesel, T.N. (1982). Postnatal development of the visual cortex and the influence of environment. *Nature*, **299**, 583–591.

Wikkelsö, C., Andersson, H., Blomstrand, C., Lindqvist, G., and Svendsen, P. (1986). Normal Pressure Hydrocephalus. *Acta Neurologica Scandinavica*, **73**, 566–573.

Wilby, M., Sinclair, S.R., Muir, E.M., Zietlow, R., Adcock, K.H., Horellou, P., Dunnett, S.B., and Fawcett, J.W. (1999). A GDNF-secreting clone of the Schwann cell line SCTM41 enhances survival and fibre outgrowth from embryonic nigral neurones grafted to the striatum and the lesioned substantia nigra. *Journal of Neuroscience*, **19**, 2301–2312.

Wilcock, G.K., Esiri, M.M., Bowen, D.M., and Smith, C.C.T. (1982). Correlation of cortical choline acetyltransferase activity with the severity of dementia and histological abnormalities. *Journal of the Neurological Sciences*, **57**, 407–417.

Wilcox, J.A. and Nasrallah, H.A. (1987). Childhood head trauma and psychosis. *Psychiatry Res.*, **21**, 303–306.

Wilkinson, G.W.G., Darley, R.L., and Lowenstein, P.R. (1994). Viral vectors for gene therapy. In *From Genetics to Gene Therapy: the Molecular Pathology of Human Disease* (ed. D.S. Latchman), pp. 161–192. Bios Scientific, London.

Will, B. and Kelche, C. (1992). Environmental approaches to recovery of function from brain damage: a review of animal studies (1981 to 1991). In *Recovery from Brain Damage: Reflections and Directions* (ed. F.D. Rose and D.A. Johnson), pp. 79–103. Plenum, New York.

Williams, L.R., Varon, S., Peterson, G.M., Wictorin, K., Fischer, W., Björklund, A. *et al.* (1986). Continuous infusion of nerve growth factor prevents basal forebrain neuronal death after fimbria fornix transection. *Proceedings of the National Academy of Sciences of the United States of America*, **83**, 9231–9235.

Wilson, B.A. (1991). Long-term prognosis of patients with severe memory disorders. *Neuropsychological Rehabilitation*, **1**, 117–134.

Wilson, B.A. (1992). Memory therapy in practice. In *Clinical Management of Memory Problems* (ed. B.A. Wilson and N. Moffat), pp. 120–153. Chapman and Hall, London.

Wilson, B.A. (1995a). Management and remediation of memory problems in brain-injured adults. In *Handbook of Memory Disorders* (ed. A.D. Baddeley, B.A. Wilson and F.N. Watts), pp. 451–479. John Wiley, Chichester.

Wilson, B.A. (1995b). Memory rehabilitation: Compensating for memory problems. In *Psychological Compensation* (ed. L. Bäckman and R. Dixon), Lawrence Erlbaum Associates, Hillsdale,NJ.

Wilson, B.A. (1997). Cognitive rehabilitation: how it is and how it might be. *Journal of the International Neuropsychological Society*, **3**, 487–496.

Wilson, B.A. (1998). Recovery of cognitive functions following nonprogressive brain injury. *Current Opinion in Neurobiology*, **8**, 281–287.

Wilson, B.A. and Davidoff, J. (1993). Partial recovery from visual object agnosia: a 10 year follow-up study. *Cortex*, **29**, 529–542.

Wilson, B.A. and Watson, P.C. (1996). A practical framework for understanding compensatory behaviour in people with organic memory impairment. *Memory*, **4**, 465–486.

Wilson, B., Cockburn, J., and Baddeley, A. (1985). *The Rivermead Behavioural Memory Test*. Thames Valley Test Company, Bury St Edmunds.

Wilson, B.A., Baddeley, A.D., Evans, J.J., and Shiel, A. (1994a). Errorless learning in the rehabilitation of memory impaired people. *Neuropsychological Rehabilitation*, **4**, 307–326.

Wilson, B.A., Shiel, A., Watson, M., Horn, S., and McLellan, D.L. (1994b). Monitoring behaviour during coma and post traumatic amnesia. In *Progress in the Rehabilitation of Brain-Injured People* (ed. A.L. Christensen and B. Uzzell), pp. 85–98. Lawrence Erlbaum Associates, Hillsdale.

Wilson, B.A., Evans, J.J., Emslie, H., and Malinek, V. (1997). Evaluation of NeuroPage: a new memory aid. *Journal of Neurology, Neurosurgery and Psychiatry*, 63, 113–115.

Wilson, B.A., Evans, J.J., Emslie, H., Balleny, H., Watson, P.C., and Baddeley, A.D. (1999). Measuring recovery from post traumatic amnesia. *Brain Injury*, 13, 505–520.

Windhager, E., Reisecker, F., Huber, H.D., Trenkler, J., Witzmann, A., Proll, S. *et al.* (1988). Chronic subdural haematoma in the elderly: diagnostic problems. *Deutsche Medicinischen Wochenschrift*, 113, 883–888.

Windl, O., Dempster, M., Estibeiro, J.P., Lathe, R., deSilva, R., Esmonde, T. *et al.* (1996). Genetic basis of Creutzfeldt-Jakob disease in the United Kingdom: a systematic analysis of predisposing mutations and allelic variation in the PRNP gene. *Human Genetics*, 98, 259–264.

Winkler, C., Fricker, R.A., Gates, M.A., Olsson, M., Hammang, J.P., Carpenter, M.K. *et al.* (1998). Incorporation and glial differentiation of mouse EGF-responsive neural progenitor cells after transplantation into the embryonic rat brain. *Molecular and Cellular Neuroscience*, 11, 99–116.

Winn, S.R., Wahlberg, L., Tresco, P.A., and Aebischer, P. (1989). An encapsulated dopamine-releasing polymer alleviates experimental parkinsonism in rats. *Experimental Neurology*, 105, 244–250.

Wischik, C.M., Crowther, R.A., Stewart, M., and Roth, M. (1985). Subunit structure of paired helical filaments in Alzheimer's disease. *Journal of Cell Biology*, 100, 1905–1912.

Wold, W.S.M. and Gooding, L.R. (1991). Region e3 of adenovirus — a cassette of genes involved in host immunosurveillance and virus-cell interactions. *Virology*, 184, 1–8.

Woldorff, M.G., Gallen, C.C., Hampson, S.A., Hillyard, S.R., Pantev, C., Sobel, D. *et al.* (1993). Modulation of early sensory processing in human auditory cortex during auditory selective attention. *Proceedings of the National Academy of Sciences of the United States of America*, 90, 8722–8726.

Wolf, S.L., Lecraw, D.E., Barton, L.A., and Jann, B.B. (1989). Forced use of hemiplegic upper extremity to reverse the effect of learned nonuse among chronic stroke and head injured patients. *Experimental Neurology*, 104, 125–132.

Wolff, J.R. and Frotscher, M. (1985). Neurogenesis of GABAergic neurons in the rat dentate gyrus: a combined autoradiographic and immunocytochemical study. *Neuroscience Letters*, 62, 317–322.

Wolff, J.A., Fisher, L.J., Xu, L., Jinnah, H.A., Langlais, P.J., Iuvone, P.M. *et al.* (1989). Grafting fibroblasts genetically modified to produce l-DOPA in a rat model of Parkinson disease. *Proceedings of the National Academy of Sciences of the United States of America*, 86, 9011–9014.

Wolswijk, G. and Noble, M. (1992). Cooperation between PDGF and FGF converts slowly dividing O-2A (adult) progenitor cells to rapidly dividing cells with characteristics of O-2A (perinatal) progenitor cells. *Journal of Cell Biology*, 118, 889–900.

Wong, P.C., Pardo, C.A., Borchelt, D.R., Lee, M.K., Copeland, N.G., Jenkins, N.A. *et al.* (1995). An adverse property of a familial ALS-linked SOD1 mutation causes motor neuron disease characterized by vacuolar degeneration of mitochondria. *Neuron*, 14, 1105–1116.

Wood, P.M. and Bunge, R.P. (1991). The origin of remyelinating cells in the adult central nervous system — the role of the mature oligodendrocyte. *Glia*, 4, 225–232.

Wood, M.J.A. and Charlton, H.M. (1994). Hypothalamic grafts and neuroendocrine function. In *Functional Neural Transplantation* (ed. S.B. Dunnett and A. Björklund), pp. 451–466. Raven Press, New York.

Wood, R.L., Winowski, T., and Miller, J. (1993). Sensory regulation as a method to promote recovery in patients with altered states of consciousness. *Neuropsychological Rehabilitation*, 3, 177–190.

Woolf, C.J., Shortland, P., and Coggeshall, R.E. (1992). Peripheral nerve injury triggers central sprouting of myelinated afferents. *Nature*, 355, 75–78.

Woolley, C.S. (1998). Estrogen-mediated structural and functional synaptic plasticity in the female rat hippocampus. *Hormones and Behavior*, 34, 140–148.

Woolsey, T.A. and Van der Loos, H. (1970). The structural organisation of layer IV in the somatosensory region (SI) of mouse cerebral cortex. The description of a cortical field composed of discrete cytoarchitectonic units. *Brain Research*, 17, 205–242.

Wu, N.X., Watkins, S.C., Schaffer, P.A., and Deluca, N.A. (1996). Prolonged gene expression and cell survival after infection by a herpes simplex virus mutant defective in the immediate-early genes encoding ICP4, ICP27, and ICP22. *Journal of Virology*, 70, 6358–6369.

Wunner, W.H. and Dietzschold, B. (1987). Rabies virus infection: genetic mutations and the impact on viral pathogenicity and immunity. *Contributions in Microbiology and Immunology*, 8, 103–124.

Wyllie, A.H. (1999). Apoptosis: an overview. *British Medical Bulletin*, 53, 451–465.

Xiao, X., Li, J., and Samulski, R.J. (1998). Production of high titer recombinant adeno-associated virus vectors in the absence of helper adenovirus. *Journal of Virology*, 72, 2224–2232.

Xu, X.M., Guenard, V., Kleitman, N., Aebischer, P., and Bunge, M.B. (1995). Combination of BDNF and NT-3 promotes supraspinal axonal regeneration into Schwann cell grafts in adult rat thoracic spinal cord. *Experimental Neurology*, 134, 261–272.

Yang, Y., Nunes, F.A., Berencsi, K., Gonczol, E., Engelhardt, J.F., and Wilson, J.M. (1994a). Inactivation of E2a in recombinant adenoviruses improves the prospect of gene therapy in cystic fibrosis. *Nature Genetics*, 7, 362–369.

Yang, Y.P., Ertl, H.C.J., and Wilson, J.M. (1994b). MHC class 1-restricted cytotoxic T lymphocytes to viral antigens destroy hepatocytes in mice infected with E1-deleted recombinant adenoviruses. *Immunity*, 1, 433–442.

Yankner, B.A., Duffy, L.K., and Kirschner, D.A. (1990). Neurotrophic and neurotoxic effects of amyloid $\beta$ protein: reversal by tachykinin neuropeptides. *Science*, 250, 279–282.

Yao, D.L., Liu, X., Hudson, L.D., and Webster, H.D. (1995). Insulin-like growth-factor-I treatment reduces demyelination and up-regulates gene expression of myelin related proteins in experimental autoimmune encephalomyelitis. *Proceedings of the National Academy of Sciences of the United States of America*, **92**, 6190–6194.

Yip, H.K., Rich, K.M., Lampe, P.A., and Johnson, E.M. (1984). The effects of nerve growth factor and its antiserum on the postnatal development and survival after injury of sensory neurons in rat dorsal root ganglia. *Journal of Neuroscience*, **4**, 2986–2992.

York, A.D., Breedlove, S.M., Diamond, M.C., and Greer, E.R. (1989). Housing adult male rats in enriched conditions increases neurogenesis in the dentate gyrus. *Society for Neuroscience Abstracts*, **15**, 962.

Yoshimoto, Y., Lin, Q., Collier, T.J., Frim, D.M., Breakefield, X.O., and Bohn, M.C. (1995). Astrocytes retrovirally transduced with BDNF elicit behavioral improvement in a rat model of Parkinson's disease. *Brain Research*, **691**, 25–36.

Youl, B.D., Turano, G., Miller, D.H., Towell, A.D., MacManus, D.G., Moore, S.G. *et al.* (1991). The pathophysiology of acute optic neuritis. An association of gadolinium leakage with clinical and electrophysiological deficits. *Brain*, **114**, 2437–2450.

Youl, B.D., Turano, G., Towell, A.D., Barrett, G., MacManus, D.G., Moore, S.G. *et al.* (1996). Optic neuritis: swelling and atrophy. *Electroencephalography Clinical Neurophysiology Supplement*, **46**, 173–179.

Young, A.W., Robertson, I.H., Hellawell, D.J., de-Pauw, K.W., and Pentland, B. (1992). Cotard delusion after brain injury. *Psychological Medicine*, **22**, 799–804.

Yu, C.S. and Crutcher, K.A. (1995). Nerve growth factor immunoreactivity and sympathetic sprouting in the rat hippocampal formation. *Brain Research*, **672**, 55–67.

Yudkin, P.L., Ellison, G.W., Ghezzi, A., Goodkin, D.E., Hughes, R.A.C., McPherson, K. *et al.* (1991). Overview of azathioprine treatment in multiple sclerosis. *Lancet*, **338**, 1051–1055.

Yuen, E.C. and Mobley, W.C. (1996). Therapeutic potential of neurotrophic factors for neurological disorders. *Annals of Neurology*, **40**, 346–354.

Yule, W. and Carr, J. (1987). *Behaviour Modification for People with Mental Handicaps*. Croom Helm, London.

Zagrebelsky, M., Buffo, A., Skerra, A., Schwab, M.E., Strata, P., and Rossi, F. (1998). Retrograde regulation of growth-associated gene expression in adult rat Purkinje cells by myelin-associated neurite growth inhibitory proteins. *Journal of Neuroscience*, **18**, 7912–7929.

Zajicek, J.P., Scolding, N.J., Foster, O., Rovaris, M., Evanson, J., Moseley, I. *et al.* (1999). Central nervous system sarcoidosis — diagnosis and management based oin a large series. *Q.J.Med.*, **92**, 103–117.

Zangwill, O.L. (1975). Excision of Broca's area without persistant aphasia. In *Cerebral Localization* (ed. K.J. Zulch, O. Creutzfeldt and G.C. Galbraith), Springer-Verlag, Berlin.

Zangwill, O.L. (1947). Psychological aspects of rehabilitation in cases of brain injury. *British Journal of Psychology*, **37**, 60–69.

Zappacosta, B., Monza, D., Meoni, C., Austoni, L., Soliveri, P., Gellera, C. *et al.* (1996). Psychiatric symptoms do not correlate with cognitive decline, motor symptoms, or CAG repeat length in Huntington's disease. *Archives of Neurology*, **53**, 493–497.

Zelena, J. and Zacharova, G. (1997). Reinnervation of cat pacinian corpuscles after nerve crush. *Acta Neuropathologica*, **93**, 285–293.

Zerfass, R., Kretzschmar, K., and Förstl, H. (1992). Depressive Störungen nach Hirininfarkt. Beziehungen zu Infarktlage, Hirnatrophie und kognitiven Defiziten. *Nervenarzt*, **63**, 163–168.

Z'Graggen, W.J., Metz, G.A.S., Kartje, G.L., Thallmair, M., and Schwab, M.E. (1998). Functional recovery and enhanced corticofugal plasticity after unilateral pyramidal tract lesion and blockade of myelin-associated neurite growth inhibitors in adult rats. *Journal of Neuroscience*, **18**, 4744–4757.

Zhang, L., Jayne, D.R., Zhao, M.H., Lockwood, C.M., and Oliveira, D.B. (1995). Distribution of MHC class II alleles in primary systemic vasculitis. *Kidney Int.*, **47**, 294–298.

Zhao, W., Richardson, J.S., Mombourquette, M.J., Weil, J.A., Ijaz, S., and Shuaib, A. (1996). Neuroprotective effects of hypothermia and U-78517F in cerebral ischemia are due to reducing oxygen-based free radicals: an electron paramagnetic resonance study with gerbils. *Journal of Neuroscience Research*, **45**, 282–288.

Zhou, H.S., O'Neal, W., Morral, N., and Beaudet, A.L. (1996). Development of a complementing cell line and a system for construction of adenovirus vectors with E1 and E2a deleted. *Journal of Virology*, **70**, 7030–7038.

Ziemann, U., Hallett, M., and Cohen, L.G. (1998). Mechanisms of deafferentation-induced plasticity in human motor cortex. *Journal of Neuroscience*, **18**, 7000–7007.

Zigmond, M.J. and Stricker, E.M. (1972). Deficits in feeding behavior after intraventricular injection of 6-hydroxydopamine in rats. *Science*, **177**, 1211–1214.

Zigmond, M.J. and Stricker, E.M. (1973). Recovery of feeding and drinking by rats after intraventricular 6-hydroxydopamine or lateral hypothalamic lesions. *Science*, **182**, 717–720.

Zigmond, M.J. and Stricker, E.M. (1984). Parkinson's disease: studies with an animal model. *Life Sciences*, **35**, 5–18.

Zigmond, M.J., Acheson, A.L., Stachowiak, M.K., and Stricker, E.M. (1984). Neurochemical compensation after nigrostriatal bundle injury in an animal model of preclinical parkinsonism. *Archives of Neurology*, **41**, 856–861.

Zimmer, J. (1973). Extended commissural and ipsilateral projections in postnatally de-entorhinated hippocampus and fascia dentate. *Brain Research*, **64**, 293–311.

# Index

Aβ amyloid protein
  and Down syndrome 80–1
  and familial Alzheimer's disease 81
  formation of 80, 81*(fig.)*
  neurotoxicity 81
  and senile plaques 80
acute disseminated encephalomyelitis
    (ADEM) 48–9
acute haemorragic leukoencephalitis
    (AHLE) 48–9
adeno-associated virus vectors, for gene
    transfer into cells 358*(table)*,
    361–4
adenovirus vectors, for gene transfer
    into cells 358*(table)*, 360–1,
    363*(fig.)*
adhesion molecules, and axon
    regeneration 148
  gene therapy 376–7
  ICAM-1, expression after injury 24
  N-CAM 306
adrenal grafts, in Parkinson's disease
    326
affective disorders 256*(table)*
  and cerebrovascular disorder 262–3
  and Huntington's disease 264–5
  and traumatic brain damage 260–1
agrin, and axon regeneration 150,
    152*(fig.)*
AIDS dementia complex 69–71
Akt, and signalling pathways in
    apoptosis 11, 12*(fig.)*
alcohol abuse, and Huntington's disease
    268
ALS (amyotrophic lateral sclerosis) *see*
    motor neurone disease
Alzheimer's disease
  cholinergic pathology 386
  classical pathology 385–6
  genetics
    Apo E 85–6
    familial Alzheimer's disease 85
    presenilins 86
  history 385–6
  link with prion disease 102
  molecular biology 386
  pathology
    neurofibrillary tangles 79
    senile plaques 79, 80–3
  role of neurotrophins 135–6
aminooxyacetic acid (AOAA), as
    metabolic toxin 33
AMPA
  chemical structure 26*(fig.)*
  for experimental lesions 27
  selective neurotoxicity 30*(fig.)*

AMPA receptor
  and calcium-mediated cell death 31
  properties 28*(table)*, 29
amyloid precursor protein (APP) *see*
    APP (amyloid precursor protein)
amyotrophic lateral sclerosis (ALS) *see*
    motor neurone disease
anatomical plasticity 171
  after stroke 183
  in auditory cortex 182–3
  functional plasticity
    in rodent barrel fields 176–7
    in visual system 177–81
  in hippocampus 183–7
  in motor cortex 181–2
  and neurogenesis 190–5
  in sensory cortex 172–6
  in spinal cord 187–90
  types of regeneration 171–2
animal models
  glial transplantation 336–8
  ischaemia 39
  Parkinson's disease, MPTP 89–90
animals, prion diseases 98
anoxia, and ischaemia 40–1
anti-cholinergic drugs, in Parkinson's
    disease 277
anti-coagulants, in autoimmune disease
    treatment 141
anti-Hu/ANNA-1 antibodies, in
    paraneoplastic syndromes
    55*(table)*, 56
anti-inflammatory treatment, for
    neuroprotection 114, 116
anti-Yo/APCA antibodies, in
    paraneoplastic cerebellar
    degeneration 54–6
antigen presentation 46–7
antioxidants
  as neuroprotectants 112–13
  and Parkinson's disease 38
apaf-1, and apoptotic cell death
    10–11
apathy, and Huntington's disease 269
apo E (apolipoprotein E), and
    Alzheimer's disease 85–6
apomorphine 201–2
apoptosis
  in adult neurones and glia 8
  anti-apoptotic treatment, for
    neuroprotection 114, 115*(fig.)*
  characteristics 4–6
  control 6–8
  measurement 5
  molecular pathways
    calcium and free radical damage

10–11
  DNA damage 13–14
  Fas and TNFα 9–10
  role of caspases 8–9
  trophic factor withdrawal 11–13
  types 5
APP (amyloid precursor protein)
  βAPP 82, 85
  and familial Alzheimer's disease 85
  senile plaques 80, 81*(fig.)*
artificial vascular beds, and
    intracerebral grafts 316–17
ascorbic acid (vitamin C), as free
    radical scavenger 111
astrocytes
  astrocyte scars 23, 24*(fig.)*
  cell lineage 346–7
  for gene therapy 369–70
  and inhibition of axon regeneration
    in CNS 158–9, 159–61, 162,
    168*(fig.)*
  removal, and axon regeneration in
    CNS 309
  and remyelination by Schwann cells
    214
  response to injury 23–4
attention and psychomotor speed tests
    251
auditory cortex
  and language-based learning
    impairment 182–3
  tonotopic remapping 182
autoimmune CNS damage
  endothelial damage 51–3
  glial damage 48–51
  neural damage 53–6
autoimmune diseases, therapies 139–41
autonomic nervous system
  characteristic deficits 235–6
  clinical assessment 236*(box)*
  organisation 234–5
autonomic neuropathy 55*(table)*
axon degeneration, mechanism 15–16
axon regeneration
  cellular interactions 146–8
  inhibition by scar tissue 149
  molecular interactions 148–9
  structural responses to axotomy
    146
axon regeneration in CNS
  astrocyte depletion 309
  CNS environment effects 156–61
  CNS glial cell removal 308
  effects of neuronal age 165,
    167*(fig.)*, 168–9
  effects of neurotrophins 310–11

axon regeneration in CNS (*cont.*):
  embryonic grafts 306–7
  events following axon lesions 155–6
  GAP-43 effects 19*(fig.)*, 146, 164–5,
    166–7*(box)*, 310
  gene therapy 376–7
  glial cell replacement strategies
    301–2
  and IN-1 monoclonal antibody
    309–10, 311*(fig.)*
  inhibitory molecules 161–3
  MAG (myelin-associated
    glycoprotein) effects 310
  and microglia 311–12
  nerve transection site effects 163–5
  neurone type effects 169–70
  olfactory ensheathing cells 304–6
  oligodendrocyte removal 308–9
  peripheral nerve grafts 301–4
  Schwann cell grafts 301–4
    molecules involved 303–4
axotomy
  and axon degeneration 15–16
  glial responses 19–23
  macroglial reaction to injury 23–5
  neuronal death 17–19
  neuronal responses 16–17
azathioprine, in autoimmune disease
  treatment 140

B lymphocytes 45, 46*(fig.)*
baclofen, for spasticity 281
bacterial meningitis 60
  disease stages 60–3, 64*(fig.)*
ballism 276*(table)*
  drug therapies 278, 286*(table)*
band of Büngner 145–6, 147*(fig.)*
  and specificity of axon regeneration
    150–3
basal ganglia
  characteristic deficits 228–9,
    230*(fig.)*
  clinical assessment of disorders
    239–42
basal lamina sheath, of nerves, and
  nerve regeneration 145–6,
    147*(fig.)*
Bcl-2, and control of apoptosis 11*(fig.)*,
  12–13
  Bcl-2/Bax family 12–13
BDNF
  and axon regeneration in CNS
    310–11
  distribution 128–9
  and dopaminergic neurone survival
    133
  effect on retinal ganglion cells 132
  in motor neurone disease treatment
    131–2
  and neuronal survival 6
  and peripheral nerve damage
    129–30
  and visual cortex plasticity 180–1
BDNF receptors, changes after
  axotomy 17

biochemical plasticity
  in dopamine pathways 197–202
  neurotransmitter plasticity 202–4
  and pain 204
birds, learning and neurogenesis 192,
    193*(fig.)*
bladder
  dysfunction, in neurological disease
    282–3
    drug therapies 283, 287*(table)*
  innervation, and autonomic nervous
    system damage 235–6, 237*(fig.)*
blood–brain barrier, and immune
  response 47–8
*Borrelia burgdorferi*, and Lyme disease
    75–7
Boston Naming Test (short form), for
  language assessment 251
botulinum toxin, for spasticity 282
botulism, and exotoxin-induced
  damage 74–5, 76*(fig.)*
bovine spongiform encephalopathy
  (BSE) 97, 98
  and prion disease pathology 101
bowel disturbance, in neurological
  disease, treatment 284
brain damage assessment
  autonomic nervous system 234–6
  coma 217–22
  motor function 223–9
  psychiatric methods 256–61,
    259*(table)*
  research tools 236–42
  sensory function 229–34
brain derived neurotrophic factor *see*
  BDNF
brainstem death, diagnosis 219*(box)*
breathing problems, in
  neurodegenerative conditions
    285
bridge grafts, for nerve repair
    149–50
bulbar dysfunction, therapies 279–80
bulbar palsy, therapies 279–80

c-jun, and axon regeneration in CNS
    304
*Caenorhabditis elegans*
  ced mutations 8, 12
  cell lineage 345, 346*(fig.)*
  and developmental cell death 6
calcium
  and glutamate toxicity 31–2
  and mechanisms of cell death 10–11,
    32
  and necrosis 3–4
calcium antagonists, as
  neuroprotectants
    anti-excitotoxic treatments 107–9
    calcium-channel antagonists
      109–11
Cambridge Multiple Sclerosis Basic
  Score (CAMBS), in clinical
  assessment of multiple sclerosis
    238

Cambridge Neuropsychological Test
  Automated Battery (CANTAB),
  for executive function 252–4
CAP-23, and axon regeneration in CNS
    310
CAPIT-HD programme
  full battery 248–54
  for Huntington's disease assessment
    240–2
  short battery 254
CAPIT-PD programme, for Parkinson's
  disease assessment 240–2
cardiovascular problems, in
  neurodegenerative conditions
    285, 288
caspase inhibitors, as neuroprotectants
    114, 115*(fig.)*
caspases, role in apoptosis 8–9
catalase
  in antioxidant therapy 112
  and defence against free radical
    damage 37
ced-9, and control of apoptosis 12
cell death
  apoptosis
    characteristics 4–6
    control 6–8
    molecular pathways 8–14
  calcium involvement 31–2
  developmental 6–8
  from metabolic toxins 32–5
  from oxidative stress 35–8
  in ischaemia 39–44
  mechanisms 3
  mechanisms of excitotoxicity 30–1,
    32*(fig.)*
  necrosis 3–4
cell lines, for neuronal transplantation
    328–9
cell-suspension transplants 317,
    318*(fig.)*
cellular energy metabolism, and
  metabolic toxins 32–5
cerebellar degeneration, subacute 53,
    55*(table)*
cerebellar disorders, therapies 279
cerebellar lesions
  characteristic deficits 227–8
  in multiple sclerosis 238–9
cholinergic forebrain neurone damage,
  role of neurotrophins 135–6
chondroitin sulphate proteoglycans,
  and inhibition of axon
  regeneration in CNS 162, 310
chorea 276*(table)*
  drug therapies 278, 286*(table)*
clonal cell lines, from progenitor cells
    350–2
*Clostridium*, *C. botulinum* and *C.
  tetani*, exotoxin-induced damage
    74–5, 76*(fig.)*
clouding of consciousness, definition
    217
CNS infection *see* infection
CNTF 128*(table)*

and axon regeneration 149
distribution 129
effect on retinal ganglion cells 132
in gene therapy 374–5
and Huntington's disease model 136,
137*(fig.)*
in motor neurone disease treatment
131–2
and peripheral nerve damage 129–30
CNTF receptor, and signalling
pathways in apoptosis 11,
12*(fig.)*
co-polymer-1, in autoimmune disease
treatment 141
coenzyme Q/p110/p0, as
neuroprotectant 113–14
cognitive assessment tools
for attention and psychomotor speed
251
criteria for 244–8
for executive function 251–4
for global cognitive functions 248–9
for IQ 249–50
for language 250–1
for memory 250
validity of tests 244–5
for visuo-perceptual function 251
cognitive deficits
behavioural strategies for
management 275–6
drug therapies 276
collateral sprouting, in CNS 171–2
coma
assessment 218–20
prediction of outcome 220
causes 218
definition 217–18
management of patients
learning ability 221–2
physical management 221
rehabilitation 221–2
sensory stimulation programmes
221
compensatory behaviour, after brain
injury 293–5
Conditional Associative Learning Test
(CALT), for memory assessment
250
confusion, definition 217
consciousness, and coma definition 217
Controlled Oral Word Association test,
of verbal fluency 251–2
cortical mapping
and normal brain function 175
reorganisation after nerve lesion
172–4
use-dependent mapping 175–6
corticoid receptors 121–2
corticoids
in autoimmune disease treatment
139–40
and brain damage
clinical evidence 123
mechanisms 122
and neurogenesis in hippocampus

123
brain entry 121
diurnal variations 121
and neurogenesis 190–1
synthetic pathway 124*(fig.)*
corticosteroids *see* corticoids
*Corynebacterium diphtheriae*, and
exotoxin-induced damage 74–5
CPP, as neuroprotectant 108
Creutzfeldt–Jakob disease (CJD)
96–8
genetics 99–100, 390
history 389
immune response 77
neuropathology 389–90
new variant form (nvCJD) 97–8
pathogenesis 100–1, 390
symptoms 389
cultured cells, as alternatives to foetal
graft tissue 328–9
cuprizone, in remyelination model
206*(table)*
cyclin-dependent kinases, and apoptotic
cell death 13
cyclins, and signalling pathways in
apoptosis 13
cyclophosphamide, in autoimmune
disease treatment 140
cyclosporin, in autoimmune disease
treatment 140
cysteine-S-sulfonic acid, and focal
neuronal degeneration 27
cytochrome c, and apoptotic cell death
10–11
cytokines, changes after axotomy 17
cytoskeletal proteins, changes after
axotomy 17

dantrolene, for spasticity 281
DATATOP trial, of Parkinson's disease
treatment 90
dehydroepiandrosterone (DHEA and
DHEAS) 123–4
and Alzheimer's disease 126
anti-glucocorticoid action 124
and brain damage 125
brain entry 124–5
effects on GABA and glutamate
receptors 124
dementia
CAPIT-HD programme for
assessment 248–54
chromosome 17 linked 86
classification 243–4
cognitive assessment tools, criteria
for 244–8
types 79–80
*see also* Alzheimer's disease
dentate gyrus, neurogenesis of granule
cells 190–1
dentorubral-pallido-luysian atrophy
(DRPLA), as trinucleotide repeat
disease 95
deprenyl, in Parkinson's disease
treatment, DATATOP trial 90,

119
desmopressin, for bladder dysfunction
treatment 283
developmental cell death 6–8
dextromorphan, as neuroprotectant
108
digit span test, for memory assessment
250
dihydroxyphenylacetic acid (DOPAC),
changes in nigro-striatal lesion
model 198
diphtheria, and exotoxin-induced
damage 74–5
dizocilpine *see* MK-801
DNA damage, and apoptotic cell death
13–14
DNA fragmentation, and apoptosis
determination 5
L-dopa, Parkinson's disease treatment
87–8, 200–2, 276–7
dopamine
changes in nigro-striatal lesion model
197–8
hydroxydopamine (6-OHDA), in
nigro-striatal lesion model
196–200
metabolism 117
neurotrophin effects on dopaminergic
neurones 133–5
and Parkinson's disease 38, 86–8
plasticity 200–2
redundancy in nigro-striatal pathway
200
synthetic pathway 87*(fig.)*
dopamine receptor agonists, in
Parkinson's disease treatment
277
dopamine receptors, supersensitivity
and /c1L/c0-DOPA side effects
201–2
in nigro-striatal lesion model
198–200
dorsal root entry zone, and inhibition
of axon regeneration in CNS
156, 157*(fig.)*, 158–9
Down syndrome, and dementia
80–1
dystonia 276*(table)*
drug therapies 278–9, 286–7*(table)*

embryonic neuronal grafts, and axon
regeneration 165, 167*(fig.)*,
168–9, 306–7
encapsulation, of cells for implantation
371–3
encephalomyelitis 48–9, 53, 55*(table)*
endothelial cells
antibodies against, in vasculitis 52
in blood–brain barrier 47
energy metabolism in cells, and
metabolic toxins 32–5
environmental toxins, and Parkinson's
disease-like symptoms 88
ependymal cells, of spinal cord,
progenitor cells 194

epilepsy
  cellular pathology and pathogenesis
    391
  drug therapies 276, 285–6(table)
  genetics 392
  history 391
  neuropathology 391–2
  symptoms 391
  treatments 392
Erk kinase, and signalling pathways in
    apoptosis 11, 12(fig.)
ethical guidelines, for foetal tissue
    transplantation 322(box)
ethidium bromide, in remyelination
    model 206(table)
ethidium bromide-induced
    demyelination model, as model
    for glial transplantation 338,
    339(fig.), 340(fig.)
excitatory amino acids
  and cell death 26–7, 30–1
  chemical structure 26(fig.)
excitotoxicity
  anti-excitotoxic treatments 107–11
  excitatory amino acids and cell death
    26–7, 30–1
  and glutamate receptors 27–30
  and ischaemia 42–4
excitotoxins, selective neurotoxicity
    29–30
executive function tests 251–4
expanded disability status scale (EDSS),
    in clinical assessment of multiple
    sclerosis 238, 239(box)
expanded precursor cells
  clonal cell lines 350–2
  for neuronal transplantation
    328–9
  neurospheres 348–50
  transplantation 352–6
extracellular matrix, changes after
    injury 24
extrapyramidal disorders 228–9,
    230(fig.)

facial nerve nucleus, glial response to
    axotomy 21–2
familial Alzheimer's disease 81
  genetics 85
Fas, and apoptotic cell death 9–10
fatal familial insomnia (FFI) 96,
    98(table)
  immune response 77
ferritin, and defence against free radical
    damage 37
fibroblast growth factors (FGFs)
    128(table)
  distribution 129
  FGF-5, and peripheral nerve damage
    130
fibroblasts
  for gene therapy 367, 370(fig.)
  and inhibition of axon regeneration
    149
flaccid paralysis, therapies 282

FLIP protein, and apoptotic cell death
    10
focal ischaemia 39, 40, 41(fig.)
foetal tissue transplantation, ethical
    issues 322(box), 323
fragile X syndrome, as trinucleotide
    repeat disease 95(table)
free radicals
  cellular defences against 36–7
  free radical scavengers, as
    neuroprotectants 111–12
  generation, and oxidative stress 36
  and ischaemia 41
  and mechanisms of cell death 37–8
  and necrosis 4
  in Parkinson's disease 38
functional plasticity
  in rodent barrel fields 176–7
  in visual system 177–81
functional recovery
  experience-dependent plasticity 291
  mechanisms 291–3
  following lesion, effectiveness of
    rehabilitation 289–91

GABA receptors
  effects of neurosteroids 124
  and plasticity in motor cortex 181
GAP-43
  and axon regeneration 146,
    166–7(box)
    effect of nerve transection site
    164–5
  mechanisms of action 165
  and axon regeneration in CNS
    19(fig.), 304, 310
  changes after axotomy 17, 18,
    19(fig.)
GDNF 128(table)
  distribution 129
  effects on dopaminergic neurones
    133–5
  in gene therapy for Parkinson's
    disease 380–1
  in motor neurone disease treatment
    131
  and neuronal survival 6
  and peripheral nerve damage 128–9
gene therapy
  encapsulation of cells 371–3
  ex vivo gene transfer
    astrocytes 369–70
    cell lines 370
    choice of cells 367
    conditionally immortalised cells
    370–1
    fibroblasts 367, 370(fig.)
    methods 367, 369(fig.)
    myoblasts 369
    primary neuronal cells 370
    uses for 357, 365–7
  in vivo gene therapy 377–9
  neurotrophins 373–5
  Parkinson's disease 379–81
  reporter genes 368–9(box)

to promote axon regeneration 376–7
  vectors
    adeno-associated virus vectors
    358(table), 361–4
    adenovirus vectors 358(table),
    360–1, 362(fig.)
    herpes simplex virus vectors
    358(table), 364–6
    retrovirus vectors 358–60
Gerstmann–Strässler–Scheinker
    syndrome (GSS) 96, 98(table),
    102
  genetics 99
  immune response 77
GFAP (glial fibrillary acidic protein),
    expression after injury 23
Glasgow Coma Scale (GCS) 218–20
glatirimer acetate, in autoimmune
    disease treatment 141
glia
  autoimmune damage 48–51
  glial scars 23, 24(fig.)
  removal, and axon regeneration in
    CNS 308
  response to axotomy
    inflammatory response 19–20
    macrophage effects 20–1
    metabolic changes 22–3
    microglia effects 21–2
    neutrophil effects 20
  and trophic factors 7–8
  see also microglia
glial transplantation
  and axon regeneration 156–7,
    158(fig.)
  experimental models 336–8
  and failure of spontaneous
    remyelination 335–6
  myelinogenic cell requirements
    338–9
  olfactory glia 343
  oligodendrocyte progenitor
    transplants 339–41
    sources of cells 341–2
  oligosphere transplantation 342
  and promotion of endogenous
    remyelination 336
  Schwann cells 342–3
global cognitive assessment tools
  Mattis Dementia Rating Scale (DRS)
    249
  Mini Mental State Exam (MMSE)
    248–9
global ischaemia 39
glucocorticoid receptors (GR) 121–2
glutamate
  and cell death 26, 27(fig.), 30–1,
    32(fig.)
  chemical structure 26(fig.)
  levels, after ischaemia 42–4
  toxicity
    and apoptosis 4, 5(fig.)
    and necrosis 3–4, 5(fig.)
glutamate receptors
  classification 28–9

effects of neurosteroids 124
and excitotoxicity 27–8
molecular structures 29–30
glutamic acid, and cell death 26
glutathione, as free radical scavenger
111
glutathione peroxidase
in antioxidant therapy 112
defence against free radical damage
37
neuroprotection in Parkinson's
disease 117, 118*(fig.)*
grafts, adrenal grafts 326
growth cones, in axon regeneration
146
growth factors 128*(table)*
and axon regeneration 149
and developmental control 6–8
for neurones, loss after axotomy
17–19
in remyelination 210*(box)*, 212
withdrawal, and apoptotic cell death
11–13
Guy's Neurological disability Scale, in
clinical assessment of multiple
sclerosis 238

*Haemophilus influenzae*, and bacterial
menginitis 60
haemopoietic factors 128*(table)*
head injury, psychiatric assessment
258–62
Hebbian synapse rules
and plasticity in ocular dominance
columns 179–80
synaptic mechanisms 180–1
and use-dependent cortical mapping
175–6
herpes simplex encephalitis (HSVE)
64–5, 66*(fig.)*
herpes simplex virus vectors, for gene
transfer into cells 358*(table)*,
364–6
hippocampus
compensatory collateral sprouting
186–7
kainic acid toxicity 26, 27*(fig.)*
neurogenesis and steroids 123
sprouting after entorhinal cortex
lesion 183–5
sympathetic sprouting 185–6
control by NGF 186
HIV infection 69–71
homocysteic acid, and focal neuronal
degeneration 27
Hopkins Verbal Learning Test (HVLT),
for memory assessment 250
HTLV-1 associated myelopathy (HAM)
68–9
Huntington's disease
and basal ganglia pathology 228–9,
230*(fig.)*
cellular pathology and pathogenesis
394
clinical assessment 239–42, 393

genetics 394
history 393
molecular genetics 93–4, 95*(table)*
neuropathology 393–4
pathology 92–3
psychiatric symptoms 263–4
affective disorders 264–5
alcohol abuse 268
apathy 269
iatrogenic mental systems 270
irritability and aggression 268–9
obsessive-compulsive disorder 267
personality disorder 267–8
prevalence 264
schizophrenia-like states 266–7
sexual dysfunction 269
sleep disorder 269–70
suicide 266
and trinucleotide repeats 270–1
symptoms 393
treatments 394
Huntington's disease model
aminooxyacetic acid (AOAA) 33
role of neurotrophins 136, 137*(fig.)*
hydrogen peroxide
as free radical 36
and mechanism of free radical
toxicity 37
and neuroprotection in Parkinson's
disease 117
hydroxydopamine (6-OHDA), in nigro-
striatal lesion model 196–200
hydroxyl radical
as free radical 36
and mechanism of free radical
toxicity 37
and neuroprotection in Parkinson's
disease 117–19
hypothalamus, and glutamate toxicity
26, 27*(fig.)*
hypoxia, and ischaemia 40–1

ibotenic acid
chemical structure 26*(fig.)*
as excitotoxin 26
for experimental lesions 27
NMDA receptor agonist 28*(table)*,
29
ICAM-1, expression after injury 24
IGF (insulin-like growth factor)
128*(table)*
IGF-1
and axon regeneration 149
and axon remyelination 336
in motor neurone disease treatment
132
in motor neurone disease treatment
131
and peripheral nerve damage 129
immune complexes, and vasculitis
52
immune system
immune privilege of brain, and
xenografts 327
immune response 45–7

immunotherapies 139–41
immunoglobulins
and axon remyelination 336
intravenous therapy in autoimmune
diseases 140
infection
and age of host 58, 60
and blood–brain barrier 57
direct damage from infective
organism
progressive multifocal
leukoencephalopathy (PML)
73–4
rabies 72–3
exotoxin-induced damage
botulism 74–5
diphtheria 74–5
tetanus 74–5
immune-mediated disease
AIDS dementia complex 69–71
bacterial meningitis 60–3,
64*(fig.)*
herpes simplex encephalitis 64–5,
66*(fig.)*
HTLV-1 associated myelopathy
68–9
leprosy 65–7
subacute sclerosing panencephalitis
(SSPE) 71
Sydenham's chorea 67–8
latent period and presentation 57,
59*(fig.)*
and MHC expression 57–8, 59*(fig.)*
polyphasic infections 75–7
routes and mechanisms 57, 58*(fig.)*
spongiform encephalopathies 77
inflammatory cells, response to
axotomy 19–20
inflammatory diseases, therapies
139–41
integrins, and axon regeneration 148
interferons, in autoimmune disease
treatment 141
interleukins
IL-1β, changes after axotomy 17
IL-6 17
IL-11 11, 12*(fig.)*
signalling pathways in apoptosis 11,
12*(fig.)*
intracerebral grafts
and artificial vascular beds 316–17
and cell-suspension transplants 317,
318*(fig.)*
implantation sites 315–16
intraocular grafts, as model
transplantation site 314–15
ionotropic glutamate receptors,
classification 28
IQ assessment
National Adult Reading Test (NART)
249
Wechsler Adult Intelligence Scale-
Revised (WAIS-R) 249–50
iron chelators, and neuroprotection in
Parkinson's disease 117

ischaemia
  animal models 39
  mechanisms of cell death 39–40
    anoxia 40–1
    excitotoxicity 42–4
    and free radical generation 41
    neutrophil and macrophage effects
      41–2
    oedema 41
    plasminogen activators and
      proteases 42
    vasoconstriction 41
  and necrosis 3
  NMDA receptor antagonists as
    neuroprotectants 107–9
  types 38–9

Jak kinases, and signalling pathways in
    apoptosis 11, 12*(fig.)*
JC virus, and progressive multifocal
    leukoencephalopathy 73–4

kainate receptor, properties 28*(table)*,
    29
kainic acid
  chemical structure 26*(fig.)*
  and focal neuronal degeneration
    26–7
  hippocampal toxicity 26, 27*(fig.)*
  selective neurotoxicity 30*(fig.)*
Kennard principle, and plasticity 202
kuru 96

L1 adhesion molecule
  and axon regeneration in CNS
    303–4
  and peripheral nerve regeneration
    148
Lambert–Eaton myasthaenic syndrome
    (LEMS), and autoimmune
    damage 54
laminin, and axon regeneration
    148–50, 152*(fig.)*
language assessment tests 250–1
language-based learning impairment,
    and auditory cortex 182–3
lazaroids, as free radical scavengers
    111
lentivirus (LV), for gene transfer into
    cells 358*(table)*
leprosy 65–7
leukaemia inhibitory factor (LIF)
  and control of sympathetic
    phenotype 203–4
  signalling pathways in apoptosis 11,
    12*(fig.)*
Lewy bodies
  and α-synuclein 91–2
  in Parkinson's disease 91
Lewy body dementias 92
limbic encephalomyelitis 53, 55*(table)*
Lou Gehrig's disease *see* motor neurone
    disease
lower motor neurone (LMN) lesions,
    characteristic deficits 224–5

Lyme disease 75–7
lymphocyte monoclonal antibodies, in
    autoimmune disease treatment
    141
lysolecithin-induced demyelination
    model 206*(table)*
  as model for glial transplantation
    338, 339*(fig.)*

Machado–Joseph disease (MJD), as
    trinucleotide repeat disease 95
macroglia, response to injury 23–5
macrophages
  and axon regeneration 148
  in immune response 45–6
  response to PNS injury 20–1
MAG (myelin-associated glycoprotein),
    and inhibition of axon
    regeneration in CNS 162, 309,
    310
MAPK (mitogen-activated protein
    kinase), and signalling pathways
    in apoptosis 11, 12*(fig.)*
Mattis Dementia Rating Scale (DRS),
    as global cognitive assessment
    tool 249
measles infection, and subacute
    sclerosing panencephalitis 71
MEK, and signalling pathways in
    apoptosis 11, 12*(fig.)*
memory
  assessment tests 250–1
  types 250
meningeal cells, and inhibition of axon
    regeneration in CNS 161
meningitis, disease stages 60–3, 64*(fig.)*
metabolic damage
  calcium effects 31–2
  excitotoxicity 26–31
  in ischaemia 38–44
  and metabolic toxins 32–5
  and oxidative stress 35–8
  in Parkinson's disease 38
metabotropic glutamate receptors
  classification 28
  properties 28*(table)*, 29
MHC class II, expression after injury
    24
microglia
  and axon regeneration in CNS 311
  and inhibition of axon regeneration
    in CNS 161
  response to CNS injury 21–2
  *see also* glia
microtubule associated proteins
    (MAPs), changes after axotomy
    17
mineralocorticoid receptors (MR)
    121–2
Mini Mental State Exam (MMSE), as
    global cognitive assessment tool
    248–9
mitochondria
  and apoptotic cell death 10–11
  electron transport complexes 33*(fig.)*

and metabolic toxins 32–4
mitochondrial function enhancers as
    neuroprotectants 113–14
and necrosis 4
MK-801
  blocking of excitotoxic cell death 30,
    31*(fig.)*
  as neuroprotectant 107–9
  as NMDA receptor antagonist 28
monoamine oxidase inhibitors, in
    Parkinson's disease treatment,
    DATATOP trial 90, 119
monoamine oxidase, and MPTP
    toxicity 90
monoclonal antibodies, in autoimmune
    disease treatment 141
monocytes, in immune response 45–6
MORT-1/FADD adapter protein, and
    apoptotic cell death 9–10
motor cortex
  plasticity after injury 181–2
  plasticity in response to motor tasks
    182
motor function
  basal ganglia disorders 228–9,
    230*(fig.)*
  and cerebellar lesions 227–8
  clinical assessment 223, 229,
    231*(fig.)*, 234*(box)*
  and motor neurone lesions 224–7
  motor system organisation 223–4
motor neurone disease
  cellular pathology and pathogenesis
    388
  genetics 388
  history 387
  neuropathology 388
  role of neurotrophins 130–2
  symptoms 387
  treatments 388
motor neurone lesions, characteristic
    deficits 224–7
movement disorders
  drug therapies 276–9, 286–7*(table)*
  types 276*(table)*
MPTP
  in humans, and Parkinson's disease
    89
  in monkeys, animal model of
    Parkinson's disease 89–90
  in rats and mice, mechanisms of
    neurotoxicity 90
multiple sclerosis
  and autoimmune damage 49–51
  clinical assessment 237–9
  diagnosis 395–6
  disease progression 395
  epidemiology 395
  genetics 395
  pathology 396
  remyelination in 214
  treatment 139–41, 396
  types 236–7
muscle end-plates, axon regeneration to
    150, 151*(fig.)*

myasthenia gravis, and autoimmune damage 54
*Mycobacterium leprae*, and leprosy 65–7
myelin sheaths, changes with remyelination 205–6, 208*(fig.)*, 209*(fig.)*
myelin-deficient mutant animals, as model for glial transplantation 336–8
myoblasts, for gene therapy 369
myoclonus 276*(table)*
  drug therapies 279, 287*(table)*
myotonic dystrophy, as trinucleotide repeat disease 95*(table)*

N-acetyl cysteine (NAC)
  as antioxidant 112
  and neuroprotection in Parkinson's disease 117, 118*(fig.)*
N-cadherin, and axon regeneration 148
N-CAM, and axon regeneration in CNS 306
N-methyl-aspartic acid, and focal neuronal degeneration 27
N-methyl-glutamic acid, as excitotoxin 26
National Adult Reading Test (NART), for IQ assessment 249
necrosis 3–4
  after axotomy 17
*Neisseria meningitidis*, and bacterial menginitis 60
neoplasms, paraneoplastic conditions, and autoimmune damage 53–6
neostriatum, focal damage by 3-nitropropionic acid (3-NP) 33–4
nerve conduction, restoration after remyelination 205, 206*(fig.)*
nerve growth factor (NGF) *see* NGF (nerve growth factor)
nerve regeneration *see* axon regeneration; axon regeneration in CNS; peripheral nerve regeneration
nerve repair
  bridge grafts 149–50
  and specificity of axon regeneration 153
nervous system infection *see* infection
neurocan, and inhibition of axon regeneration in CNS 162
neurodegeneration, 'cycle of' 37, 38*(fig.)*
neurodegenerative disease
  Alzheimer's disease 79–86
  common mechanisms of neurodegeneration 102–3
  Lewy body dementias 92
  Parkinson's disease 86–92
  prion diseases 96–102
  trinucleotide repeat diseases 92–6
neurofibrillary tangles
  in Alzheimer's disease 79, 82–4

and tau protein 84–5
neurogenesis
  in adult mammals 190–1
    progenitor cell differentiation 192–3
    progenitor cells 191–2
    progenitor cells in damaged CNS 193–5
  in hippocampus, and steroids 123
  and song bird learning 192, 194*(fig.)*
neurological disorders
  autoimmune disorders 53–6
  research tools 236–42
neuronal age, effects on axon regeneration 165, 167*(fig.)*, 168–9
neuronal transplantation
  alternatives to foetal graft tissue 323
    adrenal grafts 326
    cultured cells 328–9
    xenografts 326–8
  bridge grafts for nerve repair 149–50
  and circuit reconstruction 330*(table)*, 333–4
  embryonic neuronal grafts, and axon regeneration 165, 167*(fig.)*, 168–9, 306–7
  ethical issues 322*(box)*, 323
  expanded precursor cells 352–6
  and formation of functional connections 330*(table)*, 332, 333*(fig.)*
  graft preparation techniques 324
  growth factor treatments for graft survival 324, 325*(fig.)*
  improved use of foetal tissues 323
  intracerebral grafts 315–17, 318*(fig.)*
  intraocular graft model 314–15
  mechanisms of graft function 329–34
  neuro-endocrine mechanism of action 329–30
  neuroprotection of implanted cells 324–5
  neurospheres 353, 354*(fig.)*
  nigral grafts
    model 318–20
    Parkinson's disease 320–1, 323
  non-specific mechanisms of action 329, 330–1
  olfactory ensheathing cells 304–6
  patient assessment programs 240–2
  peripheral nerve grafts 301–4
  requirements for 313–14
  trophic mechanisms of action 330*(table)*, 331–2
  xenografts 326–8
neurones
  connections between neural graft and host 314–15
  death after axotomy 17–19
  for gene therapy 370
  responses to axotomy 16–17
neuropathies 55, 231, 233
neuropeptides 128*(table)*

neuropoietic factors 128*(table)*
neuroprotection
  anti-apoptotic treatment 114, 115*(fig.)*
  anti-inflammatory treatment 114–16
  antioxidants 112–13
  calcium antagonists 107–11
  free radical scavengers 111–12
  mitochondrial function enhancers 113–14
  in Parkinson's disease 117–19
  therapeutic trials 116–17
  use of neurotrophins 137–8
neuropsychological rehabilitation
  compensation and recovery of function 293–5
  environmental adaptations 295
  evidence for effectiveness 289–91
  functional adaptations 295–6
  guidelines for 297
  learning improvements 296
  restitution of function 291–3
  use of residual skills 296
neuroses 256*(table)*
neurospheres
  cell differentiation 349–50
  formation 348–9
  grafts 353, 354*(fig.)*
neurosteroids 123–4
  and Alzheimer's disease 126
  anti-glucocorticoid action 124
  and brain damage 125
  brain entry 124–5
  effects on GABA and glutamate receptors 124
neurotransmitters, plasticity in sympathetic neurones 202–4
neurotrophin receptors
  changes after axotomy 17
  distribution 128–9
  and signalling pathways in apoptosis 11, 12*(fig.)*
neurotrophins
  and axon regeneration 310–11
  changes after axotomy 17
  distribution 128–9
  and dopaminergic neurone survival 133–5
  effects on cholinergic forebrain neurones 135–6
  effects in Huntington's disease model 136, 137*(fig.)*
  effects on retinal ganglion cells 132
  in gene therapy 373–5, 376
  and motor neurone disease 130–2
  and neuronal survival 6, 6–7, 127–8
  for neuroprotection 137–8
NT-3
  and axon regeneration in CNS 311
  distribution 128–9
  and neuronal survival 6
  and peripheral nerve damage 129–30

neurotrophins (*cont.*):
  NT-3 receptors, changes after
      axotomy 17
  NT-4/5
      distribution 128
      and neuronal survival 6
      and visual cortex plasticity 180–1
      and peripheral nerve damage 129–30
      and visual cortex plasticity 180–1
      withdrawal, and apoptotic cell death
          11–13
neurturin 128(*table*), 129
  and dopaminergic neurone survival
      133–4
neutrophils, response to axotomy 20
NF-κB, and apoptotic cell death 10
NG2 proteoglycan, and inhibition of
      axon regeneration in CNS 162
NGF (nerve growth factor)
  and axon regeneration 149
  distribution 128
  effects on cholinergic forebrain
      neurones 135–6
  in gene therapy 373–4
  and neuronal survival 6, 6–7, 127–8
  and peripheral nerve damage 129–30
NGF (nerve growth factor) receptors,
      changes after axotomy 17
NI250 (NogoA) *see* NogoA (NI250)
nigral grafts
  nigral graft model 318–20
  in Parkinson's disease 320–1, 323
nigro-striatal lesion model
  and biochemical plasticity 196–200
  mechanisms of recovery 200
  plasticity in dopamine pathways
      197–200
  recovery from 6-OHDA lesions
      196–7
  role of neurotrophins 133–5
  unilateral lesion model 318–20
nigro-striatal pathway
  axotomy-induced changes 18
  and Parkinson's disease 86–7
nitric oxide
  and neuroprotection in Parkinson's
      disease 118–19
  and oxidative stress 35–6
  and signalling pathways in apoptosis
      13
nitropropionic acid (3-NP), as
      metabolic toxin 33–4
NMDA
  chemical structure 26(*fig.*)
  as excitotoxin 26
  for experimental lesions 27
  selective neurotoxicity 30(*fig.*)
NMDA channels *see* NMDA receptors
NMDA receptor antagonists
  blocking of excitotoxic cell death 30,
      31(*fig.*)
  and cortical plasticity 176
  and ischaemia-induced degeneration
      42, 43(*fig.*)
  as neuroprotectants 107–9

NMDA receptors
  and calcium-mediated cell death 31
  and cortical plasticity 176, 181
  and ischaemia-induced degeneration
      43(*fig.*), 44
  properties 28(*table*), 29
NogoA (NI250)
  and axon regeneration in CNS
      161–2, 309–10, 311(*fig.*)
  effects on sprouting in spinal cord
      189–90

O-2A cell lineage 346–7
obsessive–compulsive disorder, and
      Huntington's disease 267
ocular dominance columns, and
      functional plasticity 178–80
oedema, and ischaemia 41
oestrogens, and brain damage 126
Ola mouse
  and axon degeneration 15
  and axon regeneration 148
olfactory bulb, neurogenesis in 190
olfactory ensheathing cells
  axon regeneration in CNS 304–6
  for transplantation 343
oligodendrocyte progenitors
  inhibition of axon regeneration in
      CNS 161, 162
  remyelination 208–9, 210–11
  response to injury 24
  sources of cells for transplantation
      341–2
  transplantation 339–41
oligodendrocytes
  apoptosis 7–8
  inhibition of axon regeneration in
      CNS 159, 160(*fig.*), 161–2
  lineage 210(*box*)
  O-2A cell lineage 346–7
  removal, axon regeneration in CNS
      308–9
  remyelination 209–10, 212
oligospheres, for transplantation 342
opsoclonus–myoclonus 53, 55(*table*)
optic nerve lesions, in multiple sclerosis
      238
oxidative stress *see* free radicals
oxybutinin, for bladder dysfunction
      treatment 283
oxygen free radicals, toxicity *see* free
      radicals

p53, and apoptotic cell death 13
p75
  and apoptotic cell death 9–10
  changes after axotomy 17
  distribution 128
pain
  and biochemical plasticity 204
  and plasticity in spinal cord 187–9
  and somatosensory pathway damage
      234
paraneoplastic neurological conditions,
      and autoimmune damage 53–6

paranoid states 256(*table*)
parasympathetic nervous system 234–5
Parkinson's disease
  and α-synuclein 91–2
  aetiology 398
  basal ganglia pathology 228,
      230(*fig.*)
  clinical assessment 239–42
  diagnostic tests 397
  disease progression 397
  dopamine loss 86–7
  dopaminergic system plasticity
      200–2
  drug therapies 276–7, 286(*table*)
  epidemiology 88–9, 398
  free radicals 38
  gene therapy for 379–81
  genetics 398
  history 397
  incidence 88
  L-DOPA therapy 87–8
  Lewy bodies 91
  MPTP 89–90
  neuropathology 397–8
  neuroprotection 117–19
  nigral grafts 320–1, 323
  symptoms 397
  treatment 398
Parkinson's disease models, role of
      neurotrophins 133–5
peripheral nerve damage, role of
      neurotrophins 129–30
peripheral nerve grafts, axon
      regeneration in CNS 301–4
peripheral nerve regeneration
  axon regeneration 146–9
    inhibition by scar tissue 149
  bridge grafts for nerve repair 149–50
  environment for regeneration 145–6,
      147(*fig.*)
  specificity of connections 150–4
  target re-innervation 150
persephin 128(*table*)
  distribution 129
  and dopaminergic neurone survival
      133–4
persistent vegetative state (PVS),
      definition 217
personality disorders 256(*table*)
  Huntington's disease 267–8
pharmacotherapy 276–88
phenyl-*tert*-butyl-nitrone (PBN) (α-
      PBN), as free radical scavenger
      111
PI3 kinase, signalling pathways in
      apoptosis 11, 12(*fig.*)
plasma exchange, in autoimmune
      disease treatment 140–1
plasminogen activators, and ischaemia
      42
plasticity *see* anatomical plasticity;
      biochemical plasticity
polyneuropathies 230–1
polysialyated N-CAM (PSA-N-CAM),
      axon regeneration in CNS 306

presenilins, Alzheimer's disease 86
prion diseases 96–102
  in animals 98
  atypical (APD) 96, 98*(table)*
  diagnosis 98
  genetics 99–100
  in humans
    acquired cases 96–7
    familial cases 96, 98*(table)*
    sporadic cases 96–7
  pathogenesis 100–2
  prion proteins 96
  *see also* Creutzfeldt–Jakob disease;
    fatal familial insomnia;
    Gerstmann–Straussler–Scheinker
    syndrome
prion protein (PrP) *see* PrP (prion
  protein)
progenitor cells
  in adult CNS 347–8
  brain location 191–2
  cell expansion *in vitro* 348–52
  in damaged CNS 193–5
  definition 344, 345*(fig.)*
  differentiation 192–3
  nerve cell specification 345–6,
    347*(fig.)*
  neurogenesis in adults 190–1
  O-2A cell lineage 346–7
  song bird learning 192
  transplantation of expanded
    precursor cells 352–6
programmed cell death *see* apoptosis
progressive multifocal
  leukoencephalopathy (PML), as
  glial infection 73–4
proteases, and ischaemia 42
proteoglycans, inhibition of axon
  regeneration in CNS 162–3, 310
PrP gene, mutations 99–100
PrP (prion protein) 98–100
  pathogenesis of prion disease 96,
    100–2
  PrP$_1$ 96, 98, 100–2
pseudobulbar palsy, therapies
  279–80
psychiatric assessment 255–8,
  259*(table)*, 271–2
  brain disease, methods 256–7
  cerebrovascular disorder 262–3
  Huntington's disease *see*
    Huntington's disease, psychiatric
    symptoms
  traumatic brain damage
    affective symptoms 260–1
    behavioural and personality
      changes 261–2
    course of recovery 259–60
    schizophrenia-like states 261
    types of injury 258–9, 260*(box)*
psychiatric disorders 256*(table)*
  drug therapies 285, 287*(table)*

quinolinic acid, for experimental lesions
  27

quinone reductase, defence against free
  radical damage 37
quisqualic acid
  AMPA receptor agonist 28*(table)*, 29
  chemical structure 26*(fig.)*
  as excitotoxin 26
  for experimental lesions 27

rabies, as neurone-targeted infection
  72–3
Raf and Ras, signalling pathways in
  apoptosis 11, 12*(fig.)*
regenerative sprouting, in CNS 171–2
rehabilitation, functional recovery
  following lesion 289–91
Reitan Trail Making Test (TMT), for
  attention and psychomotor
  speed assessment 251
remyelination
  by Schwann cells 209*(fig.)*, 212–14
  cellular mechanisms 207–12
  failure of spontaneous remyelination
    335–6
  and functional recovery 205,
    207*(fig.)*
  identification 205–6, 208*(fig.)*,
    209*(fig.)*
  molecular mechanisms 210*(box)*,
    212
  and nerve conduction 205, 206*(fig.)*
  promotion of endogenous
    remyelination 336
reporter genes 368–9*(box)*
research tools, for assessment of
  neurological disorders
  236–42
retinal ganglion cell damage, role of
  neurotrophins 132
retino–tectal system, and formation of
  functional connections 332,
  333*(fig.)*
retinopathy 54, 55*(table)*
retrovirus vectors, for gene transfer into
  cells 358–60
Rivermead Behavioural Memory Tests
  (RBMT), for memory assessment
  250
rodent barrel fields, and functional
  plasticity 176–7
rotation response, in nigral graft model
  318–20
rubrospinal pathway
  and axon regeneration 164
  axotomy-induced changes 18

scar tissue, and inhibition of axon
  regeneration 149
schizophrenia 256*(table)*
  and head injury 261, 262*(box)*
  schizophrenia-like states, and
    Huntington's disease 266–7
Schwann cells
  and axon regeneration 146–8
  in environment for nerve
    regeneration 145–6, 147*(fig.)*

in multiple sclerosis 214
  and remyelination 209*(fig.)*, 212–14
  for transplantation 342–3
    and axon regeneration in CNS
      301–4
scrapie 98
senile dementia, Alzheimer's type 385
senile plaques, Alzheimer's disease 79,
  80
sensory cortex
  plasticity and sprouting 172–4
    age effects 174
    location of changes 175
    and normal brain function 175
    pharmacological manipulation 176
    use-dependent mapping 175–6
  rodent barrel fields, and functional
    plasticity 176–7
sensory function
  characteristic deficits 230–4
  clinical assessment 234*(box)*
  somatosensory pathways 229–30,
    232*(fig.)*
sensory neurones, survival, and
  neurotrophins 6
sensory neuronopathy 53, 55*(table)*
sensory symptoms, in neurological
  disease, drug therapies 284–5,
  287*(table)*
sexual dysfunction
  and Huntington's disease 269
  in neurological disease, drug
    therapies 283, 287*(table)*
sleep disorder, and Huntington's disease
  269–70
somatosensory cortex
  damage, and sensory deficits 233–4
  reorganisation 172–4
somatosensory pathways 232*(fig.)*
  characteristic effects of lesions 230–4
song birds, learning and neurogenesis
  192, 193*(fig.)*
spasticity 280–1
  drug therapies 281–2, 287*(table)*
  physiotherapy 281
speech *see* language assessment
spinal and bulbar muscular atrophy
  (SBMA), as trinucleotide repeat
  disease 95
spinal cord
  effect of age on plasticity 189
  ependymal (progenitor) cells 194
  GAP-43 effects on sprouting
    188*(fig.)*, 198
  NI-250 (NogoA) effects on sprouting
    189–90
  plasticity in sensory projections
    collateral sprouting 188–9
    regenerative sprouting 188
    unmasking of silent synapses
      187–8
  sprouting of corticospinal axons 189
spinal cord lesions
  and axon regeneration
    embryonic grafts 306–7

spinal cord lesions (*cont.*):
  IN-1 monoclonal antibody 309–10
  olfactory ensheathing cells 304–5
  oligodendrocyte removal 308
  peripheral nerve grafts 302, 303, 304
  characteristic deficits 233
  injury
    disease progression 399–400
    epidemiology 399
    symptoms and diagnosis 399
    treatment 400
  in multiple sclerosis 238
  repair model, and axon regeneration in CNS 303(*fig.*), 304–5
spinocerebellar atrophy 1 (SCA1), as trinucleotide repeat disease 95
spirochetal infections 75
spongiform encephalopathies, immune response 77
STAT transcription factors, and signalling pathways in apoptosis 11, 12(*fig.*)
stem cells
  cell expansion *in vitro* 348–52
  definition 344, 345(*fig.*)
  progenitor cells in CNS 345–8
  transplantation of expanded precursor cells 352–6
steroids *see* corticoids; neurosteroids
streptococcal infection, and Sydenham's chorea 67–8
*Streptococcus pneumoniae*, and bacterial menginitis 60
striatal grafts, and circuit reconstruction 333–4
stroke
  and CNS plasticity 183
  genetics 401
  neuropathology 401
  pathogenesis 401
  psychiatric symptoms 262–3
  symptoms 401
  treatments 402
Stroop colour-word test, for executive function 252
stupor, definition 217
subacute cerebellar degeneration 53, 55(*table*)
subacute sclerosing panencephalitis (SSPE) 71
subependymal cells, of ventricles, progenitor cells 191–2
subgranular layer cells, of hippocampus, progenitor cells 191
suicide, and Huntington's disease 266
superoxide anion, as free radical 36
superoxide dismutase (SOD)
  in antioxidant therapy 112
  and defence against free radical damage 36–7

in motor neurone disease 130–1
and neuroprotection in Parkinson's disease 118
sweat glands, and control of sympathetic phenotype 202–4
Sydenham's chorea 67–8
Symbol Digit Modalities Test (SDMT), for attention and psychomotor speed assessment 251
sympathetic nervous system 234–5
sympathetic neurones, and neurotransmitter plasticity 202–4
synuclein (α-synuclein), and familial Parkinson's disease 91–2

T lymphocytes 45–7
  classification 55(*box*)
tau protein
  in Alzheimer's disease initiation 85
  and neurofibrillary tangles 84–5
tauopathies, and chromosome-17 86
tenascin R, and inhibition of axon regeneration in CNS 162
tetanus, and exotoxin-induced damage 74–5, 76(*fig.*)
TGFβ 128(*table*)
  distribution 129
tics 276(*table*)
  drug therapies 287(*table*)
tight junctions, changes after injury 23
tirilazad, as free radical scavenger 111–12
tissue plasminogen activator (tPA), and ischaemia 42
tizanidine, for spasticity 282
TNFα, changes after axotomy 17
TNFα receptor, and apoptotic cell death 9–10
tocopherol (α-tocopherol) *see* vitamin E (α-tocopherol)
Token Test (short form), for language assessment 250–1
transcription factors, changes after axotomy 16, 16–17
transferrin, and defence against free radical damage 37
transplantation *see* glial transplantation; neuronal transplantation
traumatic brain damage
  psychiatric assessment 259–62
  types of injury 258–9
tremor 276(*table*)
  drug therapies 277–8, 286(*table*)
trinucleotide repeat diseases 92–6
  Huntington's disease 92–4
  and psychiatric symptoms 270–1
trk receptors
  changes after axotomy 17
  distribution 128–9

and signalling pathways in apoptosis 11, 12(*fig.*)
trophic factors *see* growth factors; neurotrophins
tropical spastic paraparesis *see* HTLV-1 associated myelopathy (HAM)
tyrosine hydroxylase (TH)
  changes in nigro-striatal lesion model 198
  in gene therapy for Parkinson's disease 379–80

Ungerstedt rotation model 198–200
Unified Huntington's disease Rating Scale (UHDRS) 239–40
Unified Parkinson's disease Rating Scale (UPDRS) 239
upper motor neurone (UMN) lesions, characteristic deficits 224, 225–7
uric acid, and defence against free radical damage 37

vascular beds, artificial, and intracerebral grafts 316–17
vasculitis, and autoimmune damage 51–3
vasoconstriction, and ischaemia 41
verbal fluency tests, for executive function 251–2
virus vectors, for gene transfer into cells
  adeno-associated viruses 358(*table*), 361–4
  adenoviruses 358(*table*), 360–1
  herpes simplex virus 358(*table*), 364–6
  retroviruses 358–60
Visual Object and Space Perception battery (VOSP) 251
visual system
  functional plasticity 177–8
    control by impulse activity 179–81
    ocular dominance columns 178–9
visuo–perceptual function tests 251
vitamin C (ascorbic acid), as free radical scavenger 111
vitamin E (α-tocopherol)
  as free radical scavenger 37, 111
  in Parkinson's disease treatment, DATATOP trial 90, 119

Wallerian degeneration, mechanism 15–16
Wechsler Adult Intelligence Scale-Revised (WAIS-R), for IQ assessment 249–50
Wisconsin Card Scoring Test (WCST), for executive function 252

xenografts, as alternatives to foetal graft tissue 326–8